# EPIDEMIOLOGY
## STUDY DESIGN
## AND DATA ANALYSIS

# CHAPMAN & HALL/CRC TEXTS IN STATISTICAL SCIENCE SERIES

Editors:

**Dr. Chris Chatfield**
Reader in Statistics
School of Mathematical Sciences
University of Bath, UK

**Professor Jim V. Zidek**
Department of Statistics
University of British Columbia
Canada

---

**The Analysis of Time Series –
An introduction**
Fifth edition
C. Chatfield

**Applied Bayesian Forecasting and
Time Series Analysis**
A. Pole, M. West and J. Harrison

**Applied Non-parametric
Statistical Methods**
Second Edition
P. Sprent

**Applied Statistics – A handbook of
BMDP analyses**
E.J. Snell

**Applied Statistics – Principles and
examples**
D.R. Cox and E.J. Snell

**Bayesian Data Analysis**
A. Gelman, J. Carlin, H. Stern and
D. Rubin

**Beyond ANOVA - Basics of applied
statistics**
R.G. Miller, Jr.

**Computer-Aided Multivariate
Analysis**
Third Edition
A.A. Afifi and V.A. Clark

**A Course in Large Sample Theory**
T.S. Ferguson

**Data Driven Statistical Methods**
P. Sprent

**Decision Analysis – A Bayesian
approach**
J.Q. Smith

**Elementary Applications of
Probability Theory**
Second edition
H.C. Tuckwell

**Elements of Simulation**
B.J.T. Morgan

**Epidemiology – Study design and
data analysis**
M. Woodward

**Essential Statistics**
Third edition
D.G. Rees

**Interpreting Data – A first course in
statistics**
A.J.B. Anderson

**An Introduction to Generalized
Linear Models**
A.J. Dobson

**Introduction to Multivariate Analysis**
C. Chatfield and A.J. Collins

**Introduction to Optimization
Methods and their Applications in
Statistics**
B.S. Everitt

**Large Sample Methods in Statistics**
P.K. Sen and J. da Motta Singer

**Markov Chain Monte Carlo –
Stochastic simulation for Bayesian
inference**
D. Gamerman

**Modeling and Analysis of Stochastic
Systems**
V. Kulkarni

**Modelling Binary Data**
D. Collett

**Modelling Survival Data in Medical Research**
D. Collett

**Multivariate Analysis of Variance and Repeated Measures – A practical approach for behavioural scientists**
D.J. Hand and C.C. Taylor

**Multivariate Statistics – A practical approach**
B. Flury and H. Riedwyl

**Practical Data Analysis for Designed Experiments**
B.S. Yandell

**Practical Longitudinal Data Analysis**
D.J. Hand and M. Crosder

**Practical Statistics for Medical Research**
D.G. Altman

**Probability – Methods and measurement**
A. O'Hagan

**Problem Solving – A statistician's guide**
Second edition
C. Chatfield

**Randomization, Bootstrap and Monte Carlo Methods in Biology**
Second edition
B.F.J. Manly

**Readings in Decision Analysis**
S. French

**Statistical Analysis of Reliability Data**
M.J. Crowder, A.C. Kimber, T.J. Sweeting and R.L. Smith

**Statistical Methods for SPC and TQM**
D. Bissell

**Statistical Methods in Agriculture and Experimental Biology**
Second edition
R. Mead, R.N. Curnow and A.M. Hasted

**Statistical Process control – Theory and practice**
Third edition
G.B. Wetherill and D.W. Brown

**Statistical Theory**
Fourth edition

**Statistics for Accountants**
S. Letchford

**Statistics for Technology – A course in applied statistics**
Third edition
C. Chatfield

**Statistics in Engineering – A practical approach**
A.V. Metcalfe

**Statistics in Research and Development**
Second edition
R. Caulcutt

**The Theory of Linear Models**
B. Jørgensen

*Full information on the complete range of Chapman & Hall/CRC statistics books is available from the publishers.*

# EPIDEMIOLOGY
## STUDY DESIGN
## AND DATA ANALYSIS

## Mark Woodward

*Senior Lecturer in Statistical Epidemiology*
*Department of Applied Statistics*
*University of Reading*
*United Kingdom*

## CHAPMAN & HALL/CRC
**Boca Raton   London   New York   Washington, D.C.**

**Library of Congress Cataloging-in-Publication Data**

Woodward, M. (Mark)
      Epidemiology : study design and data analysis / M. Woodward.
         p.  cm. -- (Chapman & Hall texts in statistical science
      series)
      Includes bibliographical references and index.
      ISBN 1-58488-009-0 (alk. paper)
      1. Epidemiology--Statistical methods. I. Title. II. Series:
      Tests in statistical science.
      RA652.2.M3W66 1999
      614.4'07'27—dc21                        99-13286
                                           CIP

No claim to original U.S. Government works
International Standard Book Number 1-58488-009-0
Library of Congress Card Number 99-13286
Printed in the United States of America     1  2 3 4 5 6 7 8 9 0
Printed on acid-free paper

To Lesley

# Contents

# Preface

This book is about the quantitative aspects of epidemiological research. I have written it with two audiences in mind: the researcher who wishes to understand how statistical principles and techniques may be used to solve epidemiological problems, and the statistician who wishes to find out how to apply his or her subject in this field. A practical approach is used; although a complete set of formulae are included where hand calculation is viable, mathematical proofs are omitted and statistical nicety has largely been avoided. The techniques described are illustrated by example, and results of the applications of the techniques are interpreted in a practical way. Extensive references are listed for further reading. To reinforce understanding, exercises (with solutions) are included and several substantial data sets are either listed within the book or made available electronically for the reader to explore using his or her own computer software. Sometimes hypothetical data sets have been constructed to produce clear examples of epidemiological concepts and methodology. However, the majority of the data are taken from real epidemiological investigations, drawn from past publications or my own collaborative research.

I have assumed that the reader has some basic knowledge of statistics, such as might be assimilated from a medical degree course, or a first-year course in statistics as part of a science degree. Even so, this book is self-contained in that all the standard methods necessary to the rest of the book are reviewed in Chapter 2. From this base, the text goes through analytical methods for general and specific epidemiological study designs, leading to a discussion of statistical modelling in epidemiology in the final three chapters. As the title suggests, this book is concerned with how to design an epidemiological study, as well as how to analyse the data from such a study. Chapter 1 includes a broad introduction to study design, and later chapters are dedicated to particular types of design (cohort, case–control and intervention studies). Chapter 8 is concerned with the problem of determining the appropriate size for a study.

Much of the material in this book is taken from my course notes. These courses were given to undergraduate students and students studying the MSc in Biometry in the Department of Applied Statistics, University of Reading, UK, and to medical and biological students at the Prince Leopold Institute of Tropical Medicine in Antwerp, Belgium. Some of the exercises are based (with permission) on questions that I had previously written for the Medical Statistics examination paper of the Royal Statistical Society.

My thanks go to all the authors who gave me permission to present data that they had already published; my apologies to the few authors whom I was unable to contact. Thanks also to the following colleagues who allowed me to show data I have been working with, that are not published elsewhere: Howard Bird, Edel Daly, Gordon Lowe, Caroline Morrison, Hugh Tunstall-Pedoe and Ewan Walters. I am grateful to Iain Crombie and Charles Florey for providing the data given in Table 7.1, to John Whitehead for providing the data given in Table C.13, to Dr D.J. Jussawalla and Dr B.B. Yeole for allowing me to use the data given in Table C.1 and to Sir Richard Doll for correcting an earlier draft of Table 1.2.

Special thanks go to Alex Owen, who typed most of this and still managed to keep smiling. Joan Knock wrote the programs to generate the statistical tables in Appendix B, for which I am very grateful. This book would not have been written without the love and understanding of my wife, Lesley, and my children, Philip and Robert. Thanks to them for putting up with all the hours I spent with my head down in some remote corner of our house.

M.W.
Sonning Common, Oxfordshire

# 1

# Fundamental issues

## 1.1 What is epidemiology?

**Epidemiology** is the study of the distribution and determinants of disease in human populations. The term derives from the word 'epidemic' which itself appears to have been derived from *epidemeion*, a word used by Hippocrates when describing a disease that was 'visiting the people'. Modern use of the term retains the restriction to human populations, but has broadened the scope to include any type of disease, including those that are far from transient. Thus epidemiologists study chronic (long-duration) diseases, such as asthma, as well as such infectious diseases as cholera that might be inferred from the idea of an 'epidemic'.

The **distribution** of disease studied is often a geographical one, but distributions by age, sex, social class, marital status, racial group and occupation (amongst others) are also often of interest. Sometimes the same geographical population is compared at different times to investigate trends in the disease. As an example, consider breast cancer as the disease of interest. This is one of the leading causes of death amongst women in industrialized countries, but epidemiological studies have shown it to be much more common in northern latitudes than in other parts of the world. However, this geographical differential seems to have been decreasing in the 1990s; for instance, studies in the USA suggest a decline in deaths due to breast cancer, whilst studies in Japan suggest an increase. In general, breast cancer rates have been found to increase with age and to be highest in those women of high socio-economic status who have never married.

The **determinants** of disease are the factors that precipitate disease. Study of the distribution of disease is essentially a descriptive exercise; study of determinants considers the aetiology of the disease. For example, the descriptive finding that those women who have never married are more prone to breast cancer leads to investigation of why this should be so. Perhaps the causal factors are features of reproduction, such as a lack of some type of protection that would be conferred by breast feeding. Several studies to address such questions in the epidemiology of breast cancer have been carried out. In general, the factors studied depend upon the particular disease in question and upon prior hypotheses. Typical examples would be exposure to atmospheric pollutants, lifestyle characteristics (such as smoking and diet) and biological characteristics (such as cholesterol and blood pressure). We shall refer to any potential aetiological agent under study as a **risk factor** for the disease of interest; sometimes this term is used in the more restricted sense of being a proven determinant of the disease.

The essential aim of epidemiology is to inform health professionals and the public at large in order for improvements in general health status to be made. Both descriptive and aetiological analyses help in this regard. Descriptive analyses give a guide to the optimal allocation of health services and the targeting of health promotion. Aetiological analyses can tell us what to do to lessen our (or, sometimes, other people's) chance of developing the disease in question. Epidemiological data are essential for the planning and evaluation of health services.

Epidemiology is usually regarded as a branch of medicine that deals with populations rather than individuals. Whereas the hospital clinician considers the best treatment and advice to give to each individual patient, so as to enable him or her to get better, the epidemiologist considers what advice to give to the general population, so as to lessen the overall burden of disease. However, due to its dealings with aggregations (of people), epidemiology is also an applied branch of statistics. Advances in epidemiological research have generally been achieved through interaction of the disciplines of medicine and statistics. Other professions frequently represented in epidemiological research groups are biochemists, sociologists and computing specialists. In specific instances other professions might be included, such as nutritionists and economists.

The fascinating history of epidemiology is illustrated by Stolley and Lasky (1995) in their non-technical account of the subject. Several of the pioneer works are reproduced in Buck *et al.* (1988), which gives a commentary on the development of epidemiological thinking. An alternative (but less comprehensive) annotated collection of key papers is provided by Ashton (1994). See Last (1995) for a dictionary of terms in common usage by epidemiologists.

## 1.2    Case studies: the work of Doll and Hill

In this book we shall concentrate on modern applications of epidemiological research. However, as an illustration of the essential ideas, purposes and practice of epidemiology, we shall now consider the innovative work on smoking and lung cancer instigated by Sir Richard Doll and Sir Austin Bradford Hill shortly after the Second World War.

In the period up to 1945 there had been a huge increase in the number of deaths due to lung cancer in England and Wales, as well as in other industrialized countries. For instance, the lung cancer death rate amongst men aged 45 and over increased sixfold between 1921–30 and 1940–44 in England and Wales (Doll and Hill, 1950); see Figure 1.1. This brought attention to a disease which had previously received scant attention in medical journals. A search was on to find the major cause of the disease.

Various factors could have explained the increase, including the possibility that it was an artefact of improved standards of diagnosis. Aetiological explanations put forward included increases in atmospheric pollutants and smoking. Certainly both pollution (such as from diesel fuel) and smoking were known to have increased such that the corresponding increase in lung cancer mortality came later – necessary for the relationship to be causal (Section 1.6). Figure 1.1 shows data on lung cancer deaths from 1906 to 1945, taken from government health publications, and industrial records of cigarette sales from 1885 to 1924. Apart from short-term fluctuations in the sales data due to the First World War, there is a close relationship between these variables, but with

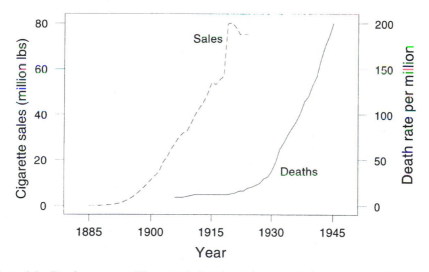

**Figure 1.1**   Death rate per million population due to lung cancer in England and Wales and cigarette sales in the United Kingdom over selected time periods.

a time delay. These data come from Peace (1985), who showed a 21-year time lag when relating the two series. Historical evidence of relationships between snuff use and nasal cancer and between pipe smoking and lip cancer gave extra credence to the smoking hypothesis.

*Example 1.1*   By 1948 only very limited evidence, of the kind just related, of a link between smoking and lung cancer was available. Smoking was a commonly enjoyed pastime backed by a lucrative industry, and thus there was reluctance to accept the hypothesis of a link. Consequently Doll and Hill, a medic and a statistician, instigated a formal scientific study. Between April 1948 and October 1949 they questioned 709 lung cancer patients in 20 hospitals in London (described in Doll and Hill, 1950). These were all the patients admitted to these hospitals with lung cancer, over the period of study, who satisfied certain practical requirements (below 75 years of age, still alive in hospital and able to respond). All cases were asked a set of smoking questions: whether they had smoked at any time, the age at which they started and stopped, the amount they smoked before the onset of their illness, the main changes in their smoking history, the maximum they had ever smoked, the various proportions smoked in pipes and cigarettes and whether or not they inhaled.

Doll and Hill realized that any results obtained from the lung cancer cases would need to be put into context if they were to provide evidence of causality. For instance, a finding that most of the lung cancer cases smoked would not, by itself, show anything conclusive because it may merely have reflected the norm in general society. Hence they decided to study a corresponding set of 709 controls. For each case they sought a non-cancer patient, of the same sex and five-year age group from the same hospital at about the same time, to act as a control. Each control was asked the same questions about smoking habits as was each case.

Table 1.1 gives some basic results from the study (taken from Doll and Hill, 1950). Here 'never-smokers' are people who have never smoked as much as one cigarette each day for as long as a year. The non-zero consumptions show the amount smoked immediately prior to the onset of illness or to quitting smoking altogether. The impact of smoking upon lung cancer may be evaluated by comparing the smoking distributions for cases and controls within each sex group. For men, whereas the percentage of controls that are in the 'never' and the 1–4 and 5–14 per day groups exceeds the corresponding percentages of cases, the opposite is true in the higher-consumption groups. Thus cases are more likely to be heavy smokers. A similar pattern is seen for women, although they tend to smoke less and have a more concentrated smoking distribution.

Doll and Hill were aware that the study just described was not ideal for demonstrating causality. In particular, there were several potential sources of **bias** – uncontrolled features in the data leading to distorted results and thus, possibly, misleading conclusions. For example, bias could have arisen from inaccuracies in recall of smoking history. It could be that lung cancer patients tended to exaggerate their consumption because they were aware that their illness may be related to smoking. A second possibility is that the control group were not sufficiently compatible with the cases so as to provide a 'fair' comparison. For instance, lung cancer cases were known to arise from a wider catchment area than did the predominantly city-dwelling controls. This could have led to some important differences in lifestyle or environmental exposures which might have explained the different patterns shown in Table 1.1. In fact, Doll and Hill (1950) provide evidence to show that these particular forms of bias were unlikely to have fully explained Table 1.1. Nevertheless, other types of bias may not

**Table 1.1**  Tobacco consumption[a] by case/control status by sex (showing percentages in brackets) for patients in London hospitals. Cases are patients with carcinoma of the lung; controls are patients without cancer

| No. of cigarettes/day | Males Cases | Males Controls | Females Cases | Females Controls |
|---|---|---|---|---|
| Never-smokers | 2 (0%) | 27 (4%) | 19 (32%) | 32 (53%) |
| 1–4 | 33 (5%) | 55 (8%) | 7 (12%) | 12 (20%) |
| 5–14 | 250 (39%) | 293 (45%) | 19 (32%) | 10 (17%) |
| 15–24 | 196 (30%) | 190 (29%) | 9 (15%) | 6 (10%) |
| 25–49 | 136 (21%) | 71 (11%) | 6 (10%) | 0 |
| 50 or more | 32 (5%) | 13 (2%) | 0 | 0 |
| Total | 649 (100%) | 649 (100%) | 60 (100%) | 60 (100%) |

[a]Ounces of tobacco are expressed in equivalent cigarette numbers; ex-smokers are attributed with the amount they smoked before giving up.

have been recognized. Interestingly, one source of bias, not obvious in 1950, will have led to an underestimate of the effect of smoking. This was the use of control patients who themselves had diseases which are now known to be associated with smoking.

*Example 1.2*  Partially to address concerns regarding their earlier study, Doll and Hill began a much larger study in November 1951. They sent a questionnaire on smoking to all those listed on the British medical register. Altogether there were almost 60 000 on this register; of these 69% of men and 60% of women responded. These subjects were followed up in succeeding years, leading to a string of published reports from 1954 onwards. This follow-up mainly took the form of recording deaths. Automatic notification was received from death registrations (Section 1.7.2) of anyone who was medically qualified, and obituary notices for the profession were regularly perused. Causes of death were recorded in each case, except in the small number of instances where this proved impossible to ascertain.

Doll and Hill (1964) report lung cancer rates according to smoking habit, over the first 10 years of the study. These are presented separately for each sex, although there were insufficient numbers of female smokers to provide a precise picture of the effect of smoking amongst women. Table 1.2 gives a small extract from the 10-year results for men. Here the definition of a 'never-smoker' is as in Example 1.1. These data provide firm evidence of a relationship between smoking and lung cancer. Not only are never-smokers much less likely to die from lung cancer, but the chance of death increases as the amount smoked goes up. Heavy (25 or more per day) cigarette smokers have over 30 times the chance of death due to lung cancer compared to never-smokers. This evidence alone does not imply causality; for instance, it could still be that lung cancer symptoms preceded smoking. However, Doll and Hill (1964) were also able to demonstrate a degree of reversibility of effect: those who had given up smoking had a lower lung cancer death rate than continuing smokers, with lower rates for those who had a longer period of abstinence.

**Table 1.2**  Lung cancer mortality rates[a] per thousand for male British doctors

| Length of follow-up | Never-smokers | Cigarette smokers (number/day) | | |
| --- | --- | --- | --- | --- |
| | | 1–14 | 5–24 | 25 or more |
| 10 years[b] | 0.07 | 0.57 | 1.39 | 2.27 |
| 40 years[c] | 0.14 | 1.05 | 2.08 | 3.55 |

[a]The 10-year data are standardized for age on the England and Wales population. The 40-year data are indirectly standardized from the whole data set (see Section 4.5 for explanations of terms).
[b]Smoking habit as at 1951 (or last recorded before death).
[c]Smoking habit as at 1990 (or last recorded before death).


The other aspect of the continuing monitoring of the doctors was a succession of mailed questionnaires to produce updated records of smoking habits. Further substantial reports on the progress of male doctors give the results of 20 years (Doll and Peto, 1976) and 40 years (Doll et al., 1994) of follow-up of deaths, related to the updated smoking habits. Table 1.2 gives some results from the 40-year follow-up. At this stage the 34 339 men recruited in 1951 had been reduced by 20 523 deaths, 2530 migrations abroad and 265 who had been lost to follow-up, leaving 11 121 alive at 1 November 1991. In Table 1.2 the smoking habit shown is that last reported (the last questionnaire had been posted in 1990). Clearly the relative patterns are the same as in the 10-year results, despite the fact that the percentage who were smoking had reduced from 62% overall in 1951 to 18% in the survivors at 1990.

Since all deaths, due to any cause, were recorded, deaths from diseases other than lung cancer could also be studied and each of the three publications cited look at deaths by cause. Indeed, having already established some evidence of an effect of smoking on lung cancer, one of the original aims of the study was to relate smoking to a range of diseases. Table 1.3 shows some results, within broad disease groupings, from the 40-year analyses; these are taken from Doll et al. (1994), who give detailed information on the constituent diseases. Again, the smoking habit is that reported on the last questionnaire returned: at 1990 or just before death. The relative sizes of the mortality rates for each disease group show the consistency of the effect of smoking. Never-smokers have the lowest death rate (except in the 'unknown' category) and heavy cigarette smokers have the highest rate for each disease group. Former cigarette smokers always have a rate that is intermediate to the never and light (1–14 per day) cigarette smokers. Other smokers, a mixed bag, are generally comparable with former cigarette smokers. The overall conclusion is that smoking has an effect which is detrimental to general health, this effect being partially reversible by quitting.

The results of this British Doctors Study could lack general applicability on account of the rather special subject group used. Doctors are certain to be more aware of health issues than are most others, and hence may act and be treated rather differently than the common man. However, the results are consistent with the very many other studies of smoking and health carried out since the Second World War, including Example 1.1. Coupled with a reasonable biological explanation of the causal pathway (carcinogens in tobacco smoke causing a neoplastic transformation), the epidemiological evidence proves, to any reasonable degree, a causal effect of smoking on the development of lung cancer.

**Table 1.3** Number of deaths (showing annual mortality rate[a] per 100 000 in parentheses) during 40 years' observation of male British doctors, by cause of death and last reported smoking habit

| Disease group | Never-smokers | Cigarette smokers (number/day) | | | | Other smokers | |
|---|---|---|---|---|---|---|---|
| | | Ex | 1–14 | 15–24 | 25 or more | Ex | Current |
| Neoplastic | 414 | 885 | 317 | 416 | 406 | 565 | 1081 |
| | (305) | (384) | (482) | (645) | (936) | (369) | (474) |
| Respiratory | 131 | 455 | 161 | 170 | 159 | 290 | 392 |
| | (107) | (192) | (237) | (310) | (471) | (176) | (164) |
| Vascular | 1304 | 2761 | 1026 | 1045 | 799 | 1878 | 2896 |
| | (1037) | (1221) | (1447) | (1671) | (1938) | (1226) | (1201) |
| Other medical | 225 | 458 | 169 | 171 | 149 | 330 | 429 |
| | (170) | (202) | (242) | (277) | (382) | (212) | (182) |
| Trauma and poisoning | 114 | 165 | 81 | 80 | 93 | 95 | 196 |
| | (72) | (84) | (103) | (90) | (172) | (79) | (88) |
| Unknown | 27 | 78 | 13 | 13 | 12 | 29 | 45 |
| | (17) | (29) | (33) | (30) | (41) | (16) | (24) |
| Total | 2215 | 4802 | 1767 | 1895 | 1618 | 3187 | 5039 |
| | (1706) | (2113) | (2542) | (3004) | (3928) | (2078) | (2130) |

[a]Standardized for age and calendar period.

## 1.3 Populations and samples

### 1.3.1 Populations

An epidemiological study involves the collection, analysis and interpretation of data from a human population. The population about which we wish to draw conclusions is called the **target population**. In many cases this is defined according to geographical criteria; for example, all men in Britain. The specific population from which data are collected is called the **study population**. Thus the British Doctors Study (Example 1.2) has all British doctors in 1951 as the study population. It is a question of judgement whether results for the study population may be used to draw accurate conclusions about the target population; possible problems with making generalizations from the British Doctors Study have already been mentioned. The ultimate target population is all human beings.

Most epidemiological investigations use study populations that are based on geographical, institutional or occupational definitions. Besides questions of generalization, the study population must also be a suitable base for exploring the hypotheses being studied. For instance, a study of the effects of smoking needs to be set in a study population where there are a reasonable number of both smokers and non-smokers. In 1951 this was true amongst British doctors, but would not have been true in a manual occupation group where virtually everyone was a smoker. The optimal study population for comparing smokers and non-smokers would have equal numbers of each (Section 8.4.3). The British population of doctors was also big enough for any effects to be estimated reliably.

Another way of classifying the study population is by the stage of the disease. We might choose a population that is diseased, disease-free or a mixture. If recommendations for the primary prevention of disease are our ultimate aim then a study population that is initially disease-free would be an ideal choice in a follow-up investigation. Often such a population is impossible or too expensive to identify; for example, the study population in Example 1.2 is a mixture of those with and without existing lung cancer in 1951 (although the seriously ill would not have been able to reply to the questionnaire in any case). If the study population is a set of people with the disease who are then monitored through time, we will only be able to study determinants of progressive (or some entirely different) disease.

If the study population is not readily available then costs will rise and non-response may be more likely. Doll and Hill no doubt chose British doctors as their study population in Example 1.2 because they were easily identifiable and likely to be co-operative. However, the issue of availability is often in conflict with that of generalizability.

## 1.3.2   Samples

If the study requires collection of new data we shall usually need to sample from our study population. Generalizability is then a two-stage procedure: we want to be able to generalize from the sample to the study population and then from the study population to the target population.

Again, there is often a conflict between availability and generalizability (cost and accuracy) at the sampling stage. An extreme example is where a volunteer sample is used. Rarely are volunteers typical of the whole. For instance, people who reply to a newspaper advertisement asking them to undergo a physical examination may well differ from the general population in several important ways that could have a bearing upon the results of the epidemiological investigation. They might be predominantly health-conscious, so that their vital signs are relatively superior. Alternatively, most of them might be out of work (and thus available for daytime mid-week screening), and getting relatively little exercise or eating a relatively poor diet as a consequence. These two scenarios may each lead to biased results, although they will lead to bias in opposite directions. In many instances we may suspect the direction of bias but have no way of quantifying it. Sampling is most reliable when done randomly, and this will always be the preferred option (Section 1.8.2).

Sometimes medical epidemiologists use the term 'study population' to refer to the group of people from whom data are collected. The rationale for this is that this group is the totality of those being studied, perhaps by monitoring for ill health during a follow-up period. However, use of the term in this way can be extremely confusing because it conflicts with the general statistical definitions of 'study population' and 'sample' (used here): the medical epidemiologist's 'study population' may be the statistical epidemiologist's 'sample'. A better term for the total group being questioned, examined or followed up would be the 'study group', although 'sample' is often perfectly adequate and technically correct.

## 1.4    Measuring disease

A typical epidemiological study will require the number of disease outcomes to be counted (as in Example 1.2) or subjects to be selected according to disease status (as in Example 1.1). Thus we require a definition of what is meant by 'disease' in each specific context. Ideally, we should like to have a clinical definition which can be tested by objective evidence. Frequently we have to rely upon less definitive criteria, if only to keep costs down. Often epidemiologists are involved in studies of the validity and consistency of diagnostic criteria.

One clear choice in several situations is whether to measure **mortality** (death due to the disease in question) or **morbidity** (being sick with the disease in question). In Example 1.1 lung cancer morbidity was used as a selection criterion and in Example 1.2 lung cancer mortality was used as the major outcome measure. In general, given two similar studies of the same disease but where one measures morbidity and the other measures mortality, the determinants of disease identified in one of the studies may differ from those found in the other. This may be a true finding; some factors may cause only relatively minor forms of a disease. Alternatively, the difference may be an artefact of the way in which data were collected. For instance, a survey of post-mortems may find a strong relationship between a particular risk factor and a given disease, but a survey of morbidity amongst live people might find no relationship simply because most of those with the risk factor have already died.

Morbidity itself may be subdivided into degrees of severity, so that comparability of results may still be a problem even within the restricted class of morbidity studies. Often severity is closely linked to the source of information used. Thus, since a family doctor or general practitioner (GP) will usually refer only his or her most serious cases to a hospital, we can expect 'disease' to mean something rather more serious when we use hospital, rather than GP, records. Sometimes sickness may be identified from self-reports, primarily sickness absence notifications to employees. Generally only the worst cases will have seen a GP. There may also be unreported cases of disease, such as those who do not feel ill enough to stay away from work. We might only be able to uncover such 'hidden' disease by screening the general population.

The hierarchy of severity of disease (including death) is sometimes represented by analogy with an iceberg that is partially submerged. In the situation illustrated by Figure 1.2, data have been derived from death certificates and hospital records; cases of disease that could have been identified by other means (usually only the less severe cases) remain unidentified.

Thus the decision about how to define disease is bound up with the source of information to be used. Generally we can expect to find more cases of disease as we move 'down' the disease iceberg. This may seem like a good thing to do, especially when the disease is very rare. However, this will normally correspond

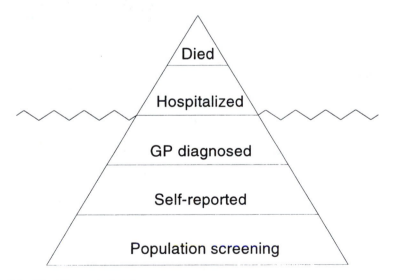

**Figure 1.2**  The 'disease iceberg'.

with a dilution of the epidemiological essence of the disease, that is, the importance of the condition to the population at large. Mild disease, leading to a quick recovery, or hidden disease, which shows no outward symptoms and has no discernible effect on its host, may have little impact on general health or the use of health services. Furthermore, we risk losing specificity as we broaden our information base; GP diagnoses may lack objective clinical confirmation, and sickness absence reports will be necessarily simplistic and thus relatively vague.

For some diseases the iceberg of Figure 1.2 has too many layers. Any disease that does not lead to death, or at least not in the normal course of events, will not require the top layer; for example, eczema. Similarly, people with serious accidental injuries will go straight to hospital for attention, missing out the GP stage. Another, less obvious, caveat to the iceberg analogy is that certain types of serious cases of disease may not be routinely reported to any recording system. This would happen if members of some minority ethnic group were reluctant to use the official health service. Under-reporting of disease, or a biased view of the relationship between disease and some risk factor that is very common (or very unusual) amongst the particular ethnic group, may result. General population screening may be the only answer to this problem.

### 1.4.1   Incidence and prevalence

As well as deciding how to define disease, we also need to decide how to count it. This leads to consideration of the most important dichotomy in epidemi-ology: incidence and prevalence of disease. **Incidence** is the number of new cases of the disease within a specified period of time. **Prevalence** is the number of existing cases of disease at a particular point in time. For example, in Table 1.3 we see the incidence of death, overall and by broad cause, over the 40-year period from 1 November 1951. If Doll and Hill had recorded the number of British doctors with lung cancer in 1951 they would have measured the prevalence of this disease. Prevalence is a measure of morbidity, whereas incidence can measure both morbidity and mortality.

Incidence and prevalence are often very different for the same disease in the same population. The prevalence certainly depends upon the incidence, but also depends upon the duration of the disease. A chronic disease which is rarely cured will have a much greater prevalence than incidence, whereas a disease which leads to death soon after it is diagnosed may have a higher incidence than prevalence. If the incidence and the average duration of the disease are constant over time, then

$$P = ID,$$

where $P$ is prevalence, $I$ is incidence and $D$ is the average duration.

In practice, the assumption of constancy may well be untrue. For many diseases, incidence is not static over successive years. If incidence is dropping, perhaps due to preventive measures consequent to epidemiological research, there may eventually be a very small annual incidence in a population where the prevalence is high (principally amongst older adults). This effect will be compounded if the preventive measures also serve to increase the chance of survival for those who already have the disease (here the average duration is also changing).

Normally incidence and prevalence are measured on a relative scale. A simple example is where counts of disease are related to the size of the study population (from census results or projections) at the middle of that year. Then we have the following definitions for a specific population and a specific year:

$$\frac{\text{Prevalence rate}}{\text{at mid-year}} = \frac{\text{Number of people with disease at mid-year}}{\text{Mid-year population}}; \quad (1.1)$$

$$\frac{\text{Incidence rate}}{\text{for the year}} = \frac{\text{Number of new cases of disease in the year}}{\text{Mid-year population}}. \quad (1.2)$$

In (1.1) and (1.2) the choices of the middle of the year for counting the at-risk population and the prevalence, and the year as the time period for counting the incidence, are arbitrary. Often incidence is averaged over several successive years to obtain an average annual rate. Sometimes the time point used in the numerator and denominator of the prevalence rate are different, although they will usually be in the same calendar year. We shall consider issues of relative measures of incidence and prevalence more fully in Chapter 3. Somewhat confusingly, epidemiologists sometimes refer to both the absolute counts of disease and their relative measures, such as (1.1) and (1.2), as prevalence or incidence (as the case may be), although the meaning is usually clear from the context.

As an example of how incidence and prevalence differ, we shall consider *Helicobacter pylori*, a chronic bacterial disease identified in the 1980s. After establishment, the organism responsible generally persists for life unless treatment is given, which is rarely the case at present. Infection seems to be associated with poor social conditions so that, in industrialized countries, many adults will have been infected in childhood, whereas children now (living in better conditions than did their parents) tend to have a low chance of infection. Hence the overall incidence should be low and the prevalence high. Epidemiological studies in developed countries have shown this to be the case; amongst adults the incidence rate is estimated to be about 0.5% per year

(Parsonnet, 1995) but the prevalence rate is between 37% and 80%, depending upon the ages of the people studied (Pounder and Ng, 1995).

Generally speaking, prevalence measures are better suited to descriptive studies. For instance, comparison of disease prevalence by region suggests how the burden of disease is distributed in a country, which leads to appropriate plans for allocation of resources. Whilst such analyses may *suggest* possible causal factors for the disease, they cannot provide convincing proof. Incidence studies are much better for studying aetiology both because they can better establish the sequence of events (Sections 1.6 and 3.4) and because they are not susceptible to bias by survival. To explain this latter point using an extreme example, suppose that everyone with a certain disease who does not take large daily doses of vitamins dies very quickly. Those who have the disease but do take large daily doses of vitamins survive for several years. Prevalence may then be positively related to vitamin consumption, making it seem as though this is a risky, rather than a healthy, habit.

Most epidemiological investigations are studies of either incidence or prevalence. Lack of identification or consideration of which has been studied is a common source of misconception when interpreting results. There are, however, some situations where some other way of counting disease is used. One example is where the number of hospital admissions with a particular disease is counted over a period of time. This gives a record of **case incidence**, which will be equal to true incidence only when there are no re-admissions of the same patient. Such data may require careful scrutiny and interpretation in any aetiological analysis.

## 1.5   Measuring the risk factor

Very many different types of attribute can be investigated, even for a single disease. Consequently there are few general comments that may be made about how to measure risk factors. However, many risk factors have the common feature that they can be measured in several different ways, and this aspect is worthy of consideration.

As an example, we shall consider the risk factor of Section 1.2, tobacco consumption. Doll and Hill asked their subjects to state their smoking habits for themselves. Since there may be a possibility of misreporting (most probably under-reporting of smoking consumption in a modern setting) an objective biochemical test may be preferable. There are many of these available, including breath tests and tests on blood, saliva or urine samples, which seek to identify the constituents of tobacco smoke or their metabolites. To select a method the epidemiologist needs to balance the issues of accuracy, cost and intrusion or distress to the subjects. Self-reporting is almost certainly the cheapest option, but could give misleading inferences if a particular pattern of misreporting prevails. Tests on blood samples may be most accurate, but are invasive and require trained personnel and expensive equipment. Note that a method which causes distress, or is difficult to carry out in the laboratory, may lead to several missing values which will reduce the accuracy of any final inferences that are drawn.

Another issue that arises in many applications is that of reproducibility. Some methods for determining the value of a particular risk factor may be deemed to be unreliable due to variation within the patient over time, between observers, or in the laboratory. It may then be decided to take multiple readings. For instance, duplicate serum cholesterol readings might be taken from any one subject and averaged to determine the value of this risk factor for the subject. Sometimes the setting within which the risk factor is measured may have an effect. A female subject, for example, may be unwilling to divulge details of her contraceptive practice if the interviewer is male. Similarly, a subject's blood pressure may increase well above its norm when a doctor measures it in a clinic setting (so-called 'white coat hypertension'). These types of problem can lead to bias error, and can only be avoided by careful planning.

When we wish to have a historical record of a subject's risk factor status we generally have to rely upon the subject's recall. This issue arose in Doll and Hill's studies (Section 1.2) when they wanted to know previous smoking habits. Exceptions are where records have been kept automatically (for example, records of atmospheric pollution) or can be arranged to be recorded prospectively. Of course, the latter is only complete when subjects are followed up from birth.

## 1.6   Causality

Epidemiological research often seeks to identify whether there is a causal relationship between the risk factor and the disease. For instance, we have already considered how far the studies described in Section 1.2 may be interpreted as showing a causal effect of smoking upon lung cancer. As there, the first stage in investigating causality is to establish an association; then we go on to consider what the particular association seems to imply.

### 1.6.1   Association

A straightforward example of an association between risk factor and disease is where a group of people have attended a conference dinner, and a proportion of them become sick overnight. If it happened that everyone who had eaten a particular food became sick, and everyone who avoided that food remained well, then the food would clearly be associated with the sickness. Indeed, it would be difficult to argue that it was not causally associated, especially if left-overs were found to be contaminated.

This type of situation is illustrated by the Venn diagram in Figure 1.3(a). In this, and other parts of this figure, the area within the rectangle represents the study population or the sample taken from it. The area within the ellipse containing the letter $E$ represents those exposed to the risk factor (the contaminated food in the example) and the shaded area represents those who have the disease (sickness in the example). In Figure 1.3(a) the exposed and diseased subgroups are conterminous.

Most epidemiological problems are not as straightforward. Even when a truly causal factor is investigated we may well find that not everyone exposed

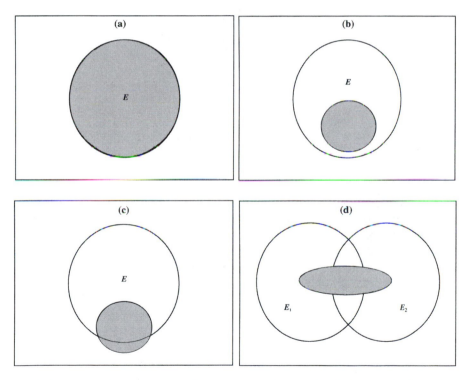

**Figure 1.3**  Venn diagrams to illustrate some possible relationships between risk factor exposure and disease status.

to it becomes diseased. Thus, anecdotal stories of hundred-year-old men who have smoked a packet of cigarettes each day since their youth have to be accounted for when discussing the causal effects of smoking. It may be that the situation illustrated by Figure 1.3(b) is encountered: disease only occurs when exposure occurs, but some of those exposed are disease-free. There is still an association here: exposure is a necessary but not a sufficient condition for disease. We may be able to build a theory of causation around such an association. Going back to the example of the conference meal, perhaps some people ate too little of the food for there to be any discernible reaction, or perhaps some people have a natural immunity.

More complex still is the situation of Figure 1.3(c). Now a proportion of those exposed are diseased, but a proportion of the unexposed are also diseased. Exposure is now neither necessary nor sufficient for disease to occur. Yet there is still an association between risk factor and disease provided the two proportions just mentioned are very different: in Figure 1.3(c) there is a much higher chance of disease amongst those exposed than amongst those unexposed. Again, we may be able to suggest a causal explanation for the findings. Related to the previous example, some people may have eaten the contaminated food at some other time, eaten other contaminated food or have some disease with symptoms that are similar to the general sickness observed. Most modern-day epidemiological analyses of a single risk factor encounter the situation of Figure 1.3(c).

Figure 1.3(d) illustrates a situation where there are two risk factors: exposures are now represented as $E_1$ and $E_2$. Some people have been exposed to only one, some have been exposed to both and some have been exposed to neither risk factor. It is only in the latter subgroup that disease does not occur. This diagram could be generalized to admit several risk factors, thus having several overlapping ellipses. Any one risk factor is associated with disease if exposure to it coincides with an excess of disease. This is the type of situation for most of the diseases studied by epidemiologists today. For instance, well over 200 risk factors have been shown to be associated with coronary heart disease (CHD). The generalized version of Figure 1.3(d) represents reality; the epidemiologist seeks to fill in the names of the risk factors involved, and ultimately to provide a causal explanation where appropriate. In this sense, Figure 1.3(c) could be a special case of Figure 1.3(d) where there are two factors associated with the disease, one of which has not yet been identified. Figure 1.3(b) could be another special case where it is only in the presence of both risk factors (one of which is currently unknown) that disease occurs (a rather special example of an **interaction**; see Chapter 4).

*1.6.2   Problems with establishing causality*

The establishment of an association is a necessary, but certainly not a sufficient, condition to establish causation. For instance, consider a study of dog ownership and blindness. A survey may well find that a greater proportion of blind people own dogs, but it would be bizarre to cite this as evidence of causation. This example shows that we need to establish which came first. If it could be shown that children born to families with dogs are more likely to go blind in later life, then there is a basis for a causal relationship. We might argue that these children have come into contact with dog faeces and thus contracted toxoplasmosis.

Another problem in establishing causality in epidemiology is that of refuting other plausible explanations of the association observed. This is an inherent problem due to the nature of epidemiological data: observational rather than experimental (Section 1.8). Consider a study that finds CHD to be much more prevalent amongst people with at least one parent who has had CHD (alive or deceased). This is interpreted as showing that a genetic factor must predispose towards CHD. On the face of it, this seems a reasonable interpretation, but are there alternative theories? Those with CHD are probably older than those without, since the disease is progressive and thus age-related. Older people will, on the whole, have older parents who thus have an increased chance of CHD. Also, people from the same family tend to have the same lifestyle, for instance in terms of smoking, diet and exercise, each of which is known to have some effect on the chance of CHD. Age and the lifestyle variables may thus explain the link with parental CHD. These variables are then said to be **confounding** factors; the effect of parental history of CHD is *confounded* by these other variables. This important topic is looked at in detail in Chapter 4. One of the greatest challenges in epidemiological research is the unravelling of overlapping associations and causal pathways, made more difficult by the fact that many lifestyle and biological risk factors are strongly interrelated (for example, many people who smoke heavily also have low intakes of vitamins and fibre). Looking at the results of the hypothetical study in another way, they could be said to promote the theory that CHD is an infectious disease. Unless the data are more detailed than we have so far supposed, the only thing against this causal theory is the lack of a convincing biological explanation.

The foregoing gives examples where data collection and analysis alone are unable to establish causality. We could even adopt the philosophical stance that causality can never be proven absolutely through epidemiological investigation, simply because it is impossible to completely control all the other factors that may be important. Whether or not a causal effect has been established by common consent is a question of the quality of the evidence available. As has already been said in Section 1.2, there is sufficient evidence from many studies to be able to state that smoking causes lung cancer. The jury is still out for many other epidemiological associations.

### 1.6.3   Principles of causality

A helpful set of principles for judging whether or not the information available is of sufficient quality to warrant a conclusion of causality were suggested by Sir Austin Bradford Hill. These have been adapted to produce the seven points below. Most of these have already been mentioned or illustrated by example. It is not suggested that any of these points is either necessary or sufficient for causality to be declared, but each will strengthen the evidence in its favour.

1. There should be evidence of a strong association between the risk factor and the disease. Weak relationships may be due to chance occurrence and are more likely to be explainable by confounding.
2. There should be evidence that exposure to the risk factor preceded the onset of disease.
3. There should be a plausible biological explanation.
4. The association should be supported by other investigations in different study settings. This is to protect against chance findings and bias caused by a particular choice of study population or study design.
5. There should be evidence of reversibility of the effect. That is, if the 'cause' is removed the 'effect' should also disappear, or at least be less likely.
6. There should be evidence of a dose–response effect. That is, the greater the amount of exposure to the risk factor, the greater the chance of disease.
7. There should be no convincing alternative explanation. For instance, the association should not be explainable by confounding.

### 1.7   Studies using routine data

The simplest type of epidemiological study is that which uses routine data, the sources of which will be reviewed in Sections 1.7.2 and 1.7.3. Studies on routine data are generally not especially useful for demonstrating causality, but are useful for descriptive purposes. Often such analyses will suggest hypotheses that more complex studies, using special data collection (Section 1.8), will then address.

The advantages of using routine data are their low cost, ready accessibility and (where official sources are used) authoritative nature. A major disadvantage is that the data are often not adequate for the purposes of the investigation. Several risk factors are not included in any routine collection and the data may not be sufficiently comprehensive, for example when they arise from several small-scale samples or relate only to special types of people. It is likely that risk factor and disease data derive from different sources, in which case differences in definition may be a problem. For instance, Figure 1.1 compares risk factor data for the UK with disease data from England and Wales, and would be misleading if increases in cigarette sales had been restricted to parts of the UK outside England and Wales. These problems are made greater when we want to allow for confounding factors, because we will need comparable data on these variables also.

## 1.7.1   Ecological data

Routine data are almost invariably grouped, typically being average values, percentages or totals for geographical regions, or for the same region at different times (as in Figure 1.1). Whenever we have grouped (or **ecological**) data we may encounter the **ecological fallacy**: the assumption that an observed relationship in aggregated data will hold at the individual level. For instance, consider a study using routine data that shows a relationship between the death rate due to AIDS and the percentage who are heavy drinkers for 20 different countries. Drinking is then certainly related to AIDS at the national level, but can we necessarily infer that the relationship will hold amongst individual people? We have no means to answer this question from the aggregate analysis; even a situation where no one who drinks heavily has AIDS may well not be incompatible with the data.

A concrete example of the fallacy is given by Morgenstern (1982). He gives data from the study of suicides by Durkheim (1951), illustrated by Figure 1.4. Here the suicide rate between 1883 and 1890 is related to the percentage of the population who were Protestant in each of four Prussian provinces. The obvious inference is that those of the Protestant religion are more likely to commit suicide. However, this is not necessarily true. An alternative explanation is that members of minority religious groups were the ones committing suicide, and the more they were in the minority, the greater was the chance of suicide. This is a completely opposite aetiological interpretation of the same data! In fact, Morgenstern (1982) shows that there was still an excess suicide rate amongst Protestants at the individual level, but the relative excess was of

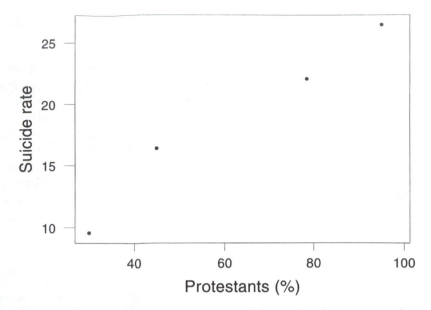

**Figure 1.4**  Suicide rate per hundred thousand population against the percentage who were Protestant in four Prussian provinces, 1883–1890.

the order of 2 rather than the 7.6 calculated using the ecological data shown in Figure 1.4.

Ecological analyses may be advantageous when risk factor measurement at the individual level is particularly prone to error. In this situation, we may only be able to see a true association at the ecological level. For example, it is notoriously difficult to measure the consumption of specific nutrients accurately, for any particular individual. This is due to variations in the nutritional content of foods, person-to-person variations in cooking practice and portion size, and day-to-day differences in the eating habits of a given person. When people are grouped, we would expect a reasonably accurate estimate of average consumption to be found, since we would anticipate that under- and overestimation would cancel out. This comment is not restricted to routine data; such a situation may arise with dedicated data collection also.

### 1.7.2   Sources of data on disease

Routine mortality data derive from death certificates. By law, a certificate is completed whenever a death occurs. This is usually done by a relative or friend of the deceased at a local registration centre where births and marriages will also be recorded. Information is then compiled at a national registration centre. Registration is thought to be close to 100% complete in most industrialized countries, but is very incomplete in many developing countries where there is poor compliance in rural areas.

On the death certificate demographic characteristics, such as age at death, sex, occupation and place of residence, are recorded along with the cause of death. The latter uses the International Classification of Diseases (ICD) codes, which are revised periodically – see, for example, World Health Organization (1992). Both the underlying and associated causes of death are recorded. Comparisons of mortality by geographical areas, or over time within the same geographical area, may be compromised by differing diagnostic practices, particularly use of different ICD revisions or different fashions for ascribing precedence when multiple causes are involved.

Routine morbidity data, as shown in Section 1.4, come from different sources. The range available, and the degree of comprehensiveness, vary from country to country. All over the world, hospitals keep detailed records which, in normal circumstances, are summarized and aggregated for official use. Routine coverage of primary health facilities is much more variable. In countries where there is a national web of local health centres, data reporting may be as regular as from hospitals. Private health care systems, which are widespread in the USA both at the primary and hospital level, usually have complete records. In the UK, where GPs are effectively self-employed, routine primary care data in a useful form for epidemiological purposes comes from occasional National Morbidity Surveys, regular returns to a national study centre from volunteer practices and local initiatives to link computerized databases.

Another source of data that is common throughout the world is notifications of infectious diseases, such as cholera and typhoid. Such data are useful for studying trends over time as well as for flagging up when and where a new outbreak of disease occurs, often leading to a special epidemiological study to discover the cause. The World Health Organization (WHO) deems certain diseases to be notifiable within all member states, whilst national governments often add other diseases when compiling their national list of notifiable diseases. Health officials will have a statutory responsibility to report each case of a notifiable disease to a local, and thus ultimately a national, registration centre. Some countries have, additionally, disease registers, such as for tuberculosis, cancer or congenital malformations. Sometimes such registration is voluntary.

Other possible sources of routine morbidity data include the sickness benefit forms already mentioned in Section 1.4, school health reports and accident statistics. Records of immunizations and vaccinations can also be of relevance.

A further source of important routine data is the population census, typically carried out every 10 years. This does not give data on the number with disease, but does tell us how many are at risk of disease in the general population. This enables routine disease counts to be put into perspective: see (1.1) and (1.2). Census reports, derived statistics and consequent projections are usually published by the national statistics office. This office often carries out additional household surveys at regular intervals, and these will sometimes have questions relating to health issues. Other national surveys that are sometimes relevant include general health and lifestyle surveys, such as the National Health and Nutrition Examination Survey (NHANES) in the USA, and oral health surveys which may be carried out every few years in any particular country.

International statistics on population and disease are published regularly by WHO. Subgroups within WHO often publish international disease data of specific interest, such as data on cardiovascular disease (see, for example, WHO MONICA Project, 1994) and data from dental surveys of children (see, for example, Table 9.8).

### 1.7.3   Sources of data on the risk factor

For some particular risk factors, data are obtainable from official or other routine sources. For instance, Figure 1.1 uses data from industrial sources on cigarette sales. Household, consumer, nutritional and lifestyle surveys are often useful sources of data, particularly on exercise, smoking, drinking and general diet. Biological measures, such as cholesterol and blood pressure, are unlikely to appear in such data compilations, but data on such commonly considered risk factors will be available from previous epidemiological studies. Such information is useful when planning new data collection exercises (see Chapter 8). Library and database searches may be required to unearth such data.

## 1.8   Study design

There are several ways in which an epidemiological study could be designed so as to collect new data. Two basic principles should always be followed: the study should be comparative and we should seek to avoid all potential causes of bias. As in Example 1.1, where Doll and Hill included controls as well as cases, we will not be able to make judgements about association unless we can make comparisons. Consider also Table 1.3; we would get completely the wrong idea about the effect of smoking from looking at the *numbers* of deaths (which lack the element of comparison to the number at risk) in each smoking category. Bias error, as we have seen by example already, can lead to erroneous conclusions about association and causation.

Two main classes of study type may be identified: observational and intervention. By far the vast majority of epidemiological studies are **observational**, meaning that data are collected simply to see what is happening, as in Examples 1.1 and 1.2. By contrast, an **intervention** study is an experiment, that is, things are made to happen. We shall start our discussion with intervention studies because these are the gold standard, as far as aetiological investigations are concerned. The brief details given here are, where indicated, expanded upon in later chapters. Other discussions on study design appear in the textbooks by Lilienfeld and Stolley (1994) and MacMahon and Trichopoulos (1996).

### 1.8.1    Intervention studies

In Section 1.2 we saw that, in the late 1940s, Doll and Hill and others were interested in the effects on health of smoking. An excellent way of studying this would be to take two groups of people, who were identical in every conceivable way, who had never smoked and had no evidence of disease, and to ask half to smoke heavily and the rest to continue to abstain. After several years their disease experience would be compared. Results from such a study would give very strong evidence of a causal effect (or otherwise) of smoking.

This is an example of an intervention study, the essential characteristics of which are that the investigators initially assign the 'treatment' (risk factor status) to whomever they wish and then observe what happens prospectively. They can manipulate the allocation so that the groups are absolutely 'fair' and so avoid any possible problem due to confounding factors. To be more specific, suppose we are studying a certain disease and its risk factor that are both known to be more common amongst old people and amongst men. We could then arrange the intervention study so that the group allocated to be exposed to the risk factor and the group allocated to be unexposed have the same age and sex make-up. This way any comparison between the groups using follow-up outcomes cannot be influenced by age or sex differences.

This design seems to be able to remove the problem of confounding, that was said to be so important in Section 1.6. So why are most epidemiological studies not done this way? The major reason is an ethical one: it is rarely ethically acceptable to force people to be exposed (or unexposed) to a risk factor. For instance, Doll and Hill would not have found it ethically acceptable to force some people to smoke, especially since they suspected smoking to have a detrimental effect. Other reasons for avoiding the intervention approach include the impossibility of allocating biological risk factors, such as hypertension, and the difficulty of avoiding 'contamination' during what is usually a long period of follow-up (for example, people allocated to smoke may quit because they are influenced by health education).

We should note that intervention studies can only control those potential confounding factors that have been identified and can be measured. However, if after allowing for these factors, the remaining allocation to risk factor groups is performed randomly then we would expect any other important confounding effects to be 'averaged out', provided that the sample is large.

Intervention studies in medical research are most commonly encountered as animal experiments or as the clinical trials on patients conducted or financed by pharmaceutical companies. Animal experiments, which are themselves a topic of ethical debate, are not the subject of this book. Neither are pharmaceutical trials, although a few examples of their practice will be included where the ideas are of use to epidemiologists, or the data illustrate a technical point particularly well. Several specialist books on clinical trials have been published, such as Pocock (1983). In this book, intervention studies are described in Chapter 7.

### 1.8.2   Observational studies

Because of their predominance in practical epidemiology, observational studies have provided most of the examples used in this book.

The simplest kind of observational study is the epidemiological **survey**. This is where a set of people (usually a sample) are observed or questioned to seek information on their risk factor exposure and/or disease status. Epidemiologists often refer to such investigations as **cross-sectional**, because they provide a snapshot in time (for example, of the relationship between risk factor and disease). These studies can only measure the prevalence of disease (Section 1.4.1) and must rely upon recall to establish which of risk factor exposure and disease came first. This is frequently unreliable, both due to a long time-lag and restricted lay knowledge of disease. Consequently, cross-sectional studies are most useful for description. They are better than studies based on routine data because we can collect just what we want and can link the data items person-by-person.

If sampling is necessary, we prefer a large sample (assuming that bias can be controlled) in order to improve the precision of our estimates. This inevitably pushes up costs, of special concern when trained field staff must be utilized. To protect against bias we should draw the sample randomly from the study population, that is, so that everyone has a known non-zero probability of being sampled. In a **simple random sampling** scheme, everyone has an equal chance of selection. Often precision may be improved by **stratification**, that is, drawing separate samples from separate subgroups of the population. For instance, if we believe that the prevalence of the disease in question varies with age and sex then we would be well advised to take separate samples from separate age and sex groups of the study population. Clearly this spreads the sample across the different types of people concerned. In practice, the sample is often drawn in a **clustered** way; for instance, we may randomly select a sample of hospitals within a county or state from which to collect our data on hospital patients. This is done to save costs (for example, travelling expenses) but, unfortunately, tends to decrease the accuracy of estimates made from the data. This happens because the sample is concentrated upon a particular group of people (so that we only obtain a picture of the communities served by our chosen hospitals).

The fundamental methodology of surveys (sample or otherwise) is well understood and has wide applications. Many books on the topic exist, such as the descriptive text by Moser and Kalton (1971) and the predominantly mathematical text by Cochran (1977).

A second type of observational study is the **case–control study**. Here the investigators identify a set of people with the disease (the **cases**) and a set without (the **controls**). These two groups are compared with regard to the risk factor. We have already seen an example of a case–control study (Example 1.1). Chapter 6 considers the method in detail. Briefly, we note here that these studies are able to study many risk factors (for example in Example 1.1, Doll and Hill could have asked their subjects about, say, alcohol habits as well as smoking), but cannot study more than one disease. They cannot be used to measure the chance of disease (in terms of incidence or prevalence) because they pre-specify that a certain number of diseased and undiseased people are being studied. Also, they are highly susceptible to bias error (see Example 1.1), sources of which are not always obvious. For these reasons case–control studies, whilst often superior to surveys or routine data examinations, are far from ideal for aetiological investigations. There are occasions when they are, nevertheless, the best choice in practice. This is where the disease in question is very rare or takes a long time to develop.

The best type of observational study for aetiological purposes is the **cohort study**, where people are followed up through time to record instances of disease (and thus measure incidence). Example 1.2, the British Doctors Study, is an example. Their superiority stems from their ability to establish the order of happenings, especially when a disease-free study population is used at the outset. In principle, they can mimic the conditions of an intervention study; for instance, the British Doctors Study could be thought of (in simple terms) as prolonged observation of two groups, smokers and non-smokers. Smoking then acts like the 'treatment' in an intervention study. However, in the cohort design people are not assigned to their groups; instead there is self-selection of risk factor status. Confounding is not controlled and is, therefore, much more likely to be a problem.

As with intervention studies, cohort studies have the disadvantage that they may require many years of observation, causing considerable expense and probable problems of loss to follow-up. Hence they are not suitable for diseases with a long latency. They are also not suitable for rare diseases because a large cohort would then be needed in order to obtain a reasonable number of positive disease outcomes to study. Unlike case–control studies, they can study many diseases (see, for example, Table 1.3). Further details are given in Chapter 5.

Perhaps the most famous cohort study is the Framingham Study, a follow-up of 5209 adults resident in Framingham, Massachusetts, begun in 1948. The subjects have been monitored through routine records, surveillance of hospital admissions and a biennial cardiovascular examination. Although primarily designed as a study of the epidemiology of cardiovascular disease, some of the many publications from the study have looked at other diseases. The Framingham Study has shown the great potential of epidemiology; its results have guided public health policy, especially in the USA where it is frequently quoted in national statements about cardiovascular disease and how to avoid it.

The foregoing describes the three major types of observational study used in epidemiological research. Variations on these themes are sometimes used. The use of repeated cross-sectional surveys (as when the population census is carried out every 10 years) and specially created disease registers are examples. Both of these methods have been used in the WHO MONICA Project (multinational monitoring of trends and determinants in cardiovascular disease) carried out in several different study populations. Sample surveys were conducted in each study population at various times within the 10-year time-span of the study. These surveys give a picture of the changing risk factor profiles (for example, for lipids, blood pressure and smoking) within each geographically defined population. Specimen data from one of the cross-sectional surveys carried out by the Scottish MONICA centre appear in Tables C.2 and C.3 in Appendix C, and elsewhere in this book. Throughout the 10 years, the MONICA centres maintained case registers so as to record every coronary event (morbid and mortal) for every member of the particular study population, thus establishing the overall disease load. Some case register data from the Scottish MONICA centre appear in Tables 4.9 and 4.10.

## 1.9    Data analysis

The analytical techniques applied to epidemiological data include general statistical methods and special methods which have been developed to fit the needs of specific epidemiological study designs. Here we will consider separately analytical methods which do and do not explicitly use a statistical model. Broadly speaking, the former do not require the use of a computer, but the latter do.

The first part of the remainder of this book (Chapters 2–8) is concerned with the first category identified above, and no assumption of the use of a computer is made. In Chapter 2 the basic statistical techniques applied widely in medical science are reviewed. Chapter 3 covers the most basic methodological tools used in quantitative epidemiology. Chapter 4 discusses the important concepts of confounding and interaction in more detail, and presents computational procedures for their detection or control. As we have seen, Chapters 5–7 deal with particular study designs. In each of these chapters we shall see how far the techniques already developed may be applied and then develop special analytical techniques, most suitable for the particular design. Chapter 8 is concerned with the fundamentals of sample size calculation, an analytical tool which is a crucial part of epidemiological study design.

The second part of the book (Chapters 9–11) describes statistical models and their application to epidemiological studies of all kinds. A great advantage of statistical models is that they provide a general framework within which most of the usual data-based epidemiological questions may be answered. This precludes the need for special formulae, such as several of those given in the earlier chapters, that are only applicable in specific situations. Disadvantages are that they make assumptions that may not be true and can lead the epidemiologist to lose the 'feel' for the data, leading to unthinking analyses. Hence the need for associated descriptive procedures and model checking will be stressed. From a small way into Chapter 9 onwards, it will be assumed that a statistical computer package will be used to generate results. This is necessary due to the sheer complexity of the computations required.

### 1.9.1    Computer packages

Although the techniques described in Chapters 2–8 may be applied without a computer, the size of many studies and the convenience of the medium make it likely that a computer will be used in practice. These relatively simple tasks can be successfully applied using a spreadsheet package or a basic statistical computing package. Of particular interest to epidemiologists is the excellent Epi Info package (Dean et al., 1996), which has been written especially for their needs. This may be downloaded electronically free of charge: see

ftp://ftp.unaids.org/inet/ftp/epi/index.html

for access. Epi Info study materials, available through

http://who.unep.ch/geenet/epidoc/module.html

could provide an accompaniment to this book.

More sophisticated analyses, including those introduced towards the end of this book, require specialist statistical software. Again, there are packages which specialize in epidemiological applications, including Stata (Stata Corp., 1997) which is popular amongst academic statisticians working in this field.

Although other packages are mentioned, results and program listings (in Appendix A) given in this book will only relate to the SAS package (SAS Institute Inc., 1992). This is due to limitations of space. No one package is used by all who work in epidemiology, and each major package has its adherents. SAS was chosen because it is so comprehensive in all aspects of data handling and analysis, is widely available and is so well established that it is likely to be around, and in development, for many years. Insofar as the computer is only used to produce illustrative results, the choice of package is largely irrelevant. Any of the leading software packages will be able to produce similar results. Where there are fundamental differences, these will be indicated in the text. The reader who does not use SAS is urged to run the data sets provided through his or her own package, and to compare results with those here. Most modern packages have a 'point and click' facility to make the selection of a particular technique fairly easy.

## Exercises

1.1 In a study of risk factors for angina (a chronic condition) subjects were asked the question, 'Do you smoke cigarettes?'. Answers were used to classify each respondent as a smoker or non-smoker. Furthermore, subjects were classified as positive for angina if they had, at some time in the past, been told by a doctor that they had angina.
   When the resultant data were analysed no association was found between cigarette smoking status and angina status.
   (i) Has the study measured incidence or prevalence of angina?
   (ii) There is a considerable body of past evidence to suggest that the risk of angina increases with increasing tobacco consumption. Suggest reasons why the study described above failed to find an association.

(iii) Suggest an alternative design of study which would be more suitable for investigating whether smoking causes angina. Consider the question(s) that you would ask the chosen subjects about their smoking habits.

1.2  A certain general hospital serves a population of half a million people. Over the past five years it has treated 20 patients with hairy cell leukaemia. Several of these patients have worked in the petrochemical industry, and hence the hospital physicians wonder if there may be a causal link. In order to explore this possibility they propose to send a questionnaire to all the survivors from the 20 patients. The questionnaire will ask about lifestyle, including diet and smoking, as well as employment history. Is this a suitable research strategy? If not, suggest an alternative plan.

1.3  A programme is to be developed to study the effects of alcohol consumption on health in a community. The study team in charge of the programme is interested in a number of medical end-points, including coronary heart and liver disease, but results must be obtained within the next two years.

   Describe a suitable study design for this problem. Give the reasons for your particular choice, and discuss the problems that have led you to reject other possible designs. Your description should include details of the sampling procedure that would be used in the data collection phase. You should also consider which variables you would wish to collect data about.

1.4  Epidemiological studies of coronary heart disease usually include measurement of each subject's blood pressure. Sometimes this is done by doctors, perhaps in their surgery, and sometimes by nurses, perhaps in the subject's home. It is thought that comparisons of blood pressure between different studies might be compromised by 'white coat hypertension': a temporary raising of blood pressure due to anxiety. The phenomenon is likely to be a greater problem in some settings than in others. How would you design a study to investigate the effect of white coat hypertension in the two settings used as examples above?

1.5  Figure 1.5 shows the results of an epidemiological investigation into the relationship between the number of decayed, missing and filled teeth (DMFT) and sugar consumption in 29 industrialized nations (Woodward and Walker, 1994). DMFT scores were obtained from WHO's oral health database. These scores are mean values from surveys of 12-year-old children. The surveys were administered within each country, and the results later compiled by WHO. National sugar consumption was estimated from government and/or industrial sources within each country. The horizontal axis on the graph shows the annual consumption divided by the estimated total population of the country (obtained from census results).

   Since the points on the graph show no evidence whatsoever of an increase of DMFT with sugar consumption, the study has been cited (by some people) as evidence that sugar is not harmful to teeth.

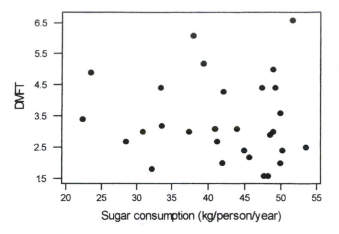

**Figure 1.5**   Dental health and sugar consumption in 29 industrialized countries.

(i) Comment upon any shortcomings that you can see in this investigation, so far as the above conclusion is concerned.

(ii) Given a limited budget and a short time in which to work, how would you design a study to investigate the relationship between sugar consumption and dental health? Describe the data you would record in your study.

# 2

# Basic analytical procedures

## 2.1  Introduction

The purpose of this chapter is to summarize the most fundamental analytical techniques that are frequently applied to epidemiological data. This is to serve both as a guide to how basic analytical procedures should be used in epidemiology, particularly in written presentations, and as a reference when more advanced, or more subject-specific, techniques are developed in later chapters. Further details on basic statistical procedures may be found in any of the introductory textbooks with medical applications, such as Altman (1991), Armitage and Berry (1994), Bland (1995), Campbell and Machin (1993) and Rosner (1994).

In this chapter we discuss both descriptive and inferential techniques, introduced through examples. A **descriptive** analysis is restricted to statements about the data that have been collected (assumed to be a sample from a larger population). **Inferential** analyses go further: they use the observed data to make general statements about the parent population from which the sample data were collected.

### 2.1.1  Inferential procedures

The two major topics in inferential analysis are hypothesis tests and estimation.

A **hypothesis test** seeks to discover whether an assertion about the population appears (on the basis of the sample data) to be unreasonable. Formally, we set up a **null hypothesis** (sometimes denoted by $H_0$) and seek information (sample data) to try to reject it. If the data do not support rejection then we say that the null hypothesis fails to be rejected, meaning that it may be true *or* that we just may not have enough data to be able to detect that it is false. The null hypothesis is taken to be that of 'no effect'; for example, that a high-fat diet has no effect on the chance of developing breast cancer. Hypothesis tests are first met in Section 2.5.1, where the remaining general definitions are given.

Criticisms of hypothesis tests are deferred to Section 3.5.5, where they are developed within a particularly important epidemiological context.

**Estimation** involves the use of some measure derived from the sample to act as a representative measure for the parent population. For example, the average height of a sample of schoolchildren might be used to estimate the average height of all schoolchildren in the country. Estimation also includes the specification of a **confidence interval**, a range of values which we are fairly confident will contain the true value of the measure of interest in the overall population. Generally 95% confidence intervals will be specified; we are 95% sure that a 95% confidence interval will contain the true value. To interpret this, we need to imagine that the sampling process is repeated very many times, for instance 10 000 times. Each time a 95% confidence interval is calculated from the resultant sample data. We then expect that 9500 (that is, 95%) of these intervals will contain the true (population) measure, such as the average height of all schoolchildren. Confidence intervals are first met in Section 2.5.2.

Generally estimation is much more useful than hypothesis testing because the estimate gives precise information on the magnitude and direction of an effect. Also, the confidence interval can often be used to make the same decision as would an associated hypothesis test: examples are given in Sections 2.5 and 2.7.

## 2.2   Case study

In order to provide a focus, a further epidemiological case study is now introduced. Data from this study are used to illustrate the various techniques presented in this and subsequent chapters.

### 2.2.1   The Scottish Heart Health Study

Scotland's annual mortality rate from coronary heart disease (CHD) is one of the highest in the world, although there is considerable variation in the CHD mortality rates between regions of the country. Concern about the high overall CHD mortality rate led to the establishment of a Cardiovascular Epidemiology Unit at the University of Dundee, with the remit to undertake a range of epidemiological studies in order to understand the factors associated with CHD prevalence across Scotland.

The Scottish Heart Health Study (SHHS) was one of these epidemiological studies, with the following objectives (Smith *et al.*, 1987):

(a) to establish the levels of CHD risk factors in a cross-sectional sample of Scottish men and women aged 40–59 years drawn from different localities;

(b) to determine the extent to which the geographical variation in CHD can be explained in terms of the geographical variation in risk factor levels;

(c) to assess the relative contribution of the established risk factors, and some more recently described ones, to the prediction of CHD within a cohort of men and women in Scotland.

Subjects were sampled from 22 of the 56 mainland Scottish local government districts, as defined in the mid-1980s. In each district a number of general practitioners were randomly selected. From their lists of patients, an equal number of people were selected in the four age/sex groups: male, 40–49 years old; female, 40–49 years old; male, 50–59 years old; female, 50–59 years old. Each selected subject was sent a questionnaire to complete and an invitation, jointly signed by the general practitioner and the study leader, to attend at a local clinic.

The questionnaire included questions on socio-demographic status (age, sex, marital status, employment, etc.), past medical history, exercise, diet, health knowledge and smoking. Also included was the Rose chest pain questionnaire (Rose et al., 1977) which is used in the determination of prevalent CHD.

The subjects took the completed questionnaires with them to the clinic where they were checked. Height, weight and blood pressure were then recorded and a 12-lead electrocardiogram was administered by trained nurses. A blood sample was taken, from which serum total cholesterol, fibrinogen and several other biochemical variables were subsequently measured. From a urine sample, sodium and potassium were evaluated. Clinic sessions were held across the country between 1984 and 1986.

Some selected respondents failed to attend for their clinic appointment. These were invited a second time but, again, not everyone responded. Altogether, information was obtained from 74% of those who received postal question-naires and invitations, giving a total sample size of 10 359 (5123 men and 5236 women). In very many cases the information received was not complete; for instance, blood samples were not obtained for 10.6% of the sample.

The resulting data set comprised 315 variables, representing many aspects of personal circumstances, lifestyle, diet and health which may be related to CHD, and three measures of prevalent CHD (self-reported previous doctor diagnosis, appropriate answers to the self-reported Rose chest pain question-naire and electrocardiogram indications). In the following years, scores of articles were written from this cross-sectional data set. These were of three major types: descriptions of the state of health of the subjects (e.g. Tunstall-Pedoe et al., 1989); investigations into the relationships between two or more of the variables that are potential risk factors for CHD (e.g. smoking and diet:

Woodward *et al.*, 1994); and comparisons of CHD prevalence between specific subgroups (e.g. occupational social class groups: Woodward *et al.*, 1992).

However, prevalence data are not ideal to demonstrate causality. For example, smokers who develop CHD could quit because of their illness, so that by the time they are surveyed they are recorded as non-smokers with CHD. Clearly this will tend to produce a misleading inference regarding the smoking–CHD relationship. Consequently the SHHS was designed as a two-phase study: the cross-sectional 'baseline' study just described, followed by a follow-up cohort study of at least 8 years' duration. During this period a copy of the death registration certificate was collected for any member of the study population who died. Furthermore, Scottish hospital records were examined to identify whenever each of the study population underwent coronary artery surgery (coronary artery bypass graft or percutaneous coronary angioplasty) or was discharged with a coronary diagnosis. After an average of around 8 years' follow-up this CHD incidence information was collated and a second series of articles began, relating baseline risk factor information to CHD outcome. In these articles the basic (initial phase) SHHS sample was combined with identical databases from three further Scottish districts collected in 1987, giving a total of 11 718 subjects (see Tunstall-Pedoe *et al.*, 1997).

In Sections 2.4 and 2.5 we shall consider the subset of 8681 people in the SHHS from whom complete information was received from the baseline study for all the variables that will subsequently be analysed. For example, anyone who failed to provide a blood sample will not be considered. We will consider these 8681 as a simple random sample (that is, a sample drawn entirely at random, where everyone has an equal chance of selection) of middle-aged Scots. In fact the sample is not strictly random, both because of the variable rates of selection by geographical area, age and sex and, possibly, because of the missing values, that might be more common in specific types of individuals. For a discussion of the problems of differential sampling rates and missing values, see Cochran (1977) and Little and Rubin (1987), respectively.

In further sections and chapters other subsets of the SHHS will be analysed. In Section 2.6 a small subset of only 50 people is introduced, in order to provide a tractable example.

## 2.3   Types of variables

Epidemiological data, such as those collected in the SHHS, consist of a number of observations, generally from different people, on a number of **variables** of interest. Variables are classified into a number of different types, and it is of some importance to recognize the type before deciding which analytical methods to apply. The first tier of classification is into the types qualitative and quantitative.

## 2.3.1   Qualitative variables

**Qualitative** variables are usually recorded (like quantitative variables) as a set of numbers, but (unlike quantitative variables) the numbers are merely convenient codes. This is best understood by considering one of the qualitative sub-types, **categorical** (or **nominative**) variables. These variables use arbitrary numbers to represent the names for each of their outcomes (**levels**). Examples are 'cause of death' and 'area of residence'. In the latter case there might be four areas of residence defined, given codes of 1, 2, 3, 4, respectively. As with any categorical variable, these codes are not unique; the codes 10, 20, 30, 40 would do equally well, as would 4, 1, 2, 3. All that matters is that we know the key for deciphering the codes. A special, very simple, kind of categorical variable is that which can only have two possible outcomes, such as the variable 'sex'. Such variables are called **binary** variables. These arise frequently in epidemiological research, to represent disease outcome (disease/no disease) or survival status (died/survived).

The other type of qualitative variable is the ordinal type. **Ordinal** variables differ from categorical variables by virtue of having a natural order to their outcomes. Common examples are responses recorded as poor/satisfactory/good (or similar), where there is an underlying order in the responses. These are sometimes called **ordered categorical** variables. We might well wish to account for the order when analysing such a variable. Data in the form of ranks, where items are classified in order of preference or desirability, are a special, and most obvious, case of ordinal data.

Descriptive techniques for qualitative data are described in Section 2.4. Some inferential techniques are described in Section 2.5.

## 2.3.2   Quantitative variables

**Quantitative** variables are similarly divided into two sub-types: discrete and continuous variables. **Discrete** variables are those which may only increase in steps, usually of whole numbers. Examples are the number of patients operated upon in a month and the number of births in a year. **Continuous** variables have no such limitation: they may take any value (subject to possible constraints on the minimum and maximum allowable). Most body measurements take continuous values, such as cholesterol, body mass index and blood pressure.

Notice that blood pressure is continuous even though it may only have been recorded as a whole number. This is because it is only the recording convention which has 'chopped off' the decimal places: they are merely hidden, not non-existent. The essential thing which makes all the variables mentioned in this paragraph quantitative (rather than qualitative) is that the numbers have a unique meaning (subject to the units of measurement adopted). If we were to add, say, one to all the cholesterol measurements this would give rise to totally different conclusions about the hypercholesterolaemic status of the sample.

Descriptive techniques for quantitative data are given in Section 2.6. Some inferential techniques are described in Sections 2.7 and 2.8.

### 2.3.3   The hierarchy of type

With regard to their use, variable types form a hierarchy in the sense that a variable can always be analysed as if it were of a type further down the hierarchy, but not vice versa:

$$\text{continuous} \rightarrow \text{ordinal} \rightarrow \text{categorical} \rightarrow \text{binary}.$$

For instance, we could use the continuous variable 'diastolic blood pressure' to define a new variable, 'hypertension status', which takes value 2 (yes, hypertensive) if diastolic blood pressure is 105 mmHg or greater, and 1 (no) otherwise. We could then analyse this new (binary) representation of diastolic blood pressure. This would not, however, be an efficient use of the data: such grouping must inevitably throw away information. Furthermore, the use of 105 as a cut-point in the example is somewhat arbitrary, and in general we may get totally different conclusions when we vary the definitions of the groups. Hence use of each variable in its original recorded type is generally to be recommended. Exceptions are in descriptive statistics where grouping may be acceptable as an aid to interpretation, and where the assumptions of a statistical method are (possibly) violated unless we 'step down' the hierarchy. The most common example of this latter exception is where **non-parametric** methods, developed for ordinal data, are used with a continuous outcome variable (Section 2.8.2).

Discrete variables are generally analysed as if they were continuous, possibly after a transformation (see Section 2.8.1) or a continuity correction (see Section 3.5.3). If a continuous analogue is not acceptable, then methods for ordinal variables would usually be the most appropriate.

## 2.4    Tables and charts

The major descriptive tools for a single qualitative variable are the **frequency table**, **bar chart** and **pie chart**. These are illustrated by Table 2.1 and Figures 2.1 and 2.2, respectively; all show SHHS data on social class. Social class is measured according to occupation, using standard classifications (Office of Population Censuses and Surveys, 1980) to form an ordinal variable.

In the bar chart the bars are drawn of equal width, but the heights are proportional to the percentages. Other possible scales for the vertical axis are

**Table 2.1**   Occupational social class in the SHHS

| Social class | | Number | (%) |
|---|---|---|---|
| I | Non-manual, professional | 592 | (7) |
| II | Non-manual, intermediate | 2254 | (26) |
| IIIn | Non-manual, skilled | 1017 | (12) |
| IIIm | Manual, skilled | 3150 | (36) |
| IV | Manual, partially skilled | 1253 | (14) |
| V | Manual, unskilled | 415 | (5) |
| Total | | 8681 | |

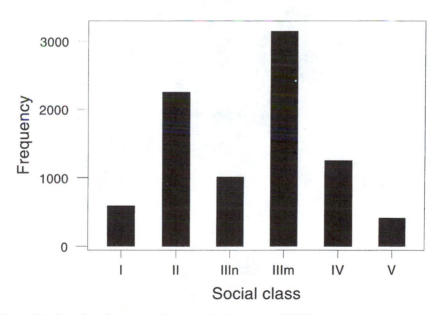

**Figure 2.1**   Bar chart for occupational social class in the SHHS.

the frequencies or **relative frequencies** (percentages divided by 100), both of which leave the shape of the bar chart unaltered. In a pie chart the areas of the slices are drawn in proportion to the frequencies by simply dividing the entire 360° of the circle into separate angles of the correct relative size.

Table 2.1 and Figures 2.1 and 2.2 all clearly show that there are relatively few in the extreme classification groups and most in social class IIIm. This gives a useful demographic profile of the sample chosen. Other useful descriptive variables in epidemiological studies are age and sex, although in the case of the SHHS the distribution by age and sex were determined by the sampling method used. If the SHHS were a true simple random sample – that is, where everyone has an equal chance of entering the sample – Table 2.1 would provide an estimated profile by social class of middle-aged Scots. Percentages are, of course, optional in Table 2.1, but they provide an extremely useful summary.

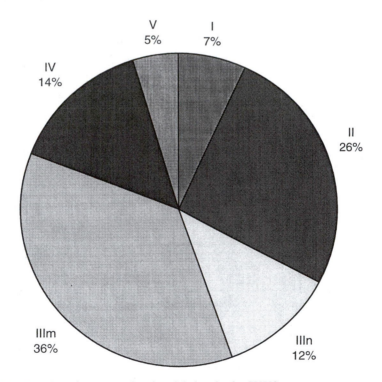

**Figure 2.2**   Pie chart for occupational social class in the SHHS.

Table 2.1 is factually exact, but lacking in visual appeal. Both the pie chart and bar chart look attractive, but the pie chart is harder to interpret because wedge-shaped areas are difficult to compare. Bar charts are also much easier to draw by hand and are far easier to adapt to more complex situations.

The next most complex situation is where there are two qualitative variables to be compared. For example, Table 2.2 shows the relationship between social class and prevalent CHD (identified by the three methods described in Section 2.2.1) in the SHHS. Of most interest here is the percentage with CHD in each social class; hence Table 2.2 gives percentages, and Figure 2.3 goes to the extreme of ignoring the actual numbers by fixing each bar to be of the same length. Instead, we could divide each bar in Figure 2.1 into two sections to represent the CHD and no CHD groups, or give separate 'CHD' and 'no CHD' bars grouped together in pairs for each social class. These have the advantage of showing raw numbers, but make relative CHD composition very difficult to judge. From Figure 2.3 we can easily see that CHD is more common as we go up the bars; that is, there is a gradient such that CHD prevalence is always higher in the more deprived social group. Another element of choice is the orientation, which has been reversed in Figure 2.3 (compared with Figure 2.1).

### 2.4.1   Tables in reports

Although tables are simple to understand and to produce, careful thought regarding layout is essential to draw attention to the most useful and interesting features of the data. Many epidemiological reports (such as papers submitted for publication) fail to get over their message due to inadequate attention to such simple descriptive techniques. For ease of reference,

**Table 2.2**   Social class by prevalent CHD status in the SHHS

| Social class | Prevalent CHD | | | |
| | Yes   (%) | No | Total |
| --- | --- | --- | --- |
| I | 100  (16.9) | 492 | 592 |
| II | 382  (17.0) | 1872 | 2254 |
| IIIn | 183  (18.0) | 834 | 1017 |
| IIIm | 668  (21.2) | 2482 | 3150 |
| IV | 279  (22.3) | 974 | 1253 |
| V | 109  (26.3) | 306 | 415 |
| Total | 1721  (19.8) | 6960 | 8681 |

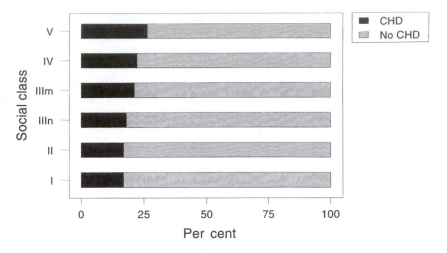

**Figure 2.3**  Bar chart for occupational social class in the SHHS, showing percentage by CHD status.

recommendations are given here in note form. Tables are also useful to present summary information from quantitative variables. Although discussion of such variables is deferred to Section 2.6, this is the appropriate place to consider the presentation of their tables, and consequently an example is included here (Example 2.1).

1.  Each table should be self-explanatory; that is, the reader should be able to understand it without reference to the text in the body of the report. This can be achieved by using complete, meaningful labels for the rows and columns and giving a complete, meaningful title. Footnotes should be used to enhance the explanation.
2.  Each table should have an attractive appearance. Sensible use of white space helps enormously: use equal spacing except where large spaces are left to separate distinct parts of the table. Vertical lines should be avoided since these clutter the presentation. Different typefaces (or fonts) may be used to provide discrimination; for example, use of **bold** type or *italics*.
3.  The rows and columns of each table should be arranged in a natural order. This is a great help in interpretation. For instance, when rows are ordered by the size of the numbers they contain it is immediately obvious where relatively big and small contributions come from. Without rank ordering, questions of size may be hard to address.
4.  Numbers are easier to compare when the table has a vertical orientation. For example, suppose that we have data on several variables for several

hospitals. We then want to compare each variable between hospitals. To achieve this it is best to have rows labelled by the name of the hospital and columns labelled by the subject of the variables. The eye can make comparisons more easily when reading down the page than when reading across. This is especially true when the variables are recorded to varying numbers of significant digits (see Example 2.1). Sometimes vertical orientation may be impossible to achieve because of limitations due to the size of the page. Occasionally such limitations can be overcome by turning the page sideways. Pages written in upright fashion (such as this page) are said to be in portrait format; pages to be read after turning through a right angle are in landscape format. See Table 2.12 for an example.

5. Tables should have consistent appearance throughout the report. Conventions for labelling and ordering rows and columns, for example, should remain the same, as far as possible. This makes the presentation easier to follow, promoting easy comparison of different tables, and reduces the chance of misinterpretation. A common fault is to interchange the rows and columns of tables within the report; for instance, when one table in the report has sex labelling the rows and age group labelling the columns, whilst another table has sex labelling the columns and age group labelling the rows (see Example 2.2).

*Example 2.1*    Tables 2.3 and 2.4 show the same information. Whereas Table 2.3 has the related figures running across the table, Table 2.4 has a vertical orientation. Notice how figures with differing numbers of decimal places are easier to incorporate within a vertical orientation.

Frequently the first draft of a report will contain many more tables than the final version. Revision will usually result in some tables being combined, perhaps because they have common row and column headings, and some tables being removed altogether, because the information they contain is not necessary to the report, or because the results can be merely included in the written text (usually true only for small tables). On the other hand, revision often increases the size of the tables that remain, either by concatenation of two or more of the original tables or because extra information, such as percentages or averages, is added to some tables. Tables from the first draft are often replaced by diagrams in the final report, usually because diagrams are easier to understand.

*Example 2.2*    In an investigation of the relationship between smoking habit and CHD in the SHHS an initial draft publication with seven tables was produced. Two of these are shown as Tables 2.5 and 2.6. In both tables the 'diagnosed' are those who have been told that they have CHD by a doctor sometime in the past, whilst the 'undiagnosed' are those who have no previous doctor diagnosis of CHD, but nevertheless appear to have CHD according to

**Table 2.3**  Minimum, median and maximum values for selected variables in developed countries, 1970

| Variable | Minimum | Median | Maximum |
|---|---|---|---|
| Gross national product per person | 1949 | 4236 | 6652 |
| Population per km$^2$ | 1.6 | 77.2 | 324.2 |
| Cigarette consumption per person per year | 630 | 2440 | 3810 |
| Infant mortality per 1000 births | 11.0 | 18.2 | 29.6 |

Source: Cochrane *et al.* (1978).

**Table 2.4**  Minimum, median and maximum values for selected variables in developed countries, 1970

| | Gross national product per person | Population density per km$^2$ | Cigarette consumption per person/per year | Infant mortality rate per 1000 births |
|---|---|---|---|---|
| Maximum | 6652 | 324.2 | 3810 | 29.6 |
| Median | 4236 | 77.2 | 2440 | 18.2 |
| Minimum | 1949 | 1.6 | 630 | 11.0 |

Source: Cochrane *et al.* (1978).

**Table 2.5**  Smoking habit by diagnosis group by sex

| Sex/ smoking habit | CHD diagnosis group | | | |
|---|---|---|---|---|
| | Diagnosed | Control | Undiagnosed | Total |
| **Males** | | | | |
| Solely cigarette | 125 (8%) | 1175 (77%) | 226 (15%) | 1526 |
| Solely cigar | 25 (7%) | 313 (83%) | 40 (10%) | 378 |
| Solely pipe | 9 (8%) | 80 (72%) | 22 (20%) | 111 |
| Mixed smokers | 39 (8%) | 379 (75%) | 89 (17%) | 507 |
| All smokers | 198 (8%) | 1947 (77%) | 377 (15%) | 2522 |
| **Females**[a] | | | | |
| Solely cigarette | 105 (6%) | 1410 (78%) | 297 (16%) | 1812 |
| Solely cigar | 0 | 12 (100%) | 0 | 12 |
| Mixed smokers | 2 (8%) | 20 (77%) | 4 (15%) | 26 |
| All smokers | 107 (6%) | 1442 (78%) | 301 (16%) | 1850 |

[a] No females smoked a pipe.

**Table 2.6**  Diagnosis group by previous smoking habit by sex for non-smokers

| CHD diagnosis group | Males | | Females | |
|---|---|---|---|---|
| | Ex-smokers | Never smokers | Ex-smokers | Never smokers |
| Diagnosed | 142 (11%) | 45 (4%) | 58 (6%) | 75 (4%) |
| Control | 993 (76%) | 888 (83%) | 767 (80%) | 1581 (78%) |
| Undiagnosed | 164 (13%) | 143 (13%) | 137 (14%) | 375 (18%) |

medical tests (Rose questionnaire or electrocardiogram). Those without any CHD problems at all are called 'controls'. Table 2.5 describes the CHD status of current smokers, whilst Table 2.6 considers those who currently do not smoke any form of tobacco.

When the investigators, and their colleagues, carefully considered Tables 2.5 and 2.6 they realized that they were hard to compare because of inconsistency: whilst Table 2.5 labels 'diagnosis group' across the columns (that is, along the top), Table 2.6 has it across the rows (down the side). More importantly, why do the tables need to be separate? Table 2.7 shows how to combine the two by simply adding the columns of Table 2.6 to the rows of Table 2.5.

Three further modifications were made to produce Table 2.7, which appeared in the subsequent publication. First, it was decided to reverse the percentages. Thus, whereas in Table 2.5 the percentages sum across the rows, in Table 2.7 they sum down the columns. A set of 100% values are shown in Table 2.7 to make it clear to the reader how the percentages

**Table 2.7**  Men and women classified by self-declared smoking habit and diagnosis group

| Sex/smoking habit | CHD diagnosis group | | |
|---|---|---|---|
| | Diagnosed | Undiagnosed | Control |
| **Males** | | | |
| Solely cigarettes | 125 (32%) | 226 (33%) | 1175 (31%) |
| Solely cigars | 25 (7%) | 40 (6%) | 313 (8%) |
| Solely pipes | 9 (2%) | 22 (3%) | 80 (2%) |
| Mixed smokers | 39 (10%) | 89 (13%) | 379 (10%) |
| Ex-smokers (of any) | 142 (37%) | 164 (24%) | 993 (26%) |
| Never smokers (of any) | 45 (12%) | 143 (21%) | 888 (23%) |
| Total | 385 (100%) | 684 (100%) | 3828 (100%) |
| **Females** | | | |
| Solely cigarettes | 105 (44%) | 297 (37%) | 1410 (37%) |
| Solely cigars | 0 | 0 | 12 (0%[a]) |
| Mixed smokers | 2 (1%) | 4 (0%[a]) | 20 (1%) |
| Ex-smokers (of any) | 58 (24%) | 137 (17%) | 767 (20%) |
| Never smokers (of any) | 75 (31%) | 375 (46%) | 1581 (42%) |
| Total | 240 (100%) | 813 (100%) | 3790 (100%) |

[a]Less than 0.5%.
Source: Woodward and Tunstall-Pedoe (1992a).

were calculated. Of course there is no 'correct' way to show percentages in a table such as this. What is best depends upon what is important to bring to the reader's attention; in this example the investigators changed their initial opinion. It is possible to include both row and column percentages in a table, but the table is then difficult to read and interpret. Since the numbers are given, as well as percentages, the reader can always calculate the row percentages for him or herself, should this be necessary.

The second major change is that the diagnosis groups are reordered. It was decided to do this because there is a natural order: someone is first disease-free (control), then gets the symptoms but is not aware of having CHD (undiagnosed) and then is diagnosed by a doctor. The table is more meaningful when this natural order is used. The third change was to omit the 'total' column from Table 2.5 but include a grand total for each sex, merely to keep the table simple, without detail that was unnecessary to the essential points.

In the final publication the initial seven draft tables were reduced to four. Despite the reduction in the number of tables, new information was added even as the reduction was made. The compact final report is easier to read and interpret.

### 2.4.2    Diagrams in reports

The table is the simplest way to present numerical data. Diagrams cannot show numerical information as precisely, but they may be easier to understand, and thus more powerful as a descriptive tool. Modern computer software makes it easy to produce most standard diagrams, even in a form suitable for publication.

Most of the recommendations given for the presentation of tables in Section 2.4.1 are equally suitable for diagrams. In particular, diagrams should be self-explanatory, of an attractive appearance and consistently presented throughout the report. Natural ordering is sometimes possible; for instance, the bars of a bar chart may be arranged according to size.

### 2.5    Inferential techniques for categorical variables

### 2.5.1    Contingency tables

When there are two categorical variables to be compared, a natural question is whether there is any evidence of an association between the two. For example, Table 2.8 shows the types of tobacco consumed by each sex in the SHHS. This table uses the same SHHS subset (that with no missing values) as in Tables 2.1 and 2.2. Note that Table 2.7, which considers a similar problem, is taken from a publication that used only the initial (22 districts) phase of the SHHS. A cross-classification table, such as Table 2.8, is known as a **contingency table**.

Does Table 2.8 provide evidence of a sex–tobacco relationship? In other words, are the patterns of tobacco consumption different for men and women? If that were not so, then the percentages within each tobacco group would be the same for men and women. We can see that they are not exactly the same in Table 2.8,

**Table 2.8**   Sex against smoking habit in the SHHS

|  | Smoking habit | | | | | |
|---|---|---|---|---|---|---|
| Sex | Non-smoker | Cigarettes | Pipes | Cigars | Mixed | Total |
| Male | 2241 (50%) | 1400 (31%) | 103 (2%) | 352 (8%) | 424 (9%) | 4520 (100%) |
| Female | 2599 (63%) | 1551 (37%) | 0 (0%) | 9 (0%) | 2 (0%) | 4161 (100%) |
| Total | 4840 | 2951 | 103 | 361 | 426 | 8681 |

where these percentages have been added as an aid to interpretation. However, they may be similar enough for these observed differences to have arisen merely by chance selection of the actual sample obtained. What is required is a test of the statistical significance of the relationship: the **chi-square test**.

To compute the chi-square test statistic by hand we must first calculate the expected frequencies within each cell of the table under the null hypothesis of no association. These are

$$E_{ij} = \frac{R_i C_j}{T},$$

where $i$ denotes the row, $j$ the column, $R_i$ the $i$th row total, $C_j$ the $j$th column total and $T$ the grand total. Hence, for Table 2.8, the expected value in, for example, cell (1,3), the third column in the first row (male pipe smokers), is

$$E_{13} = \frac{4520 \times 103}{8681} = 53.6$$

The complete set of expected values is

$$\begin{matrix} 2520.1 & 1536.5 & 53.6 & 188.0 & 221.8 \\ 2319.9 & 1414.5 & 49.4 & 173.0 & 204.2 \end{matrix}$$

The chi-square test statistic is

$$\sum_i \sum_j \frac{\left(O_{ij} - E_{ij}\right)^2}{E_{ij}}, \qquad (2.1)$$

where $O_{ij}$ is the observed value in the cell $(i,j)$. In the example $i$ ranges from 1 to 2 and $j$ from 1 to 5 and the test statistic is

$$\frac{(2241 - 2520.1)^2}{2520.1} + \cdots + \frac{(2 - 204.2)^2}{204.2} = 867.8.$$

The test statistic is to be compared to chi-square with $(r-1)(c-1)$ degrees of freedom, written $\chi^2_{(r-1)(c-1)}$. The concept of degrees of freedom is discussed in Section 2.6.3.

As with all hypothesis tests (sometimes called **significance tests**) we reject the null hypothesis whenever the test statistic exceeds the cut-point, known as the

**critical value**, at a predetermined level of significance. Otherwise we fail to reject the null hypothesis and conclude that there is insufficient evidence that the null hypothesis is incorrect at this particular level of significance. The critical values can be found from statistical tables, such as those in Appendix B, or the more complete tables by Fisher and Yates (1957). Table B.3 gives critical values for the chi-square distribution at different degrees of freedom and different levels of significance.

The **significance level** represents the chance that the null hypothesis is rejected when it is actually true. Thus it represents the chance that a particular kind of error (called **type I error**) occurs, and we should consequently wish the significance level to be small. Traditionally the significance level is given as a percentage, and the 5% level of significance is generally accepted to be a reasonable yardstick to use. When a test is significant at the 5% level, this means that the chance of observing a value as extreme as that observed for the test statistic, when the null hypothesis is true, is below 0.05. In, say, 10 000 repetitions of the sampling procedure we would expect to wrongly reject the null hypothesis 500 times. The argument goes that this is small enough to be an acceptable rate of error.

Although the basic idea of a hypothesis test is to make a decision, results of tests are often given in such a way that the reader can judge the strength of information against the null hypothesis. A simple device is to consider a few different significance levels, and report the strongest one at which the test is significant. Most often the following convention is used:

n.s.    not significant at 5%;
*       significant at 5% (but not at 1%);
**      significant at 1% (but not at 0.1%);
***     significant at 0.1%.

The idea is that, because smaller significant levels are more stringent, the number of asterisks defines the strength of evidence against the null hypothesis. Such a demarcation scheme is easy to employ using statistical tables, such as Table B.3. For example the 5%, 1% and 0.1% critical values for $\chi_4^2$ are 9.49, 13.3 and 18.5 (a few other critical values are also given in Table B.3). If the null hypothesis is true, then there is a 5% chance of observing a chi-square value of 9.49 or above, a 1% chance of 13.3 or above and a 0.1% chance of 18.5 or above. Hence, if the chi-square test statistic, (2.1), is less than 9.49 we fail to reject the null hypothesis at the 5% level of significance; we reject at 5% but not at 1% if it is greater than 9.49 but less than 13.3; we reject at 1% but not at 0.1% if it is greater than 13.3 but less than 18.5; we reject at 0.1% if it is 18.5 or more.

A major drawback with this idea is that, say, significance levels of 4.9% and 1.1% are treated equally. It is preferable to give the exact significance level, the level at which the test is just significant. Traditionally this is given as a probability, rather than a percentage, and is called the **p value**. The p value is the exact probability of getting a result as extreme as that observed for the test statistic when the null hypothesis is true. Most statistical computer packages will automatically produce p values to several decimal places. We can easily use p values to make decisions at the common significance 'cut-points': for instance, if p is below 0.05 we reject the null hypothesis at the 5% level of significance. Whenever we reject at the $X\%$ level we automatically reject at the $Y\%$ level for all $Y > X$. If we fail to reject at the $X\%$ level we automatically fail to reject at the $Y\%$ level for all $Y < X$.

Returning to the example, the test statistic is 867.8 which is to be compared to $\chi^2$ with $(2 - 1)(5 - 1) = 4$ degrees of freedom. Since $\chi_4^2 = 18.5$ at the 0.1% level we can conclude that the result is significant at the 0.1% level. In fact, since 867.8 is much greater than 18.5 we would certainly be able to reject the null hypothesis, of equal smoking habits for the two sexes, at a much more extreme (smaller) level of significance. Thus there is substantial evidence of a real difference, not explainable by chance variation associated with sampling. From Table 2.8 we can see that men are much more likely to smoke pipes and/ or cigars (possibly together with cigarettes).

One word of warning about the chi-square test is appropriate. The test is really only an approximate one (see Section 3.5.3) and the approximation is poor whenever there are small expected ($E$) values. Small expected values may be avoided by pooling rows or columns, provided that the combined classes make sense. If the table has some kind of natural ordering, then adjacent columns or rows are pooled when necessary. A rule of thumb is that no more than 20% of expected values should be below 5 and none should be below 1. If this cannot be achieved an exact method, such as is provided by many statistical computer packages, should be used. Section 3.5.4 gives an exact method for a table with two rows and two columns, a $2 \times 2$ table. Note that it is small *expected* values that cause problems; small *observed* values, such as in Table 2.8 (female pipes and mixed smoking) are not a problem in themselves, although they are a good indication that small expected values may follow.

## 2.5.2  *Binary variables: proportions and percentages*

Binary variables are, as with other categorical variables, generally summarized by proportions or the equivalent percentages, that is, proportions multiplied by 100. For example, consider the binary variable 'smoker' with the outcomes

**Table 2.9**  Sex against smoking status in the SHHS

|  | Smoking status | | |
|---|---|---|---|
| Sex | Non-smoker | Smoker | Total |
| Male | 2241 | 2279 | 4520 |
| Female | 2559 | 1562 | 4161 |
| Total | 4840 | 3841 | 8681 |

'yes' and 'no'. Suppose that we are interested in the proportion of female smokers. In Table 2.8 we have details on specific smoking habits. Table 2.9 is a collapsed version of this table. From this we can easily see that the proportion of female smokers is $1562/4161 = 0.3754$; equivalently, the percentage is 37.54%.

With sample data the proportion found is an estimate of the true proportion in the parent population. Assuming that we have a simple random sample, we can find a 95% confidence interval for this true proportion from

$$p \pm 1.96\sqrt{p(1-p)/n}, \tag{2.2}$$

where $p$ is the sample proportion and $n$ is the sample size. As explained in Section 2.1.1, this gives us limits which we are very confident will contain the true proportion. To be precise, we know that, in the long run, 95% of all such intervals, each calculated from a new simple random sample of the population, will contain the true proportion.

As an example, and taking the female portion of the SHHS as a simple random sample of middle-aged Scotswomen, a 95% confidence interval for the proportion of middle-aged Scotswomen who smoke is

$$0.3754 \pm 1.96\sqrt{\frac{0.3754(1-0.3754)}{4161}},$$

that is,

$$0.3754 \pm 0.0147,$$

which might otherwise be written as (0.361, 0.390) to three decimal places. We are 95% confident that this interval contains the unknown true proportion of smokers.

The value 1.96 appears in (2.2) because we have chosen 95% confidence and because we have assumed that the distribution of the sample proportion may be approximated by a normal distribution (Section 2.7). For a standard normal distribution (defined in Section 2.7) the middle 95% lies between $-1.96$ and 1.96 (see Table B.2). Hence 97.5% of the standard normal lies below 1.96, and 2.5% lies below $-1.96$, as can be seen, approximately, from Table B.1. Here

1.96 is the critical value for the complementary hypothesis test at the $100 - 95 = 5\%$ level of significance which rejects the null hypothesis in either the lower or upper portions ('tails') of the standard normal distribution. Such a test is said to be **two-sided**. The value $-1.96$ is called the lower $2\frac{1}{2}\%$ **percentage point**, whilst 1.96 is the upper $2\frac{1}{2}\%$ percentage point.

There is no reason to use 95% confidence except that this is most often used in practice, tying in with the common use of the complementary 5% significance level in hypothesis tests. Any other high percentage of confidence could be used instead of 95%; Table B.2 gives some useful critical values for confidence intervals and their complementary tests. All that is necessary in order to change the percentage of confidence is to replace 1.96 in (2.2) by the required critical value. Hence the width (upper minus lower limit) of the confidence interval will be

$$2V\sqrt{p(1-p)/n}, \tag{2.3}$$

where $V$ is the critical value. For example, from Table B.2, $V = 1.6449$ for a 90% confidence interval. Table B.2 shows that increasing the percentage of confidence increases $V$ and thus widens the confidence interval (probabilistic limits of error). We can only have greater confidence if we pay the price of having a wider interval of error. Precision would, on the other hand, be increased by increasing $n$ because (2.3) decreases as $n$ increases. So it is a good idea to increase sample size (all else being equal).

The number of female smokers in Scotland is quite high by international standards. Suppose (hypothetically) that the government decreed that the percentage of women smoking should be 39%, this figure being derived as the highest found from a number of population surveys world-wide. We could, then, use the sample data to test the null hypothesis that the true proportion of female smokers is 39% at the time of data collection.

The hypothesis test for the null hypothesis that the population proportion is some fixed amount, say $\Pi_0$, involves calculation of the test statistic

$$\frac{p - \Pi_0}{\sqrt{\Pi_0(1 - \Pi_0)/n}} \tag{2.4}$$

which is compared to the standard normal distribution (Table B.1 or B.2).

For the example quoted the test statistic is, from (2.4),

$$\frac{0.3754 - 0.39}{\sqrt{0.39(1 - 0.39)/4161}} = -1.93.$$

Since the absolute value of this, 1.93, is below the 5% critical value, 1.96, we fail to reject the null hypothesis (true percentage is 39%), against the alternative that it is some other value. This is what we might expect, anyway, since $\Pi_0 = 0.39$ is inside the complementary 95% confidence interval found earlier and is, therefore, a likely value for the true proportion.

This is a particular example of a general procedure: we reject the null hypothesis at the $X\%$ level only if the value under the null hypothesis lies outside the $(100 - X)\%$ confidence interval. In the case of proportions, in contrast to that for means (see Section 2.7), it is just possible, if unlikely, that we get a different result from a hypothesis test compared with using the complementary confidence interval to ascertain significance. This is due to the slightly different approximations that are used in the two procedures.

One advantage of the test procedure is that it enables us to calculate the $p$ value. From a computer package, $p = 0.054$ for the example. Quoting this figure in a report alerts the reader to the fact that the null hypothesis would, after all, be rejected if a significance level of 5.4%, or some round figure just above it, such as 6%, were used instead of 5%. When we use 5% significance we shall wrongly reject the null hypothesis one time in 20. Perhaps we are prepared to accept a slightly higher error rate. If we are prepared to be wrong 5.4% of the time (less than one chance in 18) then we could adopt 5.4% significance, and thus reject the null hypothesis in the example. If we intend to use the test to actually make a decision, it is clearly important to fix the significance level *before* data analysis begins.

So far we have not considered the **alternative hypothesis** critically; that is, we have taken it simply to be the negation of the null. In the example used the alternative hypothesis, denoted $H_1$, is that the population proportion is not equal to 0.39. This led to a two-sided test, where we reject $H_0$ if the observed proportion is sufficiently large or sufficiently small. Is this appropriate in the example? Suppose the government target was specified precisely as *less* than 39% of women should be smokers. In this situation we no longer wish to have a two-sided test; we have the hypotheses

$$H_0 : \Pi = 0.39 \text{ versus } H_1 : \Pi < 0.39,$$

where $\Pi$ is the population proportion, and we only wish to reject the null hypothesis, $H_0$, in favour of $H_1$ when the observed sample proportion is sufficiently *small*. Notice that $H_0$ is as for the two-sided test, only $H_1$ has changed (previously it was $\Pi \neq 0.39$). We now have a **one-sided** test with a single critical value in the lower tail of the standard normal distribution. Precisely, we have a one-sided 'less than' test. In another situation $H_1$ might be formulated as $\Pi > 0.39$; then we have a single critical value in the upper tail. By the symmetry of the normal distribution, this will be the negative of the critical value for the 'less than' test. Since Table B.2 gives two-sided critical values we shall need to double the required one-sided significance level before using this table for a one-sided test (of either type). Otherwise we can use Table B.1 more directly.

For a 5% test applied to our example the critical value is $-1.6449$ (Table B.1 tells us that it is slightly bigger than $-1.65$; Table B.2 gives the result to four decimal places when we look up double the required significance level). The test statistic, $-1.93$, is less than $-1.6449$, so it is a more extreme value. Hence we reject $H_0$ in favour of the one-sided $H_1$ at the 5% level. Note that this is the opposite decision to that taken after the two-sided test earlier. The $p$ value is 0.027, half of the $p$ value for the earlier two-sided test. The government's target appears to have been met.

This example shows that we should decide not only on the significance level, but also on the alternative hypothesis, before data analysis begins. In most cases the two-sided alternative is the appropriate one, and should be used unless there is a good reason to do otherwise. Consequently Appendix B gives critical values for the normal (Table B.2) and $t$ (Table B.4) distributions that are appropriate for two-sided tests.

The chi-square test of Section 2.5.1 requires one-sided critical values of chi-square in order to perform a two-sided test. As observed values move away from expected values in *either* direction (2.1) will always increase, and so it is only very large values of (2.1), in the upper tail, that are inconsistent with the null hypothesis. Similar comments can be made for the $F$ test from an analysis of variance (Section 9.2.3). Since these are the most common situations where the distributions are used, Appendix B gives one-sided critical values for the $\chi^2$ and $F$ tests.

### 2.5.3   *Comparing two proportions or percentages*

The problems described in Section 2.5.2 arise from a **one-sample** situation; that is, only one sample of data is analysed. More often, in epidemiological studies, we are interested in comparing two samples, or one sample split into two sub-samples in some meaningful way. For instance, we have so far looked at the proportion (or the percentage) of female smokers. Now we consider comparing smoking rates between the two sexes, this being a *two-sample* problem.

We obtain a 95% confidence interval for the difference between two population proportions as

$$p_1 - p_2 \pm 1.96\sqrt{\frac{p_1(1-p_1)}{n_1} + \frac{p_2(1-p_2)}{n_2}}, \qquad (2.5)$$

where $p_1$ is the sample proportion from the first sample (of size $n_1$) and $p_2$ and $n_2$ are the corresponding values for the second sample.

For the difference between male and female smoking proportions we have, from Table 2.9,

$$p_1 = 2279/4520 = 0.5042, \qquad p_2 = 0.3754,$$
$$n_1 = 4520, \qquad n_2 = 4161.$$

Hence the 95% confidence interval, from (2.5), is

$$0.5042 - 0.3754 \pm 1.96\sqrt{\frac{0.5042(1 - 0.5042)}{4520} + \frac{0.3754(1 - 0.3754)}{4161}}$$

which is $0.1288 \pm 0.0207$ or $(0.108, 0.150)$. We are 95% confident that the male percentage of smokers exceeds the female percentage by between 10.8% and 15.0%. Notice that zero is well outside these limits, suggesting that the male excess has not arisen just by chance. We may wish to test this formally.

The test statistic for testing the null hypothesis that the true difference between two population proportions is zero is

$$\frac{p_1 - p_2}{\sqrt{p_c(1 - p_c)\left(\dfrac{1}{n_1} + \dfrac{1}{n_2}\right)}}, \tag{2.6}$$

where

$$p_c = \frac{n_1 p_1 + n_2 p_2}{n_1 + n_2}. \tag{2.7}$$

We compare (2.6) with the standard normal distribution. In (2.7) $p_c$ is the 'combined proportion', a weighted average of the two individual sample proportions. An alternative definition is that $p_c$ is the sample proportion for the combined sample, created by pooling samples 1 and 2.

Suppose that we now wish formally to test the hypothesis that the same percentage of middle-aged Scottish men and women smoke. From (2.7) we have

$$p_c = \frac{4520 \times 0.5042 + 4161 \times 0.3754}{4520 + 4161} = 0.4425.$$

Note that we could get this result from Table 2.8 as the proportion of smokers for the sex groups combined. Then, from (2.6), the test statistic is

$$\frac{0.5042 - 0.3754}{\sqrt{0.4425(1 - 0.4425)\left(\dfrac{1}{4520} + \dfrac{1}{4161}\right)}} = 12.07.$$

Since this is above 1.96 we reject the null hypothesis of equal proportions at the 5% level of significance and conclude that the sexes have different proportions of smokers. In fact we have very strong evidence to reject $H_0$ since the $p$ value is below 0.0001; that is, we would reject $H_0$ even if we used a significance level as small as 0.01%. Note that there was no reason to use anything other than the general two-sided alternative hypothesis (proportions unequal) here. Even so, the sample evidence suggests that more men smoke, rather than more women, and our test, like our confidence interval, suggests that this is a 'real' difference.

Another way of looking at the problem of testing the hypothesis that the prevalence of smoking is the same for men and women is to consider the equivalent hypothesis that there is no relationship between smoking and the person's sex. Reference to Section 2.5.1 shows that we test the hypothesis of no relationship through the chi-square test applied to Table 2.9. In fact this is an equivalent procedure to that used in this section. The only difference when the chi-square test is applied to a $2 \times 2$ table is that the test statistic, (2.1), is the square of that introduced here, (2.6). The $p$ value will be exactly the same, because the critical values of $\chi_1^2$ are also the squares of those for the standard normal. Further details of how to analyse $2 \times 2$ tables are given in Section 3.5.

## 2.6   Descriptive techniques for quantitative variables

In this section we shall consider descriptive techniques for epidemiological data on a quantitative variable. We shall look at two descriptive techniques: numerical summarization and pictorial shape investigation. In an initial exploration of quantitative data, shape investigation would normally be most important because many analytical techniques are only suitable for data of a certain shape, while summarization might inadvertently obscure some interesting aspects of the data. In report writing, summarizing is generally more important because it is economical in space and easier for the reader to assimilate. It will be convenient to take summarization first in what follows.

The techniques will be illustrated using Scottish Heart Health Study data, as before, but now a small subset of these data, for 50 subjects, will be used. This is done because the complete set would be unwieldy in the present context, and the results derived here would be hard to reproduce. However, results from the subset may not, of course, necessarily approximate to results from analysis of the whole. Results of eight variables recorded on these 50 are given in Table 2.10.

**Table 2.10**   Results for 50 subjects sampled from the Scottish Heart Health Study

| Serum total cholesterol (mmol/l) | Diastolic blood pressure (mmHg) | Systolic blood pressure (mmHg) | Alcohol (g/day) | Cigarettes (no./day) | Carbon monoxide (ppm) | Cotinine (ng/ml) | CHD (1 = yes, 2 = no) |
|---|---|---|---|---|---|---|---|
| 5.75 | 80 | 121 | 5.4 | 0 | 6 | 13 | 2 |
| 6.76 | 83 | 139 | 64.6 | 0 | 4 | 3 | 2 |
| 6.47 | 76 | 113 | 21.5 | 20 | 21 | 284 | 2 |
| 7.11 | 79 | 124 | 8.2 | 40 | 57 | 395 | 2 |
| 5.42 | 79 | 127 | 24.4 | 20 | 29 | 283 | 2 |
| 7.04 | 100 | 148 | 13.6 | 0 | 3 | 0 | 2 |
| 5.75 | 79 | 124 | 54.6 | 0 | 3 | 1 | 2 |
| 7.14 | 85 | 127 | 6.2 | 0 | 1 | 0 | 2 |
| 6.10 | 76 | 138 | 0.0 | 0 | 1 | 3 | 2 |
| 6.55 | 82 | 133 | 2.4 | 0 | 2 | 0 | 2 |
| 6.29 | 92 | 141 | 0.0 | 0 | 7 | 0 | 2 |
| 5.98 | 100 | 183 | 21.5 | 20 | 55 | 245 | 1 |
| 5.71 | 78 | 119 | 50.2 | 0 | 14 | 424 | 2 |
| 6.89 | 90 | 143 | 16.7 | 0 | 4 | 0 | 1 |
| 4.90 | 85 | 132 | 40.6 | 4 | 7 | 82 | 2 |
| 6.23 | 88 | 139 | 16.7 | 25 | 24 | 324 | 2 |
| 7.71 | 109 | 154 | 7.2 | 1 | 3 | 11 | 1 |
| 5.73 | 93 | 136 | 10.8 | 0 | 2 | 0 | 2 |
| 6.54 | 100 | 149 | 26.0 | 0 | 3 | 0 | 2 |
| 7.16 | 73 | 107 | 2.9 | 25 | 29 | 315 | 1 |
| 6.13 | 92 | 132 | 23.9 | 0 | 2 | 2 | 2 |
| 6.25 | 87 | 123 | 31.1 | 0 | 7 | 10 | 2 |
| 5.19 | 97 | 141 | 12.0 | 0 | 3 | 4 | 1 |
| 6.05 | 74 | 118 | 23.9 | 0 | 3 | 0 | 2 |
| 7.12 | 85 | 133 | 24.4 | 0 | 2 | 0 | 2 |
| 5.71 | 88 | 121 | 45.4 | 0 | 8 | 2 | 2 |
| 6.19 | 69 | 129 | 24.8 | 15 | 40 | 367 | 1 |
| 6.73 | 98 | 129 | 52.6 | 15 | 21 | 233 | 2 |
| 5.34 | 70 | 123 | 38.3 | 1 | 2 | 7 | 2 |
| 4.79 | 82 | 127 | 23.9 | 0 | 2 | 1 | 2 |
| 6.78 | 74 | 104 | 4.8 | 0 | 4 | 7 | 2 |
| 6.10 | 88 | 123 | 86.1 | 0 | 3 | 1 | 1 |
| 4.35 | 88 | 128 | 15.5 | 20 | 11 | 554 | 2 |
| 7.10 | 79 | 136 | 7.4 | 10 | 9 | 189 | 1 |
| 5.85 | 102 | 150 | 4.1 | 0 | 6 | 0 | 2 |
| 6.74 | 68 | 109 | 1.2 | 15 | 15 | 230 | 2 |
| 7.55 | 80 | 135 | 92.1 | 25 | 29 | 472 | 2 |
| 7.86 | 78 | 131 | 23.9 | 6 | 55 | 407 | 1 |
| 6.92 | 101 | 137 | 2.5 | 0 | 3 | 0 | 2 |
| 6.64 | 97 | 139 | 119.6 | 40 | 16 | 298 | 2 |

**Table 2.10**  *cont.*

| Serum total cholesterol (mmol/l) | Diastolic blood pressure (mmHg) | Systolic blood pressure (mmHg) | Alcohol (g/day) | Cigarettes (no./day) | Carbon monoxide (ppm) | Cotinine (ng/ml) | CHD (1 = yes, 2 = no) |
|---|---|---|---|---|---|---|---|
| 6.46 | 76 | 142 | 62.2 | 40 | 31 | 404 | 1 |
| 5.99 | 73 | 108 | 0.0 | 0 | 2 | 4 | 2 |
| 5.39 | 77 | 112 | 11.0 | 30 | 11 | 251 | 2 |
| 6.35 | 81 | 133 | 16.2 | 0 | 3 | 0 | 2 |
| 5.86 | 88 | 147 | 88.5 | 0 | 3 | 0 | 2 |
| 5.64 | 65 | 111 | 0.0 | 20 | 16 | 271 | 2 |
| 6.60 | 102 | 149 | 65.8 | 0 | 3 | 1 | 2 |
| 6.76 | 75 | 140 | 12.4 | 0 | 2 | 0 | 2 |
| 5.51 | 75 | 125 | 0.0 | 25 | 16 | 441 | 2 |
| 7.15 | 92 | 131 | 31.1 | 20 | 36 | 434 | 1 |

Note: These data are available electronically (see Appendix C).

### 2.6.1   The five-number summary

The basic idea of summarization is to present a small number of key statistics that may be used to represent the data as a whole. If we want to use only one summary statistic, the obvious choice would be some measure of average. This is usually too great a summarization, except for very simple uses, since it says nothing about how the data are distributed about the average, that is how well the average represents the whole. In epidemiological research we would normally find it much more informative to present either the five-number summary given here, or the more succinct two-number summary of Section 2.6.3 (or possibly a selection from both).

The five-number summary comprises the following:
- the minimum value;
- the first quartile: 25% of the data are below, 75% above;
- the median (or second quartile): 50% of the data are below, 50% above;
- the third quartile: 75% of the data are below, 25% above;
- the maximum value.

Interpretation (and evaluation) of the extreme values (minimum and maximum) is obvious. The quartiles are the numbers which divide the data into four equal portions. Their derivation is very straightforward when there are, say, nine observations as in the next example.

*Example 2.3*   To find the five-number summary of the numbers

$$15, \ 3, \ 9, \ 3, \ 14, \ 20, \ 7, \ 8, \ 11$$

first we sort the data, giving:

$$3, \ 3, \ 7, \ 8, \ 9, \ 11, \ 14, \ 15, \ 20.$$

The minimum is 3 and the maximum is 20. The median, or second quartile ($Q_2$), is the middle number, which is 9 (this has four below and four above). The first quartile ($Q_1$) is 7, since this has two below and six above, giving the correct split in the ratio of 1 : 3. Similarly the third quartile ($Q_3$) is 14 since three-quarters of the remaining data are below, and one-quarter above this value.

Consider, now, the data on the 'cholesterol' variable in Table 2.10. To apply the same logic, we first need to sort the data. This has been done to produce Table 2.11. From this table the minimum and maximum are easy enough to find, but there is an immediate problem when we try to find the median. Since there are an even number (50) of observations, there is no 'middle' value. It seems reasonable to take the 25th or 26th value, or some summary of the two, as the median, but there is no single 'right' answer. Another problem arises when we try to find $Q_1$, since no number can possibly have a quarter of the remaining observations ($49/4 = 12.25$) below it. In fact, since $50/4 = 12.5$ the 'position' of $Q_1$ ought to be 12.5, so it would seem reasonable to take the 12th or 13th value, or some summary of the two.

Unfortunately there is no universally agreed rule as to which choice to take in these situations. For this reason different computer packages may give different answers for the quartiles from the same data, although the differences should be small and, usually, unimportant. When the position of a quartile is a whole number, $r$ (say), we shall take the average of the $r$th and $(r + 1)$th observations in rank order to be the median. For our data, $50/2 = 25$, which is a whole number, so we should evaluate the median as half the sum of the 25th and 26th values. On the other hand, if the position of a quartile is not a whole

**Table 2.11**  Total serum cholesterol (mmol/l) in rank order

| Rank | Value | Rank | Value | Rank | Value | Rank | Value | Rank | Value |
|------|-------|------|-------|------|-------|------|-------|------|-------|
| 1 | 4.35 | 11 | 5.71 | 21 | 6.10 | 31 | 6.55 | 41 | 7.04 |
| 2 | 4.79 | 12 | 5.73 | 22 | 6.13 | 32 | 6.60 | 42 | 7.10 |
| 3 | 4.90 | 13 | 5.75 | 23 | 6.19 | 33 | 6.64 | 43 | 7.11 |
| 4 | 5.19 | 14 | 5.75 | 24 | 6.23 | 34 | 6.73 | 44 | 7.12 |
| 5 | 5.34 | 15 | 5.85 | 25 | 6.25 | 35 | 6.74 | 45 | 7.14 |
| 6 | 5.39 | 16 | 5.86 | 26 | 6.29 | 36 | 6.76 | 46 | 7.15 |
| 7 | 5.42 | 17 | 5.98 | 27 | 6.35 | 37 | 6.76 | 47 | 7.16 |
| 8 | 5.51 | 18 | 5.99 | 28 | 6.46 | 38 | 6.78 | 48 | 7.55 |
| 9 | 5.64 | 19 | 6.05 | 29 | 6.47 | 39 | 6.89 | 49 | 7.71 |
| 10 | 5.71 | 20 | 6.10 | 30 | 6.54 | 40 | 6.92 | 50 | 7.86 |

number, then we shall take the number in the *next highest* whole number position within the ranked data set. Since the position for our $Q_1$ ought to be 12.5, which is not a whole number, we will take the 13th value in rank order to be $Q_1$. Similarly $Q_3$ will be the 38th value. Hence the five-number summary of the cholesterol data is

$$4.35 \quad 5.75 \quad 6.27 \quad 6.78 \quad 7.86$$
$$\text{min.} \quad Q_1 \quad Q_2 \quad Q_3 \quad \text{max.}$$

The blocks between these five numbers are called the **quarters** of the data.

What does the five-number summary tell us about the data? We can see that no one has a cholesterol value of more than 7.86 or less than 4.35 mmol/l; these are important and interesting findings from the epidemiological investigation. Their difference $(7.86 - 4.35 = 3.51 \text{ mmol/l})$ is called the **range**, which measures the entire spread (**variation** or **dispersion**) of the data. We can also see the middle value (6.27 mmol/l), which is a measure of **average** for the data. Perhaps not so obvious is the use of $Q_1$ and $Q_3$. In many data sets there are a small number of unusually low or unusually high values, which we will term **outliers**. Such values may distort the range, since they make it much bigger than would be expected if all the data were 'typical'. The range also has an unfortunate tendency to increase as sample size increases: the more people we observe the more chance we have of including the rare 'extreme' person. Certainly the range cannot decrease when we include more observations. The first and third quartiles are not affected by outliers, nor are they sensitive to sample size. Hence their difference $(6.78 - 5.75 = 1.03 \text{ mmol/l})$, called the **inter-quartile range**, often gives a more representative measure of the dispersion, which may be meaningfully compared with other data sets. Sometimes the semi-inter-quartile range, or **quartile deviation** is used instead. This is simply half the inter-quartile range, $(Q_3 - Q_1)/2$.

*Example 2.4* Consider Example 2.3 again, but now suppose that the nine numbers are (in rank order)

$$3, \ 3, \ 7, \ 8, \ 9, \ 11, \ 14, \ 15, \ 200;$$

that is, as before except that the maximum is now 200 rather than 20. Compared with Example 2.3 the range has increased from $20 - 3 = 17$ to $200 - 3 = 197$. The inter-quartile range, however, remains $14 - 7 = 7$. Also the median is unchanged (at the value 9). The number 200 is an outlier because it is more than 10 times larger than any other value. Notice that it could be argued that we cannot claim to know what is 'typical' on the strength of only eight other observations, but the principle behind this simplistic example clearly holds with more appropriate sample sizes.

As well as average and dispersion, the five-number summary gives an impression of the other important feature of observational data, the degree of

**symmetry**. Data are symmetrical if each value below the median is perfectly counterbalanced by another value exactly equidistant from, but above, the median (as in a mirror image). We are very unlikely to find such perfect symmetry in observational data, so instead we might look for 'quartile symmetry'. That is where

$$Q_1 - \text{minimum} = \text{maximum} - Q_3$$

and

$$Q_2 - Q_1 = Q_3 - Q_2$$

For the cholesterol data these four differences are 1.40, 1.08, 0.52 and 0.51, respectively, showing that there is almost perfect symmetry between the middle quarters of the data, but some lack of symmetry between the outer quarters.

The degree of symmetry is best judged from a diagram of the five-number summary called a **boxplot** (or **box-and-whisker plot**). Figure 2.4 is a boxplot for the cholesterol data. The line in the box marks the median, the edges of the box mark the quartiles, and the arrows (or 'whiskers') go out to the extremes.

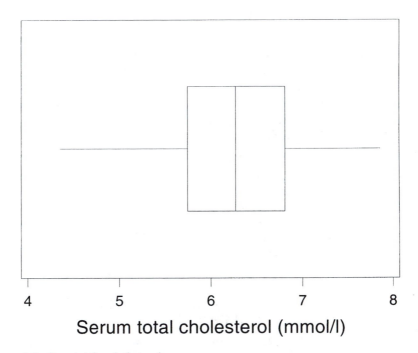

**Serum total cholesterol (mmol/l)**

**Figure 2.4**   Boxplot for cholesterol.

The cholesterol data have no obvious outliers, but when outliers are present it is best to isolate them on the boxplot. To do this we need to impose a definition of an outlier and, just as with the definition of 'quartile', there is no universally agreed rule, with the consequence that different statistical computer packages may give different results. We will define an outlier in a boxplot by conceptually placing 'fences' at the positions $1\frac{1}{2}$ times the length of the box below $Q_1$ and above $Q_3$. The left arrow will then terminate at the smallest observation inside the fences and the right arrow will terminate at the largest observation inside the fences. Any observation outside the fences will be termed an outlier and identified with an asterisk. Figure 2.5 shows a boxplot for alcohol (from Table 2.10) where there are three outliers. When outliers occur we may prefer to change our five-number summary so that the minimum and maximum are replaced by fairly extreme percentiles, such as the 1st and 99th percentiles (Section 2.6.2).

By eye, from Figures 2.4 and 2.5, we can see that cholesterol is reasonably symmetrical but alcohol is not. Non-symmetric data are said to be **skewed**. If there is a bigger portion of the boxplot to the right of the median, we say that

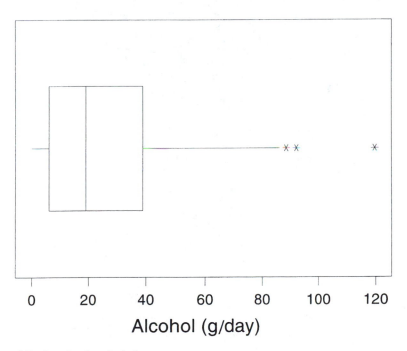

**Figure 2.5**   Boxplot for alcohol.

the data are **right-skewed** or **positively skewed**. Otherwise they are **left-skewed** or **negatively skewed**. Alcohol is right-skewed, from Figure 2.5.

Identification of skew is one of the most important parts of an initial examination of epidemiological data, since it points to what is appropriate at further stages of analysis (as we shall see). However, identification of what is *important* skew is not always straightforward since it naturally depends upon what we propose to do with the data. To some extent it also depends upon the sample size. Although our cholesterol data are not entirely symmetrical, for most practical purposes the slight lack of symmetry is not important. The alcohol data are quite different, with pronounced skew which must be accounted for in any further analysis. Notice that the symmetry of cholesterol and skewness of alcohol are properties of the *data* rather than the variables. We cannot, for example, be sure that another sample of cholesterol data will not be skewed, although if it was of the same size and taken from a similar parent population we would anticipate near-symmetry on the basis of our findings.

Boxplots are useful for comparing the same quantitative variable in different populations, or sub-populations. For example, Figure 2.6 shows cholesterol for those men with and without CHD, from Table 2.10. Since the same (horizontal) scale has been used we can see that cholesterol tends to be higher

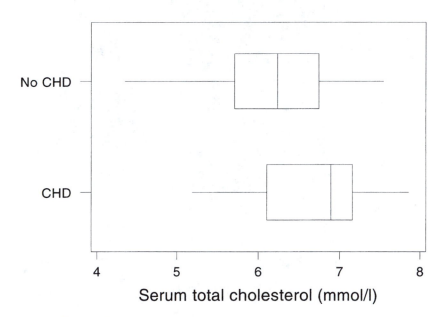

**Figure 2.6**   Boxplot for cholesterol data by CHD group.

for those with CHD. The dispersion (as measured by the inter-quartile range) is much the same in each group, although the range is slightly larger for those with CHD. Each distribution shows some evidence of left skew, notably within the first and third quartiles for those with CHD.

## 2.6.2   Quantiles

**Quantiles** are values which divide data into portions of equal size. The quartiles provide an example: they divide the data into four equal parts. Other divisions may be useful to explore how the data are distributed. Tertiles divide into three, quintiles into five, deciles into 10 and percentiles into a 100 equal parts, and so on. They may be calculated by extending the methodology used in Section 2.6.1, as the following example shows.

*Example 2.5*   Using the data of Example 2.3 (where $n = 9$), the position for the first tertile should be $\frac{1}{3} \times 9 = 3$. Since this is a whole number, we take the mean of the 3rd and 4th observations in rank order. Similarly the second tertile has position $\frac{2}{3} \times 9 = 6$, so that we take the mean of the 6th and 7th observations in rank order. Since the ordered data are

$$3, \ 3, \ 7, \ 8, \ 9, \ 11, \ 14, \ 15, \ 20,$$

the first tertile is $(7 + 8)/2 = 7.5$ and the second is $(11 + 14)/2 = 12.5$. Notice that these numbers split the data 3 : 6 (i.e. 1 : 2) and 6 : 3 (i.e. 2 : 1) respectively, as we would expect of tertiles.

Sometimes a particular quantile is of interest. For instance we may wish to find the 90th percentile of cholesterol from a national population survey such as the SHHS, since this tells us what value we can expect the highest 10% of the national population to exceed. Often the entire set of quantiles (of a particular degree) are required. For example, infant growth curves may have each percentile-for-age of weight marked, these having been calculated from extensive sample data.

When we have data on the same variable from two different sources, a **quantile–quantile plot** is a useful descriptive tool. As the name suggests, this is a plot of the quantiles (for example, deciles) from one source against the same quantiles from the other source. If the two distributions are similar then we expect to see a straight line on the quantile–quantile plot. This would provide an alternative to the two-sample boxplot (for example, Figure 2.6).

## 2.6.3   The two-number summary

If the data are reasonably symmetric, then a better measure of their average is the **mean**, rather than the median. The mean is defined as the sum of all the observations divided by the sample size, which is written mathematically as

$$\bar{x} = \frac{1}{n}\sum_{i=1}^{n} x_i, \tag{2.8}$$

where $x_1, x_2, \ldots, x_n$ are the observations (the sample is of size $n$).

To calculate the mean for the cholesterol data we simply sum up the cholesterol values in Table 2.10 and divide by 50. This gives

$$\bar{x} = \frac{1}{50} \times 314.33 = 6.287 \, \text{mmol/l}.$$

Similarly, a better measure of spread for symmetric data is the **standard deviation**, rather than the inter-quartile range (or the range). This is conceived as a mean of the differences between each observation and their mean, that is, it should tell us the average deviation of the mean from the observations themselves. In fact we cannot use quite such a simple approach because we would find that this mean of differences would always be zero. This is simply due to the definition of the mean as the arithmetic centre of the data, and is easy to prove algebraically. Here we will simply use an example to illustrate the problem.

*Example 2.6*    Consider the simple data set of size 9 from Example 2.3 again. Here the mean is from (2.8),

$$\bar{x} = \frac{1}{9}(15 + 3 + 9 + 3 + 14 + 20 + 7 + 8 + 11) = 90/9 = 10.0.$$

The differences from this mean, $x_i - \bar{x}$, are thus

$$5, \ -7, \ -1, \ -7, \ 4, \ 10, \ -3, \ -2, \ 1.$$

The sum of these differences is zero and hence the mean difference is zero, as predicted.

The problem is caused by the positive and negative contributions to the mean difference exactly cancelling each other out. One way of getting over this problem is to square each difference before averaging (since squared values are always positive). This gives rise to the **variance** (denoted $s^2$), the average of the *squared* differences between each observation and the mean. However, the variance is not very meaningful for practical purposes because it is measured in square units (e.g. squared mmol/l for cholesterol). The standard deviation, $s$, is hence defined as the square root of the variance.

One final complication is that the averaging process to arrive at the variance should be to add up the squared differences and divide by $n - 1$ rather than the sample size, $n$. This is necessary to make the variance **unbiased** – that is, to ensure that the mean value of $s^2$ over many samples equals the true variance. Another explanation is that $s^2$ uses the divisor $n - 1$ because there are only $n - 1$ independent pieces of information in the data once $\bar{x}$ is known. Look at Example

2.6 again. Once we know $\bar{x}$ and the first eight data items we automatically know what the ninth item must be. The sum of the first eight numbers is

$$15 + 3 + 9 + 3 + 14 + 20 + 7 + 8 = 79.$$

Since $\bar{x} = 10$ the sum of all nine numbers must be $9 \times 10 = 90$. Hence the ninth number must be $90 - 79 = 11$, which indeed it is. As in the chi-square test (Section 2.5.1), the term degrees of freedom (d.f.) is used to refer to the number of independent pieces of information. Hence $s^2$ has $n - 1$ d.f.

When we use a computer package to calculate $s^2$ (or $s$) we must check that it has used the $n - 1$ rather than the $n$ divisor (some do not). Many calculators will allow for division by $n$ or $n - 1$. Division by $n$ is only correct if we have a 100% sample (a **census**) of the population of interest, which is hardly ever the case.

The formula for the variance is thus

$$s^2 = \frac{1}{n-1} S_{xx} \tag{2.9}$$

where

$$S_{xx} = \sum_{i=1}^{n}(x_i - \bar{x})^2. \tag{2.10}$$

*Example 2.7*   Using (2.10) with the data of Example 2.3 gives

$$S_{xx} = 254.$$

Hence, by (2.9), the variance is $s^2 = 254/8 = 31.75$ and the standard deviation, $s = \sqrt{31.75} = 5.63$.

For the cholesterol data of Table 2.10, $S_{xx} = 28.0765$, whence the variance is, $s^2 = 0.5730$ and the standard deviation $s = 0.757 \, \text{mmol/l}$.

With symmetric or near-symmetric data the mean and standard deviation provide a **two-number summary** of the two major features of the data, their average and their dispersion about this average.

With right-skewed data the mean will tend to be pulled upwards (above the median) by the few large observations. With left-skewed data the reverse is true, the mean will be pulled down below the median. Either type of skewness inflates the standard deviation. By contrast, the median and inter-quartile range are largely unaffected by skewness. We can see this contrast by considering, again, the effect of a single outlier, a particular case of skewness.

*Example 2.8*   Consider the data of Examples 2.3 and 2.4 (in rank order):

$$3, \ 3, \ 7, \ 8, \ 9, \ 11, \ 14, \ 15, \ 20$$

and

$$3, \ 3, \ 7, \ 8, \ 9, \ 11, \ 14, \ 15, \ 200.$$

For the first set of data $\bar{x} = 10.0$ (as shown in Example 2.6). For the second (with the outlier) it is 30.0. The first mean is a reasonable measure of average for its data, the second certainly is not, since it is by no means typical. However, in Examples 2.3 and 2.4 we saw that the median is 9 for both sets of data. Similarly, when 20 is replaced by 200 the standard deviation changes from 5.63 to 63.89, but the inter-quartile range is unaltered (see Example 2.4).

The mean is thus not a suitable measure of average for highly skewed data, but the question remains as to why we should prefer it to the median for symmetric or near-symmetric data. One reason is that the mean uses every observation in the data, which is not true of the median which only uses the middle value or values. A second reason is that the mean is what most people think of as 'the average'. Third, the mean has a mathematical expression, (2.8), but the median does not. This allows us to manipulate the mean mathematically, and thus enables powerful, more complex, methods of analysis to be devised. So we should use the mean if we can, but not when it is unrepresentative of the average, in which case we either transform the data (see Section 2.8.1) or use the median. The standard deviation should always be used with the mean, since it has a similar derivation and its advantages are much the same.

### 2.6.4   Further summary statistics

Here we present three further summary statistics. In each case, examples appear subsequently in Table 2.12.

Sometimes a quantitative variable is summarized by showing the **standard error** of the mean, rather than the standard deviation alongside the mean. The standard error of the mean is a measure of the inaccuracy of the sample mean as a representative of the mean of the entire parent population from which the sample was drawn. In fact, it is the standard deviation of the distribution of sample means (the means of repeated samples of the same size from the same population). The standard error of the mean is $s/\sqrt{n}$. Notice that this will decrease as the sample size, $n$, increases. Standard errors may be defined for other summary statistics besides the mean; for instance, the standard error of the difference between two means will be used in Section 2.7.3.

The **coefficient of variation** is defined as the standard deviation divided by the mean. This is a standardized measure of variation, often used to compare dispersion for variables with different units of measurement. Sometimes it is multiplied by 100 so as to give a percentage measure.

Finally, the **coefficient of skewness** is a numerical measure of skewness. It is defined as

$$\frac{k\sum(x-\bar{x})^3}{s^3},$$

where $k$ is some function of the sample size, $n$. If the distribution of the $x$ variable is perfectly symmetrical, the coefficient of skewness will be zero. Negative values imply left skewness; positive values imply right skewness. Different textbooks and computer packages use different forms for $k$. For this, and other reasons, it is not possible to give general rules regarding how big this coefficient should be so as to conclude that the skewness is important. In any case, reference to a boxplot will be more informative. The coefficient of skewness is most useful to provide summary comparisons, say before and after a variable is transformed (see Section 2.8.1).

However $k$ is defined, the coefficient of skewness summarizes the cubed deviations from the overall mean, standardized by the process of division by the cube of the standard deviation. Due to this standardization the coefficient of skewness is, like the coefficient of variation, unit-free. In Table 2.12 we shall take

$$k = n/(n-1)(n-2).$$

### 2.6.5    Assessing symmetry

We have already seen how the boxplot may be used to assess symmetry. Here we consider how summary statistics, including those represented on the boxplot, may be used to determine whether a variable is symmetric, or (more likely in practice) reasonably so. This not only determines whether the mean and standard deviation (or standard error) are suitable summary measures, but is also a first step to determining whether inferential techniques based upon the normal distribution are appropriate (Section 2.7).

Table 2.12 shows several summary statistics for each of the quantitative variables in Table 2.10. Boxplots of the five variables not so far presented appear in Figure 2.7. The '2' on the boxplot for carbon monoxide indicates two outliers with the same value. In this 'compound boxplot' each variable has been standardized so as to avoid the gross differences in magnitude which occur when the original variables are plotted on a common scale. For each variable, its median was subtracted from all its values, followed by division by its inter-quartile range. This standardization ensures that the boxes are all of equal width and the median line occurs in the same position for all standardized variables. Hence Figure 2.7 may not be used to compare averages or dispersions. In any case such comparisons would be meaningless.

**Table 2.12**  Summary statistics for variables from Table 2.10 (IQR = inter-quartile range, CV = coefficient of variation), sample size $n = 50$

| Summary statistic | Serum total cholesterol (mmol/l) | Diastolic blood pressure (mmHg) | Systolic blood pressure (mmHg) | Alcohol (g/day) | Cigarettes (no./day) | Carbon monoxide (ppm) | Cotinine (ng/ml) |
|---|---|---|---|---|---|---|---|
| Mean | 6.287 | 84.6 | 131.3 | 26.76 | 8.7 | 12.8 | 139.5 |
| Median | 6.27 | 82.5 | 131.5 | 19.1 | 0 | 6 | 7 |
| Std deviation | 0.757 | 10.5 | 14.3 | 27.75 | 12.5 | 14.9 | 177.3 |
| Std error | 0.107 | 1.5 | 2.0 | 3.92 | 1.8 | 2.1 | 25.1 |
| $Q_1$ | 5.75 | 76 | 123 | 6.2 | 0 | 3 | 0 |
| $Q_3$ | 6.78 | 92 | 139 | 38.3 | 20 | 16 | 284 |
| IQR | 1.03 | 16 | 16 | 32.1 | 20 | 13 | 284 |
| Minimum | 4.35 | 65 | 104 | 0 | 0 | 1 | 0 |
| Maximum | 7.86 | 109 | 183 | 119.6 | 40 | 57 | 554 |
| Range | 3.51 | 44 | 79 | 119.6 | 40 | 56 | 554 |
| Skewness | -0.23 | 0.36 | 0.69 | 1.50 | 1.19 | 1.68 | 0.78 |
| CV | 12% | 12% | 11% | 104% | 143% | 117% | 127% |

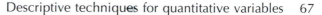

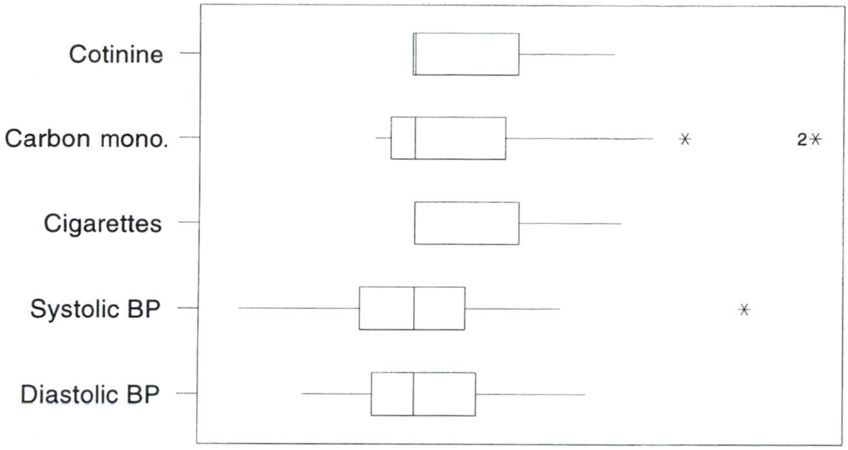

**Figure 2.7**  Boxplots (using standardized scales) for several variables from Table 2.10.

From Figure 2.7, diastolic and systolic blood pressure are reasonably symmetrical, although the outlier in systolic blood pressure might usefully be reported separately (without the outlier the mean becomes 130.2). The other three variables are right-skewed. 'Cigarettes' is so skewed that the minimum, first quartile and median are all equal (to zero). Cotinine is almost as badly skewed; its minimum and first quartile are both zero. Recall that Figures 2.4 and 2.5 show that cholesterol has a slight, but unimportant, left skew and that alcohol is highly right-skewed.

From Table 2.12, notice that the mean is bigger than the median in all four cases where skewness is apparent in the boxplots, as we would expect. In these cases the relatively few large values distort the mean as a measure of centre of the data. For perfectly symmetric data the mean and median would be equal since then there is only one 'centre'. There is no reason for the standard deviation and inter-quartile range to be related since the standard deviation does not involve the concept of 'quarters'. Unless there are several negative values, a variable will usually (although not necessarily) be skewed when the standard deviation is of a similar size to, or exceeds, the mean. This will happen when the coefficient of variation approaches or exceeds 100%, which happens for all four highly skewed variables in Table 2.12. The coefficient of skewness is, as anticipated, positive except in the case of the left-skewed variable, cholesterol. Notice how the outlier has inflated the quantitative measure of skewness for systolic blood pressure. Otherwise the coefficients of skewness tend to follow the relative magnitudes anticipated from the boxplots. Values above about 0.7 seem to be associated with severe skewness.

### 2.6.6  Investigating shape

The summary statistics shown in Table 2.12 (or some subset of them) provide a short, informative description of the data for a quantitative variable. In some instances the summary is too extreme and we would wish to show more about the overall shape of the data.

The first step when investigating shape is to create a **grouped frequency table** (or **grouped frequency distribution**), such as Table 2.13 created from the cholesterol data in Table 2.10. As in Table 2.1, the percentages (and cumulative percentages) are optional, but informative.

Figure 2.8 is a **histogram** drawn from Table 2.13; this gives a visual impression of the shape which is apparent, but more difficult to assimilate, from the table. Boxplots also give an impression of some aspects of shape, but histograms show much more: they enable symmetry/skewness to be judged but also show where the 'peaks' and 'troughs' appear (cholesterol clearly peaks in the middle and drops away to either side, but more slowly to the left). The only drawback is that the shape produced can depend very much upon the number of groups (or **classes**) used, as well as the choice of start and end of the scale.

The **class intervals** used in Table 2.13 (i.e. 4.0 to less than 4.5, etc.) and in Figure 2.8 are all of equal size (0.5) and in this situation the histogram is easy to draw: indeed, the histogram is then essentially a bar chart except that the bars have been joined to emphasize the continuous nature of the variable concerned. When the variable concerned is discrete a continuity correction is

**Table 2.13**  Grouped frequency distribution for serum total cholesterol

| Cholesterol (mmol/l) | Frequency | Percentage | Cumulative percentage |
|---|---|---|---|
| 4.0 to less than 4.5 | 1 | 2% | 2% |
| 4.5 to less than 5.0 | 2 | 4% | 6% |
| 5.0 to less than 5.5 | 4 | 8% | 14% |
| 5.5 to less than 6.0 | 11 | 22% | 36% |
| 6.0 to less than 6.5 | 11 | 22% | 58% |
| 6.5 to less than 7.0 | 11 | 22% | 80% |
| 7.0 to less than 7.5 | 7 | 14% | 94% |
| 7.5 to less than 8.0 | 3 | 6% | 100% |
| Total | 50 | 100% | |

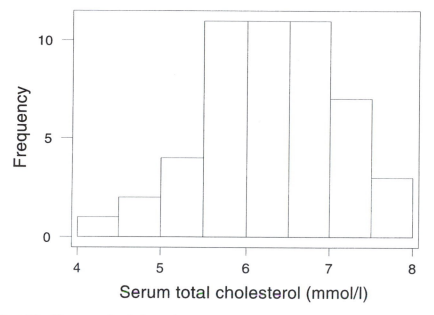

**Figure 2.8**   Histogram for cholesterol.

applied before the histogram is drawn. This simply 'joins' adjacent classes by starting each bar midway between adjacent class limits (and extending the extreme bars by half a class interval).

It is not essential, nor always very sensible, to maintain equal class sizes, particularly when the data are very bunched in a certain part of their distribution, but very sparse elsewhere. When the class sizes are unequal we should plot the **frequency density** (relative frequency divided by the class size) on the vertical axis to ensure that the areas of the bars are in the correct relative proportions. Table 2.14 and Figure 2.9 provide an example: notice how the skew, already apparent from Figure 2.5, is represented. Some computer packages produce histograms as bar charts and hence make no allowance for unequal class sizes. Sometimes histograms are plotted horizontally.

Sometimes cumulative frequencies (or percentages) are of more interest than the basic frequencies (percentages) – for example, when we wish to see the percentage of people that have serum total cholesterol less than a certain value. This is easily achieved for our data using Table 2.11, cholesterol values in sorted order. Figure 2.10 plots the percentage of cholesterol values up to and including each successive value in Table 2.11 against the values themselves; for

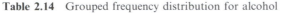

**Table 2.14**  Grouped frequency distribution for alcohol

| Alcohol (g/week) | Frequency | Relative frequency | Frequency density |
|---|---|---|---|
| 0 but less than 10 | 16 | 0.32 | 0.0320 |
| 10 but less than 20 | 9 | 0.18 | 0.0180 |
| 20 but less than 30 | 10 | 0.20 | 0.0200 |
| 30 but less than 50 | 5 | 0.10 | 0.0050 |
| 50 but less than 70 | 6 | 0.12 | 0.0060 |
| 70 but less than 120 | 4 | 0.08 | 0.0016 |
| Total | 50 | 1 | |

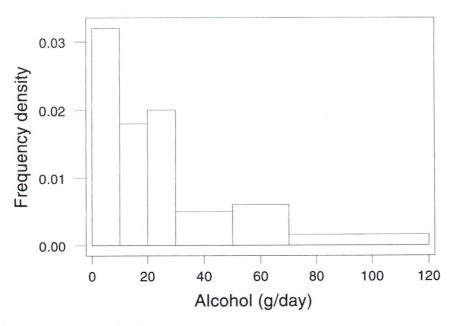

**Figure 2.9**  Histogram for alcohol.

example, 100% is plotted against the maximum value, 7.86. This is called a cumulative (percentage) frequency plot or **ogive**.

The quartiles are easily found (approximately) from an ogive. For example, we find the median by drawing a horizontal line from the 50% position on the vertical scale across to the curve. We drop a vertical line from this point down to the horizontal axis and read off the median. Look at the dotted lines on Figure 2.10, and compare the visual reading with the exact cholesterol median given in Table 2.12.

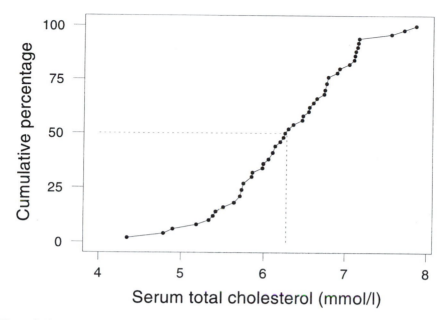

**Figure 2.10**   Ogive for cholesterol.

A less accurate ogive could be drawn from Table 2.13. The right-hand column of this table should be plotted against the upper class limits. For example, 100% is plotted against 8.0. Often the ogive (of either type) is 'smoothed out' to avoid kinks due to sampling variation (such as are apparent in Figure 2.10).

## 2.7   Inferences about means

When we wish to use quantitative data to make inferences about the wider population from which the sample was drawn, we generally prefer to use the simplest, most useful, summary measure for a quantitative variable: the measure of average. As we have seen, the mean is the most useful measure of average provided the data are reasonably symmetrical. In this section we shall take this to be the case, and develop confidence intervals and hypothesis tests for means, just as we did earlier for proportions.

In fact, to be more precise, the material in this section assumes that the mean is sampled from a **normal probability distribution**. This should be so if the data have, at least approximately, a normal shape like a long-skirted bell which is symmetric about its middle value (see Figure 2.11). This might be assessed from the histogram. The approximation must be fairly good for small samples but can be much less exact for large samples. This is because a fundamental theorem of statistics, the **central limit theorem**, says that the sampling distribution of sample means (that is, the means from repeated sampling) will tend to a normal distribution as $n$ tends to infinity. This is the justification for the use of the normal distribution when dealing with proportions in Section 2.5.2 (a proportion is a special type of sample mean). The procedures given there will only be justifiable if $n$ is reasonably big – say above 100. Convergence to the normal of the distribution of means is faster when the data themselves have a shape that is nearer to the normal. In Section 2.8 we shall consider what to do when the data on a quantitative variable do not have a normal distribution, even approximately, so that the central limit theorem cannot be invoked.

The **standard normal distribution** is that normal with mean 0 and standard deviation 1. This is the normal distribution tabulated in Tables B.1 and B.2. We can change any normal into this standard form by subtracting its mean and dividing by its standard deviation.

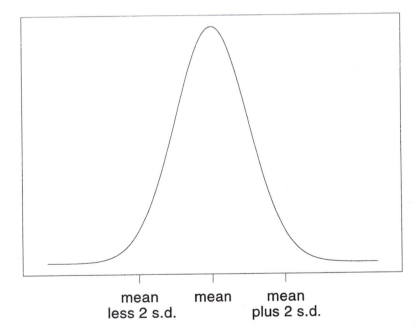

Figure 2.11    The normal curve (s.d. = standard deviation).

## 2.7.1    Checking normality

Various tests of normality have been suggested (see Stephens, 1974), including procedures based upon a measure of skewness (see Snedecor and Cochran, 1980). However, these are often too sensitive in epidemiological studies where sample sizes are generally large. That is, slight variations from normality cause rejection even when the variations have little effect on the final results of the epidemiological investigation.

Generally descriptive procedures, such as those based on histograms, boxplots and summary statistics, are more useful. One disadvantage with these procedures is that they may not be able to distinguish the normal from other symmetric shapes. For example, they may not be able to distinguish a triangular shaped distribution from the normal. A descriptive technique that is specific to the normal distribution is that of the **normal plot**. This is a plot of the data against their **normal scores**, the expected values *if* the data had a standard normal distribution. If the data do have a normal distribution then the normal plot will produce a straight line. Essentially normal plots are quantile–quantile plots (see Section 2.6.2) where one of the distributions is a theoretical one, and the quantiles plotted are determined by the data themselves.

For example, Figures 2.12 and 2.13 show normal plots for total cholesterol and alcohol respectively, using the data in Table 2.10. The points in Figure 2.12, but not in Figure 2.13, approximate a straight line fairly well: cholesterol, but not alcohol, is approximately normally distributed. For a test procedure based upon correlations from the normal plot, see Weiss (1995).

Normal scores are available from all the major statistical software packages. To calculate them by hand we would first need to rank the data. For the *i*th largest data value out of *n*, we then use Table B.1 to find that value from the standard normal distribution for which $S_i = 100(i/n)\%$ of the standard normal lies below it. For example, Table 2.11 shows that the smallest cholesterol value (with rank = 1) is 4.35. The normal score should correspond to

$$S_i = 100i/n = 100/50 = 2\%.$$

To avoid problems of computation for the highest rank, $S_i$ is often replaced by $100i/(n+1)$. Further 'corrections' are sometimes made to 'smooth' the results: both Figures 2.12 and 2.13 have normal scores computed using $S'_i = 100(i - 0.375)/(n + 0.25)$. This is a commonly used corrected formula for normal scores. For the cholesterol value of 4.35 considered above,

$$S'_i = 100(1 - 0.375)/(50 + 0.25) = 1.24\%.$$

From Table B.1 the corresponding $z$ value (normal score) is about $-2.25$, since the chance of a standard normal value below $-2.25$ is 0.0122 which is as near as this table gets to $1.24/100 = 0.0124$.

The same technique may be used for probability distributions other than the normal, for instance to check whether the data have a binomial distribution.

### 2.7.2    Inferences for a single mean

A confidence interval for a population mean is given by

$$\bar{x} \pm t_{n-1} s/\sqrt{n}, \tag{2.11}$$

where $t_{n-1}$ is the critical value, at some prescribed level, from Student's $t$ distribution with $n - 1$ degrees of freedom (the divisor used to calculate the standard deviation). The $t$ distribution can be thought of as a small-sample analogue of the standard normal distribution ($t$ has a rather wider peak, but otherwise looks much the same). For large $n$, the standard normal and $t$ are identical, for all practical purposes. Table B.4 gives critical values for $t$; for example, the 5% critical value ranges from 12.7 for 1 d.f. to 1.96 for infinite

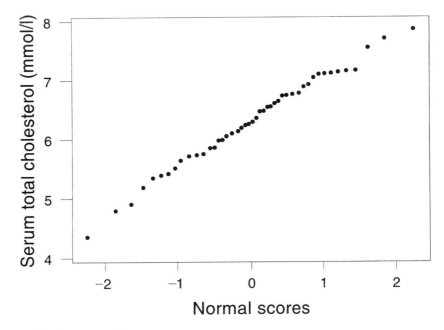

**Figure 2.12**    Normal plot for cholesterol.

degrees of freedom. The value 1.96 is also the 5% critical value for the standard normal (see Table B.2), thus demonstrating how the $t$ converges to the standard normal.

We can use the cholesterol data in Table 2.10 to find a 95% confidence interval for the mean cholesterol of all middle-aged Scotsmen, assuming the sample to be a simple random sample of such people. In previous sections we have seen that these data are quite symmetrical and reasonably near-normal in shape. For these data $\bar{x} = 6.287$ and standard error is $s/\sqrt{n} = 0.107$. From Table B.4 we can see that the 5% critical value for $t_{49}$ must be 2.01 to two decimal places. Using these results in (2.11) we get

$$6.287 \pm 2.01 \times 0.107,$$

which is $6.287 \pm 0.215\,\text{mmol/l}$. Hence we are 95% confident that the interval (6.072, 6.502) contains the true mean cholesterol level of middle-aged Scotsmen.

The population mean is represented symbolically by $\mu$. A hypothesis test for the null hypothesis $H_0 : \mu = \mu_0$ comes from calculating

$$\frac{\bar{x} - \mu_0}{s/\sqrt{n}} \tag{2.12}$$

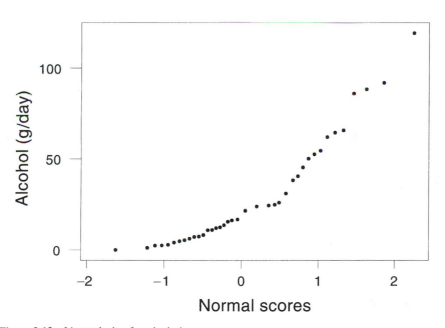

**Figure 2.13**   Normal plot for alcohol.

and comparing the result with $t_{n-1}$. This is known as **Student's *t* test** or simply the *t* **test**.

*Example 2.9*  Suppose that we hypothesize that the mean male cholesterol in Scotland is 6.0 mmol/l. We then collect the data shown in Table 2.10. Do these data suggest that our assertion is false?

From (2.12), our test statistic is

$$\frac{6.287 - 6.0}{0.107} = 2.68.$$

Since $n - 1 = 49$ we should compare this to $t$ with 49 d.f. The nearest we can get to this using Table B.4 is 50 d.f., showing that this is significant at approximately the 1% level. From a computer package the exact $p$ value was found to be 0.010 – exactly at the 1% level, to three decimal places. Hence there is strong evidence to suggest that the average cholesterol of Scotsmen is not 6.0; in fact it seems to be higher.

This result is consistent with the 95% confidence interval we found earlier. Since 6.0 is outside the 95% confidence interval we would expect to reject $H_0 : \mu = 6.0$ at the 5% level of significance. Since 5% is less extreme than 1%, rejection of $H_0$ at 1% automatically implies rejection at the 5% level. Notice that a two-sided test has been assumed.

### 2.7.3  Comparing two means

Section 2.7.2 relates to a one-sample problem; that is, the data on cholesterol are taken as a whole. Often we wish to compare mean values of the same variable between two subgroups or between two separate populations. Provided the two samples are drawn independently of each other, we then use the **two-sample *t* test** and associated confidence interval, which will now be defined.

For example, we saw that serum total cholesterol seems to be different amongst those with and without prevalent CHD in the sample of 50 Scotsmen (see Figure 2.6). Since there is no great skew in these data, we could use the two-sample $t$ test to formally test the null hypothesis that the mean cholesterol is the same in the two groups; that is, the observed difference is simply due to random sampling variation.

The two-sample $t$ test requires calculation of the test statistic,

$$\frac{\bar{x}_1 - \bar{x}_2 - (\mu_1 - \mu_2)}{\hat{se}}, \qquad (2.13)$$

where $\bar{x}_1$ and $\bar{x}_2$ are the two sample means and $\mu_1$ and $\mu_2$ the corresponding values of the population means under the null hypothesis and $\hat{se}$ is the estimated standard error of the difference between the means (the 'hat' denotes that an estimate is taken). Often the null hypothesis is $H_0 : \mu_1 = \mu_2$, in which case (2.13) reduces to

$$\frac{\bar{x}_1 - \bar{x}_2}{\hat{se}}. \tag{2.14}$$

We can test $H_0$ exactly if the two population variances, denoted $\sigma_1^2$ and $\sigma_2^2$, are equal. In this case,

$$\hat{se} = s_p\sqrt{1/n_1 + 1/n_2}, \tag{2.15}$$

where $s_p^2$ is the pooled estimate of variance (pooled over the two samples drawn from populations of equal variance) defined by

$$s_p^2 = \frac{(n_1 - 1)s_1^2 + (n_2 - 1)s_2^2}{n_1 + n_2 - 2}. \tag{2.16}$$

This is a weighted average of the two sample variances where the weights are the degrees of freedom. With this value of $\hat{se}$ we compare (2.13) or (2.14) to $t$ with $n_1 + n_2 - 2$ d.f. The procedure is then called a **pooled $t$ test**.

On the other hand, if we have evidence that $\sigma_1^2$ and $\sigma_2^2$ are unequal we have no reason to consider a pooled estimate of variance. Instead, we calculate

$$\hat{se} = \sqrt{s_1^2/n_1 + s_2^2/n_2}. \tag{2.17}$$

Unfortunately there is no exact test in this circumstance, although various approximate tests have been suggested (see Armitage and Berry, 1994). One approximation is given by Ryan and Joiner (1994): compare (2.13) or (2.14), using (2.17) against $t$ with $f$ degrees of freedom where

$$f = \frac{\left[(s_1^2/n_1) + (s_2^2/n_2)\right]^2}{\left((s_1^2/n_1)^2/(n_1 - 1)\right) + \left((s_2^2/n_2)^2/(n_2 - 1)\right)},$$

rounded to the nearest whole number.

We may calculate a confidence interval for the difference between two population means, $\mu_1 - \mu_2$, as

$$\bar{x}_1 - \bar{x}_2 \pm t(\hat{se}), \tag{2.18}$$

where $t$ is the value from Student's $t$ distribution with the appropriate d.f. for the required percentage confidence. For example, we need the 5% critical value from $t$ with $n_1 + n_2 - 2$ d.f. to obtain a 95% confidence interval when a pooled estimate of variance is used.

Before applying the two-sample $t$ test, or computing the associated confidence interval, we clearly need to see whether there is reason to doubt that the two population variances are equal. We can carry out another form of hypothesis test to try to refute this assertion. That is, we test

$$H_0 : \sigma_1^2 = \sigma_2^2 \quad \text{versus} \quad H_1 : \sigma_1^2 \neq \sigma_2^2,$$

which is achieved using the test statistic

$$s_1^2 / s_2^2, \tag{2.19}$$

where $s_1^2$ and $s_2^2$ are the two sample means, with $s_1^2 > s_2^2$ (this is *essential*). The test statistic is compared to the $F$ distribution with $(n_1 - 1, n_2 - 1)$ d.f.

*Example 2.10*  For the SHHS cholesterol values of Table 2.10, split into the two CHD groups, we have the following summary statistics:

| CHD | No CHD |
| --- | --- |
| $n = 11$ | $n = 39$ |
| $\bar{x} = 6.708$ | $\bar{x} = 6.168$ |
| $s = 0.803$ | $s = 0.709$ |

Since the sample standard deviation is highest in the CHD group, we shall take this group to have subscript '1'. Then the preliminary test of equal population variances, (2.19), gives

$$\frac{(0.803)^2}{(0.709)^2} = 1.28.$$

We compare this with $F_{10,38}$. Table B.5 gives one-sided critical values for 10%, 5%, 2.5%, 1% and 0.1%. We have a two-sided test, so these correspond to 20%, 10%, 5%, 2% and 0.2% critical values for our test. $F_{10,38}$ is not given, but $F_{10,35} = 1.79$ and $F_{10,40} = 1.76$ at the 20% level (two-sided) from Table B.5(a). Thus $F_{10,38}$ must be about 1.77, and we will fail to reject $H_0$ at the 20% level. From a computer package, the exact $p$ value is 0.552. There is thus no evidence to reject $H_0$: population variances equal.

Consequently we may proceed with the pooled $t$ test, that is, with $\hat{s}e$ given by (2.15). From (2.16),

$$s_p^2 = \frac{10(0.803)^2 + 38(0.709)^2}{10 + 38} = 0.532.$$

So from (2.15),

$$\hat{s}e = \sqrt{0.532}\sqrt{1/11 + 1/39} = 0.249,$$

and the test statistic, (2.13), is

$$\frac{6.708 - 6.168}{0.249} = 2.17.$$

This is to be compared to Student's $t$ with $n_1 + n_2 - 2 = 48$ d.f. From Table B.4, 5% critical values are

$$t_{45} = 2.01, \quad t_{50} = 2.01;$$

and 2% critical values are

$$t_{45} = 2.41, \quad t_{50} = 2.40.$$

Hence $t_{48}$ is 2.01 and about 2.41 at 5% and 2%, respectively. Thus we reject $H_0$ at the 5%, but not at the 2% level of significance (or at any level below 2%). The exact $p$ value is actually 0.035. We conclude that there is some evidence of a different cholesterol level in the two groups, in fact it is higher for those with CHD, but the evidence is not strong.

Suppose that we opted to calculate a 99% confidence interval for $\mu_1 - \mu_2$. Since we have accepted a pooled estimate of variance, from (2.18) this is given by

$$6.708 - 6.168 \pm 0.249 t_{48},$$

where $t_{48}$ is the 1% critical value. Again, Table B.4 does not give the exact value, but a computer package gives it as 2.682. Hence the 99% confidence interval is $0.54 \pm 0.67$ mmol/l. That is, we are 99% confident that the average extra amount of cholesterol in the blood of those with CHD is between $-0.13$ and $1.21$ mmol/l. As we would anticipate, because we have already seen that the hypothesis of no difference was not rejected at the 1% level, this confidence interval does contain zero.

### 2.7.4   Paired data

In Section 2.7.3 we assumed that the two samples are independent. One situation where this is not the case is where the data are **paired**. Pairing means that each individual selected for sample 1 is associated with a like individual, who is then selected for sample 2. For instance, an individual with CHD might be paired with another who is free of CHD, but shares important character-istics, such as being of the same age and sex. This has the advantage of balancing the age/sex composition of the two groups, and thus providing a rather fairer comparison of cholesterol levels than we might expect from purely independent samples (in Example 2.10), assuming that age and sex will influence CHD and cholesterol. One specific instance of pairing is where each individual acts as his or her own control, usually encountered where observations are taken before and after some intervention (see Example 2.11).

Analysis of paired data has to be different from the unpaired case because now the two groups are intrinsically non-independent. This problem is overcome very easily: we simply subtract one value from the other within each pair. As a result the paired two-sample problem is reduced to a one-sample problem, to be analysed according to Section 2.7.2. More precisely, let $x_{1i}$ be the first observation from the $i$th pair, and $x_{2i}$ be the second observation from the same pair (where 'first' and 'second' have some consistent definition from pair to pair). Let $d_i = x_{1i} - x_{2i}$. Then all we do is to apply the methods of Section 2.7.2 to the set of differences, $\{d_i\}$.

Let the subscript 'd' denote differenced data. We test $\mu_1 = \mu_2$ by testing for $\mu_d = 0$. From (2.12) the test statistic for $H_0 : \mu_d = 0$ is

$$\frac{\bar{x}_d}{s_d/\sqrt{n}}, \qquad (2.20)$$

which is compared with $t_{n-1}$. Here $n$ is the number of *pairs*. Also, from (2.11), a confidence interval for $\mu_1 - \mu_2 = \mu_d$ is

$$\bar{x}_d \pm t_{n-1}s_d/\sqrt{n}. \qquad (2.21)$$

The benefit of pairing, to 'remove' the effect of other variables which may influence the comparison of the two groups (a common goal in epidemiology), is clear by common sense. Another way of looking at this is that the background variation against which we have to compare our two groups is likely to be reduced. This is because we are now analysing between-pairs variation rather than person-to-person or between-subject variation (which is likely to be the bigger). Smaller background variation means, for example, a narrower confidence interval.

*Example 2.11*    Although the SHHS introduced in this chapter does not involve any paired data directly, the same basic screening protocol was used by the SHHS investigators in the town of Alloa, where a set of individuals were entered into a study to assess the effect of cholesterol screening. A sample of men and women were invited to attend a series of three clinics during which they were given dietary advice to lower their blood cholesterol and a blood sample was taken, from which total cholesterol was subsequently measured and communicated to the subject concerned. Table 2.15 shows the female data collected at the first and second clinics (three months apart). We can use these data to assess whether this type of cholesterol screening has any short-term effect on blood cholesterol levels.

The data are clearly paired because this is a 'before and after' study of the same individuals. Hence the first step is to calculate the second clinic minus first clinic differences for each woman. For example, the difference for the first woman is $3.250 - 3.795 = -0.545$. Note that differences may be positive or negative and the sign must be retained. The summary statistics for the differences are

$$\bar{x}_d = -0.1700, \quad s_d = 0.5587, \quad n = 44.$$

Substituting into (2.21) gives the 95% confidence interval for the true difference as

$$-0.1700 \pm 0.5587 t_{43}/\sqrt{44}.$$

From a computer package, $t_{43} = 2.0167$ at the 5% level. This gives the 95% confidence interval, $-0.1700 \pm 0.1699$, which is the interval from $-0.3399$ to $-0.0001$ mmol/l. Since 0 is just outside the 95% confidence interval, we know that the null hypothesis of no difference will be rejected with a $p$ value of just under 0.05. Hence there is evidence that cholesterol screening has reduced cholesterol.

It is interesting to compare the results of the valid paired procedure with what we would get if we used the incorrect two-sample approach. Applying (2.18) with either (2.15) or (2.17) to the data in Table 2.15 gives the 95% confidence interval as $-0.17 \pm 0.53$. This has exactly the same centre as the interval calculated in Example 2.11, as it must since $\bar{x}_d = \bar{x}_1 - \bar{x}_2$ (the mean of the differences is the difference of the means). It is, however, substantially wider than the correct interval, reflecting the fact that here we have failed to take account of the reduction in random variation brought about by pairing.

**Table 2.15**   Serum total cholesterol (mmol/l) at clinic visits 1 and 2 for 44 women in the Alloa Study

| 1st Visit | 2nd Visit | 1st Visit | 2nd Visit | 1st Visit | 2nd Visit |
|---|---|---|---|---|---|
| 3.795 | 3.250 | 7.480 | 6.955 | 5.410 | 5.280 |
| 6.225 | 6.935 | 4.970 | 5.100 | 5.220 | 5.175 |
| 5.210 | 4.750 | 6.710 | 7.480 | 4.700 | 4.815 |
| 7.040 | 5.080 | 4.765 | 4.530 | 4.215 | 3.610 |
| 7.550 | 8.685 | 6.695 | 6.160 | 5.395 | 5.705 |
| 7.715 | 7.775 | 4.025 | 4.160 | 7.475 | 6.580 |
| 6.555 | 6.005 | 5.510 | 6.010 | 4.925 | 5.190 |
| 5.360 | 4.940 | 5.495 | 5.010 | 7.115 | 6.150 |
| 5.285 | 5.620 | 5.435 | 5.975 | 7.020 | 6.395 |
| 6.230 | 5.870 | 5.350 | 4.705 | 5.365 | 5.805 |
| 6.475 | 6.620 | 5.905 | 5.465 | 3.665 | 3.710 |
| 5.680 | 5.635 | 6.895 | 6.925 | 6.130 | 5.160 |
| 5.490 | 5.080 | 4.350 | 4.260 | 4.895 | 5.145 |
| 9.865 | 9.465 | 5.950 | 5.325 | 7.000 | 7.425 |
| 4.625 | 4.120 | 5.855 | 5.505 | | |

Note: each value shown is the average of two biochemical assays.

Similarly, the $p$ value from a paired $t$ test (the correct procedure) applied to the data in Table 2.15 is (to two decimal places) 0.05, using (2.20), whereas an incorrect two-sample $t$ test gives a $p$ value of 0.52, using (2.14) with either (2.15) or (2.17). Hence, again, we get entirely the wrong result (in fact a 'less significant' result) if we ignore the pairing.

## 2.8   Inferential techniques for non-normal data

As explained in Section 2.6.3, the two-number summary is only appropriate when the data are reasonably symmetrical in shape. As explained in Section 2.7, for $t$ tests we require rather more: the data must also be approximately normally distributed. Just what degree of approximation is acceptable cannot be stated in absolute terms. Certainly we require a single-peak distribution with no great skew, so that the mean is similar to the median. The larger the sample, the less precise the approximation needs to be, although we must be careful when analyses by subsets are performed subsequently. Several other statistical procedures that are common in epidemiological analysis, such as regression and analysis of variance, assume normality (Chapter 9).

As we have already seen, epidemiological data do not always have even an approximately normal shape. Discrete variables, such as counts (for example, the number of cigarettes per day in Table 2.12) rarely have a near-normal shape. Severe skewness is possible even with data on a continuous variable (e.g. cotinine in Table 2.12). As we have seen, medians and allied statistics are more appropriate summaries for such variables. If we wish to consider formal inferential procedures (estimation and testing) with non-normal data we have two basic choices. Either we try to **transform** the raw data into a form which is near-normal or we use **non-parametric** methods of analysis. Both approaches will be described.

### 2.8.1   Transformations

Table 2.16 gives a range of transformations that are often successful with forms of data that are common in epidemiology. Of all the transformations, the logarithmic (log) is probably the most used. As with all the other transformations, it defines a new variable, $y$ (say), from the original observed variable, $x$ (say). In this particular case,

$$y = \log(x),$$

where the base of the logarithm may be anything we choose. Problems in applying this arise when $x$ can take values of zero. In such cases we add a small constant to all data values so as to avoid this problem. A similar ruse could be used when $x$ can go negative.

Often proportionate data are reported as percentages, in which case we should divide by 100 before applying the arcsine square root transformation suggested in Table 2.16. This transformation defines

$$y = \sin^{-1}\left(\sqrt{x}\right),$$

where $x$ is a proportion.

The reciprocal transformation,

$$y = 1/x$$

**Table 2.16**   Transformations which are often successful in removing skew and making the data better approximated by the normal curve

| Form of the data | Transformation |
| --- | --- |
| Slightly right-skewed | Square root |
| Moderately right-skewed | Logarithmic |
| Very right-skewed | Reciprocal |
| Left-skewed | Square |
| Counts | Square root |
| Proportions | Arcsine square root |

has the unfortunate property of reversing the original ordering of the variables (so that the smallest on the original scale becomes the largest on the transformed scale). To maintain the original order the negative reciprocal

$$y = -1/x$$

may be used instead.

It is fairly easy to see why the suggested transformations will be useful for skewed data; for example, square roots of small numbers are fairly close to their original numbers (for example, $\sqrt{4} = 2$) whereas taking square roots of large numbers leads to considerable reduction (for example, $\sqrt{144} = 12$). Hence the upper part of the scale is pulled in. The transformations for counts and proportions arise from theoretical considerations; in the case of proportions the arcsine square root is only strictly justifiable in theory when all proportions arise from a constant sample size, which is rare in practice.

There is no guarantee that any of the transformations suggested in Table 2.16 will work on any specific set of data. All we can do is to try them out and see what happens. This trial and error approach is not too labour-intensive should a statistics or spreadsheet computer package be available.

Some statistical packages implement the Box–Cox (Box and Cox, 1964) method of searching for the most appropriate **power transformation** – that is, a transformation which takes the form

$$y = x^{\theta},$$

for some value of $\theta$. This includes some of the transformations we have already seen; for example $\theta = -1$ gives the reciprocal transformation.

Theoretical details and recommendations for choosing transformations are given by Snedecor and Cochran (1980). A case study using the SHHS data is provided by Millns et al. (1995).

For the highly skewed data in Table 2.10, the square root transformation for alcohol and log transformation for carbon monoxide are quite successful in removing skew (see Figure 2.14) and improving approximate normality. Cigarette consumption and cotinine do not seem to be amenable to normalizing transformations; certainly none of the basic transformations is at all successful. However, cigarette consumption is really a 'mixture' variable: a mixture of data from non-smokers (all of whom have a consumption of zero) and smokers. Hence it may be sensible to split the cigarette data by smoking status. In fact, the smokers' data on cigarette consumption (mean = 19.9, median = 20) is very close to perfect 'quartile symmetry', as Figure 2.15 shows. The non-smokers' data has no variation and so all we can do is to report the proportion (or percentage) of non-smokers, $28/50 = 0.56$ (56%). Cotinine (which is a biochemical measure of tobacco consumption) could also be split

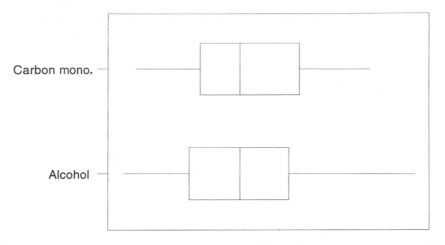

**Figure 2.14**  Boxplot (using standardized scales) for $\sqrt{}$(alcohol) and $\log_e$ (carbon monoxide).

by smoking status, but this may not be appropriate since several non-smokers have non-zero cotinine values: indeed, one non-smoker has a cotinine value of 424 ng/ml. This may seem strange, but smoking status in Table 2.10 is self-reported and deception may occur. Small non-zero values of cotinine may also be due to other factors such as passive (secondary) smoking, dietary intake of cotinine and inaccuracies in the assay. So we may decide not to split cotinine data, and conclude that we cannot transform to a near-normal shape. In general, we should not expect transformations to be successful whenever the data have more than one peak (unless the data are split), or when the data are very sparsely distributed.

As well as not always being successful, transformations have the disadvantage that they inevitably produce answers on the transformed scale. For instance, it is perfectly reasonable to use the mean to summarize the square root alcohol data, but the mean (4.42 for the example) is for the square root of daily consumption in $\sqrt{}$(gram) units. Similarly, inferences about differences between means will only be valid on the square root scale. Hence we find a 95% confidence interval for the difference between mean $\sqrt{}$(alcohol) consumption for smokers and non-smokers, but not for the difference between the true mean consumptions.

It may be useful, when presenting results, to back-transform estimates at the last stage of analysis to return to the original scale. For instance, from (2.11), a 95% confidence interval for $\sqrt{}$(alcohol) using the data in Table 2.10 turns out to be $4.417 \pm 0.773$, that is (3.644, 5.190). Back-transforming (that is, squaring) the mean and the lower and upper confidence limits gives a back-transformed

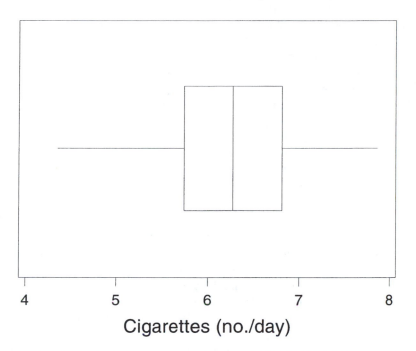

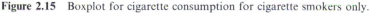

Figure 2.15  Boxplot for cigarette consumption for cigarette smokers only.

mean for alcohol of 19.5 g with a 95% confidence interval of (13.3, 26.9)g. Notice that, unlike cases we have seen earlier, the estimate (mean) is not in the middle of this confidence interval.

Back-transformed results should be appropriately labelled so as to avoid ambiguity. For instance, 19.5 is certainly not an estimate of mean alcohol consumption (see Table 2.12 for a valid estimate). Similarly, the transformed results for the difference in mean $\sqrt{}$(alcohol) between smokers and non-smokers cannot be squared to define limits for the difference in alcohol itself, because

$$\sqrt{x_1} - \sqrt{x_2} \neq \sqrt{x_1 - x_2}.$$

## 2.8.2  Non-parametric methods

When transformations fail, or are thought to be inappropriate, non-parametric methods may be applied. Non-parametric methods are sometimes said to be **distribution-free** because they make no assumption about the shape, or distribution, of the data. Most, if not all, **parametric** procedures, such as those based on the normal distribution, have a non-parametric analogue. For example, the **one-sample Wilcoxon test** (or **signed-rank sum test**) is sometimes used in place of the one-sample $t$ test. Similarly, the **two-sample Wilcoxon test** could replace the two-sample $t$ test.

When non-parametric methods are used in place of parametric methods we will be treating the variable as of a lower type than it really is (see Section 2.3.3). Hence they ignore some of the information in the data; not surprisingly, this makes them rather less powerful than their parametric alternatives. For instance, we have less chance of rejecting an incorrect null hypothesis using the two-sample Wilcoxon test than using the $t$ test. For this reason parametric procedures (based, for example, on the normal distribution) are usually to be preferred, even if a prior data transformation is necessary. ('Power' is formally defined in Section 8.2.)

There is insufficient space to provide a full account of non-parametric methods here: see Conover (1980) for an extensive exposition. Instead, we shall look at the most useful one in basic epidemiological analysis, the two-sample Wilcoxon test and associated confidence interval. This test treats the data as ordinal, that is, the precise distance between numbers is ignored, only their relative order is used. In some situations, such as clinicians' ranking of severity of disease between patients, the raw data are ordinal and this would be the (two-sample) method of choice at the outset.

The Wilcoxon test procedure begins by ranking the combined data set from the two samples to be compared. Consider the null hypothesis that the two populations have equal medians. If $H_0$ is true, then the ranks for either sample are equally likely to fall anywhere in the list of all possible ranks. Consider now the sum of the ranks for one of the two samples, say sample 1,

$$T = \sum_{i=1}^{n_1} R_{1i}, \qquad (2.22)$$

where $R_{11}$ is the first rank in sample 1, $R_{12}$ is the second rank, etc., and sample 1 has $n_1$ observations. The idea is then to find all conceivable rank sums should sample 1 take any of the possible $n_1$ of the combined set of $n_1 + n_2$ ranks. The one-sided $p$ value for the test is then the probability of obtaining a rank sum at least as big as that actually observed, that is, (2.22). This probability is the number of possible rank sums as big as that observed, divided by the total number of possible rank sums. Two-sided $p$ values are obtained simply by doubling.

Unfortunately, the process is very cumbersome for hand calculation. Some work can be saved by taking sample 1 in (2.22) to be the smaller of the two samples. Tables of critical values are available, for example in Conover (1980), but provided either sample size is above 20 a normal approximation may be used. This requires calculation of

$$\frac{T - \dfrac{n_1(n+1)}{2}}{\sqrt{\dfrac{n_1 n_2 (n+1)}{12}}}, \tag{2.23}$$

where $n = n_1 + n_2$. This is to be compared with the standard normal distribution.

Sometimes there are **tied ranks**; that is, two or more identical numbers in the combined data set. In this situation we assign the average rank in the tied range to each member of the tie. For instance, if there are three values which are all equal 10th largest, then the tied range is 10 to 12 and the rank assigned to each is $(10 + 11 + 12)/3 = 11$. The procedure based upon (2.23) works well provided there are just a few ties. Otherwise (2.23) should be replaced by

$$\frac{T - \dfrac{n_1(n+1)}{2}}{\sqrt{\dfrac{n_1 n_2}{n(n-1)} \sum R^2 - \dfrac{(n+1)^2 n_1 n_2}{4(n-1)}}}, \tag{2.24}$$

where $\sum R^2$ is the sum of all the squared ranks.

*Example 2.12*   Consider the cholesterol data appearing in Table 2.11 once again. Suppose we wish to consider the null hypothesis that the median cholesterol is the same for those with and without CHD.

First we rank the combined data. The result is given as Table 2.17, which differs from Table 2.11 only by the way ties are expressed and by denoting those with CHD. Here there are four pairs of tied ranks: the average rank is given for each pair.

We will take, for ease of computation, sample 1 to be the smaller group, $n_1 = 11$ and $n_2 = 39$ (big enough for a normal approximation). Using (2.22),

$$T = 4 + 17 + 20.5 + 23 + 28 + 39 + 42 + 46 + 47 + 49 + 50 = 365.5$$

Hence the test statistic, (2.23), is

$$\frac{365.5 - \dfrac{11 \times 51}{2}}{\sqrt{\dfrac{11 \times 39 \times 51}{12}}} = 1.99.$$

Here there are few ties, so we should expect (2.23) to be acceptable. To check, we use the more complex formula (2.24). This requires

$$\sum R^2 = \text{sum of squares of all 50 ranks} = 42\,923.$$

Substituting this into (2.24) gives

$$\frac{365.5 - \dfrac{11 \times 51}{2}}{\sqrt{\dfrac{11 \times 39}{50 \times 49} 42\,923 - \dfrac{51^2 \times 11 \times 39}{4 \times 49}}} = 1.99,$$

which is the same result as from (2.23) to two decimal places.

**Table 2.17** Serum total cholesterol (mmol/l) in rank order with average tied ranks (* indicates that the individual concerned has CHD)

| Rank | Obs. | Rank | Obs. | Rank | Obs. | Rank | Obs. | Rank | Obs. |
|------|------|------|------|------|------|------|------|------|------|
| 1    | 4.35 | 10.5 | 5.71 | 20.5 | 6.10* | 31 | 6.55 | 41 | 7.04 |
| 2    | 4.79 | 12   | 5.73 | 22   | 6.13 | 32 | 6.60 | 42 | 7.10* |
| 3    | 4.90 | 13.5 | 5.75 | 23   | 6.19* | 33 | 6.64 | 43 | 7.11 |
| 4    | 5.19* | 13.5 | 5.75 | 24  | 6.23 | 34 | 6.73 | 44 | 7.12 |
| 5    | 5.34 | 15   | 5.85 | 25   | 6.25 | 35 | 6.74 | 45 | 7.14 |
| 6    | 5.39 | 16   | 5.86 | 26   | 6.29 | 36.5 | 6.76 | 46 | 7.15* |
| 7    | 5.42 | 17   | 5.98* | 27  | 6.35 | 36.5 | 6.76 | 47 | 7.16* |
| 8    | 5.51 | 18   | 5.99 | 28   | 6.46* | 38 | 6.78 | 48 | 7.55 |
| 9    | 5.64 | 19   | 6.05 | 29   | 6.47 | 39 | 6.89* | 49 | 7.71* |
| 10.5 | 5.71 | 20.5 | 6.10 | 30   | 6.54 | 40 | 6.92 | 50 | 7.86* |

The 5% two-sided critical value is 1.96, and hence we just reject the null hypothesis of equal medians at the 5% level (the $p$ value is actually 0.048).

Sometimes the Wilcoxon test is said to be a non-parametric test of the equality of two **means**. This is reasonable if the two populations differ only in location, not in spread or shape, because then all differences between corresponding points of location in the two populations will be equal. Hence the similarity between the results of Examples 2.10 and 2.12 is not unexpected. As discussed already, the distribution of cholesterol approximates a normal curve reasonably well and the sample is moderately big, so that Example 2.10 provides the preferred analysis in this case.

Most statistical computer packages will carry out the Wilcoxon test, although some only use the large-sample approximation, (2.23). Sometimes the equivalent **Mann–Whitney test** is used instead. See Altman (1991) for comments on the relationship between the Wilcoxon and Mann–Whitney approaches.

Similar theory may be used to create a confidence interval for the median difference. This requires all the differences between each observation in the first group and each observation in the second group to be found and then ranked, which is an extremely tedious procedure to follow by hand. Statistical computer packages may be used to produce confidence intervals for median differences with no effort. If hand calculation is necessary, then see Gardner and Altman (1989) for details.

## 2.9   Measuring agreement

The chi-square test, two-sample $t$ test and two-sample Wilcoxon test all provide tests of relationships. Sometimes we wish to go further and investigate whether two sets of data are entirely the same, or at least reasonably similar. Such a problem arises frequently in laboratory testing. For instance, as mentioned in Section 2.2.1, fibrinogen was measured from blood samples of participants in the SHHS. There are several different fibrinogen assays available, and hence the question of agreement between pairs of assays is of epidemiological importance, particularly when comparisons between studies that use different methods are envisaged.

### 2.9.1    Quantitative variables

When the variable is quantitative, as in the fibrinogen example above, no new methodology is necessary. To generate appropriate data we should apply the two methods to be compared to the same subjects; for instance, the blood plasma from any one individual would need to be split and a different fibrinogen assay applied to each part, in our example. This generates paired data, which are analysed as described in Section 2.7.4, unless the normal assumption fails entirely so that the one-sample Wilcoxon test on the differences is necessary.

Sometimes this problem is incorrectly tackled by measuring the correlation (Section 9.3.2) between the two sets of results. This is inappropriate because correlation measures association (in fact, linear association), rather than agreement. Bland and Altman (1986) discuss this problem in a medical setting. They suggest that the most suitable pictorial representation of the data is a plot of the differences against the mean results from the two methods.

### 2.9.2    Categorical variables

When the variable, assessed by the two methods in question, is categorical the data would typically be presented as a square contingency table (see Table 2.18). Perfect agreement would give entries only in the diagonal cells of the table. A common situation where the issue of agreement arises is where two observers are each asked to assess a subject independently for illness. For instance, two nurses might each be asked to decide whether a person has anaemia based on observation of clinical signs, such as pallor of the eyes and nails. The issue is then one of **inter-observer** (or **inter-rater**) **agreement**.

Given a categorical variable with $\ell$ outcomes (for example, $\ell = 4$ in Table 2.18), we can construct a measure of agreement based upon the difference between the number observed and expected in the $\ell$ diagonal cells. The numbers expected are the $E$ values in the chi-square test statistic, (2.1). Using the notation of Table 2.18,

**Table 2.18**  Display of data for an agreement problem with four categorical outcomes (A–D)

| Method two | Method one | | | | |
| | A | B | C | D | Total |
| --- | --- | --- | --- | --- | --- |
| A | $O_{11}$ | $O_{12}$ | $O_{13}$ | $O_{14}$ | $R_1$ |
| B | $O_{21}$ | $O_{22}$ | $O_{23}$ | $O_{24}$ | $R_2$ |
| C | $O_{31}$ | $O_{32}$ | $O_{33}$ | $O_{34}$ | $R_3$ |
| D | $O_{41}$ | $O_{42}$ | $O_{43}$ | $O_{44}$ | $R_4$ |
| Total | $C_1$ | $C_2$ | $C_3$ | $C_4$ | $n$ |

Note: $O$ is the observed number, $R$ is the row total and $C$ is the column total.

$$E_{ii} = \frac{R_i C_i}{n}$$

is the expected value in cell $(i, i)$, that cell which is in both row $i$ and column $i$. Hence agreement may be measured using the observed minus expected differences summed over all the diagonals, that is

$$\sum_{i=1}^{\ell}(O_{ii} - E_{ii}).$$

If there are just as many observed agreements in classification as would be expected by chance, this sum will be zero. High positive values represent a high degree of agreement.

In this application it is traditional to compare proportions rather than numbers. The observed proportion that agree, $p_O$, is the sum of the observed diagonal elements in the contingency table divided by the number of subjects classified, that is

$$p_O = \left(\sum_{i=1}^{\ell} O_{ii}\right)\bigg/ n \qquad (2.25)$$

The corresponding expected proportion is

$$p_E = \left(\sum_{i=1}^{\ell} E_{ii}\right)\bigg/ n$$

$$= \left(\sum_{i=1}^{\ell} R_i C_i\right)\bigg/ n^2. \qquad (2.26)$$

The extent of agreement is now measured by the difference $p_O - p_E$. It is convenient to standardize this difference, and thus use

$$\kappa = \frac{p_O - p_E}{1 - p_E} \qquad (2.27)$$

as the measure of agreement. This is known as **Cohen's kappa** statistic. It takes the value 1 if the agreement is perfect (that is, when $p_O = 1$) and 0 if the amount of agreement is entirely attributable to chance. If $\kappa < 0$ then the amount of agreement is less than would be expected by chance. If $\kappa > 0$ then there is more than chance agreement. Following the suggestions of Fleiss (1981), we shall conclude

$$\begin{cases} \text{excellent agreement} & \text{if} & \kappa \geq 0.75, \\ \text{good agreement} & \text{if} & 0.4 < \kappa < 0.75, \\ \text{poor agreement} & \text{if} & \kappa \leq 0.4, \end{cases}$$

although other 'scoring' systems have been suggested. Fleiss (1981) also suggests an approximate objective test of randomness, that is a test of

$$\mathrm{H}_0 : \kappa = 0 \text{ versus } \mathrm{H}_1 : \kappa \neq 0.$$

This requires calculation of

$$\left( \frac{\kappa}{\hat{\mathrm{se}}(\kappa)} \right)^2, \qquad (2.28)$$

which is compared to chi-square with 1 d.f. In (2.28) the estimated standard error of $\kappa$ is

$$\hat{\mathrm{se}}(\kappa) = \sqrt{\frac{1}{(1 - p_E)^2 n} \left\{ p_E^2 + p_E - \sum_{i=1}^{\ell} \frac{R_i C_i}{n^3} (R_i + C_i) \right\}}. \qquad (2.29)$$

Since we are normally only interested in agreement that is better than chance, a one-sided test is often used in this application.

An approximate 95% confidence interval for the true measure of agreement is

$$\kappa \pm 1.96 \hat{\mathrm{se}}(\kappa). \qquad (2.30)$$

This uses a normal approximation; the values $\pm 1.96$ are derived from Table B.2 as the cut-points within which 95% of the standard normal lies. For other percentages of confidence we replace 1.96 by the corresponding critical value from the normal distribution.

*Example 2.13* In Table 2.1, and elsewhere in this chapter, we have seen the occupational social class distribution of the SHHS subjects. In keeping with the decision made by the study investigators, married women were classified according to their husband's occupation. It is of interest to compare the social classification by this method and when all women are classified according to their own occupation. Table 2.19 gives the data from the same selection criteria that gave rise to Table 2.1, showing all women for whom a classification could be made by both methods.

**Table 2.19**   Social class according to husband's and own occupation for women in the SHHS

| Husband's occupation | Own occupation | | | | | | |
|---|---|---|---|---|---|---|---|
| | *I* | *II* | *IIIn* | *IIIm* | *IV* | *V* | *Total* |
| I | 22 | 80 | 73 | 6 | 9 | 4 | 194 |
| II | 11 | 471 | 241 | 31 | 60 | 12 | 826 |
| IIIn | 3 | 61 | 379 | 20 | 29 | 15 | 507 |
| IIIm | 0 | 159 | 326 | 197 | 263 | 152 | 1097 |
| IV | 0 | 60 | 92 | 43 | 266 | 64 | 525 |
| V | 0 | 10 | 26 | 11 | 41 | 97 | 185 |
| Total | 36 | 841 | 1137 | 308 | 668 | 344 | 3334 |

In this case the number of categories $\ell = 6$. From (2.25),

$$p_O = (22 + 471 + 379 + 197 + 266 + 97)/3334 = 0.4295.$$

From (2.26),

$$p_E = (36 \times 194 + 841 \times 826 + 1137 \times 507 + 308 \times 1097$$
$$+ 668 \times 525 + 344 \times 185)/3334^2$$
$$= 0.1827$$

Hence, from (2.27),

$$\kappa = \frac{0.4295 - 0.1827}{1 - 0.1827} = 0.302.$$

Also, using (2.28), the estimated standard error of kappa turns out to be $\hat{se}(\kappa) = 0.0078$.

Here the degree of agreement is poor. Notice that this does not imply that either way of classifying a woman's social class is, in any way, 'wrong', but it does signify that we might anticipate different results in epidemiological analyses that use the different methods.

### 2.9.3   Ordered categorical variables

In many instances the outcomes of the categorical variable have a rank order. For instance, the classification of anaemia in the example of Section 2.9.2 might be unlikely/possible/probable/definite, rather than just no/yes. In this situation there is a worse discrepancy when the two methods give results two ordinal categories apart than when they are only one apart, for example.

To allow for such problems, Cohen (1968) suggested a weighted version of the kappa statistic. The **weighted kappa** statistic is given by (2.27) again, but with (2.25) and (2.26) replaced by

$$p_O = \left( \sum_{i=1}^{\ell} \sum_{j=1}^{\ell} w_{ij} O_{ij} \right) \Big/ n \qquad (2.31)$$

$$p_E = \left( \sum_{i=1}^{\ell} \sum_{j=1}^{\ell} w_{ij} R_i C_j \right) \Big/ n^2, \qquad (2.32)$$

where the weight for cell $(i,j)$ is

$$w_{ij} = 1 - \frac{|i - j|}{\ell - 1}, \qquad (2.33)$$

in which $|i - j|$ means the absolute value (with sign ignored) of $(i - j)$. The test for $\kappa = 0$ and 95% confidence interval follow from (2.28) and (2.30) as before, but now using the estimated standard error of weighted kappa, which is

$$\hat{s}e(\kappa_w) = \sqrt{\frac{1}{(1 - p_E)^2 n} \left\{ \sum_{i=1}^{\ell} \sum_{j=1}^{\ell} \frac{R_i C_j}{n^2} \left( w_{ij} - w_i - w_j' \right)^2 - p_E^2 \right\}}, \qquad (2.34)$$

where

$$w_i = \sum_{j=1}^{\ell} \frac{C_j w_{ij}}{n} \qquad (2.35)$$

and

$$w_j' = \sum_{i=1}^{\ell} \frac{R_i w_{ij}}{n}. \qquad (2.36)$$

*Example 2.14*   In the problem of Example 2.13 social class is graded, and a discrepancy of several social classifications is more important than one of only a few. Hence it seems reasonable to weight the measure of concordance. The weights given by (2.33) are shown in Table 2.20; as required, we weight (for agreement) more strongly as we approach the diagonals.

**Table 2.20**   Weights for Example 2.14

| Husband's occupation | Own occupation | | | | | |
|---|---|---|---|---|---|---|
| | *I* | *II* | *IIIn* | *IIIm* | *IV* | *V* |
| I | 1 | 0.8 | 0.6 | 0.4 | 0.2 | 0 |
| II | 0.8 | 1 | 0.8 | 0.6 | 0.4 | 0.2 |
| IIIn | 0.6 | 0.8 | 1 | 0.8 | 0.6 | 0.4 |
| IIIm | 0.4 | 0.6 | 0.8 | 1 | 0.8 | 0.6 |
| IV | 0.2 | 0.4 | 0.6 | 0.8 | 1 | 0.8 |
| V | 0 | 0.2 | 0.4 | 0.6 | 0.8 | 1 |

From (2.31) and Tables 2.19 and 2.20,

$$p_O = (1 \times 22 + 0.8 \times 80 + \cdots + 1 \times 97)/3334 = 0.8263.$$

From (2.32) and Tables 2.19 and 2.20,

$$p_E = (1 \times 194 \times 36 + 0.8 \times 194 \times 841 + \cdots + 1 \times 185 \times 344)/3334^2 = 0.6962.$$

Hence, by (2.27), the weighted kappa is

$$\kappa_w = \frac{0.8263 - 0.6962}{1 - 0.6962} = 0.428.$$

This is now just inside the 'good' agreement range. Inspection of Table 2.19 shows why the weighted kappa is larger than the unweighted: the discrepancies which do occur tend not to be extreme.

We can obtain the estimated standard error of the weighted kappa using (2.34). This requires prior evaluation of the six equations specified by (2.35) and the six equations specified by (2.36). For illustration, one of each of these will be evaluated.

From (2.35) when $i = 3$,

$$w_3 = (36 \times 0.6 + 841 \times 0.8 + \cdots + 344 \times 0.4)/3334 = 0.7847.$$

From (2.36) when $j = 5$,

$$w'_5 = (194 \times 0.2 + 826 \times 0.4 + \cdots + 185 \times 0.8)/3334 = 0.6671.$$

Substituting these, together with other components, into (2.34) gives $\hat{se}(\kappa) = 0.0110$. From (2.30) a 95% confidence interval for the true weighted kappa, relating self to husband's occupational social classification for middle-aged Scotswomen, is $0.428 \pm 1.96 \times 0.0110$, that is, (0.41, 0.45).

## 2.10    Assessing diagnostic tests

Epidemiological investigations often require classification of each individual studied according to some binary outcome variable, the most important example of which is disease status (yes/no). These classification procedures will be called **diagnostic tests**. In some situations there will be no question about the accuracy of the diagnosis, most obviously where the 'disease' is death from any cause. Sometimes the state of affairs may be less certain. In particular, clinical and laboratory procedures are often used for diagnosis. Examples include cancer screening clinics and analysis of blood samples for signs of an illness. Such tests may not be 100% reliable, and it is of interest to quantify just how reliable any particular test really is. This may be achieved by applying the test to a number of individuals whose true disease status is known and interpreting the results. Notice the contrast to the situation of Section 2.9: here we will also be comparing two sets of results, but now one set of results provides the standard. The problem is one of calibration rather than investigating equivalence.

**Table 2.21**   Display of data from a diagnostic test

|  | True disease status | | |
|---|---|---|---|
| Test result | Positive | Negative | Total |
| Positive | a | b | a + b |
| Negative | c | d | c + d |
| Total | a + c | b + d | n |

There are two types of error that can occur during diagnostic testing. Consider the problem of classifying disease status once more. First, the test could wrongly decide that a person with the disease does not have it. Second, the test could wrongly decide that a person without the disease does have it. Clearly we would wish for the probabilities of each type of error to be small.

Consider data from a test of $n$ subjects presented in the form of Table 2.21, showing the test decision (the rows) and the true state of affairs (the columns). Notice that this assumes that we are testing for the presence of disease; in some applications 'disease' would not be the appropriate label for the columns (for example, when assessing preparatory pregnancy testing kits). Nevertheless, we shall continue to assume this situation for simplicity.

From Table 2.21 we can see that the (estimated) probabilities of the two wrong decisions are:

(1)   for false negatives, $c/(a + c)$;

(2)   for false positives, $b/(b + d)$.

In fact the complementary probabilities are more often quoted – that is, the probability of making the right decision whenever a person has the disease, called the **sensitivity** of the test; and the probability of making the right decision whenever a person does not have the disease, called the **specificity** of the test. These are thus estimated as:

$$
\begin{aligned}
&(1) \quad \text{sensitivity} = a/(a + c); \\
&(2) \quad \text{specificity} = d/(b + d).
\end{aligned}
\tag{2.37}
$$

Notice that these are, respectively, the relative frequency of correct decisions amongst true positives and true negatives, and involve calculations using the two columns of the table.

Sometimes we may also wish to consider the probability that someone really does have the disease once the test has given a positive result. This is called the **predictive value of a positive test**. Also we may consider the probability that someone really does not have the disease once the test has given a negative result. This is called the **predictive value of a negative test**. From Table 2.21 estimated predictive values are:

$$
\begin{aligned}
&(1) \quad \text{for a positive test, } a/(a+b); \\
&(2) \quad \text{for a negative test, } d/(c+d).
\end{aligned}
\tag{2.38}
$$

Notice that these two calculations use the two rows of the table.

Since all the measures in (2.37) and (2.38) are proportions, we can use the material of Section 2.5.2 to make inferences; for instance, (2.3) may be used to attach confidence intervals to any of the results.

Although sensitivity, specificity and predictive values are defined for the case where true disease outcome is known, they are frequently used, in practice, to compare a test against some standard test which is generally assumed to be correct. Notice that this is, strictly speaking, only *relative* sensitivity, etc.

*Example 2.15* Ditchburn and Ditchburn (1990) describe a number of tests for the rapid diagnosis of urinary tract infections (UTIs). They took urine samples from over 200 patients with symptoms of UTI which were sent to a hospital microbiology laboratory for a culture test. This test is taken to be the standard against which all other tests are to be compared. All the other tests were much more immediate, and thus suitable for use in general practice. We will only consider one of the rapid tests here, a dipstick test to detect pyuria (by leucocyte-esterase estimation). The results are given in Table 2.22.

The estimated probabilities are thus, from (2.37) and (2.38),

$$
\begin{aligned}
\text{sensitivity} &= 84/94 = 0.894 \\
\text{specificity} &= 92/135 = 0.681 \\
\text{predictive value of positive test} &= 84/127 = 0.661 \\
\text{predictive value of negative test} &= 92/102 = 0.902.
\end{aligned}
$$

So, assuming the culture test to be the truth, the pyuria test is rather better at diagnosing UTI than diagnosing absence of UTI (sensitivity greater than specificity). Also more of the apparent UTI cases than apparent UTI non-cases

**Table 2.22**   Results of a dipstick test for pyuria

| Dipstick test | Culture test (standard) | | |
| --- | --- | --- | --- |
| | Positive | Negative | Total |
| Positive | 84 | 43 | 127 |
| Negative | 10 | 92 | 102 |
| Total | 94 | 135 | 229 |

(according to the pyuria test) will have been incorrectly diagnosed (predictive value greatest for the negative test).

It would be incorrect to conclude that predictive values give no useful information once sensitivity and specificity are known. Predictive values depend upon the relative numbers of true positives and negatives that have been tested. For instance, suppose the methodology described in Example 2.15 was repeated in a different population and produced the results shown in Table 2.23.

Sensitivity and specificity are just as before ($252/282 = 0.894$ and $92/135 = 0.681$, respectively). The predictive values are now $252/295 = 0.854$ (positive test) and $92/122 = 0.754$ (negative test), which are not only different in magnitude from before, but also in reverse order (positive test now bigger). This is because the sample in Table 2.23 has more true (culture) positives than negatives, whereas in Table 2.22 the opposite is true.

### 2.10.1   Weighting sensitivity and specificity

Sometimes there are several tests to compare. For example, Ditchburn and Ditchburn (1990) also give the results of another dipstick test, this time for nitrate. This test has a sensitivity of 0.57, below that for the pyuria test, but a specificity of 0.96, higher than that for the pyuria test. If we had to choose one of the two tests, which should we choose?

One criterion that is often used is the **likelihood ratio**, defined to be

$$\frac{s}{1-p},\tag{2.39}$$

where $s$ is sensitivity and $p$ is specificity, for the different tests. This will increase if either sensitivity or specificity increase with the other remaining constant, or if both sensitivity and specificity increase. Thus the largest values of (2.39) are considered best. However, (2.39) may go up or down if sensitivity and specificity move in opposite directions, as in the dipstick tests example. Consequently the likelihood ratio criterion has limited utility.

**Table 2.23**   Alternative (hypothetical) results of a dipstick test for pyuria

| Dipstick test | Culture test (standard) | | |
| --- | --- | --- | --- |
| | Positive | Negative | Total |
| Positive | 252 | 43 | 295 |
| Negative | 30 | 92 | 122 |
| Total | 282 | 135 | 417 |

In general, we need to consider the relative importance, or 'weight', that we will give to sensitivity and specificity. For instance, if the disease in question is likely to lead to death and the preferred treatment (subsequent to a positive diagnosis) has few side-effects then it will be more important to make sensitivity as large as possible. On the other hand, if the disease is not too serious and no known treatment is completely free of unpleasant side-effects then more weight might be given to specificity. The cost of the treatment given to those with positive test results could also come into consideration. If the weight, however decided, given to sensitivity is $w$ (and the weight given to specificity is thus $1 - w$) then we would seek to maximize

$$M = ws + (1 - w)p \qquad (2.40)$$

where $s$ is sensitivity and $p$ is specificity, as before.

In many situations the primary aim will be to maximize the total number of correct decisions made by the test. Here we should make a distinction between correct decisions during the test (that is, on the sample of people tested) and when the test is later applied to the whole population. These may not be the same; in particular, the sample chosen for testing may have been selected to give a particular ratio of true positives and negatives. If we take the 'sample' criterion then we maximize the number of correct decisions by taking

$$w = \frac{\text{no. of positive samples}}{\text{total no. of samples}}.$$

Applied to Example 2.15, $w = 94/229$ and so $1 - w = 1 - 94/229 = 135/229$, the number of negative samples divided by the total number of samples. Hence, from (2.40),

$$M = \frac{94}{229} \times \frac{84}{94} + \frac{135}{229} \times \frac{92}{135} = \frac{84 + 92}{229},$$

that is the overall proportion of correct test results, as we would expect. On the other hand, if we take the 'population' criterion then we maximize the number of correct decisions by taking

$$w = \frac{\text{no. of people with disease in the population}}{\text{total population size}},$$

that is, the disease prevalence in the population. Often this is not known exactly and must be estimated.

Another possibility is to give equal weight to sensitivity and specificity (after Youden, 1950), in which case $w = 0.5$. The choice of which particular value to use for $w$ may be crucial in comparative diagnostic testing.

*Example 2.16*    Carbon monoxide in expired air (CO) is often used to validate self-reported smoking habits. Consider the problem of determining the cut-point for CO which best discriminates between non-smokers and smokers. For instance, if the CO cut-point used is 6 ppm then everyone with a value of CO above 6 ppm will be 'test positive' and anyone else will be 'test negative' for being a smoker. Such a test is useful in epidemiological research when there is reason to believe that self-reported smoking may be inaccurate. But how should the best cut-point be decided?

This question was addressed by Ruth and Neaton (1991). They recorded the CO of 5621 smokers and 3274 non-smokers in the Multiple Risk Factor Intervention Trial, conducted in the USA. These values are summarized in Table 2.24. The table also gives the results of calculations of sensitivity and specificity, calculated from (2.37) repeatedly, using each possible cut-point. These are combined using (2.40) with Youden's equal weighting; the best cut-point is CO = 10 ppm.

Different weightings of sensitivity and specificity would give different results. In the extreme case where only sensitivity is important (so that $w = 1$) the optimum cut-point will be zero – that is, everyone is designated a smoker. Clearly we can never miss a smoker using this rule, although the test is unlikely to be acceptable in practice! At the opposite extreme, suppose that only specificity is important ($w = 0$). Then we should simply designate everyone as a non-smoker. Again it is difficult to envisage a situation in which this would be a useful procedure. These extreme situations illustrate the importance of considering both sensitivity and specificity.

Interpretation of the performance of different cut-points is enhanced by diagrams, such as a plot of sensitivity, specificity and their sum against the cut-point used (see Figure 2.16). A common plot in this context is that of sensitivity against (1 − specificity), called the **receiver operating characteristic (ROC) plot**. This is particularly helpful when we wish to compare two (or more) diagnostic tests. For instance, Ruth and Neaton (1991) also give data on a second test for smoking status, the level of thiocyanate (SCN) in each subject's blood. These data, together with CO data, were used to produce a simple combination test of smoking status: anyone with levels of SCN and CO below or at each cut-point was designated a non-smoker, and all others were designated a smoker. The ROC curves for the CO test (from Table 2.24) and the combined (SCN + CO) test are shown in Figure 2.17.

A test which produces a diagonal line for its ROC plot (each sensitivity matched by an equal lack of specificity) is undiscriminating in that the chance of a right decision when someone has the disease is equal to the chance of a wrong decision when someone does not. A perfect test would always have perfect sensitivity or specificity, and hence its ROC curve would go straight up the vertical axis to a sensitivity of 1 and then straight across, parallel to the horizontal axis. The test which is nearest this ideal is the best. In Figure 2.17 the combined (SCN + CO) test is best (although only marginally): for any given false positive rate it always has at least as high a true positive rate as does

**Table 2.24**   Results of a test for smoking status

| CO value (ppm) | No. of smokers above this value | No. of non-smokers at or below this value | Sensitivity (s) | Specificity (p) | 0.5s + 0.5p |
|---|---|---|---|---|---|
| LOW−1 | 5621 | 0 | 1.000 | 0.000 | 0.500 |
| 5 | 5460 | 817 | 0.971 | 0.250 | 0.610 |
| 6 | 5331 | 1403 | 0.948 | 0.429 | 0.688 |
| 7 | 5200 | 1914 | 0.925 | 0.585 | 0.755 |
| 8 | 5057 | 2360 | 0.900 | 0.721 | 0.810 |
| 9 | 4932 | 2696 | 0.877 | 0.823 | 0.850 |
| 10 | 4818 | 2972 | 0.857 | 0.908 | 0.882 |
| 20 | 3499 | 3266 | 0.622 | 0.998 | 0.810 |
| 30 | 1984 | 3273 | 0.353 | 1.000 | 0.676 |
| 40 | 874 | 3273 | 0.155 | 1.000 | 0.578 |
| HIGH | 0 | 3274 | 0.000 | 1.000 | 0.500 |

Note: LOW is the smallest CO value observed, HIGH is the largest CO value observed; these
    are not specified in the source paper.
Source: Ruth and Neaton (1991).

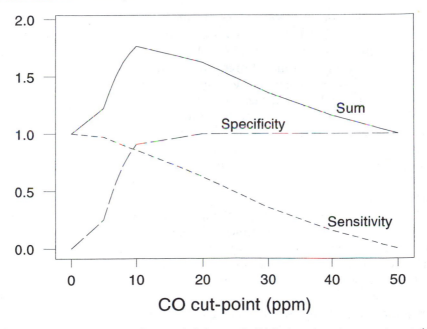

**Figure 2.16**   Sensitivity, specificity and their sum (solid line) against the cut-point used to
distinguish smokers from non-smokers for the data in Table 2.24. Here it is assumed that
LOW = 1 and HIGH = 50.

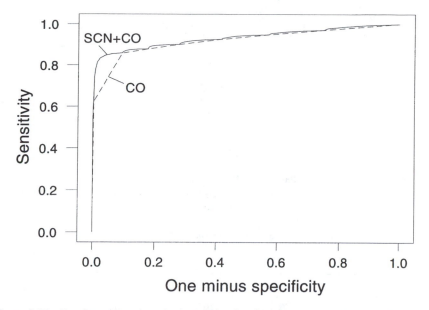

**Figure 2.17**  Receiver operating characteristic plot for two tests designed to distinguish smokers from non-smokers: the CO test (dashed line) and the SCN + CO test (solid line).

the CO test. Notice that the procedure used here for combining SCN and CO information is very crude. Ruth and Neaton (1991) give a better method, which produced a superior test, based on logistic regression modelling (see Chapter 10). For more details on ROC curves, see Hanley and McNeil (1982).

For an example that is very similar to Example 2.16 but used the SHHS data which is referred to repeatedly in this chapter, see Woodward and Tunstall-Pedoe (1992b).

**Exercises**

2.1 Mason *et al.* (1997) studied the habit of illicit drug taking by remand prisoners at the time of their arrival in Durham jail. The table below shows the number of types of illicit drug used in the past year by the unconvicted prisoners studied.
   (i)  Construct a suitable diagram and calculate a suitable summary measure of average for these data.
   (ii) Estimate the proportion of new remand prisoners in the jail who have taken illicit drugs in the year prior to entry. Calculate a 95% confidence interval for this proportion.

| No. of drugs | No. of subjects |
|---|---|
| 0 | 236 |
| 1 | 108 |
| 2 | 96 |
| 3 | 55 |
| 4 | 27 |
| 5 | 17 |
| 6 | 8 |
| 7 | 1 |

2.2 Refer to the lung cancer data in Table C.1 (Appendix C).
   (i)  Construct a table to show how the age of a lung cancer sufferer varies by sex, education and marital status. If a computer is not available to do the data analysis, a dummy table will suffice.
   (ii) The table of sex by tumour type turns out to be:

| | Type of tumour | | |
|---|---|---|---|
| Sex | Local | Regional | Advanced |
| Male | 165 | 169 | 229 |
| Female | 37 | 39 | 43 |

Test the null hypothesis that the distribution of tumour types is the same for men and women. Find a 95% confidence interval for the percentage of advanced tumours (both sexes combined).

2.3 For the Scottish Heart Health Study data on carbon monoxide in Table 2.10, draw a histogram and ogive and construct a normal plot. Compare these with results for carbon monoxide given in Table 2.12 and Figure 2.7.

2.4 Refer to the Glasgow MONICA data in Table C.2.
   (i)   Draw histograms for both protein C and protein S.
   (ii)  Find the five-number summaries of both the protein C and protein S data. Draw boxplots for each variable.
   (iii) Find the two-number summaries of both the protein C and protein S data.
   (iv)  Find the coefficients of skewness of both the protein C and protein S data.
   (v)   Are data for either of the variables highly skewed? If so, try suitable transformations to obtain a reasonably symmetric form, repeating the operations in (i)–(iv), as necessary, on the transformed data.
   (vi)  Produce normal plots for protein C and protein S in their raw state and in whatever transformed state you decided upon in (v). Do these plots confirm your findings in (v)?
   (vii) Find a 95% confidence interval for the mean protein C and another for the mean protein S. Use back-transformations where necessary.

(viii)   Divide the subjects into two groups: those who drank alcohol in the past week (alcohol status = 1 or 2) and those who did not (alcohol status = 3, 4 or 5). Find a 95% confidence interval for the proportion who have drunk in the past week.

(ix)     An interesting question is whether protein S varies with drinking in the past week. Construct a pair of boxplots, on the same scale, to compare drinkers and non-drinkers (in the past week).

(x)      Test whether mean protein S is the same for drinkers in the past week and non-drinkers using a $t$ test. Note that a preliminary test of the equality of variances is required.

(xi)     Use a Wilcoxon test to compare the average values of protein S for drinkers and non-drinkers (in the past week).

(xii)    Repeat (ix) – (xi) for protein C, using an appropriate transformation when required.

(xiii)   Summarize your findings from (ix) – (xii) in words.

(xiv)    Find a 95% confidence interval for the difference in mean protein S for drinkers compared with non-drinkers. Does this agree with your result in (x)?

(xv)     For the full data set the mean protein S is 108.9. Test the null hypothesis that the mean of the subset of 40 observations given in Table C.2 is 108.9 against the two-sided alternative that it is not.

2.5  Oats are an important source of fibre and nutrients, but are often avoided by people with coeliac disease. Srinivasan *et al.* (1996) gave ten patients with the disease an 'oats challenge': 50 g of oats per day for 12 weeks. Results for enterocyte height (μm) before and after the challenge were:

| Patient | 1 | 2 | 3 | 4 | 5 | 6 | 7 | 8 | 9 | 10 |
|---------|------|------|------|------|------|------|------|------|------|------|
| Before  | 36.3 | 36.0 | 40.8 | 44.9 | 32.8 | 28.8 | 38.4 | 31.1 | 29.8 | 30.2 |
| After   | 35.3 | 38.3 | 37.9 | 37.6 | 28.8 | 27.1 | 42.6 | 34.7 | 30.6 | 36.8 |

(i)    Test the null hypothesis that the oats challenge had no effect on enterocyte heights.

(ii)   Find a 90% confidence interval for the difference in mean values after and before the challenge.

(iii)  What conclusion do you draw?

2.6  Sugar, derived from the diet, is classified into three types:
- extrinsic sugar – derived from sweets, puddings, etc.;
- intrinsic sugar – naturally occurring in fresh fruit, vegetables and grain;
- lactose sugar – derived from milk.

Bolton-Smith and Woodward (1995) compared the dietary intake (expressed as a percentage of total dietary consumption of energy from all foods) of each sugar type to the body mass index (BMI) for subjects in the Scottish Heart Health Study and First Scottish MONICA Survey. Results from the study are given below.

Draw a diagram or diagrams to illustrate these data, so as to show comparisons between BMI groups for each specific sugar type. Comment on the major features of the data.

| BMI group $(kg/m^2)$ | Type of sugar | | | |
|---|---|---|---|---|
| | Extrinsic | Intrinsic | Lactose | Total |
| Males | | | | |
| < 20 | 14.2 | 1.5 | 3.3 | 19.0 |
| 20–25 | 12.5 | 1.9 | 3.3 | 17.6 |
| 25–30 | 10.4 | 2.1 | 3.4 | 15.9 |
| > 30 | 8.8 | 2.2 | 3.4 | 14.4 |
| Females | | | | |
| < 20 | 12.2 | 2.8 | 4.0 | 19.1 |
| 20–25 | 9.4 | 3.2 | 4.2 | 16.8 |
| 25–30 | 8.0 | 3.3 | 4.2 | 15.4 |
| > 30 | 7.5 | 3.4 | 4.0 | 14.8 |

2.7 McKinney *et al.* (1991) compared mothers' reports of childhood vaccinations with the records of the children's general practitioners. For the first whooping cough vaccination the concordance between the two sources of data (neither of which can be considered to represent 'the truth', according to the authors) can be judged from the table below. Use this table to estimate the kappa statistic, together with an approximate 95% confidence interval.

| GPs record | Mothers' report | | |
|---|---|---|---|
| | No vaccination | Vaccination | Total |
| No vaccination | 79 | 37 | 116 |
| Vaccination | 11 | 167 | 178 |
| Total | 90 | 204 | 294 |

2.8 In the study of Mason *et al.* (1997), already used in Exercise 2.1, all unconvicted men remanded into custody in Durham jail from 1 October 1995 to 30 April 1996 were given a detailed interview. From this, the researchers were able to ascertain who did and did not take drugs at the time of incarceration. The table below shows the research findings for cannabis, showing also whether or not the prison's own reception screening programme had detected cannabis use.

| Screening finding | Research finding | |
|---|---|---|
| | User | Non-user |
| User | 49 | 6 |
| Non-user | 201 | 118 |

Treating the research finding as the truth, estimate (i) the sensitivity, (ii) the specificity, and the predictive values of (iii) a positive test and (iv) a negative test. Give confidence intervals corresponding to each estimate. Interpret your findings.

2.9 The table below shows the results of the thiocyanate (SCN) test for smoking reported by Ruth and Neaton (1991). Find the sensitivity and specificity for each SCN cut-point. Find the optimum cut-point according to each of the following criteria:

(i)   Youden's equal weighting of sensitivity and specificity.
(ii)  To maximize the number of correct decisions for the sample data.
(iii) To maximize the number of correct decisions in a population where 25% of people smoke.

| SCN value | No. of smokers above this value | No. of non-smokers below or at this value |
|---|---|---|
| LOW−1 | 5621 | 0 |
| 20 | 5602 | 149 |
| 40 | 5502 | 1279 |
| 60 | 5294 | 2271 |
| 80 | 5030 | 2806 |
| 100 | 4750 | 3057 |
| 120 | 4315 | 3185 |
| 140 | 3741 | 3240 |
| 160 | 2993 | 3259 |
| 180 | 2166 | 3268 |
| 200 | 1417 | 3271 |
| 220 | 823 | 3274 |
| HIGH | 0 | 3274 |

Note: LOW is the smallest observed SCN value; HIGH is the largest observed SCN value.

2.10 Suppose that you were asked to write a report on the studies of Doll and Hill described in Section 1.2. Assuming that you could obtain access to the raw data, how (if at all) would you redesign Tables 1.1–1.3 for inclusion in your report?

# 3

# Assessing risk factors

## 3.1 Risk and relative risk

In epidemiology, we are often interested in evaluating the chance that an individual who possesses a certain attribute also has a specific disease. The most basic epidemiological measure is the probability of an individual becoming newly diseased given that the individual has the particular attribute under consideration. This is called the **risk** of disease; as defined in Section 1.1, the attribute considered is called the **risk factor**. Hence risk measures the probability of disease incidence.

Although risk is a useful summary of the relationship between risk factor and disease, it is not sufficient by itself for assessing the importance of the risk factor to disease outcome. For instance, we may find that 30% of a sample of women who use a particular type of contraceptive pill develop breast cancer, so that the risk of breast cancer is 0.3 for pill users. This would seem impressive evidence implicating the pill, unless it transpired that a similar percentage of pill non-users have also developed breast cancer. As in most procedures in epidemiology, a comparison group is required, and the simplest one to take here is the group without the risk factor. This leads to the definition of the **relative risk** (or **risk ratio**) as the ratio of the risk of disease for those with the risk factor to the risk of disease for those without the risk factor. If the relative risk is above 1 then the factor under investigation increases risk; if less than 1 it reduces risk. A factor which has a relative risk less than 1 is sometimes referred to as a **protective factor**. In most cases we shall use the general term 'risk factor' without specifying the direction of its effect.

Computation of the risk and relative risk is particularly simple from a $2 \times 2$ table (two rows by two columns) of risk factor status against disease status, designated algebraically by Table 3.1. This represents data from $n$ subjects, free from disease at the outset of the study (the **baseline**). Each individual's risk factor status at baseline was recorded, as was whether or not he or she went on to develop the disease during the study.

**Table 3.1**   Display of data from an incidence study

| Risk factor status | Disease status | | |
| --- | --- | --- | --- |
| | Disease | No disease | Total |
| Exposed | a | b | a + b |
| Not exposed | c | d | c + d |
| Total | a + c | b + d | n |

From Table 3.1 we see that, for example, the number of people with the risk factor but without the disease is $b$. Note that $n = a + b + c + d$. In general,

$$\text{risk} = \text{number of cases of disease/number of people at risk.} \qquad (3.1)$$

From Table 3.1, the exposure-specific risks are, for those with the risk factor, $a/(a+b)$; and for those without the risk factor, $c/(c+d)$. The relative risk for those with the risk factor, compared to those without, is given by

$$\frac{a/(a+b)}{c/(c+d)} = \frac{a(c+d)}{c(a+b)}. \qquad (3.2)$$

In most real-life situations the data collected in an epidemiological study will be a sample of data on the subject of interest. Hence the risk and relative risk calculated from the data are estimates for the equivalent entities in the population as a whole; for instance, all pre-menopausal women in the earlier example relating to use of the pill. In fact we shall see, in Section 6.2, that the sample values are not appropriate estimates for the population equivalents for case–control studies. As a consequence, risk and relative risk should *not* be calculated from case–control studies.

We should specify the sampling error inherent in our sample-based estimates of the true (population) risk and relative risk. As in other cases, this is best done by specifying either the standard error (sample-to-sample variation in the value of the estimate) or a confidence interval. We shall use the symbol $R$ to represent the population risk and $r$ to represent the sample risk.

By definition, the population risk is simply a probability, and the standard error is estimated by

$$\hat{se}(r) = \sqrt{r(1-r)/n}. \qquad (3.3)$$

Using a normal approximation, as was used to define (2.2), the 95% confidence interval for $R$ is

$$r \pm 1.96\hat{se}(r). \qquad (3.4)$$

The value 1.96 appears because this is the 5% critical value for the normal distribution. As usual, should we require a different percentage confidence interval we simply alter this value: see (2.3). As with (3.1), we could use (3.3) and (3.4) for the risk amongst those exposed or amongst those unexposed or, indeed, for everyone (both groups combined).

The confidence interval for the relative risk is slightly more difficult to compute. The distribution of the sample relative risk is skewed and a log transformation is necessary to ensure approximate normality. On the log scale, Katz *et al.* (1978) showed that, in the notation of Table 3.1,

$$\hat{se}(\log_e \hat{\lambda}) = \sqrt{\frac{1}{a} - \frac{1}{a+b} + \frac{1}{c} - \frac{1}{c+d}}, \tag{3.5}$$

where $\lambda$ is the population relative risk and $\hat{\lambda}$ is its estimate in the sample, defined by (3.2). Hence the 95% confidence interval for $\log_e \lambda$ is

$$\log_e \hat{\lambda} \pm 1.96\hat{se}(\log_e \hat{\lambda}),$$

with lower and upper limits of

$$\begin{aligned} L_{\log} &= \log_e \hat{\lambda} - 1.96\hat{se}(\log_e \hat{\lambda}), \\ U_{\log} &= \log_e \hat{\lambda} + 1.96\hat{se}(\log_e \hat{\lambda}). \end{aligned} \tag{3.6}$$

We really want a 95% confidence interval for $\lambda$ itself. This is obtained by raising the two limits in (3.6) to the power e. That is, the lower and upper limits in the 95% confidence interval for the relative risk, $\lambda$, are

$$\begin{aligned} L &= \exp(L_{\log}), \\ U &= \exp(U_{\log}). \end{aligned} \tag{3.7}$$

*Example 3.1*   The Pooling Project (Pool 5) studied risk factors for coronary heart disease amongst men in Albany, Chicago, Framingham and Tecumseh (Pooling Project Research Group, 1978). Table 3.2 gives current smoking status at entry to study and whether or not a coronary event occurred within the following (approximately) 10 years for 1905 men aged 50–54 years at entry. Any man with pre-existing coronary symptoms at entry is excluded.

From (3.1), the overall risk of a coronary event is 216/1905 = 0.1134; the risk for smokers is 166/1342 = 0.1237, whilst for non-smokers it is 50/563 = 0.0888. From (3.2), the relative

**Table 3.2**   Smoking and coronary events in the Pooling Project

| Smoker at entry? | Coronary event during follow up? | | |
|---|---|---|---|
| | *Yes* | *No* | *Total* |
| Yes | 166 | 1176 | 1342 |
| No | 50 | 513 | 563 |
| Total | 216 | 1689 | 1905 |

risk is $0.1237/0.0888 = 1.393$. From (3.4), the 95% confidence interval for the risk of a coronary event for smokers is

$$0.1237 \pm 1.96\sqrt{0.1237(1 - 0.1237)/1342},$$

that is, $0.1237 \pm 0.0176$ or $(0.1061, 0.1413)$. From (3.5), the estimated standard error of the log of the relative risk is

$$\sqrt{\frac{1}{166} - \frac{1}{1342} + \frac{1}{50} - \frac{1}{563}} = 0.1533.$$

From (3.6), 95% confidence limits for the log of the relative risk are then

$$L_{\log} = \log_e(1.393) - 1.96 \times 0.1533 = 0.0310,$$
$$U_{\log} = \log_e(1.393) + 1.96 \times 0.1533 = 0.6319.$$

From (3.7), 95% confidence limits for the relative risk of a coronary event for smokers compared to non-smokers are then

$$L = \exp(0.0310) = 1.031,$$
$$U = \exp(0.6319) = 1.881.$$

Hence we estimate that the risk of a coronary event for smokers is 0.124, and we are 95% sure that the interval (0.106, 0.141) contains the true population risk. The estimated relative risk of a coronary event for smokers compared to non-smokers is 1.39, and we are 95% sure that the interval (1.03, 1.88) contains the true population relative risk. Although numbers have been calculated to several decimal places here, this is both because several results are subsequently used to derive other results and because we will wish to make comparisons with other analytical methods later. Two decimal places are usually sufficient in a presentation. In brief, we conclude that 12% of smokers experience a coronary event, this being almost 1.4 times as many as non-smokers. That is, smoking elevates the estimated risk by almost 40%.

Notice that (3.3) could have been applied to calculate a confidence interval for the overall risk (pooled over smoking status) or the risk for non-smokers, if either were required. Also, there is no theoretical necessity to calculate relative risk as smokers' risk over non-smokers' in Example 3.1. Instead the inverse, non-smokers' risk over smokers' risk, could be calculated in a similar way, should this be of practical interest. In fact it is simply the reciprocal of the relative risk found already, $1/1.393 = 0.72$. Similarly the 95% confidence limits for the relative risk of a coronary event for non-smokers compared to smokers are found as the reciprocals of the limits found already, except that the order of the two limits is reversed, that is, the lower limit is $1/1.881 = 0.53$ and the upper limit is $1/1.031 = 0.97$. There is no advantage in stating both, but this example shows that it is important to specify clearly what is being related (in the numerator) to what (in the denominator). The outcome used to define the denominator in the relative risk is called the **base** or **reference**. Generally the base is taken as absence of the risk factor in a situation akin to Example 3.1.

## 3.2   Odds and odds ratio

As we have seen, the risk is a probability. Whenever a probability is calculated it is possible to calculate an alternative specification of 'chance' called the **odds**. Whereas the probability measures the number of times the outcome of interest (for example, disease) occurs relative to the total number of observations (that is, the sample size), the odds measures the number of times the outcome occurs relative to the number of times it does not. The odds can be calculated for different groups; here we would be interested in the odds for those exposed to the risk factor and the odds for those unexposed. The ratio of these two is called the **odds ratio**. Similar to the relative risk, an odds ratio above 1 implies that exposure to the factor under investigation increases the odds of disease, whilst a value below 1 means the factor reduces the odds of disease. In general,

odds = number of cases of disease/number of non-cases of disease.   (3.8)

From Table 3.1 the exposure-specific odds are, for those with the risk factor, $a/b$; and for those without the risk factor, $c/d$. The odds ratio for those with the risk factor, compared to those without, is given by

$$\hat{\psi} = \frac{a/b}{c/d} = \frac{ad}{bc}.$$   (3.9)

The Greek letter $\psi$ (psi) is commonly used (as here) to represent the population odds ratio. In (3.9) the hat, once again, denotes a sample value that is an estimate of its population equivalent.

Another way of deriving the odds is as the ratio of the risk to its complement; for example, the odds for those with the risk factor are given by $r/(1-r)$. This can easily be justified from (3.1) and (3.8). In everyday life, odds are most often heard about in gambling situations, such as the odds of a horse winning a race. Epidemiologists take 'odds' and 'odds ratio' to refer to the chance of a disease *incidence*, just as they do 'risk' and 'relative risk'. In practice, the odds are rarely of interest, and the odds ratio is generally quoted alone (Section 3.3).

As with the relative risk, the distribution of the odds ratio is better approximated by a normal distribution if a log transformation is applied. Woolf (1955) showed that

$$\hat{se}(\log_e \hat{\psi}) = \sqrt{\frac{1}{a} + \frac{1}{b} + \frac{1}{c} + \frac{1}{d}}, \tag{3.10}$$

and hence 95% confidence limits for $\log_e \psi$ are

$$\begin{aligned}
L_{\log} &= \log_e \hat{\psi} - 1.96\hat{se}(\log_e \hat{\psi}), \\
U_{\log} &= \log_e \hat{\psi} + 1.96\hat{se}(\log_e \hat{\psi}),
\end{aligned} \tag{3.11}$$

and the 95% confidence limits for $\psi$ itself are

$$\begin{aligned}
L &= \exp(L_{\log}), \\
U &= \exp(U_{\log}).
\end{aligned} \tag{3.12}$$

*Example 3.2*    For the Pooling Project, Table 3.2 gives the following results. From (3.8), the overall odds of a coronary event are $216/1689 = 0.1279$; the odds of a coronary event for smokers are $166/1176 = 0.1412$, whilst for non-smokers they are $50/513 = 0.0975$. From (3.9), the odds ratio for a coronary event, comparing smokers to non-smokers, is

$$\frac{166/1176}{50/513} = \frac{0.1412}{0.0975} = 1.448$$

From (3.10), the estimated standard error of the log of the odds ratio is

$$\sqrt{\frac{1}{166} + \frac{1}{1176} + \frac{1}{50} + \frac{1}{513}} = 0.1698.$$

From (3.11), 95% confidence limits for the log of the odds ratio are then

$$\begin{aligned}
L_{\log} &= \log_e(1.448) - 1.96 \times 0.1698 = 0.0374, \\
U_{\log} &= \log_e(1.448) + 1.96 \times 0.1698 = 0.7030.
\end{aligned}$$

From (3.12), 95% confidence limits for the odds ratio for a coronary event, comparing smokers to non-smokers, are then

$$\begin{aligned}
L &= \exp(0.0374) = 1.038, \\
U &= \exp(0.7030) = 2.020.
\end{aligned}$$

The odds of a coronary event are estimated to be 1.45 times as great for smokers as for non-smokers, and we are 95% sure that the interval (1.04, 2.02) contains the true odds ratio. In brief, smoking is estimated to elevate the odds of a coronary event by 45%.

Although it would be unusual to want to do so, it is possible to compute the odds ratio, and its confidence interval, for non-smokers compared to smokers. As in the case of the relative risk (Section 3.1), we can do this from the results of Example 3.2 without recourse to the data. We simply take the reciprocal of the original odds ratio and its confidence limits, with order reversed: 0.69 (0.50, 0.96). As with the relative risk, it is important to specify what is being compared to what whenever an odds ratio is stated.

Note that the formulae for the limits of confidence intervals given in this section and Section 3.1 are really only approximations. For example, (3.4) uses a normal approximation to the true binomial distribution of the number who are cases out of the number at risk. See Clarke and Cooke (1992) for an introduction to the binomial distribution and Conover (1980) for details on exact binomial procedures and the normal approximation. Modern computer packages will provide more accurate results, based on exact theory. Other approximate formulae for confidence intervals commonly used are due to Cornfield (1956), for the odds ratio, and Greenland and Robins (1985), for the relative risk. Generally results will be virtually the same by the alternative approaches whenever sample sizes are large.

## 3.3   Deciding upon a measure of comparative chance

### 3.3.1   Relative risk or odds ratio?

As we have seen, both risk and odds measure the chance of disease incidence in some way, and thus the relative risk and odds ratio measure comparative chance. Risk is the preferred measure because it is a probability, and probabilities are well understood as long-run versions of proportions. Odds are less well understood, and consequently rarely used.

So why consider odds at all? The answer is that the odds ratio is often a good approximation to the relative risk, and in some cases the odds ratio is either all that we can estimate (the situation in case–control studies: see Chapter 6) or is the most convenient to calculate (in logistic regression analysis: see Chapter 10).

The odds ratio will be a good approximation to the relative risk whenever the disease in question is rare. Referring to Table 3.1, when the disease is rare it must be that

$$a + b \simeq b,$$
$$c + d \simeq d, \tag{3.13}$$

where $\simeq$ means 'approximately equal to'. Hence, from (3.2), (3.9) and (3.13),

$$\hat{\psi} = \frac{ad}{bc} \simeq \frac{a(c+d)}{(a+b)c} = \hat{\lambda}.$$

Comparison of Examples 3.1 and 3.2 shows that the relative risk (1.39) and odds ratio (1.45) for a coronary event, comparing smokers to non-smokers, are fairly similar for the Pooling Project. Inspection of Table 3.2 shows that coronary events are quite unusual, despite coronary heart disease being the major cause of premature death amongst middle-aged American men. Many other diseases will have lower overall incidence rates, suggesting even better agreement. However, the approximation is only good if incidence is relatively low amongst *both* those with and without the risk factor. For example, if few non-smokers have a coronary event, but virtually all smokers do, then the odds ratio would be substantially larger than the relative risk.

*Example 3.3*   Consider the hypothetical results of Table 3.3. An extra column of risks has been added to enhance interpretation; this is often useful in written reports. In this case the disease is rare overall (only about one person in 100 has it) and yet the relative risk is

$$\hat{\lambda} = \frac{0.5}{0.00102} = 490,$$

whereas the odds ratio is

$$\hat{\psi} = \frac{9 \times 981}{1 \times 9} = 981,$$

just over twice as big. So the odds ratio does not provide a good approximation to the relative risk in this case.

Situations akin to Table 3.3, where the risk factor is virtually the sole causal agent for the disease, arise infrequently in practical epidemiological research, as do odds ratios/relative risks in the hundreds or more. Table 3.3 shows a very extreme example of how the odds ratio can overestimate the relative risk and it could be argued that exact values matter little when the direction of effect is so obvious. However, since the relative risk and odds ratio are not the same, it is appropriate to specify which of the two is being reported. Many epidemiological publications have been in error in this regard, usually by wrongly calling an odds ratio a relative risk. It would be possible to compute both in any follow-up investigation, as in Examples 3.1 and 3.2, although not in a case–control study. However, we would normally only want to report one.

### 3.3.2   Measures of difference

Both the relative risk and odds ratio are *proportionate* measures. Such measures seem the most natural when chance is being measured because chance

**Table 3.3**   Hypothetical data from an incidence study

| Risk factor status | Disease status | | | |
| --- | --- | --- | --- | --- |
| | Disease | No disease | Total | Risk |
| Exposed | 9 | 9 | 18 | 0.5 |
| Not exposed | 1 | 981 | 982 | 0.001 02 |
| Total | 10 | 990 | 1000 | 0.010 10 |

is itself measured proportionately. However, difference measures may also be used: that is, the difference between the risks or between the odds. It is generally the **risk difference** which is used whenever a difference measure is chosen. Hence for Example 3.1 the coronary risk difference, smokers compared to non-smokers, is $0.1237 - 0.0888 = 0.0349$. The risk of a coronary event is thus around 0.03 higher for smokers. This is arguably not as easy to interpret as the earlier statement, using the relative risk, that smokers have 1.39 times the risk of a coronary event. A 95% confidence interval for the risk difference may be calculated using (2.5).

## 3.4   Prevalence studies

In the preceding sections risk, relative risk, odds, odds ratio and risk difference have been defined as measures of chance in incidence studies. Technically there is no reason why the same definitions could not be used in prevalence studies: (3.1)–(3.13) could all be defined quite properly in a mathematical sense. Unlike general English usage, epidemiologists reserve all these key terms to refer to incidence. However, this is really rather unfortunate, since it is perfectly natural to want to talk about 'risk' in relation to prevalence data such as those in Table 2.2. To overcome this difficulty the prefix 'prevalence' should be used; for example, the **prevalence relative risk** of CHD for manual (classes IIIm, IV and V) compared to non-manual (classes I, II and IIIn) workers can be calculated from Table 2.2 as

$$\frac{(668 + 279 + 109)/(2482 + 974 + 306)}{(100 + 382 + 183)/(492 + 1872 + 834)} = 1.35.$$

Thus manual workers have a 35% higher chance of having CHD than do non-manual workers. If one is prepared to be less pedantic, a more elegant name for the measure in this example is the 'relative risk for prevalent CHD'.

*Example 3.4*   Smith *et al.* (1991) give the results of a cross-sectional study of peripheral vascular disease (PVD) in Scotland. Table 3.4 shows prevalent cases and non-cases of the disease classified by cigarette smoking status for men. Hence,

overall prevalence risk of PVD = $56/4956$ = 0.0113;

prevalence risk of PVD for cigarette smokers = $15/1727$ = 0.00869;

prevalence risk of PVD for non-smokers = $41/3229$ = 0.0127;

prevalence relative risk = $0.00869/0.0127$ = 0.68;

prevalence odds of PVD for cigarette smokers = $15/1712$ = 0.00876;

prevalence odds of PVD for non-smokers = $41/3188$ = 0.0129;

prevalence odds ratio = $0.00876/0.0129$ = 0.68

**Table 3.4**   Cigarette smoking and peripheral vascular disease in a sample of Scottish men

| Cigarette smoker? | Peripheral vascular disease? | | |
| | Yes | No | Total |
| --- | --- | --- | --- |
| Yes | 15 | 1712 | 1727 |
| No | 41 | 3188 | 3229 |
| Total | 56 | 4900 | 4956 |

Notice that the prevalence relative risk and odds ratio are the same (to two decimal places), as would be expected for a disease as rare as peripheral vascular disease.

The results of Example 3.4 seem to go against expectation: cigarette smoking appears to be protective (relative risk below 1). This illustrates one great drawback with prevalence studies: individuals with pre-existing disease may have altered their lifestyle, possibly due to medical advice, so that they are now no longer exposed to the risk factor. In the example a smoker may quit once he has experienced PVD or other cardiovascular symptoms.

*Example 3.5*   The original article which gave rise to Example 3.4 distinguished between ex-smokers and never-smokers when considering the non-smoking group. Table 3.5 shows the results when this more extensive classification is used. As we expect, those who have never smoked have the lowest prevalence. Ex-smokers have the highest prevalence, with current smokers somewhere in-between.

In other situations we may not be able to identify those who were previously exposed to whatever risk factor is of interest. The results may then be biased in favour of the risk factor, as in Example 3.4. Of course, even in Example 3.5 there is no guarantee that disease has caused people to give up, or indeed that disease has even preceded giving up. We can infer that this is likely, but it is not proven unless we can ascertain the sequence of events for each current non-smoker. Notice that the Pooling Project incidence study (Example 3.1) avoided

**Table 3.5**   Cigarette smoking and peripheral vascular disease in a sample of Scottish men

| Cigarette smoking status | Peripheral vascular disease? | | | |
| | Yes | No | Total | Prevalence |
| --- | --- | --- | --- | --- |
| Current smoker | 15 | 1712 | 1727 | 0.0087 |
| Ex-smoker | 33 | 1897 | 1930 | 0.0171 |
| Never smoked | 8 | 1291 | 1299 | 0.0062 |
| Total | 56 | 4900 | 4956 | 0.0113 |

the problem of disease causing smoking cessation by excluding cases of existing disease at the outset (when smoking status was recorded).

Other problems with prevalence studies are mentioned in Section 1.4.1. All these problems show that if we wish to demonstrate direct causality from risk factor to disease, we would be advised to use incidence, rather than prevalence, data.

## 3.5  Testing association

We have seen that the relative risk and odds ratio are meaningful measures of association between risk factor and disease. Both measure the relative chance of disease with the risk factor, compared to without. If the supposed risk factor has no effect, both the relative risk and odds ratio should turn out to be around unity. In practice, we take a sample of data and measure either the sample relative risk or odds ratio; we could then consider whether this sample result provides evidence that the equivalent population value is different from 1.0. If not, then we would conclude that there is no evidence of an association between the supposed risk factor and the disease in question. Such a result would cast doubt upon the theory that the supposed risk factor causes the disease.

Considering Table 3.1, it is clear that a test of no association between risk factor and disease is achieved by the chi-square test (Section 2.5.1). From Table 3.1 the expected ($E$) values when the null hypothesis of no association (equivalent to $H_0 : \lambda = 1$ or $H_0 : \psi = 1$) is true are

$$(a+b)(a+c)/n \qquad (a+b)(b+d)/n$$
$$(c+d)(a+c)/n \qquad (c+d)(b+d)/n$$

respectively. Using (2.1), a little algebraic manipulation produces the specific form of the chi-square test statistic for a $2 \times 2$ table:

$$\frac{n(ad-bc)^2}{(a+b)(c+d)(a+c)(b+d)}. \qquad (3.14)$$

Since there are two rows and two columns, the degrees of freedom associated with this chi-square statistic are $(2-1)(2-1) = 1$. Hence we compare (3.14) with $\chi_1^2$.

*Example 3.6*   Consider the Pooling Project data of Table 3.2 once again. By (3.14), the chi-square test statistic is

$$\frac{1905(166 \times 513 - 50 \times 1176)^2}{1342 \times 563 \times 216 \times 1689} = 4.80.$$

From Table B.3, $\chi_1^2 = 3.84$ at the 5% level and 5.02 at the $2\frac{1}{2}$% level. Hence the result is significant at the 5% level, but not at the more extreme $2\frac{1}{2}$% level. The exact $p$ value is 0.028, found from a computer package. We conclude that there is evidence (although not particularly strong) of an association between smoking and a coronary event. The relative risk and odds ratio are both significantly different from 1, at the 5% level of significance.

One thing to note about the above result is that we cannot use it to conclude that smoking causes coronary heart disease. Although the result certainly does not refute the idea of a causal link, the association *could* be the result of external forces. For instance, it could be that smokers are mainly older people and it is older people who experience coronary events. Smoking and coronary disease are then, perhaps, only associated because of their common causal link with age. This issue is considered further in Chapter 4.

The chi-square test is a two-sided test, so that the conclusion in Example 3.6 was that $\lambda \neq 1$, or $\psi \neq 1$. To ascertain the direction of the link between risk factor and disease we simply look at the estimate of $\lambda$ or $\psi$. From Examples 3.1 and 3.2 we see that the estimated values, $\hat{\lambda} = 1.39$ and $\hat{\psi} = 1.45$, are both greater than 1. Hence we conclude that smokers are more likely to have a coronary event, and we have evidence that the observed association between smoking and coronary disease is not simply due to chance.

We can also tie up the results of Examples 3.1 and 3.2 with Example 3.6. The 95% confidence intervals for $\lambda$ and $\psi$ were (1.03, 1.88) and (1.04, 2.02), respectively. Both exclude unity, which agrees with the result $\lambda \neq 1$ or $\psi \neq 1$, at the 5% level of significance. The lower 95% confidence limits are both only just above 1, which is reflected in the $p$ value being only just below 0.05.

### 3.5.1    Equivalent tests

As already described in Section 2.5.1, the chi-square test of no association in a $2 \times 2$ table is entirely equivalent to the test of equality of two proportions. In the current context, this implies that we can equally well test the null hypothesis of no association between risk factor and disease, $\lambda = 1$ or $\psi = 1$, by testing whether the same proportion have the disease in the risk factor positive and risk factor negative groups. In some contexts the chi-square approach is somewhat easier; in others the test of equal proportions will seem more natural. As noted in Section 2.5.3, the only difference is that everything is squared in the chi-square formulation.

*Example 3.7*   For the Pooling Project, the proportions with a coronary event in the sample are, for smokers,

$$p_1 = 166/1342 = 0.1237,$$

and for non-smokers,

$$p_2 = 50/563 = 0.0888.$$

The proportion for smokers and non-smokers combined may be obtained from (2.7) as

$$p_c = \frac{1342 \times 0.1237 + 563 \times 0.0888}{1342 + 563} = 0.1134;$$

or alternatively, and rather more easily, from Table 3.2 as $216/1905 = 0.1134$ (as given in Example 3.1). Then, from (2.6), the test statistic for testing whether the population proportions with a coronary event are the same for smokers and non-smokers is

$$\frac{0.1237 - 0.0888}{\sqrt{0.1134(1 - 0.1134)\left(\dfrac{1}{1342} + \dfrac{1}{563}\right)}} = 2.19.$$

This result is to be compared with the standard normal distribution (Table B.2). A computer package was used to obtain the exact $p$ value as 0.028 for a two-sided test (that is, when the alternative hypothesis is that the two proportions are unequal). This is the same result as that obtained in Example 3.6. Notice that the square of the test statistic in this example equals the test statistic in Example 3.6, $2.19^2 = 4.80$, as it should.

Another equivalent test is less interesting to the epidemiologist, but perfectly acceptable. This is a test of whether the same proportion have the risk factor in the diseased and non-diseased groups. In the Pooling Project example this compares the proportion smoking: $166/216$ for those with CHD and $1176/1689$ for those without CHD. The test statistic, (2.6), for this comparison is 2.19, exactly the same as in Example 3.7.

One word of caution: these tests on proportions will make practical sense only if the entire data are drawn as a random sample. For instance, if those diseased and undiseased are sampled independently, as in a case–control study, then a test that compares proportions with disease (similar to Example 3.7) would not be suitably formulated (although it would be mathematically correct). The chi-square test considered as a test of no association does not have this practical difficulty.

### 3.5.2   One-sided tests

In most cases we will wish to perform two-sided tests of no association between risk factor and disease, simply because we will still wish to identify situations where the risk factor is actually protective against the disease. To take the Pooling Project example, we certainly do not expect smoking to prevent coronary disease, but we would not want to miss such a relationship, should the data suggest it.

If we decide that a one-sided test is appropriate, in the situation where (say) only an increased risk in the presence of the risk factor ($\lambda > 1$) is of interest, the procedure is straightforward if we use the normal test of Section 3.5.1. We read off one-sided $p$ values directly from Table B.1, or an equivalent table with greater coverage. Due to the symmetry of the normal distribution, the $p$ value for a one-sided test is always half of that for the equivalent two-sided test. Hence if a one-sided alternative were sensible in Example 3.7 the $p$ value for the test of equality of risk would be $0.028/2 = 0.014$. We can obtain this result approximately from Table B.1, because it tells us that the proportion of the standard normal below 2.20 is 0.9861; hence the probability of a value above 2.19, when the null hypothesis is true, is just above $1 - 0.9861 = 0.0139$.

When the chi-square test is adopted, the one-sided procedure is not as obvious. This is because the chi-square test is a test of the null hypothesis of no association against the alternative of *some* association; in the current context it is always two-sided. Consequently Table B.3 gives two-sided $p$ values. However, since we have already seen that the two tests are equivalent when applied to a $2 \times 2$ table, the solution is very obvious: we simply halve the chi-square $p$ value whenever a one-sided test is required. The same procedure is possible whenever a chi-square test with one degree of freedom is concerned. In most other situations where chi-square tests are used (see Section 2.5.1) the concept of a one-sided test will not be meaningful and the problem does not arise.

### 3.5.3   Continuity corrections

Both the chi-square test and the equivalent normal test just described are really only approximate tests. An exact test is possible, and will be described in Section 3.5.4. One aspect of the approximation is that the data in a $2 \times 2$ table of risk factor status against disease outcome must be discrete and yet the probability distribution (chi-square or normal) used to test the data is continuous. In order to improve this continuous approximation to a discrete distribution a **continuity correction** is sometimes used. The correction generally used is **Yates's correction**, which reduces the absolute difference between the observed and (under the null hypothesis) expected numbers in the chi-square test statistic, (2.1), by a half. That is, (2.1) becomes

$$\sum_i \sum_j \frac{\left(|O_{ij} - E_{ij}| - \frac{1}{2}\right)^2}{E_{ij}} \tag{3.15}$$

which, for a $2 \times 2$ table, becomes

$$\frac{n\left(|ad - bc| - \frac{1}{2}n\right)^2}{(a+b)(c+d)(a+c)(b+d)}, \tag{3.16}$$

replacing (3.14). In (3.15) $|O_{ij} - E_{ij}|$ denotes the absolute value of $O_{ij} - E_{ij}$, that is, negative outcomes are treated as positive; similarly for $|ad - bc|$ in (3.16). Using Yates's correction in the test for equality of two proportions alters (2.6) to give

$$\frac{|p_1 - p_2| - \frac{1}{2}\left(\dfrac{1}{n_1} + \dfrac{1}{n_2}\right)}{\sqrt{p_c(1 - p_c)\left(\dfrac{1}{n_1} + \dfrac{1}{n_2}\right)}}. \tag{3.17}$$

*Example 3.8*   Reworking Example 3.6 using (3.16) rather than (3.14) gives test statistic

$$\frac{1905(|166 \times 513 - 50 \times 1176| - 1905/2)^2}{1342 \times 563 \times 216 \times 1689} = 4.46.$$

This is smaller by 0.34 than the result when Yates's correction is not used. The $p$ value for this test turns out to be 0.035, slightly larger than the 0.028 found earlier. Hence the continuity correction has made only a slight difference to the result, and leaves the conclusion unchanged: there is evidence, although not strong evidence, that smoking is associated with coronary events.

   This example could be based upon the normal test. Once again, this gives an entirely equivalent result. Using (3.17) on the Pooling Project data gives a test statistic of 2.11, the square root of the 4.46 found above.

   There is an ongoing debate as to whether Yates's correction is worthwhile. In its favour is the point that it gives a better approximation to the exact result. See Example 3.9 below and the discussion in Mantel and Greenhouse (1968). Against it is the argument that it is more complex to understand and calculate (Kleinbaum *et al.*, 1982). Provided absolute faith is not attached to significance level cut-points (Section 2.5.2), the distinction should not be important unless the numbers are small. Given its extra complexity, the continuity correction is only worthwhile when numbers are fairly small. However, if at least one of the expected numbers is very small an exact test should always be used; the continuity correction is then not sufficient.

### 3.5.4   Fisher's exact test

As already mentioned, the chi-square test is an approximate test. An exact procedure, at least under the assumption that the row and column totals (called the **marginal** totals) are fixed, is given here. This is usually used whenever any expected value in a $2 \times 2$ table is below 5.

The procedure, ascribed to Sir Ronald Fisher, works by first using probability theory to calculate the probability of the observed table, given fixed marginal totals. Referring to Table 3.1, the probability of the observed outcomes $a$, $b$, $c$ and $d$, with the marginal totals $(a + c)$, $(b + d)$, $(a + b)$ and $(c + d)$ fixed, may be shown to be

$$\frac{(a + c)!(b + d)!(a + b)!(c + d)!}{n!a!b!c!d!}, \tag{3.18}$$

where, for example, $n!$ is read as '$n$ factorial' and is defined as the product of all integers up to and including $n$. Hence $n! = n(n - 1)(n - 2)\ldots(2)(1)$. By definition, $0! = 1$. See Mood et al. (1974) for an explanation of (3.18).

Fisher's procedure then requires the probability of all more extreme tables to be computed, using (3.18) repeatedly. The sum of all these probabilities is the $p$ value for the test. By 'more extreme' here is meant all tables that provide more evidence of an association. Thinking in terms of relative risks (or odds ratios): if the observed relative risk is larger than 1, then all more extreme tables give relative risks even larger than 1. On the other hand, if the relative risk from the observed table is below 1, more extreme tables have even smaller relative risks. Due to this, Fisher's exact test, unlike the chi-square test, is fundamentally *one-sided*. However, it is possible to formulate a two-sided version: see Fleiss (1981) for details.

Example 3.9 illustrates how Fisher's exact test works. In fact the exact test should not be necessary in this example because there are no expected frequencies below 5. The example has been deliberately chosen to show the effect of the continuity correction in a situation where the chi-square test is acceptable, yet the numbers concerned are small enough to allow the exact test to be conducted easily.

*Example 3.9*    Crowther et al. (1990) describe a comparative study of hospitalization for bed rest against normal activity for 118 Zimbabwean women who were expecting twins. Around a half of the women were allocated to each of the two activity regimes. Table 3.6 gives measurements of hypertension status (where hypertension is defined as a blood pressure $\geq 140/90$ mmHg) for the mothers at the time of their deliveries. This table can be used to test the null hypothesis: pregnant women (with twins) are no more likely to develop hypertension than those left to get on with normal daily living.

Clearly bed rest tends to reduce the chance of hypertension compared to normal activity: the estimated relative risk is $0.0517/0.1500 = 0.345$. The one-sided alternative is $H_1$: bed rest reduces hypertension. Using (3.18), we can calculate the probability of the observed outcomes 3, 55, 9, 51 in Table 3.6 as

**Table 3.6**   Results of a follow-up study of women pregnant with twins in Zimbabwe

|  | Hypertension status | | | |
| Activity | Yes | No | Total | Risk |
| --- | --- | --- | --- | --- |
| Best rest | 3 | 55 | 58 | 0.0517 |
| Normal | 9 | 51 | 60 | 0.1500 |
| Total | 12 | 106 | 118 | |

$$\frac{12!106!58!60!}{118!3!55!9!51!} = 0.0535.$$

Now we have to identify all the more extreme tables. The easiest way to do this is to consider the smallest observed frequency, 3. If this were to decrease, then the risk for the bed rest group would also decrease. At the same time this would automatically cause the risk in the normal activity group to increase. This is so because the marginal totals are fixed: thus any decrease from the value 3 in Table 3.6 is balanced by an equal increase from the value 9, and so on. When the risk in the bed rest group increases and that in the normal activity group decreases, the relative risk becomes even smaller than it was originally. Hence decreasing the value 3 in Table 3.6 produces more extreme tables. Since frequencies cannot be negative, there are three more extreme tables. These are given in outline below, with the consequent relative risk (given in brackets) and probability, calculated from (3.18), shown underneath.

| 2 56 | 1 57 | 0 58 |
| 10 50 | 11 49 | 12 48 |
| (0.179) | (0.078) | (0) |
| 0.0146 | 0.0023 | 0.0002 |

The $p$ value for the test is the sum of the four probabilities

$$0.0535 + 0.0146 + 0.0023 + 0.0002 = 0.071.$$

Hence we marginally fail to reject the null hypothesis at the 5% level of significance. There is insufficient evidence to conclude that bed rest has a real effect on the chance of a pregnant woman developing hypertension. However, the $p$ value is small enough to suggest that a rather larger study would be worthwhile.

As pointed out earlier, all expected values are greater than 5 in this example; hence the chi-square test would be the natural choice, rather than the exact test, because it is easier to compute. Without the continuity correction, (3.14) gives the test statistic as 3.12. With the continuity correction, (3.16) gives the test statistic as 2.13. These results correspond to $p$ values of 0.0774 and 0.1440, respectively. Since the chi-square test is two-sided, we must halve these (Section 3.5.2) to obtain results that are comparable with the one-sided Fisher's exact test. Thus the uncorrected chi-square test gives a $p$ value of 0.039 and the continuity-corrected chi-square test has $p = 0.072$. The latter is very close to the exact result and shows the real advantage of the continuity correction when there are observed frequencies that are fairly small.

## 3.5.5    Limitations of tests

In most epidemiological analyses, hypothesis tests are less useful than estimation procedures: see Gardner and Altman (1989) for a general discussion. Specific problems include the arbitrary nature of the cut-point used to define 'significance' (for example, $p < 0.05$) and the dependence of the conclusion upon the sample size. The observed value of the test statistic, and hence the exact $p$ value, depends both upon the magnitude of the effect measured and the amount of information available to estimate the effect.

*Example 3.10*   Table 3.7 shows hypothetical data from two studies of the same relationship between risk factor and disease. In both studies the risk, relative risk, odds and odds ratio are the same, and so the estimated effect of the risk factor is the same. This should be so because study B simply has all cell contents twice as large as in study A. However, there is a significant relationship between risk factor and disease in study B but not in study A, at least using the conventional 5% level of significance.

No matter how small the effect, it is always possible to find it significant if a large enough sample is used. This is even true when we choose to take a very extreme significance level, such as $p < 0.0001$. Since epidemiological studies frequently involve several thousand subjects, this issue is of real concern. The epidemiologist must consider biological, as well as statistical, significance.

*Example 3.11*   Table 3.8 shows further hypothetical data wherein the relative risk is only 1.03 (the odds ratio is 1.06), suggestive of an effect that has little or no medical importance. However, the result is statistically significant at the conventional 5% level. Conclusions based

**Table 3.7**   Results from two hypothetical incidence studies

| Risk factor status | Study A | | | Study B | | |
|---|---|---|---|---|---|---|
| | Disease | No disease | Risk[a] | Disease | No disease | Risk[a] |
| Exposed | 10 | 15 | 0.40 | 20 | 30 | 0.40 |
| Not exposed | 5 | 20 | 0.20 | 10 | 40 | 0.20 |
| Relative risk[b] | | | 2.00 | | | 2.00 |
| Odds ratio[c] | | | 2.67 | | | 2.67 |
| $p$ value[d] | | | 0.12 | | | 0.03 |
| $n$ | | | 50 | | | 100 |

[a] Using (3.1).
[b] Using (3.2).
[c] Using (3.9).
[d] Using (3.14).

**Table 3.8**  Results from a hypothetical large incidence study

| Risk factor status | Disease status | | Risk[a] |
|---|---|---|---|
| | Disease | No disease | |
| Exposed | 4140 | 5860 | 0.414 |
| Not exposed | 4000 | 6000 | 0.400 |
| Relative risk[b] | | | 1.03 |
| Odds ratio[c] | | | 1.06 |
| p value[d] | | | 0.04 |
| n | | | 20 000 |

[a] Using (3.1).
[b] Using (3.2).
[c] Using (3.9).
[d] Using (3.14).

solely on the hypothesis test would be misleading. The large sample size (20 000) has caused the test to be extremely sensitive to small effects. Note that this order of magnitude for the sample size is not unusual in published epidemiological studies.

In conclusion, whilst hypothesis tests are useful to check whether results are attributable to chance, estimates of effects should be considered before conclusions are drawn. In many cases the confidence intervals for the estimates will encompass all the useful information of the hypothesis test. For instance, we can see that the result is (at least approximately) significant at the 5% level if the value of the effect under the null hypothesis is outside the 95% confidence interval for the effect.

## 3.6    Risk factors measured at several levels

Up to now we have assumed that the risk factor is measured only at two levels: exposed and unexposed. Sometimes we may, instead, have a set of possible categorical outcomes for the risk factor. For example, Table 2.2 shows social class, measured on an ordered six-point scale, against prevalent CHD. We may extend the ideas of relative risks and odds ratios from $2 \times 2$ tables, such as Table 3.2, to $\ell \times 2$ tables (for $\ell > 2$), such as Table 2.2, very easily. We choose one level of the risk factor to be the base level and compare all other levels to this base. For example, in Table 2.2 we could choose social class I to be the base. We can find the prevalence relative risk, for example, of social class II relative to social class I, by thinking of the two corresponding rows of Table 2.2 as the *only* rows. Ignoring all other rows leaves Table 2.2 in the form of a

$2 \times 2$ table, as shown in Table 3.9. Then, from (3.2), the relative risk of prevalent CHD for social class II compared with I is

$$\hat{\lambda}_{II} = \frac{382/2254}{100/592} = 1.003.$$

Odds, confidence intervals and tests all follow as previously described.

Notice that we must be careful how we lay out the sub-table so as to correspond with Table 3.1: the base must be the bottom row and positive disease must be the left-hand column. Similar tables to Table 3.9 can be drawn up for the other **contrasts** with social class I; for example, the relative risk for social class V compared with social class I is

$$\hat{\lambda}_V = \frac{109/415}{100/592} = 1.55.$$

Thus all five contrasts with social class I may be obtained.

It should be apparent that it is not necessary to formally draw out the five sub-tables, of which Table 3.9 is the first. Calculations may be done straight from the $6 \times 2$ table, Table 2.2, by ignoring all but the relevant rows for each contrast. Indeed the prevalence relative risks, apart from rounding error, can be found very easily as quotients of the percentage prevalences already given (in parentheses) in Table 2.2. For example,

$$\hat{\lambda}_V = \frac{26.3}{16.9} = 1.56,$$

which is only in error due to the rounding of percentages in Table 2.2.

As ever, choice of the base level is arbitrary. There is a sound statistical argument that the base level should be chosen as that level with risk, or odds, that has the smallest standard error. In practice, the base is usually taken to be either the level with the lowest risk (or odds) or, should the levels have some natural order (as in Table 2.2), the smallest level.

**Table 3.9**  A portion of Table 2.1

| Social class | Prevalent CHD | | |
| --- | --- | --- | --- |
| | Yes | No | Total |
| II | 382 | 1872 | 2254 |
| I | 100 | 492 | 592 |
| Total | 482 | 2364 | 2846 |

It is possible to have a 'moving base': for instance, we could compare social class II with I, then III with II, etc., but this is more difficult to interpret. In fact we can easily construct relative risks or odds ratios for other comparisons as quotients of the basic contrasts already derived. For instance, the relative risk for social class V relative to social class II is

$$\hat{\lambda}_V / \hat{\lambda}_{II} = 1.55/1.003 = 1.55.$$

This works because the risk for social class I in the denominator of $\hat{\lambda}_V$ and $\hat{\lambda}_{II}$ simply cancels out:

$$\frac{risk_V}{risk_I} \div \frac{risk_{II}}{risk_I} = \frac{risk_V}{risk_{II}}.$$

To test for a significant overall effect of the risk factor on disease we apply the chi-square test, (2.1), with $\ell-1$ d.f. to the $\ell \times 2$ table.

### 3.6.1    Continuous risk factors

The ideas of relative risk and odds ratio are so attractive that it is natural to want to specify one or the other for all the risk factors in an epidemiological study. Whenever the relationship between the risk factor and the disease is shown in a table this is straightforward. Should the data be continuous (or discrete with several outcomes), tables are not feasible for the raw data. Instead, tables of manageable size may be derived by grouping the continuous risk factor. Relative risks or odds ratios may then be derived from the grouped table.

There are drawbacks to the grouping. Inevitably considerable information on the risk factor is lost: for example, we do not know how risk alters within each group. Also different ways of grouping can produce quite different results and inferences. This phenomenon may easily be seen from a simple artificial example.

*Example 3.12*    Table 3.10 shows a risk factor with three levels, 1, 2 and 3, representing increasing doses. Suppose that we decide to group the three levels into two. If we combine 1 and 2 as 'low dose', leaving 3 as 'high dose' then the relative risk (high compared to low dose) is, from (3.2),

$$\frac{189/200}{197/210} = 1.01.$$

We conclude that the dose has little effect: high dose increases risk by a negligible amount.

On the other hand, if 1 is 'low' and 2 and 3 are combined to define 'high dose', then the relative risk becomes

$$\frac{385/400}{1/10} = 9.6,$$

**Table 3.10**    Hypothetical results of a study of risk factor dose

|  | Disease status | | |
| --- | --- | --- | --- |
| Risk factor dose | Disease | No disease | Total |
| 1 | 1 | 9 | 10 |
| 2 | 196 | 4 | 200 |
| 3 | 189 | 11 | 200 |
| Total | 386 | 24 | 410 |

which is almost 10 times as big as before: we now conclude that high dose increases risk. Obviously the choice of 'cut-off' for high dose has made a considerable difference. Even though this is an extreme example, the problem could arise whenever grouping is performed.

A similar problem occurs when hypothesis tests are used; one grouping system may produce a significant effect, say at the 5% level of significance, whereas another does not. In fact this happens in Example 3.12, using the chi-square test with Yates's correction and Fisher's exact test as appropriate.

So as to avoid the possibility of a biased selection (a choice that leads to the desired result), an objective method of grouping is far preferable. In some situations we may be able to use some pre-existing standard system of grouping; for example, the classification of levels of obesity made by Garrow (1981). This classifies obesity grade according to a person's body mass index: weight (in kilograms) divided by the square of height (in metres). For instance, 30 but less than 40 $kg/m^2$ is defined as 'clinically obese'.

Another objective way of grouping is to divide the data into groups of equal size. This has the statistical advantage of providing maximum power when one group is compared with another. This might be achieved by simply dividing the range of values taken by the risk factor into equal parts. In practice, this rarely gives groups of even approximately equal size because of non-uniformity in distribution of the risk factor. So, instead, the quantiles of the risk factor are found and used as the cut-points that define the groups. For example, the quartiles define four equal groups, called the **fourths** or **quarters**. A further question then arises: how many groups should be used? There is no simple answer. Taking few groups means that much information is lost; for instance, we cannot possibly discover any evidence of curvature in the relationship between risk factor and disease if we take only two groups. On the other hand, many groups will be hard to interpret and will inevitably result in wide overlapping confidence intervals (for risk, etc.), unless the sample size is large. In practical epidemiological research it is rare to find more than five groups used.

*Example 3.13*  Table 3.11 shows data from the follow-up (cohort) phase of the Scottish Heart Health Study (Tunstall-Pedoe *et al.*, 1997). Here the 4095 men who had their cholesterol measured and were free of CHD at baseline are classified by cholesterol and CHD status: whether or not they developed CHD in the six years after their cholesterol was measured. The continuous variable 'cholesterol' has been grouped into its fifths; the quintiles which define the limits of these fifths being 5.40, 6.00, 6.55, and 7.27 mmol/l. Notice that the fifths are not quite the same size due to repeated values at the quintiles.

Here the first fifth has been taken as the base group (relative risk = 1) and all other fifths are compared to this using (3.2), (3.5), (3.6) and (3.7) repeatedly. Risk clearly increases with increasing cholesterol. There is, at the 5% level, no significant difference (in risk) between the 2nd and 1st or between the 3rd and 1st fifths, but there is a significant difference between the 4th and 1st and between the 5th and 1st fifths.

### 3.6.2    A test for linear trend

When the risk factor is defined at $\ell$ levels we have seen that the chi-square test, (2.1), can be used to test association. Essentially this is a test of the null hypothesis

$$H_0 : R_1 = R_2 = R_3 = \ldots = R_\ell$$

against $H_1$ : they are not all equal, where the $R$ values represent the risks at each of the $\ell$ levels. An equivalent formulation may be made in terms of odds. Under $H_0$ all $\ell$ risks are equivalent to some overall 'average risk'. In epidemiology we are often interested in **dose-response effects**; that is, situations where an increased value of the risk factor means a greater likelihood of disease. More precisely, in the current context, the risk of disease increases as the dose of the risk factor increases. As mentioned in Section 1.6.3, this would provide meaningful evidence of a causal relationship.

**Table 3.11**    Total serum cholesterol data from the SHHS follow-up

| Cholesterol fifth | Disease status | | | Relative risk (95% CI) |
| | CHD | No CHD | Total | |
| --- | --- | --- | --- | --- |
| 1 | 15 (1.85%) | 798 | 813 | 1 |
| 2 | 20 (2.46%) | 794 | 814 | 1.33 (0.69, 2.58) |
| 3 | 26 (3.18%) | 791 | 817 | 1.72 (0.92, 3.23) |
| 4 | 41 (4.96%) | 785 | 826 | 2.69 (1.50, 4.82) |
| 5 | 48 (5.82%) | 777 | 825 | 3.15 (1.78, 5.59) |
| Total | 150 (3.66%) | 3945 | 4095 | |

It is possible to use the chi-square approach to test for a dose-response trend whenever the $\ell$ levels of the risk factor are graded. The theory behind the procedure is based upon the ideas of simple linear regression (Section 9.3.1). Consequently we should denote the result as a test of *linear* trend. See Armitage (1955) for details of the theory, and Maclure and Greenland (1992) for a general discussion of the methodology. Although the previous paragraph talked about increasing risk, the direction of trend could be either positive or negative. Negative trend means an increasing protective effect of the 'risk factor'; for instance, increasing consumption of vitamin C might be expected to give increased protection against certain cancers.

To apply the test we need, first, to assign representative scores for each level of the risk factor. These should reflect the rank ordering; for example, the social class groupings in Table 2.2 could be labelled from 1 (class I) to 6 (class V). Table 3.12 displays the theoretical form of the data. The test statistic, for the test of linear trend, is

$$X^2_{(L)} = \{T_1 - (n_1 T_2/n)\}^2/V, \tag{3.19}$$

where

$$T_1 = \sum_1^\ell a_i x_i, \qquad T_2 = \sum_1^\ell m_i x_i, \qquad T_3 = \sum_1^\ell m_i x_i^2 \tag{3.20}$$

and

$$V = n_1 n_2 (n T_3 - T_2^2)/n^2(n-1), \tag{3.21}$$

and the remaining variables are defined by Table 3.12. We compare $X^2_{(L)}$ against chi-square with 1 d.f.

**Table 3.12**   Display of data from a dose-response study

| Risk factor level ('score') | Disease status | | |
| --- | --- | --- | --- |
| | Disease | No disease | Total |
| $x_1$ | $a_1$ | $b_1$ | $m_1$ |
| $x_2$ | $a_2$ | $b_2$ | $m_2$ |
| . | . | . | . |
| . | . | . | . |
| . | . | . | . |
| $x_\ell$ | $a_\ell$ | $b_\ell$ | $m_\ell$ |
| Total | $n_1$ | $n_2$ | $n$ |

*Example 3.14*    Figure 3.1 shows the risks for prevalent CHD (with confidence intervals), calculated from (3.1) and (3.3), for the SHHS social class data of Table 2.2. There is clear indication of a trend here (see also the related Figure 2.3). Scoring social class from 1 to 6, we have, from (3.20),

$$T_1 = 100 \times 1 + 382 \times 2 + 183 \times 3 + 668 \times 4 + 279 \times 5 + 109 \times 6 = 6134$$
$$T_2 = 592 \times 1 + 2254 \times 2 + 1017 \times 3 + 3150 \times 4$$
$$+ 1253 \times 5 + 415 \times 6 = 29506$$
$$T_3 = 592 \times 1 \times 1 + 2254 \times 2 \times 2 + 1017 \times 3 \times 3 + 3150 \times 4 \times 4$$
$$+ 1253 \times 5 \times 5 + 415 \times 6 \times 6 = 115426.$$

Then, from (3.21),

$$V = \frac{1721 \times 6960(8681 \times 115426 - 29506^2)}{8681^2 \times 8680} = 2406.3357$$

Hence, (3.19) gives

$$X^2_{(L)} = \frac{(6134 - 1721 \times 29\,506/8681)^2}{2406.3357} = 33.63.$$

From Table B.3, $\chi^2_1 = 10.8$ at the 0.1% level. Hence the test is highly significant: there is evidence of a linear trend.

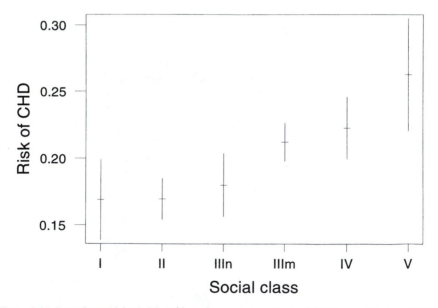

**Figure 3.1**    Prevalence risks (with 95% confidence intervals) for CHD by social class; SHHS.

When the levels are defined by groups, as in Example 3.13, the conventional epidemiological approach is to use the rank scores 1, 2, 3, ..., just as in Example 3.14. The trend in question then represents a consistent rise in risk from group to successive group (fifth to successive fifth in Example 3.13). A more meaningful test may be to test for a consistent rise across the range of the risk factor. In this case we should use a numerical summary score which represents the location of each group. The median value of the risk factor within the group is a sensible choice.

The overall chi-square test (with $\ell - 1$ d.f.) and that for linear trend (with 1 d.f.) may well give opposite results. For instance, the overall test may be not significant ($p > 0.05$) but the linear test highly significant ($p < 0.001$). All this means is that, whilst the risks in the $\ell$ groups are never very different from their overall average, they do tend to increase (or decrease). Evidence of a trend is a more powerful indication of causality than is evidence of an association.

### 3.6.3    A test for non-linearity

Sometimes the relationship between the risk factor and disease is non-linear. For example, it could be that low and high doses of the risk factor are both harmful compared with average doses. Such a U-shaped relationship has been found by several authors who have investigated the relationship between alcohol consumption and death from any cause: see, for example, Duffy (1995).

To test for a non-linear relationship, we calculate the difference between the overall chi-square test statistic, (2.1), and the trend test statistic, (3.19). This difference is compared to chi-square with d.f. given by the difference in the d.f. of these two components, $(\ell - 1) - 1 = \ell - 2$ d.f. This gives a test for *any* non-linear relationship. In Sections 9.3.3 and 10.7.3 we shall consider some specific non-linear relationships within the context of statistical modelling.

*Example 3.15*    The chi-square test statistic, (2.1), for the data in Table 2.2 turns out to be 36.40. In Example 3.14 we found the test statistic for linear trend, $X^2_{(L)} = 33.63$. Hence the test statistic for non-linearity is $36.40 - 33.63 = 2.77$. Compared to chi-square with $6 - 2 = 4$ d.f. this is not significant ($p = 0.60$). Hence there is no evidence that the risk of prevalent CHD rises in anything but a linear fashion as we go down the social scale, from highly advantaged to highly disadvantaged.

## 3.7    Attributable risk

Although the relative risk is very useful as a measure of the relative importance to the disease of the risk factor, it does not tell us the overall importance of that risk factor. For instance, Kahn and Sempos (1989) report results from the

Framingham study that show the relative risk of coronary heart disease for those with systolic blood pressure of 180 mmHg or more compared with others to be 2.8, whereas the relative risk for cigarette smoking is only 1.9. Hence, it might appear that it would be more important to target health education measures to reduce hypertension. This is not necessarily true, because we must also take account of the prevalence of the risk factors. In the population in which hypertension is very rare but smoking is common, the overall impact on heart disease of reducing the prevalence of high blood pressure will be minimal, although it would be extremely important to reduce smoking (see Example 3.17). What is required is a measure which combines relative risk and the prevalence of the risk factor: the **attributable risk** or **aetologic fraction.** This will measure the proportion of cases of disease that are attributable to the risk factor.

As with the relative risk, epidemiologists generally reserve the term 'attributable risk' to refer to disease incidence. Consider, then, Table 3.1 as the results of an incidence study; suppose that the $n$ individuals are a random sample from the background population which are followed up over time to record cases of disease. If exposure to the risk factor were removed then everyone would experience the risk of the non-exposed group, which is $c/(c+d)$. Hence we would expect to have an overall proportion of $c/(c+d)$ cases of disease; that is, we would expect $nc/(c+d)$ cases of disease amongst the $n$ people. In fact we have $a+c$ cases, so that the excess number of cases attributable to the risk factor is

$$(a+c) - \frac{nc}{c+d}. \tag{3.22}$$

The attributable risk (denoted $\theta$) is then estimated by

$$\hat{\theta} = \frac{1}{a+c}\left\{(a+c) - \frac{nc}{c+d}\right\} = \frac{r - r_{\bar{E}}}{r}. \tag{3.23}$$

Here $r$ is the overall risk of disease and $r_{\bar{E}}$ is the risk in the unexposed group for the sample data. Both are calculated by (3.1); that is, $r = (a+c)/n$ and $r_{\bar{E}} = c/(c+d)$.

Approximate 95% confidence limits for the attributable risk are given by

$$\frac{(ad-bc)\exp(\pm u)}{nc + (ad-bc)\exp(\pm u)}, \tag{3.24}$$

where $\pm$ is replaced by a minus sign for the lower limit and a plus sign for the upper limit, and

$$u = \frac{1.96(a+c)(c+d)}{ad-bc}\sqrt{\frac{ad(n-c)+c^2b}{nc(a+c)(c+d)}}. \tag{3.25}$$

As usual, we replace 1.96 by the appropriate critical value from the normal distribution in (3.25) whenever we wish to derive confidence intervals for some percentage other than 95% . As with the odds ratio and relative risk, there are other methods for calculating approximate confidence limits. The limits in (3.24) were suggested by Leung and Kupper (1981). They have been found to produce shorter confidence limits than other simple methods across the majority of likely values for $\theta$ (see Whittemore, 1983).

Notice that (3.22) is the excess number of cases in the *sample*; if we require an estimate of the excess number of cases in the *population* we should multiply $\hat{\theta}$ by the total number of cases of disease in the population (known, perhaps, from official routine statistics).

*Example 3.16*    Example 3.1 describes a random sample which should be a reasonable representation of 50–54-year-old American men at the time of sampling. Here $r = 0.1134$ and $r_{\bar{E}} = 0.0888$. The attributable risk of a coronary event for smoking is thus estimated to be, from (3.23),

$$\hat{\theta} = \frac{0.1134 - 0.0888}{0.1134} = 0.217.$$

So 22% of the risk of a coronary event is estimated to be attributable to smoking.
From (3.25) and by reference to Tables 3.1 and 3.2,

$$u = \frac{1.96 \times 216 \times 563}{166 \times 513 - 1176 \times 50} \sqrt{\frac{166 \times 513(1905 - 50) + 50^2 \times 1176}{1905 \times 50 \times 216 \times 563}} = 1.06581$$

Then, from (3.24), approximate 95% confidence limits for the attributable risk are

$$\frac{\{166 \times 513 - 1176 \times 50\} \exp(\pm 1.06581)}{1905 \times 50 + \{166 \times 513 - 1176 \times 50\} \exp(\pm 1.06581)},$$

giving the 95% confidence interval (0.087, 0.445) or, in percentage terms, 8.7% to 44.5%.

As the derivation of (3.23) suggests, the *population* (as opposed to the sample) attributable risk is

$$\theta = \frac{R - R_{\bar{E}}}{R}, \tag{3.26}$$

where $R$ and $R_{\bar{E}}$ are the population equivalents of the sample values of $r$ and $r_{\bar{E}}$, respectively. An alternative definition, derived from (3.26) using probability theory, is

$$\theta = \frac{p_E(\lambda - 1)}{1 + p_E(\lambda - 1)}, \tag{3.27}$$

where $p_E$ is the probability of exposure to the risk factor and $\lambda$ is, as usual, the relative risk (exposed versus unexposed). This definition shows explicitly how the attributable risk combines the relative risk and the prevalence of the risk factor. When we have sample data we substitute sample estimates of $p_E$ and $\lambda$ into (3.27), as usual. Note that $\theta$ is only defined when $\lambda > 1$.

Although we can always invert the numerator and denominator risks making up $\lambda$ to ensure that $\lambda > 1$, we may wish to see how many, or what proportion, of cases of disease are prevented by a protective risk factor. Kleinbaum et al. (1982) describe the appropriate methodology for this situation.

Table 3.13 illustrates how $\theta$ depends upon $p_E$ and $\lambda$, using (3.27) repeatedly. If the risk factor is rare and has little relative effect on the disease, then the attributable risk is low. If the risk factor is common and has a large relative risk, then the attributable risk is high. Within these extremes, a considerable attributable risk can occur when the relative risk is low provided the risk factor is common, or when the risk factor is fairly rare provided the relative risk is high.

Often (3.27) is used to produce an estimated $\theta$ when the procedure represented by (3.23) cannot be applied. This includes the situation where a case–control study has been carried out (Section 6.2.4). Occasionally we might combine data from other studies to estimate $\theta$. One example is an occupational health study wherein separate samples are selected from two employment groups – say, workers in a nuclear power station and workers in some other place of employment. Such a study is perfectly adequate for estimating $\lambda$ or $R_E$ but cannot estimate either $p_E$ or $R$, because we then have no overall random

**Table 3.13** Attributable risk (as a percentage) for various values of the relative risk and prevalence (expressed as a percentage) of the risk factor

| Prevalence (%) | Relative risk | | | | | | | |
|---|---|---|---|---|---|---|---|---|
| | 1.5 | 2 | 2.5 | 3 | 4 | 5 | 10 | 15 |
| 1 | 0.5 | 1.0 | 1.5 | 2.0 | 2.9 | 3.8 | 8.3 | 12.3 |
| 5 | 2.4 | 4.8 | 7.0 | 9.1 | 13.0 | 16.7 | 31.0 | 41.2 |
| 10 | 4.8 | 9.1 | 13.0 | 16.7 | 23.1 | 28.6 | 47.4 | 58.3 |
| 20 | 9.1 | 16.7 | 23.1 | 28.6 | 37.5 | 44.4 | 64.3 | 73.7 |
| 30 | 13.0 | 23.1 | 31.0 | 37.5 | 47.4 | 54.5 | 73.0 | 80.8 |
| 40 | 16.7 | 28.6 | 37.5 | 44.4 | 54.5 | 61.5 | 78.3 | 84.8 |
| 50 | 20.0 | 33.3 | 42.9 | 50.0 | 60.0 | 66.7 | 81.8 | 87.5 |
| 60 | 23.1 | 37.5 | 47.4 | 54.5 | 64.3 | 70.6 | 84.4 | 89.4 |
| 70 | 25.9 | 41.2 | 51.2 | 58.3 | 67.7 | 73.7 | 86.3 | 90.7 |
| 80 | 28.6 | 44.4 | 54.5 | 61.5 | 70.6 | 76.2 | 87.8 | 91.8 |
| 90 | 31.0 | 47.4 | 57.4 | 64.3 | 73.0 | 78.3 | 89.0 | 92.6 |
| 95 | 32.2 | 48.7 | 58.8 | 65.5 | 74.0 | 79.2 | 89.5 | 93.0 |
| 99 | 33.1 | 49.7 | 59.8 | 66.4 | 74.8 | 79.8 | 89.9 | 93.3 |

sample. We might, however, be able to obtain an estimate of either of those unknowns from published work, possibly from routine statistics or national surveys conducted by government. The confidence limits given in (3.24) would, however, no longer be valid (see Leung and Kupper, 1981).

The next example shows how prevalence data from the cross-sectional phase of the SHHS can be combined with pre-existing data to estimate the attributable risks for high blood pressure and smoking used as examples earlier. Of course, once follow-up data from the SHHS (as described in Section 5.2) are available, the SHHS can be used to estimate incidence rates and $\theta$ without regard to other studies. This example supposes that an estimate of $\theta$ is required at the time of the cross-sectional study when only prevalence risks may be estimated from the SHHS data themselves.

*Example 3.17*   Shewry *et al.* (1992) use data from the initial phase (22 districts) of the SHHS to estimate the prevalence of cigarette smoking amongst middle-aged Scotsmen to be 0.392. At the time of this publication no incidence data were available from the study. Table 3.14 shows corresponding data on systolic blood pressure. From this, the prevalence of high blood pressure (as defined here) is estimated to be 124/5084 = 0.024. If we suppose that the relative risks of 2.8 for high blood pressure and 1.9 for cigarette smoking from the Framingham study (as stated in Kahn and Sempos, 1989) are appropriate to middle-aged Scottish men, then (3.27) allows the attributable risks in Scotland to be estimated. The results are: for high blood pressure,

$$\frac{0.024(2.8 - 1)}{1 + 0.024(2.8 - 1)} = 0.04;$$

for cigarette smoking,

$$\frac{0.392(1.9 - 1)}{1 + 0.392(1.9 - 1)} = 0.26.$$

So we estimate that 26% of the male cases of CHD in Scotland are attributable to cigarette smoking, but only 4% to high (systolic) blood pressure. Notice that this contrast is despite high blood pressure having a higher relative risk.

Unfortunately the term 'attributable risk' does not have a standard meaning. For example, Schlesselman (1982), amongst others, defines it to be the

**Table 3.14**    Systolic blood pressure in the initial phase of the SHHS

| Systolic blood pressure | Number |
|---|---|
| Low (under 180 mmHg) | 4920 |
| High (180 mmHg or more) | 124 |
| Total | 5084 |

difference between the risks in the exposed and unexposed groups. Hence, caution is required when interpreting published results. Frequently it is useful to define a second type of attributable risk which only relates to those exposed to the risk factor. By the same argument as used earlier, the attributable risk amongst only those exposed to the risk factor in the population is

$$\frac{R_E - R_{\bar{E}}}{R_E} = \frac{\lambda - 1}{\lambda},$$

where $R_E$ is the risk in the exposed group, estimated by $a/(a+b)$.

Finally, notice that 'attributable' does not necessarily imply causation, even though $\theta$ will often be interpreted in this way. For instance, if smoking does cause heart disease then we may use Example 3.17 to conclude that 26% of CHD cases would be removed if cigarette smoking were to cease. If, however, there is a third factor involved, which causes both smoking and heart disease, then the conclusion will be over-optimistic. Similarly, another risk factor (such as stress) may become more important as smoking is removed, again causing the conclusion to be over-optimistic. In general, this is a problem of confounding (Chapter 4). A simple way to allow for this is to replace the relative risk in (3.27) by its confounder-adjusted estimate, although the other formulae given in this section would then be no longer hold. See Whittemore (1983) and Gefeller (1992) for discussions. A further problem is that the effect of smoking is not instantly reversible: even if someone stops smoking now a residual ill effect may persist for several years. In some situations the risk effect may not be at all reversible in the current population.

## 3.8    Rate and relative rate

Our definition of risk in Section 3.1 uses the proportion who have disease among so many individuals at risk. In some situations we know the number who have disease but do not know the exact number at risk; that is, we know the numerator but not the denominator required to find the risk. Instead, we may have an estimate of the number at risk, typically the mid-year population of the at-risk group. This gives rise to the estimate of a disease **rate**,

$$\hat{\rho} = e/p, \tag{3.28}$$

where $e$ is the number of events (a count of the number of cases of disease) and $p$ is the mid-year population. This equation generalizes the definition of the prevalence rate given by (1.1), when the disease count is at a particular time, and of the incidence rate given by (1.2), when the disease count is the number of new cases within a particular time period. In general, the rate and the risk will be different, although in many instances it is reasonable to assume that one will be a good approximation to the other.

*Example 3.18*   Table 3.15 gives data on the male population of Scotland in 1995. These data come from routine sources, including death registrations and the Census. The final two columns are calculated using (3.28), giving a cause-specific and overall mortality rate respectively, for each five-year age group. The mid-year population acts as the denominator for both of these incidence rates.

Provided that the disease events occur randomly and independently, a reasonable assumption is that their number follows a Poisson distribution (see Clarke and Cooke, 1992). Assuming that the denominator is a fixed known quantity, the estimated standard error of the disease rate is then

$$\hat{se}(\hat{\rho}) = e/\sqrt{p}.$$

We can find approximate 95% confidence limits for the number of events, $(e_L, e_U)$ from

$$e_L = \left(\frac{1.96}{2} - \sqrt{e}\right)^2,$$

$$e_U = \left(\frac{1.96}{2} + \sqrt{e+1}\right)^2,$$

(3.29)

giving 95% confidence limits for the disease rate of $(\rho_L, \rho_U)$, where

$$\rho_L = e_L/p,$$
$$\rho_U = e_U/p.$$

(3.30)

This uses a normal approximation which works well for $e > 100$. Different percentage confidence limits are, as usual, obtained by replacing 1.96 by the

**Table 3.15**   Demographic data and derived mortality rates for Scotsmen in 1995

| Age group (years) | Number of deaths | | Mid-year population | Mortality rate (per thousand) | |
|---|---|---|---|---|---|
| | CHD | Total | | CHD | Total |
| 40–44 | 81 | 419 | 166 582 | 0.5 | 2.5 |
| 45–49 | 190 | 736 | 173 587 | 1.1 | 4.2 |
| 50–54 | 294 | 1010 | 141 048 | 2.1 | 7.2 |
| 55–59 | 515 | 1613 | 131 738 | 3.9 | 12.2 |
| 60–64 | 823 | 2531 | 121 420 | 6.8 | 20.8 |
| 65–69 | 1222 | 3724 | 108 649 | 11.2 | 34.3 |

Source: General Register Office for Scotland (Crown Copyright).

appropriate percentage point in (3.29). Exact values of $(e_L, e_U)$ come from tables of the Poisson distribution: see Gardner and Altman (1989).

To compare two rates we shall use the relative rate, although the difference in rates would be another possibility. Suppose that we have data from two groups. For example, group 1 might be those exposed, and group 2 those unexposed, to some risk factor. In group 1 there are $e_1$ events, the mid-year population is $p_1$ and the estimated disease rate is $\hat{\rho}_1 = e_1/p_1$. Similarly for group 2 with '2' subscripts. The estimated relative rate, group 2 compared to group 1, is then

$$\hat{\omega} = \frac{\hat{\rho}_2}{\hat{\rho}_1} = \left(\frac{p_1}{p_2}\right)\left(\frac{e_2}{e_1}\right). \tag{3.31}$$

Consider the probability that, when an event occurs, it occurs in group 2. Call this quantity $\pi$. From sample data it is estimated by

$$\hat{\pi} = e_2/(e_1 + e_2). \tag{3.32}$$

An approximate 95% confidence interval for $\pi$ comes from (2.2). Let the 95% confidence limits be $(\pi_L, \pi_U)$. Comparing (3.31) and (3.32) shows that

$$\hat{\omega} = \left(\frac{p_1}{p_2}\right)\left(\frac{\hat{\pi}}{1 - \hat{\pi}}\right).$$

Thus the 95% confidence limits $(\omega_L, \omega_U)$ for the relative rate are

$$\omega_L = \left(\frac{p_1}{p_2}\right)\left(\frac{\pi_L}{1 - \pi_L}\right),$$
$$\omega_U = \left(\frac{p_1}{p_2}\right)\left(\frac{\pi_U}{1 - \pi_U}\right). \tag{3.33}$$

*Example 3.19*  Suppose that we wished to compare national male and female coronary death rates amongst 40–59-year-olds. This problem would be relevant to the investigators of the SHHS, which was restricted to this age range in Scotland. Table 3.16 gives relevant data (the male data may be derived from Table 3.15). Considering 1995 as a sample year, we can estimate coronary death rates by sex group and the relative rate of coronary death. From (3.28) the rate for men is $1080/612955 = 1.76$ per thousand. From (3.29) the 95% confidence limit for the number of male deaths is $(e_L, e_U)$, where

$$e_L = \left(\frac{1.96}{2} - \sqrt{1080}\right)^2 = 1016.548,$$

$$e_U = \left(\frac{1.96}{2} + \sqrt{1081}\right)^2 = 1146.402.$$

**Table 3.16**  Demographic data for Scots aged 40–59 in 1995

|        | CHD deaths | Mid-year population |
|--------|-----------|---------------------|
| Women  | 306       | 634 103             |
| Men    | 1080      | 612 955             |

Source: General Register Office for Scotland (Crown Copyright).

Hence, using (3.30), the 95% confidence interval for the male coronary death rate is obtained by dividing each of the above by 612 955: that is, (1.66, 1.87) per thousand. Similar calculations give the estimated female coronary rate (with 95% confidence interval) as 0.483 (0.430, 0.540) per thousand.

The estimated relative coronary death rate for men compared to women is, from (3.31),

$$\hat{\omega} = \frac{634103}{612955} \times \frac{1080}{306} = 3.65.$$

As expected, this is, except for rounding error, equal to the ratio of the male and female rates (that is, 1.76/0.483). Middle-aged men are thus 3.65 times as likely to die from a coronary attack as are women, in Scotland.

The estimated proportion of coronary deaths that are male is $\hat{\pi} = 1080/(1080 + 306) = 0.77922$, from (3.32). An approximate 95% confidence interval $(\pi_L, \pi_U)$, for the proportion of deaths that are male, comes from (2.2):

$$\pi_L = 0.77922 - 1.96\sqrt{0.77922(1 - 0.77922)/1386}$$
$$= 0.77922 - 0.02184 = 0.75738;$$

and so

$$\pi_U = 0.77922 + 0.02184 = 0.80106.$$

From (3.33) the 95% confidence interval for the relative coronary death rate, comparing men to women, is $(\omega_L, \omega_U)$, where

$$\omega_L = \frac{634103}{612955} \times \frac{0.75738}{1 - 0.75738} = 3.23,$$
$$\omega_U = \frac{634103}{612955} \times \frac{0.80106}{1 - 0.80106} = 4.17.$$

By analogy with (3.27), an attributable risk might be estimated from data on disease rates as

$$\frac{\hat{p}_E(\hat{\omega} - 1)}{1 + \hat{p}_E(\hat{\omega} - 1)}.$$

### 3.8.1   The general epidemiological rate

So far we have looked at rates where the denominator is the population 'at risk'. More generally, an epidemiological rate is any quotient where the denominator is assumed to be fixed and the numerator is a count of the number of events, this being a random variable. The estimated rate compares the observed value of the numerator to this fixed denominator. The denominator does not have to be in the same units of measurement as the numerator, although the comparison achieved has to have some physical interpretation to be useful. In Section 5.6 we shall see another kind of epidemiological rate where the denominator is the number of person-years of observation.

## Exercises

3.1 The table below shows data from a random sample of middle-aged men taken in Kuopio, Finland (Kauhanen *et al.*, 1997). A beer binger is defined as someone who usually drinks six or more bottles of beer per drinking session. This was recorded at the outset of the study; mortality was recorded from death certificates over an average of 7.7 years' follow-up.

| Beer binger? | Cardiovascular death? | | |
| --- | --- | --- | --- |
| | Yes | No | Total |
| Yes | 7 | 63 | 70 |
| No | 52 | 1519 | 1571 |
| Total | 59 | 1582 | 1641 |

(i) Estimate the risks of cardiovascular death for bingers and for non-bingers, together with 95% confidence intervals.

(ii) Estimate the relative risk of cardiovascular death for bingers compared to non-bingers, together with a 95% confidence interval.

(iii) Estimate the odds of cardiovascular death for bingers and for non-bingers.

(iv) Estimate the odds ratio for cardiovascular death for bingers compared to non-bingers, together with a 95% confidence interval.

(v) Test the null hypothesis that beer binging has no relationship with cardiovascular death.

(vi) Estimate the attributable risk of cardiovascular death for beer binging, together with a 95% confidence interval.

3.2 From an investigation into asthma in seven primary schools in the South of England, Storr *et al.* (1987) reported data on 55 pupils with asthma. Twenty of these pupils lost 10 days or more of schooling over the previous year. Of these 20, eight had parents who provided adequate medication. A further 35 pupils with asthma lost less than 10 days of schooling; four of these had parents who provided adequate medication. Use Fisher's exact test to see whether the time lost from school is unrelated to the provision of adequate medication. Interpret your result.

3.3 In a Danish study of healthy mothers (Tetzschner *et al.*, 1997), urinary incontinence and pudendal nerve terminal motor latency (PNTML) were recorded 12 weeks after delivery. PNTML was recorded as 'high' if it was in excess of the normal range for the relevant laboratory; otherwise it is 'low'. Of the 17 women with high PNTML, 6 were incontinent; of the women with low PNTML, 19 were incontinent and 110 were not.

   (i)   Calculate the relative risk for incontinence comparing high against low PNTML, together with a 95% confidence interval.

   (ii)  Calculate the odds ratio for incontinence comparing high against low PNTML, together with a 95% confidence interval.

   (iii) Test the null hypothesis that PNTML has no effect on incontinence.

   (iv) Calculate the attributable risk for incontinence that is ascribable to high PNTML, together with a 95% confidence interval.

3.4 Refer to the total columns of the Glasgow MONICA survey summary data given in Table C.3.

   (i)   Calculate the prevalence risks of cardiovascular disease (CVD) by factor IX status for each sex.

   (ii)  Calculate the prevalence relative risk for high compared to low factor IX, together with 95% confidence limits for each sex.

   (iii) Repeat (i), but for odds.

   (iv) Repeat (ii), but for the odds ratio.

   (v)  Test whether factor IX has an effect on CVD for men and women separately.

   (vi) Interpret all your results.

3.5 Wilson and McClure (1996) give the data shown below on the number of babies of extremely low birthweight (less than 1000 g) admitted to a regional neonatal intensive care unit on the first day of life. 'Survival' means that the baby was discharged alive; gestational age was estimated from the date of the last menstrual period, fetal ultrasonography and physical examination of the baby.

Calculate the chi-square test statistics for

   (i)   an overall effect,

   (ii)  a linear trend (dose-response) effect,

   (iii) a non-linear effect

of gestational age. Interpret your results. (*Hint*: In calculating (ii) use *x* values of 0, 1, 2, 3, 4, 5 and 8 to ease computation.)

| Gestational age (weeks) | Number of babies | Number of survivors |
|---|---|---|
| 23 | 4 | 0 |
| 24 | 12 | 5 |
| 25 | 16 | 9 |
| 26 | 17 | 10 |
| 27 | 13 | 12 |
| 28 | 5 | 4 |
| 29–33 | 10 | 10 |

3.6 In the Cancer Prevention Study II in the USA 578 027 adult women with complete reproductive histories were followed up for 7 years (Calle *et al.*, 1995). Of 425 599 women without a history of spontaneous abortions, 951 died from breast cancer. For women who had experienced one spontaneous abortion, 208 out of 101 773 died from breast cancer; for two spontaneous abortions 54/32 887 died from breast cancer; for three or more spontaneous abortions 34/17 768 died from breast cancer.

(i) Calculate the risk of death from breast cancer for women who have had at least one spontaneous abortion, together with a 99% confidence interval.

(ii) Calculate the relative risk for those who have had at least one compared to those who have had no spontaneous abortions, together with a 99% confidence interval.

(iii) Test for a significant linear trend in the percentage dying from breast cancer. To do this you need to assume some average in the 'three or more' group. In order to provide a verifiable calculation, you may take this to be four.

3.7 Pearson *et al.* (1991) studied the uptake of well woman clinics in Liverpool. The table below shows the number of attendees in 1986, together with the estimated 1986 mid-year population of Liverpool (provided by the City Council), by 10-year age groups.

| Age group (years) | Clinic attendees | Liverpool population |
|---|---|---|
| 15–24 | 36 | 40 941 |
| 25–34 | 88 | 33 350 |
| 35–44 | 95 | 29 014 |
| 45–54 | 47 | 25 381 |
| 55–64 | 27 | 28 382 |
| 65–74 | 4 | 25 750 |

(i) Find the age-specific attendance rates per thousand population.

(ii) Find a 95% confidence interval for the rate per thousand in the 35–44 age group.

(iii) Find the relative rates for each of the other age groups compared to the 15–24 age group. Interpret your results.

(iv) Find a 95% confidence interval for the relative rate comparing women aged 35–44 to women aged 15–24.

# 4

# Confounding and interaction

## 4.1 Introduction

In the previous chapter we were only concerned with two variables: the risk factor and the disease status. Often a third factor may have an important influence on the apparent relationship between these two variables. If the third factor can explain (at least partially) this relationship then **confounding** is present. For instance, a relationship between the number of children and prevalent breast cancer for a sample of mothers may be explained by the ages of the mothers: older mothers tend to have more children and also have a greater chance of having contracted breast cancer. Age is then the third factor which explains the observed relationship between number of children and breast cancer. The effect (upon breast cancer) of multiple childbearing is confounded with the effect of age.

If, instead, the third factor modifies the relationship between risk factor and the disease, then **interaction** is present. For instance, suppose that the relationship between salt consumption and cerebrovascular disease (stroke) is quite different for men and women; perhaps women have to have a very high salt intake to make any appreciable difference to their risk, whereas even a moderate intake elevates the risk substantially in men. Sex would then be the third factor which modifies the relationship between salt and stroke. Sex would be said to interact with salt consumption in determining the propensity for a stroke.

The issues of confounding and interaction need to be considered whenever an epidemiological study is designed or analysed. Consideration of likely confounding and interaction effects is necessary even before a study is begun because analytical methods to deal with confounding or interaction can only be applied if data on the specific 'third factor' can be collected. In most cases there will not be a single potential confounding variable, nor a single potential interaction variable. Thus the term 'third factor' could refer to a set of factors.

Although confounding and interaction are very different phenomena, they are often confused. Part of the reason for this is that we may be unsure, at the stage of designing a study, whether a particular variable that we decide to record has a confounding or interactive effect on the specific relationship that we wish to study. Indeed, we may have several risk factors that we decide to measure, and part of the study aims is to decide which risk factors are confounded, and which interact, with others in regard to the disease outcome of interest. Methods for detecting and dealing with confounding and interaction are described in Sections 4.2–4.6; interaction is considered in Sections 4.7–4.9.

## 4.2   The concept of confounding

A confounding variable, or **confounder**, is an extraneous factor that wholly or partially accounts for the observed effect of the risk factor on disease status. The 'effect' here could be either an apparent relationship or an apparent lack of relationship. In the first case the confounder is causing the relationship to appear; in the second the confounder is masking a true relationship. Two hypothetical examples will illustrate how these situations could arise.

*Example 4.1*  Table 4.1 shows the cross-tabulation of risk factor status (exposure/no exposure in these examples) and disease outcome for a hypothetical prospective study of 320 subjects. Using the methodology of the previous chapter, and specifically (3.1) and (3.2), we find that the relative risk of disease (risk factor present versus absent) is 5.52. This is formally significant ($p < 0.0001$), from (3.15). Hence we conclude that the risk factor does, indeed, have an effect on disease.

   However, suppose that we also have data on a third variable, a potential confounding factor denoted by $C$. Again, suppose we simply recorded whether $C$ was present or absent for each subject. Table 4.2 shows the relationship between the risk factor and disease separately for those individuals with $C$ present and those with $C$ absent. In the former case those exposed and unexposed to the risk factor both have a risk of disease of 0.1 and hence the relative risk is 1. In the latter case the two risks are 0.8 and hence the relative risk is also 1. When considered within levels of $C$, the supposed risk factor has absolutely no effect on the disease. The apparent relationship, seen in Table 4.1, is entirely explained by confounding with $C$.

**Table 4.1**  Risk factor status by disease status

| Risk factor status | Disease status | | |
| --- | --- | --- | --- |
| | *Disease* | *No disease* | *Risk* |
| Exposed | 81 | 29 | 0.7364 |
| Not exposed | 28 | 182 | 0.1333 |
| Relative risk | | | 5.52 |

**Table 4.2**   Risk factor status by disease status by confounder ($C$) status

| Risk factor status | Confounder absent | | | Confounder present | | |
|---|---|---|---|---|---|---|
| | Disease | No disease | Risk | Disease | No disease | Risk |
| Exposed | 1 | 9 | 0.1000 | 80 | 20 | 0.8000 |
| Not exposed | 20 | 180 | 0.1000 | 8 | 2 | 0.8000 |
| Relative risk | | | 1.00 | | | 1.00 |

Careful inspection of the tables shows why the confounding occurs: presence/absence of the confounder and the risk factor tend to go together. $C$ is, itself, a risk factor for the disease with a relative risk (for presence versus absence) of

$$\frac{(80 + 8)/(80 + 8 + 20 + 2)}{(1 + 20)/(1 + 20 + 9 + 180)} = 8.$$

When we think that we are seeing the effect of the 'risk factor' we may really be seeing the effect of $C$.

*Example 4.2*   Table 4.3 shows results from another hypothetical prospective study. This time, before we consider the confounder, there is absolutely no effect of the potential risk factor: the risk is the same whether it is present or absent. In Table 4.4 the three-way cross-classification identifies that, on the contrary, exposure to the risk factor is more likely to lead to disease: in fact 2.45 times as likely. Indeed, if we apply formal hypothesis tests, using (3.15), to either of the sub-tables of Table 4.4 the relative risk is significantly different from unity ($p = 0.03$ and $p < 0.0001$, respectively). This relationship is entirely masked by the confounder, $C$, in the simple analysis of Table 4.3.

In this example the presence of the confounder tends to go with the absence of the risk factor whilst the absence of the confounder tends to go with the presence of the risk factor. As in Example 4.1, $C$ is, itself, a risk factor for the disease. The relative risk, $C$ present versus $C$ absent, is

$$\frac{(105 + 195)/(105 + 195 + 5 + 305)}{(135 + 5)/(135 + 5 + 415 + 45)} = 2.11.$$

In Table 4.3 exposure to the risk factor and $C$ effectively cancel each other out.

**Table 4.3**   Risk factor status by disease status

| Risk factor status | Disease status | | |
|---|---|---|---|
| | Disease | No disease | Risk |
| Exposed | 240 | 420 | 0.3636 |
| Not exposed | 200 | 350 | 0.3636 |
| Relative risk | | | 1.00 |

**Table 4.4**    Risk factor status by disease status by confounder (*C*) status

| Risk factor status | Confounder absent | | | Confounder present | | |
|---|---|---|---|---|---|---|
| | *Disease* | *No disease* | *Risk* | *Disease* | *No disease* | *Risk* |
| Exposed | 135 | 415 | 0.2455 | 105 | 5 | 0.9545 |
| Not exposed | 5 | 45 | 0.1000 | 195 | 305 | 0.3900 |
| Relative risk | | | 2.45 | | | 2.45 |

When there is **perfect confounding** the relative risks (or other estimates of relative chance of disease) for the various levels (there need not be only two) of the confounder are all the same, and this common value is different from the relative risk when the confounding variable is ignored. Examples 4.1 and 4.2 both illustrate perfect confounding. Indeed, they are quite extreme examples of perfect confounding since in each case there appears to be either no effect of the risk factor (relative risk of 1) or a substantial effect, depending on the analysis.

Perfect confounding is extremely unlikely in real-life epidemiological data. Furthermore, approximations to perfect confounding are neither necessary nor sufficient for confounding to be present. The degree of confounding may be much more marginal or less consistent across the sub-tables, and confounding is more likely to lead to underestimation or overestimation of an effect, unless it is controlled for (as in the next example). We can, however, be sure that confounding is not an important issue whenever the estimates in the different levels, or **strata**, of the confounder are all very similar and are also not very different from the overall estimate. As we shall discover in Section 4.7, if the estimates differ substantially by strata, and no stratum has a small sample size, then interaction is present, and should be allowed for.

*Example 4.3*    Table 4.5 shows data from six years' follow-up of men in the Scottish Heart Health Study (SHHS). These data are for those with no symptoms of coronary heart disease (CHD) at the beginning of the study. The variable 'housing tenure' records whether they rent or own their accommodation. As can be seen, the chance of a CHD event is substantially higher amongst the renters.

Housing rental in Scotland is predominantly a feature of the more disadvantaged social groups. The more disadvantaged tend to have a less healthy lifestyle, and hence the question arises as to whether the risk of renting is explained by confounding with lifestyle. In particular, 57% of the renters but only 35% of the owner-occupiers smoke cigarettes, and cigarette smoking is a well-established risk factor for CHD.

Table 4.6 shows Table 4.5 split by cigarette smoking status. As before, living in rented housing seems to be a risk factor. However, its effect has been reduced (because of the smaller

**Table 4.5**   Housing tenure by CHD outcome after six years, SHHS men

|  | CHD? | | |
|---|---|---|---|
| Housing tenure | Yes | No | Risk |
| Rented | 85 | 1821 | 0.0446 |
| Owner-occupied | 77 | 2400 | 0.0311 |
| Relative risk |  |  | 1.43 |

**Table 4.6**   Housing tenure by CHD outcome after six years by cigarette smoking status, SHHS men

|  | Non-smokers | | | Smokers | | |
|---|---|---|---|---|---|---|
| Housing tenure | CHD | No CHD | Risk | CHD | No CHD | Risk |
| Rented | 33 | 923 | 0.0345 | 52 | 898 | 0.0547 |
| Owner-occupied | 48 | 1722 | 0.0271 | 29 | 678 | 0.0410 |
| Relative risk |  |  | 1.27 |  |  | 1.33 |

relative risks) once we account for smoking. There is certainly confounding here because the reduction has occurred in both strata. Since the reductions are small, we can conclude that the degree of confounding is small.

Confounding can arise in real-life data either because of an interrelationship between the variables in general, or because of the way in which the data were collected. For instance, if (antisocial) drug taking and heavy (alcoholic) drinking tend to go together then the effects of drug taking on any alcohol-related disease are sure to be confounded by the effects of heavy drinking. This is an example of a general relationship leading to confounding. On the other hand, consider an experimental study of the effect of an active prophylactic drug compared with a placebo. Suppose that the patients selected to receive the active drug, by chance, turned out to be predominantly male; patients on the placebo, by contrast, are predominantly female. Suppose that the disease is more likely in men. Then we should expect to find that the drug does not perform as well as it should because its effect is confounded with that of sex. Notice that we would not have expected this type of confounding if there had not been the sex bias in drug allocation; hence this is confounding by design. In the extreme case where everyone in one treatment group is male and everyone in the other is female, the effects of drug and sex are indistinguishable, or **aliased**. Clearly this would be a very poor study design.

**4.3   Identification of confounders**

In our discussion so far, we have only looked at the basic concepts, and some possible consequences, of confounding. Here we shall consider what conditions are necessary before a variable may be considered a confounder.

Let us denote the disease by $D$, the risk factor by $F$ and the third variable by $C$. If $C$ is to be a confounder it must:

• be related to the disease, but not be a consequence of the disease;

• be related to the risk factor, but not be a consequence of the risk factor.

After Schlesselman (1982), path diagrams will be used to illustrate situations where $C$ is, and is not, a confounder of the $F$–$D$ relationship. The arrows show relationships that exist regardless of all other relationships inherent in the path diagram. Double-sided arrows are used to denote non-causal relationships; single-sided arrows show the direction of causality.

Figure 4.1 shows three of the possible situations where $C$ is a confounder and Figure 4.2 gives particular examples. Figure 4.2(a) is an oft-quoted example of confounding (see, for example, Kahn and Sempos, 1989). Grey hair tends to be related to any disease, such as stroke, which is age-related. However, this does not mean that grey hair is an independent risk factor for such diseases, it is simply caused by the ageing process. The other two examples in Figure 4.2 were introduced earlier. In Figure 4.2(c) it is supposed that house

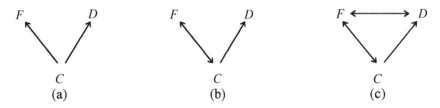

**Figure 4.1**   Some situations in which $C$ is a confounder for the $F$–$D$ relationship.

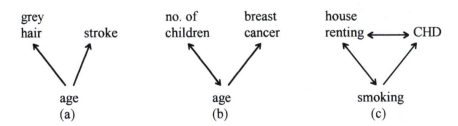

**Figure 4.2**   Some examples that may fit the situations in Figure 4.1.

renting is not causally related to CHD, but rather that there are other causal factors, besides smoking, that are also confounded with renting. If it is, indeed, the fact of renting itself that is causal then the *F–D* arrow should be single-sided, pointing at *D*. There would still be confounding with smoking.

The example of the prophylactic experimental study in Section 4.2 is of type (c), whilst the example relating antisocial drugs and alcohol is of either type (b) or type (c). In two of the three examples in Figure 4.2 the confounder is age: this is the most common confounding variable in epidemiological investigations.

Figure 4.3 illustrates four possible situations in which *C* is **not** a confounder; Figure 4.4 gives a potential example for each case. To see why *C* is not a confounder it is useful to consider the consequence of controlling, or adjusting, the *F–D* relationship for *C*. In Sections 4.4–4.6 we shall see how to carry out adjustments: the technical details are not important at this stage.

The most straightforward situation is (a), where *F* and *C* act independently. It would not be incorrect to control for *C* here, but it would serve no purpose. The example given supposes that the effects of smoking and a diet that is rich in cholesterol are independent with regard to CHD. In (b), *C* causes *D* only through the intermediate agent, *F*. Eating fruit causes a low intake of vitamin C which causes scurvy. In both (c) and (d), *F* causes *C*. Thus, in (c), smoking and fibrinogen are both risk factors for CHD, but smoking promotes increased fibrinogen. Controlling smoking for fibrinogen would not be sensible because

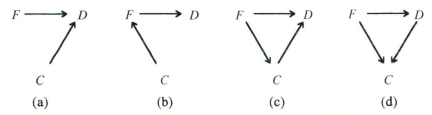

**Figure 4.3**   Some situations in which *C* is not a confounder for the *F–D* relationship.

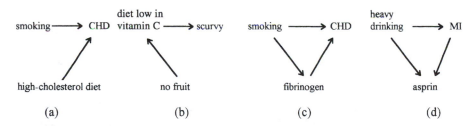

**Figure 4.4**   Some examples that may fit the situations in Figure 4.3.

this would, effectively, mean controlling the effect of smoking for part of itself. In (d), the added feature is that $D$ causes $C$. People who have had myocardial infarction (MI) are routinely advised to take aspirins, so as to help avoid a recurrence. Controlling any risk factor that is associated, causally or non-causally, with aspirin taking (such as heavy drinking) would not be sensible since this is, effectively, controlling the effect on disease for part of itself. Hence, (d) fails on two counts.

### 4.3.1    A strategy for selection

As the foregoing has shown, what makes something a confounder depends both upon data-based observed relationships and a priori knowledge of the supposed biological processes at work. In order to decide which variables are potential confounders, path diagrams need to be considered for all candidate variables. Figure 4.5 summarizes the necessary conditions: Figures 4.1 and 4.3 are special cases.

Any variable that satisfies the conditions in Figure 4.5 should be considered as a confounder. If we are not sure about the positive aspects, but know that the negative ones are false, then there is nothing wrong with proceeding as if confounding occurs and subsequently assessing whether this was really worthwhile (using the methods presented in Section 4.4). For this reason, all known risk factors for the specific disease are potential confounders; this should be borne in mind at the stage of study design. Similarly, age and sex are always worth considering, when appropriate.

## 4.4    Assessing confounding

Once the data have been collected we can use analytical methods to assess the effect of any variable that is a potential confounder. As in other problems, we can choose to use analytical techniques based upon estimation or hypothesis tests. The former is preferable, because it is both the most straightforward and the most meaningful.

### 4.4.1    Using estimation

We can assess confounding by estimating the effect of the risk factor with and without allowing for confounding. For instance, in Example 4.3 the relative risk of renting is 1.43 unadjusted, and around 1.30 (the average over the two strata) after adjustment for smoking. We would then estimate the effect of

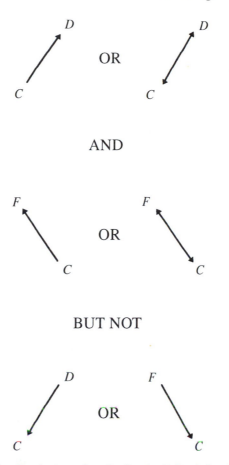

**Figure 4.5**  Conditions for $C$ to be a confounder for the $F$–$D$ relationship.

confounding as $E_C/E$, where $E$ is the unadjusted, and $E_C$ is the adjusted, estimate. In the example this is $1.30/1.43 = 0.91$; adjustment has reduced the relative risk by 9%.

One problem with this approach is that the answer will depend upon the measure of comparative chance of disease (exposed versus not exposed) that is used. An extensive description of this issue is given by Miettinen and Cook (1981). For example, consider the use of odds ratios, rather than relative risks, as the measure of comparative chance of disease in Example 4.2. The unadjusted odds ratio is 1.00, the same as the relative risk, but the odds ratios by strata are 2.93 and 32.85, which are very different from the relative risks and from each other. However, the assessment of confounding by comparing relative risks and by comparing odds ratios will be similar whenever the disease is rare (see Section 3.3). Thus, in Example 4.3, the odds ratios are 1.45 (unadjusted) and 1.28 and 1.35 in the smoking groups. As these are very similar to the relative risks, the value of $E_C/E$ will be much the same by both criteria.

The method of stratification, used in Examples 4.1–4.3, provides separate estimates (of whatever parameter is used to represent the chance of disease) by strata. The arithmetic mean, over the strata, may be used to represent $E_C$, but there are several better ways of deriving an adjusted estimate. In Sections 4.5 and 4.6 we shall discuss methods of adjustment based on tables (non-parametric methods); in Chapters 9–11 we shall see how to use statistical models for adjustment.

For simplicity, all the examples so far have considered binary confounding and risk factor variables. The methods of adjustment presented in this chapter will handle confounding variables with many levels; the modelling methods of later chapters will also cope with continuous variables. However, when the risk factor has more than two levels there is no single measure of confounding, $E_C/E$, because this will vary by the levels being compared. The best strategy is to present sets of estimates, unadjusted (or, perhaps, adjusted only for non-modifiable risk factors, such as age) and adjusted, side by side. The reader can then judge the effects of confounding for him or herself. Of course, if confounding has little effect then one set of estimates will suffice.

*Example 4.4*    Table 4.7 presents unadjusted and age-adjusted coronary event rates and risks of death subsequent to a coronary event for men in north Glasgow, 1991 by socio-economic (deprivation) group. These data will be described, and the numerical results derived, in Examples 4.6 and 4.8.

Coronary event rates not only change quite considerably after adjustment, but also change in rank order (group IV is highest after adjustment; group III was highest before). Hence adjustment has had an important effect here and it is useful to present both the unadjusted

**Table 4.7**    Coronary event rates and risk of death by deprivation group, north Glasgow men in 1991

| Deprivation group | Coronary event rate (per thousand) | | Risk of coronary death | |
|---|---|---|---|---|
| | Unadjusted | Age-adjusted | Unadjusted | Age-adjusted |
| I (most advantaged) | 2.95 | 3.28 | 0.57 | 0.59 |
| II | 4.32 | 4.20 | 0.50 | 0.50 |
| III | 6.15 | 5.30 | 0.51 | 0.52 |
| IV (least advantaged) | 5.90 | 5.75 | 0.56 | 0.56 |

and adjusted values (see also Figure 4.6). The risks of coronary death, on the other hand, remain much the same and retain the same overall pattern after adjustment. In this case there is little point in presenting both sets of values; adjustment has clearly had virtually no effect. We conclude that age is a confounder for the deprivation–event, but not the deprivation–death, relationship.

### 4.4.2   Using hypothesis tests

As in other situations (Section 3.5.5), hypothesis tests by themselves are of limited use. The situation is worse here because there is no direct test for 'successful' confounding.

What we can do is to test whether $F$ and $D$ are related after the adjustment for $C$ has been made: that is, we can test for an **adjusted relationship** between $F$ and $D$, often interpreted as an **adjusted effect** of $F$ on $D$. We might compare the result to a similar test before adjustment has been made. If, for example, $F$ is highly significantly related to $D$ before adjustment ($p < 0.001$), but not after adjustment (say, $p > 0.1$), then there is evidence that the confounder has really had an effect.

Similarly, when there is still a significant effect of $F$ on $D$ after adjustment for $C$, we may infer that $F$ has an effect on $D$ over and above any effect of $C$. Such a significant adjusted effect is often called an **independent effect** by epidemiologists, especially when the effect of $F$ has been adjusted for all (other) known risk factors for $D$ simultaneously (Section 4.4.3). Note that this is not the same as **statistical independence**, which signifies that the risk of disease given exposure to $F$ is exactly the same whether or not a person has also been exposed to $C$.

The word of caution expressed in Section 3.5.5 needs reiterating: the results of hypothesis tests depend upon sample size. Thus a significant adjusted effect could be simply a reflection of a vast study sample. The very act of allowing for the confounder has an effect on the overall estimate of unexplained (background) variation, and thus the effective sample size is different before and after adjustment. If the confounder has several missing values we may even have used different actual sample sizes for the unadjusted and adjusted tests, and hence will not even be comparing like with like when we compare the tests.

### 4.4.3   Dealing with several confounding variables

For simplicity, the foregoing examples have taken the situation where there is only one confounding variable. In practice there could be several. The analytical methods for dealing with one confounder may easily be extended to the case of several confounders: for example, stratification (as used in

Examples 4.1–4.3) would use all the confounders simultaneously. Thus if we consider both smoking (yes/no) and exercise (coded as seldom/sometimes/often/very often) as confounders for the relationship between housing tenure and CHD in Example 4.3 we would define $2 \times 4 = 8$ strata, and corresponding sub-tables (see also Example 4.12).

The interpretation of the effect of several confounders is much less straightforward. The effect of any one confounder by itself may be quite different when a second confounder is also considered. For instance, it might be that coffee drinking is a confounder for the relationship between smoking and some specific type of cancer. However, perhaps controlling for coffee drinking has no effect when the smoking–cancer relationship has already been controlled for alcohol consumption. This may be because coffee and alcohol are themselves related. On the other hand, if the smoking–cancer relationship is adjusted for, say, coffee and tea drinking simultaneously it could be that there is no (joint) effect. Coffee may be a confounder by itself, but not in conjunction with tea, possibly because coffee and tea drinking are inversely related.

In essence, the problem here is that of confounding (or interaction) of confounders, and the causes may be more subtle than the simple examples given above may suggest. In general, we cannot necessarily predict what the joint or adjusted effects of two confounders will be simply from observing their relationship to each other and their individual relationships to the disease. It is how they affect the relationship between risk factor and disease that is crucial.

As with the effect of any one confounder, the best way to assess joint confounding is to compare unadjusted and adjusted estimates. 'Adjusted' here could encompass adjustments for each single confounder, all possible pairs, all possible triples, etc. In practice this will often be too unwieldy, especially for presentation purposes. Often the most meaningful adjustment will be that for all the potential confounders simultaneously: for example, all previously well-established risk factors for the disease. However, this may include some redundant confounders and may hide some interesting and useful facts about interrelationships.

*Example 4.5*  Kaufman *et al.* (1983) describe a case–control study of cigarette smoking as a risk factor for MI, which was carried out in parts of Connecticut, Massachusetts, New York and Rhode Island. Table 4.8 gives their results for different levels of smoking: these are as reported, except that the unadjusted results have been calculated from figures supplied in their paper, using (3.9) and (3.12). This table gives data for 501 cases of MI and 827 controls (subjects with no MI).

Adjustment for age reduces the effect of smoking, but adjustment for the complete set of potential confounders identified by Kaufman *et al.* increases the effect (except amongst ex-smokers). The 'downward' effect of age as a confounder is swamped by the 'upward' effect of one or more of the other confounders. With the information available we cannot investigate

**Table 4.8** Odds ratios (with 95% confidence intervals) for myocardial infarction by cigarette smoking habit amongst men aged 30–54 living in the north-east of the USA

| Smoking habit | Unadjusted | Age-adjusted | Multiply-adjusted[a] |
|---|---|---|---|
| Never smoked | 1 | 1 | 1 |
| Ex-smoker | 1.5 (1.0, 2.2) | 1.1 (0.7, 1.7) | 1.2 (0.8, 1.9) |
| < 25 per day | 2.1 (1.4, 3.2) | 2.1 (1.4, 3.1) | 2.5 (1.6, 3.9) |
| 25–34 per day | 2.5 (1.6, 3.8) | 2.4 (1.5, 3.7) | 2.9 (1.8, 4.7) |
| 35–44 per day | 4.1 (2.7, 6.4) | 3.9 (2.5, 5.9) | 4.4 (2.8, 7.1) |
| ≥ 45 per day | 4.4 (2.8, 7.0) | 4.0 (2.5, 6.4) | 5.0 (3.1, 8.3) |

[a] Adjusted for age, geographic region, drug treatment for hypertension, history of elevated cholesterol, drug treatment for diabetes mellitus, family history of myocardial infarction or stroke, personality score, alcohol consumption, religion and marital status.

this further. Clearly we can say that current smoking has a real effect on MI, regardless of the effect of age or of the other potential confounders taken together. Kaufman *et al.* sensibly include a test of dose-response amongst current smokers. This is reported as statistically significant ($p < 0.001$) after both age and multiple adjustment.

Whenever several variables are recorded, in addition to disease status, it may be that each in turn will be considered as *the* risk factor with all the remaining variables as confounders. In different situations any specific variable may act as the risk factor or as one of the confounders (perhaps the only one).

## 4.5   Standardization

The method of **standardization** deals with confounding by choosing a **standard population**, with a known distribution of the confounding variable, and evaluating the theoretical effect of the risk factor, as observed in the study population, on the standard population. In this way the effect of the particular distribution of the confounding variable in the study population is removed.

The vast majority of practical applications of standardization occur where the confounding variable is age, leading to **age standardization**. Sometimes sex standardization is employed concurrently, leading to **age/sex standardization**. This is a standard tool in demography (see Pollard *et al.* 1990), for example, when comparing death rates between communities. The classic example of the need for age standardization in demographic analyses is the comparison of mortality rates between a seaside resort and an industrialized town. The former tends to have higher death rates despite its healthier environment, the explanation being that elderly people tend to retire to the seaside. Age standardization tends to reverse the ranking of the two death rates.

In epidemiology, standardization is often used in a very similar way. As in the above example, it is generally used to facilitate meaningful comparisons between two or more groups. Instead of all-causes death rates, cause-specific death rates, morbidity rates, hospitalization rates, referral rates etc. may be standardized. Although age standardization is most usual, standardization for any variable is possible, providing that the distribution of this variable is known.

This leads to consideration of what population to choose as the standard. The choice is essentially arbitrary, as long as the standard can be considered typical of the type of population(s) under study. Sometimes there is an appropriate universal standard, such as the World Standard Population of the United Nations (Example 4.6). Otherwise the standard population is usually chosen either to be a super-set of the study populations to be compared or as one of the study populations themselves. Hence, if we wished to compare cancer rates by towns in the USA we might choose the entire population of the USA as the standard, or we might take one of the study towns as the standard. Unfortunately, the choice of the standard can affect the results considerably, and so the use of a super-population or universal standard is preferable because these are more objective.

For simplicity the remainder of this section will deal with standardization for age. Other variables would be handled similarly. Standardization may be applied to event rates or risks. Rates are dealt with in Sections 4.5.1 and 4.5.2; risks are discussed in Section 4.5.3. Throughout we shall assume that the effect on disease of whatever risk factor is investigated is reasonably homogeneous across age groups. If not there will be interaction between the risk factor and age (Section 4.7) and standardization is inappropriate.

## 4.5.1    Direct standardization of event rates

The **direct standardized event rate** is the number of events (for example, deaths) that would be expected in the standard population if the age-specific event rates in the study population prevailed, divided by the size of the standard population. To avoid small numbers, this is usually multiplied by 1000.

Let the superscript s denote the standard population. Suppose that both the study and standard populations have been subdivided into the same set of age groups (say, 0–9, 10–19, 20–29, ...). Let $e_i$ be the number of events in the $i$th age group of the study population, $p_i$ be the size of the $i$th age group of the study population, $p_i^{(s)}$ be the size of the $i$th age group of the standard population, and $p^{(s)} = \sum p_i^{(s)}$ be the total size of the standard population. Then the (direct) age-standardized event rate per thousand is

$$dsr = \frac{1000}{p^{(s)}} \sum \left(\frac{e_i}{p_i}\right) p_i^{(s)}. \tag{4.1}$$

If we assume that the observed number of events, $e_i$, has a Poisson distribution then the standard error of the direct standardized rate is

$$se(dsr) = \frac{1000}{p^{(s)}} \left\{ \sqrt{\sum e_i \left(\frac{p_i^{(s)}}{p_i}\right)^2} \right\}. \tag{4.2}$$

An approximate 95% confidence interval for the direct standardized rate is

$$dsr \pm 1.96se(dsr).$$

An exact method for obtaining a confidence interval is given by Dobson *et al.* (1991).

*Example 4.6*    Morrison *et al.* (1997) describe an enquiry into the variation of CHD rates by social class groups in north Glasgow using data collected as part of the World Health Organization MONICA Study (WHO MONICA Project, 1994). All north Glasgow residents aged 25–64 years were included in the investigation; here we will consider only men and only one of the years covered by the study. That part of Glasgow north of the River Clyde was divided into four areas of differing degrees of deprivation but roughly equal population size. The level of deprivation was determined from 1991 Census data on key neighbourhood characteristics (McLoone, 1994).

Table 4.9 shows the number of coronary events and population size (from the Census) by age and ranked deprivation group (I = least disadvantaged; IV = most) in 1991. Also shown is the World Standard Population (extracted from Breslow and Day, 1987) for this age range. This gives a typical spread of national population, in proportionate terms. This will be used as the standard population here; reasonable alternatives would be the Scottish male population at the 1991 Census or the total male population of north Glasgow.

Table 4.9 also shows the crude event rate (the total number of events divided by the total population size) per thousand in each deprivation group. There is an increase from groups I to II to III but a drop from III to IV. It may be that this break in the pattern is due to age differences within the deprivation groups. Group III has a relatively older age structure (see Table 4.9) and CHD rates are well known to increase with age. Hence, it seems sensible to 'remove' the age effect, by standardizing each of the four rates for age, so as to produce a more meaningful comparison.

This is simple to achieve using (4.1), but quite tedious. Spreadsheet packages can handle such repeated calculations very efficiently. For illustration, consider the direct age-standardized rate per thousand for deprivation group III. From (4.1), this is

$$\frac{1000}{45} \left( \frac{0}{4351} \times 8 + \frac{0}{3232} \times 6 + \frac{1}{2438} \times 6 + \frac{9}{2241} \times 6 \right.$$
$$\left. + \frac{17}{2360} \times 6 + \frac{19}{2708} \times 5 + \frac{43}{2968} \times 4 + \frac{53}{2802} \times 4 \right) = 5.30.$$

Similar calculations give standardized rates, in increasing rank of deprivation group, of 3.28, 4.20, 5.30 and 5.75 per thousand. These increase with rank, so we can conclude that the

**Table 4.9**  Coronary events and population by age group and deprivation group, north Glasgow men in 1991, and the World Standard Population aged 25–64

| | Deprivation group | | | | | | | | World Standard |
| | I | | II | | III | | IV | | |
| Age group (years) | Events | Popn | Events | Popn | Events | Popn | Events | Popn | Popn |
|---|---|---|---|---|---|---|---|---|---|
| 25–29 | 0 | 4 784 | 0 | 4 972 | 0 | 4 351 | 0 | 4 440 | 8 |
| 30–34 | 0 | 4 210 | 0 | 4 045 | 0 | 3 232 | 1 | 3 685 | 6 |
| 35–39 | 1 | 3 396 | 4 | 3 094 | 1 | 2 438 | 5 | 2 966 | 6 |
| 40–44 | 6 | 3 226 | 7 | 2 655 | 9 | 2 241 | 10 | 2 763 | 6 |
| 45–49 | 7 | 2 391 | 13 | 2 343 | 17 | 2 360 | 15 | 2 388 | 6 |
| 50–54 | 16 | 2 156 | 11 | 2 394 | 19 | 2 708 | 24 | 2 566 | 5 |
| 55–59 | 17 | 2 182 | 28 | 2 597 | 43 | 2 968 | 28 | 2 387 | 4 |
| 60–64 | 25 | 2 054 | 44 | 2 667 | 53 | 2 802 | 56 | 2 380 | 4 |
| Total | 72 | 24 399 | 107 | 24 767 | 142 | 23 100 | 139 | 23 575 | 45 |
| Rate (per thousand) | 2.95 | | 4.32 | | 6.15 | | 5.90 | | |

chance of a male CHD event increases with worsening deprivation, once age differences taken account of.

From (4.2) the standard error of the standardized rate for deprivation group III is

$$\frac{1000}{45}\left\{ \sqrt{0\left(\frac{8}{4351}\right)^2 + 0\left(\frac{6}{3232}\right)^2 + 1\left(\frac{6}{2436}\right)^2 + 9\left(\frac{6}{2241}\right)^2}\right.$$

$$\left. + 17\left(\frac{6}{2360}\right)^2 + 19\left(\frac{5}{2708}\right)^2 + 43\left(\frac{4}{2968}\right)^2 + 53\left(\frac{4}{2802}\right)^2 \right\}$$

$$= \frac{1000}{45} \times 0.02077 = 0.462.$$

Similarly, the other standard errors are (I) 0.399, (II) 0.451 and (IV) 0.493.

Our solution to Example 4.6 has, by using (4.1) directly, bypassed a stage that is sometimes useful. As already noted, direct standardization is the application of **age-specific rates** (that is, rates for each age group) in the study population to the age structure of the standard population. Sometimes the age-specific rates are of interest in their own right, and are thus calculated as an intermediate stage. From (3.28), the age-specific rate in age group $i$ is $\hat{\rho}_i = e_i/p_i$. In Example 4.6 we obtain age-specific rates, for the four deprivation groups, by dividing adjacent columns in Table 4.9. Given the set of age-specific rates for a particular study population, (4.1) becomes

$$\text{dsr} = \frac{1000}{p^{(s)}} \sum \hat{\rho}_i p_i^{(s)},$$

and (4.2) becomes

$$\text{se(dsr)} = \frac{1000}{p^{(s)}}\left\{ \sqrt{\sum \frac{\hat{\rho}_i}{p_i}(p_i^{(s)})^2} \right\}.$$

### 4.5.2 Indirect standardization of event rates

Indirect standardization is a two-stage process. First, in contrast to the direct method, the age-specific event rates in the standard population are applied to the study population. This produces the **expected number** of events in the study population. When the observed number of events is divided by this expected number, the result is called the **standardized event ratio** (SER). When events are deaths this becomes the **standardized mortality ratio** (SMR). The SMR is multiplied by 100 for presentation purposes. An SMR of 100 indicates a study population with a mortality rate that is less than the standard, having allowed for age differentials; above 100 means above the standard. This

edure is particularly useful when the standard is the national population
d SMRs are calculated for several towns or other geographical areas.

The second stage, in calculation of the indirect standardized rate, is to multiply
the SER by the crude (that is, total) event rate in the standard population.
Consequently the standard rate is adjusted either up or down accordingly.

Adding to the notation introduced in Section 4.5.1, let $e = \sum e_i$ be the total
number of events in the study population (the observed number of events), $e_i^{(s)}$
be the number of events in the $i$th age group of the standard population,
$e^{(s)} = \sum e_i^{(s)}$ be the total number of events in the standard population,
$\rho_i^{(s)} = e_i^{(s)}/p_i^{(s)}$ be the event rate in the $i$th age group for the standard population, and $\rho^{(s)} = e^{(s)}/p^{(s)}$ be the overall event rate in the standard population.
Then the expected number of events in the study population is

$$E = \sum \rho_i^{(s)} p_i = \sum \left( \frac{e_i^{(s)}}{p_i^{(s)}} \right) p_i. \tag{4.3}$$

By definition,

$$\text{SER} = \frac{\text{observed number of events}}{\text{expected number of events}} = \frac{e}{E}. \tag{4.4}$$

Assuming a Poisson distribution for the observed number of events, $e$, the
standard error of the indirect standardized rate is

$$\text{se(SER)} = \frac{\sqrt{e}}{E}. \tag{4.5}$$

If results are to be expressed in percentage form, (4.4) and (4.5) should be
multiplied by 100.

As with the direct standardized rate, the indirect rate is often expressed per
thousand people. It is then

$$\text{isr} = 1000 \times \text{SER} \times \rho^{(s)} = 1000 \times \text{SER} \times \frac{e^{(s)}}{p^{(s)}}, \tag{4.6}$$

with standard error

$$\text{se(isr)} = 1000\rho^{(s)} \frac{\sqrt{e}}{E} = \frac{1000e^{(s)}\sqrt{e}}{p^{(s)}E}. \tag{4.7}$$

Note tha‌he SER should not be pre-multiplied by 100 when using (4.6) and
(4.7). See ‍tions 5.6.2 and 5.6.3 for more details of SERs.

*Example 4.7*
‍xample 4.6.‍ indirect method of standardization may be applied to the problem of
‍rld Standa‍ver, age-specific coronary event rates are not available for the idealized
time we s‍ulation, and so a different standard population will have to be chosen.
‍s. In fact t‍ an internal standard: the total population over the four deprivation
results. T‍mit a few with deprivation group unknown, but this has little influence
‍ary data, all obtained from Table 4.9, are given in Table 4.10.

Consider calculation of the expected number of events for deprivation group I. By (4.3), this requires multiplication of the group I population by the right-hand column of Table 4.10. That is, the expected number per thousand is

$$0 \times 4784 + 0.0659 \times 4210 + 0.9248 \times 3396 + 2.9398 \times 3226 + 5.4841 \times 2391$$
$$+ \ 7.1254 \times 2156 + 11.4466 \times 2182 + 17.9744 \times 2054 = 103273,$$

and thus $E = 103.273$. Then, from (4.4) and (4.5), the standardized event ratio is $72/103.273 = 0.6972$, with standard error $\sqrt{72}/103.272 = 0.0822$. Hence the first deprivation group (the least deprived) has coronary events at around 70% of the rate that is the local norm.

Applying (4.6) converts the SER into the indirect standardized event rate,

$$0.6972 \times 4.7996 = 3.35.$$

Notice that we did not need to multiply by 1000 here since $\rho^{(s)} = 4.7996$ is already expressed per thousand (see Table 4.10). By (4.7), the standard error of the indirect standardized rate is

$$4.7996\sqrt{72}/103.273 = 0.394.$$

Similar calculations can be made for the other deprivation groups. The four expected numbers of events are, by increasing rank, 103.273, 118.505, 125.632 and 112.590. The standardized event ratios (with standard errors) are 69.72 (8.216), 90.29 (8.729), 113.03 (9.485) and 123.46 (10.471). The indirect standardized rates (and standard errors) are a constant multiple of the above. These are 3.35 (0.394), 4.33 (0.419), 5.42 (0.455) and 5.93 (0.503)

From Example 4.6 the direct standardized equivalents are 3.28 (0.399), 4.20 (0.450), 5.30 (0.462) and 5.75 (0.493), which are very similar but always slightly smaller. Since we have used a different standard population here we would not expect identical results. In any case there are clear differences in the methods of computation.

One useful way of comparing the raw (unadjusted), direct and indirect standardized rates is through the relative rates that they define. For example, choosing deprivation group I to be the 'base' group we obtain relative indirect standardized rates of 1, 1.29, 1.62 and 1.77, by increasing deprivation rank. Figure 4.6 plots the three sets of relative rates: the two adjusted sets are virtually indistinguishable. Since deprivation group I (the base group) has the youngest age structure in north Glasgow, failure to account for age differences has exaggerated the relative rates, particularly in deprivation group III.

Although the data used in Examples 4.6 and 4.7 have permitted both direct and indirect standardization, in some situations the available data may allow only one method to be used. For instance, we may not know the age-specific numbers of events for the desired standard population (in which case the direct method is applicable) or we may not know them for the study population. The latter case sometimes occurs with demographic data from developing countries, when the number of deaths by age is not known very accurately and yet the total number of deaths is known to a reasonable degree of accuracy. Only the indirect method, using some suitable standard population, with known or assumed age-specific death rates, can be used in this context.

**Table 4.10**  Population by age and deprivation group and total number of coronary events by deprivation group, north Glasgow men in 1991

| Age group (years) | Deprivation group populations | | | | Total | | |
|---|---|---|---|---|---|---|---|
| | I | II | III | IV | Events | Popn | Rate/1000 |
| 25–29 | 4 784 | 4 972 | 4 351 | 4 440 | 0 | 18 547 | 0 |
| 30–34 | 4 210 | 4 045 | 3 232 | 3 685 | 1 | 15 172 | 0.0659 |
| 35–39 | 3 396 | 3 094 | 2 438 | 2 966 | 11 | 11 894 | 0.9248 |
| 40–44 | 3 226 | 2 655 | 2 241 | 2 763 | 32 | 10 885 | 2.9398 |
| 45–49 | 2 391 | 2 343 | 2 360 | 2 388 | 52 | 9 482 | 5.4841 |
| 50–54 | 2 156 | 2 394 | 2 708 | 2 566 | 70 | 9 824 | 7.1254 |
| 55–59 | 2 182 | 2 597 | 2 968 | 2 387 | 116 | 10 134 | 11.4466 |
| 60–64 | 2 054 | 2 667 | 2 802 | 2 380 | 178 | 9 903 | 17.9744 |
| Total | 24 399 | 24 767 | 23 100 | 23 575 | 460 | 95 841 | |
| No. of events | 72 | 107 | 142 | 139 | | | |
| Rate/1000 | 2.95 | 4.32 | 6.15 | 5.90 | | | 4.7996 |

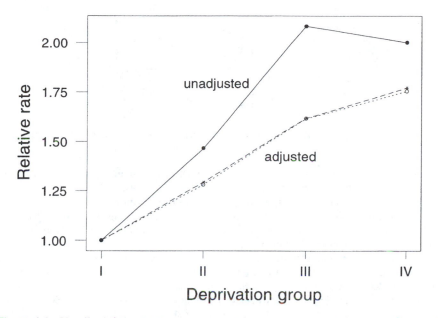

**Figure 4.6**  Unadjusted (raw) and age-adjusted coronary event relative rates for north Glasgow men in 1991. The dotted line shows adjustment by direct standardization and the dashed line shows adjustment by indirect standardization.

### 4.5.3   *Standardization of risks*

Theoretically risks could be either directly or indirectly standardized, but direct standardization will be the only method described here. Essentially the methodology is identical to that already used for rates except that the binomial probability distribution is appropriate rather than the Poisson. Similar to Section 4.5.1, age-specific values in the study population will be applied to the standard population. Hence, if $e_i$, $p_i^{(s)}$ and $p^{(s)}$ are as in Section 4.5.1, and $n_i$ is the number at risk in the $i$th age group of the study population and $r_i = e_i/n_i$ is the risk in the $i$th age group of the study population, then the age-standardized risk is

$$\mathrm{sr} = \frac{1}{p^{(s)}} \sum \left(\frac{e_i}{n_i}\right) p_i^{(s)} = \frac{1}{p^{(s)}} \sum r_i p_i^{(s)}. \tag{4.8}$$

If we assume that the number of events, $e_i$, out of the number of 'trials', $n_i$, has a binomial distribution then the standard error of the standardized risk is

$$\mathrm{se(sr)} = \frac{1}{p^{(s)}} \left\{ \sqrt{\sum \frac{(p_i^{(s)})^2}{n_i^3} e_i(n_i - e_i)} \right\} \tag{4.9}$$

$$= \frac{1}{p^{(s)}} \left\{ \sqrt{\sum \frac{r_i(1 - r_i)}{n_i} (p_i^{(s)})^2} \right\}.$$

If we wish to express the results in percentage form, (4.8) and (4.9) should be multiplied by 100.

*Example 4.8*   The study of Morrison *et al.* (1997), described in Example 4.6, recorded whether or not each coronary event led to death within 28 days. Table 4.11 shows the number of deaths, out of so many events, within each age and deprivation group. The numbers of coronary events are as in Table 4.9. Since there was only one event aged below 35, Table 4.11 does not include the 25–34-year-olds. To avoid confusion, 'events' are called 'coronaries' in Table 4.11. In this context the outcome is death.

Table 4.11 also shows the crude risks (total number of deaths divided by the total number of men experiencing a coronary attack) in each deprivation group. These show no obvious pattern by deprivation group; is this lack of effect due to confounding by age?

To answer this question we shall calculate age-standardized risks. For example, let us take deprivation group II. From (4.8), the standardized risk for this group is

$$\frac{1}{459} \left( \frac{0}{4} \times 11 + \frac{4}{7} \times 32 + \frac{8}{13} \times 52 + \frac{5}{11} \times 70 + \frac{12}{28} \times 116 + \frac{24}{44} \times 178 \right)$$

$$= \frac{228.9091}{459} = 0.499.$$

From (4.9) the standard error of this is

$$\frac{1}{459} \left\{ \sqrt{\frac{11^2}{4^3} 0(4 - 0) + \frac{32^2}{7^3} 4(7 - 4) + \frac{52^2}{13^3} 8(13 - 8)} \right.$$

$$\left. \overline{+ \frac{70^2}{11^3} 5(11 - 5) + \frac{116^2}{28^3} 12(28 - 12) + \frac{178^2}{44^3} 24(44 - 24)} \right\}$$

$$= \sqrt{491.7250}/459 = 0.04831.$$

Similar calculations for the other three groups lead to the full set of standardized risks (and standard errors) by increasing deprivation rank, 0.587 (0.0575), 0.499 (0.0483), 0.520 (0.0409) and 0.558 (0.0418). The age-standardized risks are clearly very similar to the crude risks, so that there appears to be minimal effect of age (that is, no confounding). The four standardized risks are quite similar, with no gradient by increasing deprivation. Hence, we can conclude that deprivation seems to have no systematic effect on the chance of survival after a coronary attack, having controlled for age. Deprivation seems to be a factor that affects the chance of a coronary event (see Example 4.6 or 4.7), but does not affect the subsequent survival.

**Table 4.11**  Number of coronaries, and number of coronaries leading to death within 28 days, by age group and deprivation group, north Glasgow men in 1991

| Age group (years) | Deprivation group | | | | | | | | Total coronaries |
|---|---|---|---|---|---|---|---|---|---|
| | I | | II | | III | | IV | | |
| | Deaths | Coronaries | Deaths | Coronaries | Deaths | Coronaries | Deaths | Coronaries | |
| 35–39 | 1 | 1 | 0 | 4 | 1 | 1 | 2 | 5 | 11 |
| 40–44 | 3 | 6 | 4 | 7 | 4 | 9 | 5 | 10 | 32 |
| 45–49 | 4 | 7 | 8 | 13 | 7 | 17 | 6 | 15 | 52 |
| 50–54 | 7 | 16 | 5 | 11 | 10 | 19 | 11 | 24 | 70 |
| 55–59 | 10 | 17 | 12 | 28 | 19 | 43 | 15 | 28 | 116 |
| 60–64 | 16 | 25 | 24 | 44 | 31 | 53 | 38 | 56 | 178 |
| Total | 41 | 72 | 53 | 107 | 72 | 142 | 77 | 138 | 459 |
| Risk | 0.569 | | 0.495 | | 0.507 | | 0.558 | | |

## 4.6    Mantel–Haenszel methods

In Examples 4.1–4.3 we considered stratifying the risk factor versus disease table by the levels of the confounding variable. Mantel and Haenszel (1959) took this approach, and then considered how best to calculate a summary measure of the odds ratio across the strata. The method they used assumes that there is a common true odds ratio for each stratum; differences in observed odds ratios are purely due to chance variation. Their estimate is now known as the **Mantel–Haenszel estimate** (of the odds ratio).

Consider the sub-table for any individual stratum. Table 4.12 introduces the notation that will be used here: the $i$ subscript denotes stratum $i$. We shall denote the row totals by $E_i$ (for exposure) and $\overline{E}_i$ (for non-exposure), and the column totals by $D_i$ (for disease positive) and $\overline{D}_i$ (for no disease). Other notation follows the style of Table 3.1.

The Mantel–Haenszel estimate is a weighted average of the odds ratios in the individual strata. The weight for any one stratum is chosen to be equal to the precision, measured as the inverse of the variance, of the odds ratio for that stratum. In this way, the most precise stratum-specific odds ratio gets the largest weight; generally this will tend to give greater weight to the bigger strata, that is, the strata with larger $n_i$.

It turns out (Mantel and Haenszel, 1959) that this results in an estimate of common odds ratio of

$$\hat{\psi}_{\mathrm{MH}} = \left(\sum \frac{a_i d_i}{n_i}\right) \bigg/ \left(\sum \frac{b_i c_i}{n_i}\right), \tag{4.10}$$

where both summations go over all strata.

In order to derive a confidence interval for this estimate we need to consider its standard error. In fact we will, instead, consider the standard error of the natural logarithm of $\hat{\psi}_{\mathrm{MH}}$, because this quantity has a more symmetrical distribution that is much better approximated by a normal distribution (just as for the odds ratio in a single stratum: see Section 3.2). Various estimators for

**Table 4.12**    Display of data for stratum $i$ of the confounding variable

| | Disease status | | |
|---|---|---|---|
| Risk factor status | Disease | No disease | Total |
| Exposed | $a_i$ | $b_i$ | $E_i$ |
| Not exposed | $c_i$ | $d_i$ | $\overline{E}_i$ |
| Total | $D_i$ | $\overline{D}_i$ | $n_i$ |

the standard error of $\log_e \hat{\psi}_{MH}$ have been suggested. Robins *et al.* (1986b) show that the following estimator has useful properties:

$$\hat{se}(\log_e \hat{\psi}_{MH}) = \sqrt{\frac{\sum P_i R_i}{2(\sum R_i)^2} + \frac{\sum P_i S_i + \sum Q_i R_i}{2 \sum R_i \sum S_i} + \frac{\sum Q_i S_i}{2(\sum S_i)^2}}, \qquad (4.11)$$

where, for stratum $i$,

$$\begin{aligned} P_i &= (a_i + d_i)/n_i, \quad Q_i = (b_i + c_i)/n_i, \\ R_i &= a_i d_i/n_i, \qquad\quad S_i = b_i c_i/n_i. \end{aligned} \qquad (4.12)$$

The 95% confidence limits for $\log_e \hat{\psi}_{MH}$ are then

$$\begin{aligned} L_{\log} &= \log_e \hat{\psi}_{MH} - 1.96\hat{se}(\log_e \hat{\psi}_{MH}), \\ U_{\log} &= \log_e \hat{\psi}_{MH} + 1.96\hat{se}(\log_e \hat{\psi}_{MH}); \end{aligned} \qquad (4.13)$$

and the 95% confidence limits for $\hat{\psi}_{MH}$ itself are thus

$$\begin{aligned} L &= \exp(L_{\log}), \\ U &= \exp(U_{\log}). \end{aligned} \qquad (4.14)$$

*Example 4.9* The data in Table 4.6 involve two strata for the confounder 'smoking status'. For convenience, the data are presented again in Table 4.13 with totals included. Each stratum is now in the form of Table 4.12.

Using (4.10), the common odds ratio is estimated by

$$\hat{\psi}_{MH} = \frac{\left(\dfrac{33 \times 1722}{2726}\right) + \left(\dfrac{52 \times 678}{1657}\right)}{\left(\dfrac{923 \times 48}{2726}\right) + \left(\dfrac{898 \times 29}{1657}\right)} = \frac{42.123}{31.969} = 1.32.$$

If we consider the strata individually, we can find the odds ratios from (3.9) as 1.28 (non-smokers) and 1.35 (smokers). As we would expect, the Mantel–Haenszel summary is somewhere in-between the two separate estimates: in fact, it is just about in the middle in this example, although this will not always happen.

**Table 4.13**  Data from Table 4.6, with totals

| Housing tenure | Non-smokers | | | Smokers | | |
|---|---|---|---|---|---|---|
| | CHD | No CHD | Total | CHD | No CHD | Total |
| Rented | 33 | 923 | 956 | 52 | 898 | 950 |
| Owner-occupied | 48 | 1722 | 1770 | 29 | 678 | 707 |
| Total | 81 | 2645 | 2726 | 81 | 1576 | 1657 |

We can attach confidence limits to $\hat{\psi}_{\text{MH}}$ using (4.11)–(4.14). First, we use (4.12) to find

$$P_1 = \frac{33 + 1722}{2726} = 0.6438 \qquad P_2 = \frac{52 + 678}{1657} = 0.4406,$$

$$Q_1 = \frac{923 + 48}{2726} = 0.3562 \qquad Q_2 = \frac{898 + 29}{1657} = 0.5594,$$

$$R_1 = \frac{33 \times 1722}{2726} = 20.85 \qquad R_2 = \frac{52 \times 678}{1657} = 21.28,$$

$$S_1 = \frac{923 \times 48}{2726} = 16.25 \qquad S_2 = \frac{898 \times 29}{1657} = 15.72.$$

Thus,

$$\Sigma\, P_i R_i = 0.6438 \times 20.85 + 0.4406 \times 21.28 = 22.80,$$
$$\Sigma\, P_i S_i = 0.6438 \times 16.25 + 0.4406 \times 15.72 = 17.39,$$
$$\Sigma\, Q_i R_i = 0.3562 \times 20.85 + 0.5594 \times 21.28 = 19.33,$$
$$\Sigma\, Q_i S_i = 0.3562 \times 16.25 + 0.5594 \times 15.72 = 14.58,$$
$$\Sigma\, R_i = 20.85 + 21.28 = 42.13,$$
$$\Sigma\, S_i = 16.25 + 15.72 = 31.97.$$

In (4.11), these give

$$\hat{\text{se}}(\log_e \hat{\psi}_{\text{MH}}) = \sqrt{\frac{22.80}{2 \times 42.13^2} + \frac{17.39 + 19.33}{2 \times 42.13 \times 31.97} + \frac{14.58}{2 \times 31.97^2}} = 0.1649.$$

Then, by (4.13) and (4.14), the confidence interval for $\psi_{\text{MH}}$ is

$$\exp(\log_e 1.32 \pm 1.96 \times 0.1649),$$

that is, (0.95, 1.82). The smoking-adjusted estimate of the odds ratio for CHD, comparing renters to owner-occupiers, is 1.32 with 95% confidence interval (0.95, 1.82).

### 4.6.1   The Mantel–Haenszel relative risk

Although Mantel and Haenszel sought only to produce a summary estimate of the common odds ratio, over strata, the same basic technique can be used to derive a summary estimate of the common relative risk (Tarone, 1981). The formulae that follow are taken from Greenland and Robins (1985).

The Mantel–Haenszel estimate of relative risk is

$$\hat{\lambda}_{\text{MH}} = \frac{\sum(a_i \overline{E}_i / n_i)}{\sum(c_i E_i / n_i)}. \qquad (4.15)$$

The estimated standard error of the logarithm of this is

$$\hat{\text{se}}(\log_e \hat{\lambda}_{\text{MH}}) = \sqrt{\frac{\sum (E_i \overline{E}_i D_i - a_i c_i n_i)/n_i^2}{\left(\sum (a_i \overline{E}_i / n_i)\right)\left(\sum (c_i E_i / n_i)\right)}}; \qquad (4.16)$$

hence the 95% confidence limits $(L_{\log}, U_{\log})$ for $\log_e \lambda_{MH}$ are

$$
\begin{aligned}
L_{\log} &= \log_e \hat{\lambda}_{MH} - 1.96\hat{se}(\log_e \hat{\lambda}_{MH}), \\
U_{\log} &= \log_e \hat{\lambda}_{MH} + 1.96\hat{se}(\log_e \hat{\lambda}_{MH}),
\end{aligned}
\tag{4.17}
$$

and the 95% confidence limits $(L, U)$ for $\hat{\lambda}_{MH}$ itself are

$$
\begin{aligned}
L &= \exp(L_{\log}), \\
U &= \exp(U_{\log}).
\end{aligned}
\tag{4.18}
$$

*Example 4.10*   Consider, again, the data in Table 4.13. This time we shall seek to estimate the common relative risk, $\lambda_{MH}$. From (4.15), this is estimated by

$$
\hat{\lambda}_{MH} = \frac{(33 \times 1770/2726) + (52 \times 707/1657)}{(48 \times 956/2726) + (29 \times 950/1657)} = \frac{43.614}{33.460} = 1.30.
$$

From (4.16), the standard error of the log of $\lambda_{MH}$ is estimated by

$$
\sqrt{\frac{(956 \times 1770 \times 81 - 33 \times 48 \times 2726)/2726^2 + (950 \times 707 \times 81 - 52 \times 29 \times 1657)/1657^2}{(33 \times 1770/2726 + 52 \times 707/1657)(48 \times 956/2726 + 29 \times 950/1657)}}
$$

$$
= \sqrt{\frac{19.025 + 18.904}{43.614 \times 33.460}} = 0.1612.
$$

Then, by (4.17) and (4.18), the confidence interval for $\lambda_{MH}$ is

$$
\exp(\log_e 1.30 \pm 1.96 \times 0.1612),
$$

that is, (0.95, 1.78). The smoking-adjusted estimate of the relative risk of CHD for renters compared to owner-occupiers is 1.30, with 95% confidence interval (0.95, 1.78). Note that, in this case, the Mantel–Haenszel estimate is the same as the arithmetic mean over the strata (Example 4.3). As with the Mantel–Haenszel odds ratio, this will not always be the case, and is unlikely to be even approximately true when the sample sizes, $n_l$, differ substantially across the strata.

### 4.6.2   The Cochran–Mantel–Haenszel test

Whether odds ratios or relative risks are used to estimate relative propensity for disease, the association between the risk factor and the disease, controlling for the confounder, can be tested using a test ascribed to Cochran as well as Mantel and Haenszel.

Within any stratum, when row and column totals are known, knowledge of any one cell in the $2 \times 2$ contingency table automatically fixes the other three cells. Hence, the test for no association can be based upon a test of the values in, say, the top left-hand cell of each stratum. Recall that the observed value in this cell is $a_i$ for stratum $i$. This will be a value from a hypergeometric distribution with expected (that is, mean) value $E(a_i)$ and variance $V(a_i)$, where

$$E(a_i) = \frac{D_i E_i}{n_i}, \qquad V(a_i) = \frac{D_i \overline{D}_i E_i \overline{E}_i}{n_i^2 (n_i - 1)}. \qquad (4.19)$$

Notice that the expected value is just what we would compute in the standard chi-square test of no association (Section 2.5.1). If the distribution from which each $a_i$ is derived is not very skewed, we expect the distribution of

$$\frac{(\sum a_i - \sum E(a_i))^2}{\sum V(a_i)} \qquad (4.20)$$

to be approximately chi-square with one degree of freedom. Here the summations each run over all the strata. We might, instead, use a continuity-corrected version of (4.20),

$$\frac{(|\sum a_i - \sum E(a_i)| - \frac{1}{2})^2}{\sum V(a_i)}. \qquad (4.21)$$

Hence the test for no association, confounder-corrected, is to compare either (4.20) or (4.21) with $\chi_1^2$. See Section 3.5.3 for a discussion of continuity corrections. This test is, equivalently, a test of $E_C = 1$ (Section 4.4.1) where $E_C$ might refer to the corrected relative risk or odds ratio.

*Example 4.11*   Once more, consider the data in Table 4.13. Here we have, using (4.19),

$$a_1 = 33, \qquad\qquad\qquad\qquad a_2 = 52,$$

$$E(a_1) = \frac{81 \times 956}{2726} = 28.406, \qquad E(a_2) = \frac{81 \times 950}{1657} = 46.439,$$

$$V(a_1) = \frac{81 \times 2645 \times 956 \times 1770}{2726^2 \times 2725} = 17.903, \quad V(a_2) = \frac{81 \times 1576 \times 950 \times 707}{1657^2 \times 1656} = 18.857.$$

Then, using (4.21), the continuity-corrected test statistic is

$$\frac{(|(33 + 52) - (28.406 + 46.439)| - 0.5)^2}{17.903 + 18.857} = 2.54.$$

Comparing with Table B.3, we see that this is not significant even at the 10% level. Hence we conclude that there is no evidence of an association between housing tenure and CHD, after allowing for cigarette smoking status. There is no evidence to refute the hypothesis that the adjusted odds ratio equals 1 (or that the adjusted relative risk is 1).

### 4.6.3   Further comments

The Mantel–Haenszel approach is based upon an assumption that the parameter representing the comparative chance of disease does not vary by levels of the confounding variable. See Section 4.8 for tests of this assumption.

The procedures given here for confidence intervals of Mantel–Haenszel odds ratios and relative risks behave well in a range of circumstances, but other procedures have been suggested which may have the advantage of simplicity or may be more appropriate in a specific situation. A discussion is given in Robins et al. (1986b). In particular, when the sample size is small an exact method of analysis, not employing the normal distribution approximation, will be advisable: see Thomas (1975) and Mehta et al. (1985).

The Mantel–Haenszel approach is used in various other contexts in epidemiology; for example, in the log-rank test for survival data (Section 5.5.1) in person-years analysis (Section 5.6.4) and in matched case–control studies (Section 6.6.2). It has been generalized in various ways, including situations where the risk factor is measured at several (more than two) levels: see Yanagawa et al. (1994).

To conclude the discussion of this topic here, the data analysed in the original Mantel and Haenszel (1959) paper are presented and analysed.

*Example 4.12*   Table 4.14 shows the results of a case–control study of epidermoid and undifferentiated pulmonary carcinoma. The issue of interest is whether smoking is a risk factor for this disease, having accounted for both occupation and age. Mantel and Haenszel (1959) only give data for non-smokers and heavy (one pack or more per day) smokers.

Notice that, in contrast to Examples 4.9–4.11, smoking is now the risk factor rather than the confounder. As stated in Section 4.4.3, the status of any variable depends upon the question(s) to be answered. There are two confounding variables here: employment with three levels, and age with four. There are thus $3 \times 4 = 12$ strata for the confounding variables. The resultant sub-tables, one for each stratum, are given in Table 4.15.

Since this is a case–control study, it is not appropriate to estimate the relative risk. Instead, we can use (4.10)–(4.14) to find the Mantel–Haenszel odds ratio (with 95% confidence interval) as 10.68 (4.47, 39.26). Applying the Cochran–Mantel–Haenszel test with the continuity correction, (4.21), gives a test statistic of 30.66 which is extremely significant ($p < 0.0001$). Hence there is strong evidence that smoking is associated with the disease; heavy smokers have over 10 times the odds of disease compared to non-smokers.

## 4.7   The concept of interaction

Interaction occurs between two risk factors when the effect of one risk factor upon disease is different at (at least some) different levels (outcomes, strata) of the second risk factor. Hence the equivalent term, **effect modification**. When there is no interaction the effects of each of the risk factors are consistent (homogeneous) across the levels of the other risk factor.

**Table 4.14**   Cases of epidermoid and undifferentiated pulmonary carcinoma and controls classified by occupation, age and smoking habit

|  |  | Cases (diseased) | | Controls (no disease) | |
|---|---|---|---|---|---|
| Occupation | Age (years) | Non-smokers | $\geq 1$ pack/day | Non-smokers | $\geq 1$ pack/day |
| Housewives | <45 | 2 | 0 | 7 | 0 |
|  | 45–54 | 5 | 2 | 24 | 1 |
|  | 55–64 | 6 | 3 | 49 | 0 |
|  | $\geq 65$ | 11 | 0 | 42 | 0 |
| White-collar | <45 | 0 | 3 | 6 | 2 |
| workers | 45–54 | 2 | 2 | 18 | 2 |
|  | 55–64 | 4 | 2 | 23 | 2 |
|  | $\geq 65$ | 6 | 0 | 11 | 1 |
| Other | <45 | 0 | 1 | 10 | 3 |
| occupations | 45–54 | 1 | 4 | 12 | 1 |
|  | 55–64 | 6 | 0 | 19 | 1 |
|  | $\geq 65$ | 3 | 1 | 15 | 0 |

**Table 4.15**   Strata derived from Table 4.14; each is expressed in the form of Table 4.12 with smoking as the risk factor

```
 0   0 |  0      2   1 |  3      3   0 |  3       0   0 |  0
 2   7 |  9      5  24 | 29      6  49 | 55      11  42 | 53
 2   7 |  9      7  25 | 32      9  49 | 58      11  42 | 53


 3   2 |  5      2   2 |  4      2   2 |  4       0   1 |  1
 0   6 |  6      2  18 | 20      4  23 | 27       6  11 | 17
 3   8 | 11      4  20 | 24      6  25 | 31       6  12 | 18


 1   3 |  4      4   1 |  5      0   1 |  1       1   0 |  1
 0  10 | 10      1  12 | 13      6  19 | 25       3  15 | 18
 1  13 | 14      5  13 | 18      6  20 | 26       4  15 | 19
```

An example of an interaction that has been reported in the medical literature is the study of porcelain painters by Raffn *et al.* (1988), where the effect of exposure to cobalt upon lung function was found to be worse amongst painters who smoke. Another possible interaction involving smoking is suggested by Barbash *et al.* (1993). They found that non-smokers have a worse prognosis after a myocardial infarct, both in terms of a higher chance of reinfarction and mortality within the next 6 months, than smokers. Since smoking is a well-established risk factor for a first MI, this suggests that there may be an interaction between smoking and previous MI status (yes/no).

Just as with confounding, the analysis of interaction may produce different results depending upon how the comparative chance of disease is measured. In Section 4.8 we shall see how to deal with both the relative risk and odds ratio. Until then we shall continue to leave the choice of measurement unspecified.

For simplicity, let us assume (for now) that both of the risk factors have only two outcomes: call these exposure and non-exposure. Then interaction occurs when the comparative effect of exposure compared to non-exposure for one risk factor is different for the subgroup who are, and the sub-group who are not, exposed to the second risk factor.

Figure 4.7 gives a set of **interaction diagrams** which illustrate three ways in which interaction could happen, as well as the situation of no interaction. **Antagonism** is where the effect of risk factor A works in the opposite direction when acting in the presence of exposure, to the direction in which it acts in the absence of exposure, to risk factor B. This is the strongest type of interaction, since it represents a reversal of effect. **Synergism** is where the effect of A is in the same direction, but stronger in the presence of B. **Unilateralism** is where A has no effect in the absence of B, but a considerable effect when B is present. In fact, 'presence' and 'absence' of exposure are interchangeable in these definitions. Figure 4.7 illustrates the situations when A and B (themselves interchangeable) are both risk factors, rather than protective factors, for the disease. Unilaterism could, alternatively, appear as a sideways 'V', that is, with both lines emanating from the same point. To see this, consider how Figure 4.7(b) would look if B, rather than A, was 'plotted' on the horizontal axis.

As Figure 4.7(a) shows, lack of interaction does not mean that the chance of disease (however measured) after exposure to A is the same regardless of the exposure status of B. When the chance of disease is measured by risk, this would be the situation of statistical independence. This would appear as a single line, rather than the parallel lines for no interaction. Lack of interaction means that the *comparative* chance is constant.

In practice, we are hardly likely to find exact agreements in comparative chance – that is, exactly parallel lines on the interaction diagram. Chance sampling variation may explain slight, or even (with small samples) fairly large, differences. Conversely, sampling variation may explain crossing of lines on the interaction diagram when there is no true interaction in the population. Thus it is reasonable to carry out tests of interaction so as to sift out the 'real' effects. These will be described in Section 4.8. As in other applications, these tests should be combined with consideration of estimates; for instance, through interaction diagrams.

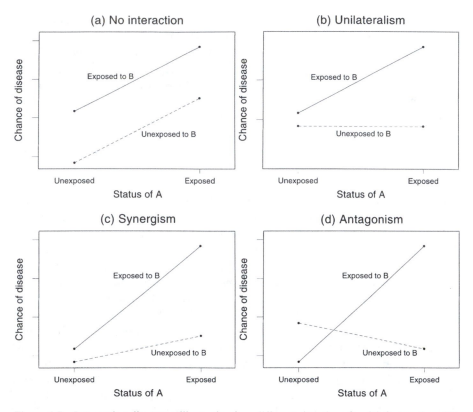

**Figure 4.7**    Interaction diagrams, illustrating four different situations for risk factors A and B.

One method of testing that is quite common, but not appropriate, is to carry out separate tests in each stratum of the 'second risk' factor. For instance, the interaction between smoking and previous MI suggested earlier might be investigated by testing the effect of smoking for those who have had a previous MI, and then repeating the procedure for those who have not. Then the respective $p$ values are compared and the lowest taken to signify the greatest effect. This is wrong, except in the situation where the sample sizes in the two subgroups (defined by previous MI status in the example) are equal. As explained in Section 3.5.5, the $p$ value depends on sample size as well as on the magnitude of the effect. A very common situation is where one subgroup is small, leading to a high $p$ value ('non-significance') even for a large effect, but the other subgroup is large, leading to a small $p$ value ('significance'), even when the size of the effect is not any larger. Unilateralism is then incorrectly inferred from this separate testing method. Notice that the absurdity of this inference would be obvious if an interaction diagram was inspected.

## 4.8   Testing for interaction

In this section we shall consider how to test for interaction in the situations where one of the most common measures of comparative chance is employed. Since a different conclusion may be forthcoming when a different measurement is adopted, it is crucial to state which convention is adopted, unless it is clear from the context.

### 4.8.1   Using the relative risk

Suppose that two risk factors (A and B) are being studied, and the relative risk of disease for exposure to A alone compared to no exposure is $\lambda_A$ and the relative risk for exposure to B alone compared to no exposure is $\lambda_B$. Take $\lambda_{AB}$ to be the relative risk for joint exposure to A and B compared to no exposure. Then interaction occurs if

$$\lambda_{AB} \neq \lambda_A \lambda_B. \tag{4.22}$$

Since products are used, this is called a **multiplicative model** of risk interaction. If we take $R_{00}$ as the risk for those unexposed to both A and B, $R_{10}$ as the risk for those exposed only to A, $R_{01}$ as the risk for those exposed only to B, and $R_{11}$ as the risk for those exposed to both A and B, then (4.22) implies that there is no interaction when

$$\frac{R_{11}}{R_{00}} = \frac{R_{10}}{R_{00}} \times \frac{R_{01}}{R_{00}}. \tag{4.23}$$

A test of the null hypothesis of no interaction is thus derived by considering the situation where the table of risk factor versus disease for one variable (say, A) is split into sub-tables by the strata of the second risk factor, B. This is the very situation described by Table 4.12, except that the confounder has now become risk factor B. For simplicity, we shall continue to assume that B has only two strata. In stratum 1 (no exposure to B) the relative risk for A is $R_{10}/R_{00}$. In stratum 2 (exposure to B) the same measure is $R_{11}/R_{01}$. Now, from (4.23), no interaction is equivalent to

$$\frac{R_{11}}{R_{01}} = \frac{R_{10}}{R_{00}}.$$

Thus there is no interaction when the relative risk is the same in both strata. When B has several, $\ell$, strata it turns out that no interaction is the same as a constant relative risk across all the strata. Since this is the very situation in which the Mantel–Haenszel summary measure of relative risk is appropriate, a test of the null hypothesis of no interaction is also a test of the suitability of application of the Mantel–Haenszel technique (assuming other requirements for confounding are met). Thus whenever we suspect that something is a confounder, we should first apply a test for interaction before using the Mantel–Haenszel procedure.

A test for a common relative risk, $\lambda_0$, across all strata is given by comparing

$$\sum \frac{(a_i - \mathrm{E}(a_i))^2}{\mathrm{V}(a_i)} \tag{4.24}$$

to chi-square with $\ell - 1$ d.f. Here the summation runs over all the $\ell$ strata and $a_i$ is (as usual) the observed value in the top left-hand cell of the $2 \times 2$ table for stratum $i$. Also

$$\mathrm{E}(a_i) = \frac{E_i D_i \lambda_0}{\bar{E}_i + E_i \lambda_0} \tag{4.25}$$

and

$$\mathrm{V}(a_i) = \left( \frac{1}{\mathrm{E}(a_i)} + \frac{1}{\mathrm{E}(b_i)} + \frac{1}{\mathrm{E}(c_i)} + \frac{1}{\mathrm{E}(d_i)} \right)^{-1}, \tag{4.26}$$

such that

$$\begin{aligned}
\mathrm{E}(b_i) &= E_i - \mathrm{E}(a_i), \\
\mathrm{E}(c_i) &= D_i - \mathrm{E}(a_i), \\
\mathrm{E}(d_i) &= n_i - \mathrm{E}(a_i) - \mathrm{E}(b_i) - \mathrm{E}(c_i),
\end{aligned} \tag{4.27}$$

using notation from Table 4.12.

To be able to evaluate (4.25) and thus, ultimately, (4.24) we need to fix a value for $\lambda_0$. One way to do this, which works reasonably well in practice, is to use the Mantel–Haenszel estimate, $\hat{\lambda}_{\mathrm{MH}}$, as defined by (4.15).

Notice also that taking logarithms of both sides of (4.23) gives

$$\log R_{11} - \log R_{00} = \log R_{10} - \log R_{00} + \log R_{01} - \log R_{00},$$

or

$$\log R_{11} - \log R_{10} = \log R_{01} - \log R_{00}.$$

That is, the differences in log(risk) in the two strata defined by exposure and non-exposure to B must be equal for there to be no interaction. This suggests that the most useful interaction diagram in this situation is one in which log(risk) is plotted on the vertical axis (see Figures 4.8 and 4.9). This is because it is easier to interpret absolute, rather than relative, differences pictorially.

*Example 4.13*   In Section 4.7 it was reported that there may be an interaction between smoking and previous MI status in the prediction of CHD. Table 4.16 gives some data from the 6-year follow-up of the SHHS which will be used to explore this suggestion. The data show cigarette smoking status at the start of the study against whether or not a CHD event (MI or death) occurred in the following 6 years, separately for those who had and had not already suffered an MI when the study began. On this occasion SHHS data are shown for women only; those women with unknown smoking or previous MI status have been excluded.

There is clearly a suggestion of interaction, since smokers have a higher risk amongst those without a previous MI and a lower risk amongst those with a previous MI. This suggests that antagonism may occur.

The relative risks are, from (3.2) or directly (as here): for no previous MI, $3.15/1.31 = 2.40$; for previous MI, $13.56/21.15 = 0.64$. Figure 4.8 gives a suitable interaction diagram for this problem. There is clear crossing of lines.

To test the null hypothesis of no interaction we first calculate the value of $\hat{\lambda}_{MH}$. From (4.15), this is

$$\hat{\lambda}_{MH} = \frac{(67 \times 3500/5628) + (8 \times 52/111)}{(46 \times 2128/5628) + (11 \times 59/111)} = 1.954.$$

Taking this to be the $\lambda_0$ in (4.25) gives, for stratum 1 (no previous MI),

$$E(a_1) = \frac{2128 \times 113 \times 1.954}{3500 + 2128 \times 1.954} = 61.355.$$

Using this to complete the expected table for the first stratum gives, as expressed by (4.27),

$$E(b_1) = 2128 - 61.355 = 2066.645,$$
$$E(c_1) = 113 - 61.355 = 51.645,$$
$$E(d_1) = 5628 - 61.355 - 2066.645 - 51.645 = 3448.355.$$

Then, in (4.26),

$$V(a_1) = \left( \frac{1}{61.355} + \frac{1}{2066.645} + \frac{1}{51.645} + \frac{1}{3448.355} \right)^{-1} = 27.446.$$

**Table 4.16**   Smoking status by CHD outcome after 6 years by previous MI status, SHHS women

| Smoking status | No previous MI | | | Previous MI | | |
|---|---|---|---|---|---|---|
| | CHD | No CHD | Total | CHD | No CHD | Total |
| Smoker | 67 (3.15%) | 2061 | 2128 | 8 (13.56%) | 51 | 59 |
| Non-smoker | 46 (1.31%) | 3454 | 3500 | 11 (21.15%) | 41 | 52 |
| Total | 113 | 5515 | 5628 | 19 | 92 | 111 |

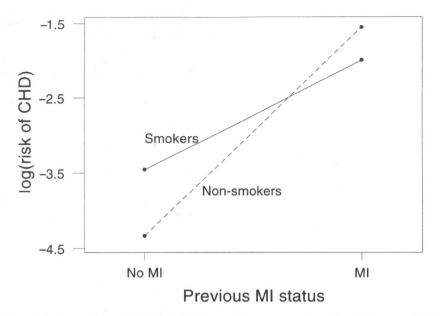

**Figure 4.8**   Logarithm of risk of CHD by smoking status and previous MI status; SHHS women.

Similar calculations for stratum 2 (those with previous MI) give

$$E(a_2) = 13.094, \qquad V(a_2) = 3.458.$$

Substituting into (4.24) gives the test statistic

$$\frac{(67 - 61.355)^2}{27.446} + \frac{(8 - 13.094)^2}{3.458} = 8.67.$$

This is to be compared with $\chi^2$ on $\ell - 1 = 2 - 1 = 1$ d.f. From Table B.3, $0.005 > p > 0.001$ and hence we have strong evidence to reject the null hypothesis: that is, we conclude that there is interaction between smoking and previous MI status.

*Example 4.14*   In Example 4.10 we assumed that there was a common relative risk in the two strata defined by smoking status in Table 4.13, and used the Mantel–Haenszel relative risk of 1.30 to estimate it. We can now test whether this assumption was reasonable. Figure 4.9 is an interaction diagram for this problem: as in Example 4.13, we will be testing whether the lines are parallel.

From (4.25)–(4.27),

$$E(a_1) = 33.41 \qquad E(a_2) = 51.51,$$
$$V(a_1) = 19.01 \qquad V(a_2) = 17.89;$$

and (4.24) then takes a value of 0.02 which is clearly not significant at any sensible significance level. Hence there is no interaction here; we are justified in using the summary relative risk.

*4.8.2   Using the odds ratio*

When the odds ratio is used (as it must be in case–control studies) in place of the relative risk, theoretical details follow in very much the same way as Section 4.8.1. Interaction occurs if

$$\psi_{AB} \neq \psi_A \psi_B,$$

where $\psi_A$ and $\psi_B$ are the odds ratios for exposure to A alone and to B alone, respectively, and $\psi_{AB}$ is the odds ratio for joint exposure compared to no exposure. This is, again, a multiplicative model for interaction.

As with relative risks, no interaction is equivalent to a constant odds ratio for A across the strata of B (or vice versa). This would be a preliminary test for the adoption of the Mantel–Haenszel odds ratio, (4.10).

A test for a constant odds ratio across the strata, as represented by Table 4.12 for stratum *i* of risk factor B, uses (4.24) again. All calculations are just as in Section 4.8.1, except that (4.25) is replaced by

$$E(a_i) = \frac{P_i \pm \sqrt{P_i^2 - 4\psi_0(\psi_0 - 1)E_i D_i}}{2(\psi_0 - 1)},  \qquad (4.28)$$

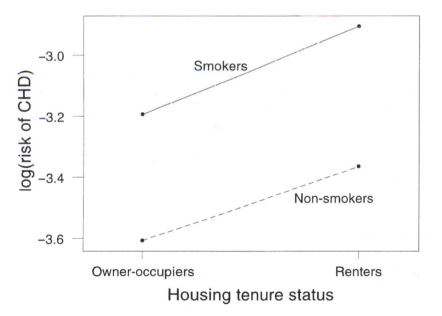

**Figure 4.9**   Logarithm of risk of CHD by smoking status and housing tenure status, SHHS men.

where

$$P_i = (\psi_0 - 1)(E_i + D_i) + n_i \qquad (4.29)$$

and $\psi_0$ is some estimate of the presumed common odds ratio, such as the Mantel–Haenszel estimate. Although (4.28) will yield two outcomes, we require only the outcome which gives positive values for all the expected cell values. We shall need to use (4.28) to calculate the result of (4.26) via (4.27) for each stratum, and so produce the test statistic, (4.24).

*Example 4.15*    Consider the problem of Example 4.13, but this time suppose that we choose to measure comparative chance by odds ratios. From (3.9), the odds ratios are 2.44 (no previous MI) and 0.58 (previous MI). Since these are substantially different, and very similar to the corresponding relative risks, we shall anticipate rejecting the null hypothesis of no interaction.

The first step, in carrying out the formal test, is to calculate $\hat{\psi}_{MH}$ from (4.10). This is

$$\hat{\psi}_{MH} = \frac{(67 \times 3454/5628) + (8 \times 41/111)}{(2061 \times 46/5628) + (51 \times 11/111)} = 2.013.$$

Then, for stratum 1 (no previous MI), when $\hat{\psi}_{MH}$ is used for the common (over all strata) value of $\psi_0$, (4.29) becomes

$$P_1 = (2.013 - 1)(2128 + 113) + 5628 = 7898.133.$$

Using (4.28), we find

$$E(a_1) = \frac{7898.133 \pm \sqrt{7898.133^2 - 4 \times 2.013 \times 1.013 \times 2128 \times 113}}{2 \times 1.013}$$

$$= \frac{7898.133 \pm 7772.973}{2.026}$$

$$= 7734.998 \quad \text{or} \quad 61.777.$$

Of these, only the smaller will give positive expected values for all the remaining cells of the first stratum: thus $E(a_1) = 61.777$ and then, by (4.27),

$$E(b_1) = 2128 - 61.777 = 2066.223,$$
$$E(c_1) = 113 - 61.777 = 51.223,$$
$$E(d_1) = 5628 - 61.777 - 2066.223 - 51.223 = 3448.777.$$

From (4.26),

$$V(a_1) = \left( \frac{1}{61.777} + \frac{1}{2066.223} + \frac{1}{51.223} + \frac{1}{3448.777} \right)^{-1} = 27.410.$$

Similar calculations for the second stratum (previous MI) give

$$E(a_2) = 12.741, \qquad V(a_2) = 3.549.$$

Substituting into (4.24) gives the test statistic

$$\frac{(67 - 61.777)^2}{27.410} + \frac{(8 - 12.741)^2}{3.549} = 7.33.$$

When compared to $\chi^2$ on $\ell - 1 = 1$ d.f. (Table B.3), we find $0.01 > p > 0.005$. There is strong evidence to reject the null hypothesis; we conclude that there is interaction, measured through odds ratios, between smoking and previous MI status in the 6-year prediction of coronary events in the SHHS.

As we would expect for a disease that is (reasonably) rare, the numerical results in Examples 4.13 and 4.15 are very similar. If we apply the test for a common odds ratio to the data of Table 4.13 we can expect similar results to those in Example 4.14.

The tests defined here and in Section 4.8.1 both involve various approximations, such as a chi-square distribution for the test statistics. These approximations will be acceptable whenever the cell numbers are large in each stratum's $2 \times 2$ table. As with single tables (see Section 2.5.1) we can expect problems whenever several expected numbers are small, say less than 5. This suggests that the number of strata may need to be restricted, perhaps by combining strata in some sensible way. For instance, application of the test for a common odds ratio given here should not be applied to the set of stratified tables in Table 4.15. Indeed, it cannot be applied since some of the expected cell values will be zero, which leads to a requirement for division by zero in (4.26). This may be avoided by combining adjacent age groups in the original table, Table 4.14. More accurate procedures for testing for a common summary parameter over stratified tables are given by Breslow and Day (1980; 1987).

### 4.8.3   Using the risk difference

When the risk difference is used to measure the comparative chance of disease, interaction between the risk factors A and B occurs when

$$R_{11} - R_{00} \neq (R_{10} - R_{00}) + (R_{01} - R_{00}) \qquad (4.30)$$

where the $R$s are the risks defined in Section 4.8.1. That is, the difference in risk from joint exposure must be different than the total difference in risk from the individual exposures, where each risk is compared to no exposure.

In this case we have an **additive model** of risk interaction. One advantage of this additive formulation is that risk can be plotted directly on the interaction diagram, allowing a more direct interpretation. Since (4.30) reduces to

$$R_{11} - R_{01} \neq R_{10} - R_{00},$$

no interaction is equivalent to a constant difference in risk, for exposure compared to non-exposure to A, across the levels of risk factor B.

One way to see that detection of interaction is very much a function of the measurement convention is to divide (4.30) by $R_{00}$. The condition for interaction, using the risk difference approach, is then

$$\frac{R_{11}}{R_{00}} - 1 \neq \left(\frac{R_{10}}{R_{00}} - 1\right) + \left(\frac{R_{01}}{R_{00}} - 1\right)$$

and, using the definitions in Section 4.8.1, this gives

$$\lambda_{AB} \neq \lambda_A + \lambda_B - 1$$

which is completely different from (4.22).

Some epidemiologists prefer to adopt additive measures of interaction; see Matthews and Altman (1996) for a simple example and Rothman and Greenland (1997) for a discussion of the merits of this approach. Our approach will be to use the same comparative measure in the analysis of interaction as is chosen to analyse chance. Relative risks seem the natural choice for comparing risks, except where odds ratios are more convenient or are used as approximate relative risks. Hence our approach will be to prefer multiplicative models when analysing incidence or prevalence.

### 4.8.4    Using statistical models

Although strictly out of sequential order, it is appropriate here to consider what kind of interaction will be assumed when statistical models are adopted (in their standard form). Of the models that will be introduced later, logistic, Cox and Poisson regression all assume multiplicative effects of interaction. The general linear model (standard regression and analysis of variance) is the only one that assumes additive effects. For example, analysis of variance compares means. Since means are not proportionate, unlike risks, the additive scale is the standard choice: we compare means through their difference (Section 2.7.3) rather than their ratio.

### 4.8.5    Which interactions to test?

Faced with a large data set, including several potential risk factors, there are many interactions that could be investigated. This could include high-order interactions (three-way or above), although these are only worth considering if the number of observations is extremely large and there is some prior reason for expecting such a complex interaction. With small data sets the chance of detecting a high-order interaction is minimal, even when it exists. On the other hand, we must beware of false positives when many hypothesis tests are carried out in order to trawl for interactions: with 5% significance tests we expect to wrongly reject the null hypothesis of no interaction five times in a hundred. Furthermore, high-order interactions are difficult to interpret. Hence, it is often reasonable to restrict to investigate two-way interactions.

When there are several variables, the false positives problem is also relevant for two-way interactions. Furthermore, there may be an unreasonable amount of work concerned with testing two-way interactions for all variables. Consequently, the approach sometimes taken in epidemiological data analysis is to test only for two-way interactions between those variables that have already been identified as true risk (or protective) factors or confounders. With this approach we have to accept that we would miss identifying an important interaction that involves two risk factors which are, by themselves, not associated with disease. There are occasions when this could be a real problem. For instance, two drugs, each taken in isolation, may be beneficial in curing a disease, whereas in combination they might cause harmful toxic effects.

## 4.9  Dealing with interaction

Whenever we have detected interaction between two risk factors it will *not* be appropriate to consider the effects of each independently of the other. So when A and B interact in determining the chance of disease, as measured through the relative risk, we should not quote the relative risk for A or the relative risk for B (the so-called **main effects** of A and B, respectively). To do so would give a misleading result.

This is most obvious when there is evidence of antagonism. For instance, the relative risk of CHD for smoking (main effect, ignoring previous MI status) from Table 4.16 is

$$\frac{75/2187}{57/3552} = 2.14.$$

Taking this as the estimate of relative risk for all people is clearly inappropriate when applied to someone with a previous history of MI, since it goes in the wrong direction (increased rather than decreased risk). Another incorrect approach is to take the average of the two relative risks, by strata of previous MI status, as a measure of overall risk. The answer would then be (from Example 4.13)

$$\frac{2.40 + 0.64}{2} = 1.52,$$

which is very misleading when used for either previous MI group. It badly underestimates the relative risk for one subgroup and is in the wrong direction for the other.

Instead of giving main effects, we should state the estimates of effect for one risk factor separately for each stratum of the second. Hence, it is appropriate to carry out separate analyses for those with and without previous MI from Table 4.16. The relative risks, with 95% confidence intervals from (3.5)–(3.7) in parentheses, for smoking compared to non-smoking, are: for no previous MI, 2.40 (1.65, 3.47); for previous MI, 0.64 (0.28, 1.47).

Since unity lies in the second, but not the first, confidence interval we would conclude that smoking certainly seems to be a risk factor for a first MI, but the evidence for a protective effect after an initial MI is inconclusive. That is, there could be unilateralism rather than antagonism.

This is not the appropriate place to investigate the (apparently bizarre) change in effect of smoking. One obvious possibility is that there is some change in smoking habit subsequent to an MI, but before smoking habits are ascertained. The great weakness in the analysis here, chosen for its simplicity rather than its scientific completeness, is the absence of any consideration of lifetime tobacco consumption.

Unlike the treatment of other problems, we have not tried to *estimate* the effect of interaction. That is, no confidence intervals for the interaction (by whatever definition) have been given. This is because the fact of interaction is generally more important than its magnitude. The only exception is where statistical models are used, in which the interaction will be one (or a set) of the terms in the model. Even then, the practical interest in the magnitude of effect of the interaction will be its contribution to the stratum-specific effects of the factor: see Section 10.9 for an example.

## Exercises

4.1 The age-standardized mortality ratios for male doctors in England and Wales in 1982–83 were 57 for lung cancer, 115 for hepatic cirrhosis (a rough measure of alcohol abuse) and 172 for suicide (Rawnsley, 1991). These results take the national population as the standard (SMR = 100). Interpret these results and speculate as to their causes; consider why it was thought necessary to standardise for age.

4.2 In each of the following situations $F$ is the risk factor, $D$ is the study disease and $C$ is a third variable. In which cases could $C$ possibly be a confounder?

(i)  $F$ = regular use of mouthwashes
     $D$ = oral cancer
     $C$ = smoking

(ii) $F$ = smoking
     $D$ = lung cancer
     $C$ = yellow staining on teeth

(iii) $F$ = dental disease
     $D$ = cardiovascular disease
     $C$ = smoking

In the cases where $C$ could be a confounder, what prior evidence would convince you that $C$ really is worth considering as a likely confounder when designing a study to relate $F$ to $D$? Search the literature to locate previous publications that contain such evidence.

4.3 In a study of risk factors for a certain disease, smoking status and average daily fat consumption were recorded. Suppose that the relative risks for the combinations of smoking status and level of fat consumption (never smoking, low fat consumers = 1) were as given below:

| Fat consumption | Smoking status | | | |
|---|---|---|---|---|
| | Never | Ex | Light | Heavy |
| Low | 1 | 1.5 | 2.0 | 3.0 |
| Medium | 1.2 | 1.8 | 2.4 | 3.6 |
| High | 1.5 | 2.3 | 3.0 | 4.5 |
| Very high | 2.0 | 3.5 | 4.0 | 6.0 |

Risk is clearly accentuated by having a relatively 'high' value of the second risk factor, whatever the value of the first, so that those who are both very high fat consumers and heavy smokers are at most risk. Does the table suggest that one of the two variables might be confounded with the other? Does it suggest that fat consumption and smoking interact in their effect upon the disease?

4.4 This question is based on the following table of demographic data from Romania in 1993 (United Nations, 1996):

| Age group (years) | Population | | Deaths | |
|---|---|---|---|---|
| | Urban | Rural | Urban | Rural |
| 0–9 | 1 800 680 | 1 359 501 | 3 526 | 4 997 |
| 10–19 | 2 128 150 | 1 642 941 | 1 010 | 1 049 |
| 20–29 | 1 967 110 | 1 450 550 | 1 599 | 1 977 |
| 30–39 | 2 118 205 | 1 019 015 | 4 333 | 3 300 |
| 40–49 | 1 691 033 | 1 139 065 | 8 312 | 6 903 |
| 50–59 | 1 200 412 | 1 396 080 | 14 896 | 16 739 |
| 60–69 | 921 072 | 1 380 709 | 24 191 | 32 443 |
| 70–79 | 404 304 | 670 133 | 23 706 | 38 872 |
| 80 and above | 175 238 | 291 062 | 25 909 | 49 561 |

(i)   Find the crude death rates (per thousand) in urban and rural areas.

(ii)  Using the overall population as the standard, find the age-standardized death rates (per thousand) for both the rural and the urban areas using the direct method.

(iii) Using the overall population as the standard, find the standardized mortality ratios for urban and rural areas. Use these to find the indirect standardized death rates (per thousand).

(iv) Interpret your results.

4.5 Cole and MacMahon (1971) present the data given below from a case–control study of bladder cancer:

| High-risk occupation? | High cigarette consumption? | No. of cases | No. of controls |
|---|---|---|---|
| No | No | 43 | 94 |
| No | Yes | 173 | 189 |
| Yes | No | 26 | 20 |
| Yes | Yes | 111 | 72 |

(i)  Calculate the odds ratio for bladder cancer comparing high-risk to other occupations (ignoring cigarette consumption).
(ii)  Test the null hypothesis that the odds ratio is the same for those who work in high-risk and in other occupations.
(iii)  Calculate the Mantel–Haenszel odds ratio for high-risk versus other occupations, adjusted for cigarette consumption.
(iv)  Test the null hypothesis that the smoking-adjusted odds ratio is one.
(v)  Interpret your results.

4.6 Refer to the following table, which gives summary results derived from the north Glasgow male coronary event registration data presented in Table 4.11.

| | Deprivation group | | | |
|---|---|---|---|---|
| | I and II | | III and IV | |
| Age group (years) | Deaths | Coronaries | Deaths | Coronaries |
| 35–44 | 8 | 18 | 12 | 25 |
| 45–54 | 24 | 47 | 34 | 75 |
| 55–64 | 62 | 114 | 103 | 180 |

(i)    Find the age-specific risks of death for coronary cases from the two deprivation groups. Find their logarithms and plot them on a graph. Does the graph suggest that there may be an effect of age or deprivation group or any interaction between age and deprivation group?
(ii)   Find the relative risk (ignoring age) of a death for coronary cases in deprivation groups III and IV compared with I and II, together with the corresponding 95% confidence interval.
(iii)  Find the Mantel–Haenszel age-adjusted relative risk and confidence interval corresponding to (ii).
(iv)   Test whether there is any evidence of a difference in the age-specific relative risks between deprivation groups (that is, test for an age-deprivation group interaction using risks).
(v)    Repeat (ii) replacing 'relative risk' by 'odds ratio'.
(vi)   Repeat (iii) replacing 'relative risk' by 'odds ratio'.
(vii)  Repeat (iv) replacing 'relative risks' by 'odds ratios' and 'risks' by 'odds'.

(viii) Test for an effect of deprivation on the chance of death, ignoring age.

(ix)   Test for an effect of deprivation on the chance of death, adjusting for age.

(x)    Interpret your results.

4.7 Refer to the MONICA data of Table C.3.

(i)     Estimate the prevalence relative risk for high versus low factor IX.

(ii)    Find the Mantel–Haenszel sex-adjusted estimate of the prevalence relative risk (high versus low).

(iii)   Find the Mantel–Haenszel age-adjusted estimate of the prevalence relative risk (high versus low).

(iv)    Find the Mantel–Haenszel age/sex-adjusted estimate of the prevalence relative risk (high versus low). This requires taking the 10 age/sex groups as strata.

(v)     Test for an interaction between sex and factor IX in determining the risk of prevalent CVD.

(vi)    Test for an interaction between age and factor IX in determining the risk of prevalent CVD.

(vii)   Test for an interaction between age, sex and factor IX in determining the risk of prevalent CVD. This requires taking the 10 age/sex groups as strata.

(viii)–(xi)  Repeat (i)–(iv) replacing 'relative risk' by 'odds ratio'.

(xii)–(xiv)  Repeat (v)–(vii) replacing 'risk' by 'odds'.

(xv)    Interpret your results and summarize your conclusion about the effect of factor IX on prevalent CVD.

# 5

# Cohort studies

## 5.1 Design considerations

A **cohort, prospective** or **longitudinal** study is one in which individuals are followed up over time to monitor their health. The simplest approach is to select two groups of people at the start of the study, the **baseline**. One group consists of people who possess some special attribute which is thought to be a possible risk factor for a disease of interest, whilst the other group does not. Both groups are followed for a set period of time and the incidence of disease is compared between the groups. Hence, in a study of the hazards of working in the coal industry, a group of coal-miners and a second group of employees in other heavy industries might be selected at baseline. Both groups would then be monitored for (say) 10 years, after which time the incidence of (say) bronchitis is compared between the groups. The non-factor group (other heavy industries in the example) is included to act as a control group for purposes of comparison – that is, to enable the excess morbidity associated with the risk factor (coal-mining) to be found. Figure 5.1 gives a schematic representation of this type of cohort study.

Sometimes we may be able to study the entire population exposed to the risk factor, such as every person who was present in a factory at the time of a radiation leakage. Most often both groups will need to be sampled. When sampling, as always, we prefer to take random samples in order to avoid possible bias.

Ideally, everyone who enters the study should be free of the disease being studied. So, in the coal-mining example, only people without symptoms of bronchitis would be included at baseline. In this situation we may show that the hypothesized cause does indeed precede the effect. During the follow-up we shall be recording disease *incidence*.

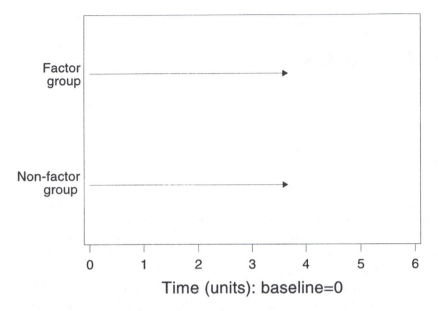

**Figure 5.1**   A representation of a cohort study.

*5.1.1   Advantages*

1. Cohort studies give direct information on the sequence of happenings. This is ideal for demonstrating causality.
2. Many diseases can be studied simultaneously. We do this by ensuring that we record episodes of all the required diseases during the follow-up.

*5.1.2   Disadvantages*

1. Cohort studies are often very expensive and time-consuming. This is because they typically require monitoring of a large set of subjects over a long time period.
2. They are not suitable for diseases with a long latency, since the time period for the study would then become unacceptably long. If, for example, young disease-free cigarette smokers and non-smokers were followed up to investigate lung cancer we might have to plan for at least a 20-year time horizon, in order to give the tumours time to grow and be identified.
3. Cohort studies are not suitable for rare diseases. If the disease is rare then we would either have to take an enormous baseline sample or have to

monitor for a very long time, both of which may be unacceptable. For instance, consider a disease which has an incidence rate of 5 cases per 100 000 population per year. Suppose we decide that we need around 100 cases before we can make any meaningful evaluation of the risk profile for the disease. We would then expect to need, for example, an initial cohort of 200 000 subjects if we wished to finish after 10 years. Alternatively, given an initial cohort of 40 000 subjects, we would expect to have to continue monitoring for 50 years!

4. There may be 'study effects'; that is, someone may act differently simply by virtue of being studied. For instance, some people may alter their dietary habits once they are entered into a study of smoking as a risk factor for heart disease, because they become more aware of current 'healthy eating' advice. This problem is reduced by the inclusion of a non-factor group, as is recommended, since this group would experience the same effects.

5. Exposure to the factor of interest may change, especially when the time horizon is long, for reasons unconnected with the investigation. The result is that someone initially classified to the factor group might have the attributes necessary to the non-factor group before the study is over. For instance, a smoker may quit within a few weeks of the baseline study and yet continue to be counted amongst the smokers in subsequent analyses. Provided that changes to risk factors are monitored, along with disease outcome, this can be accounted for by the person-years method of analysis (Section 5.6).

6. Withdrawals may occur. Provided that these are made for reasons unconnected with disease they may be accounted for using appropriate methods of analysis. Withdrawal and consequent loss to follow-up may, however, be a direct or indirect consequence of disease. Thus coal-miners with bronchitis may emigrate to a warmer climate in order to avoid further distress, or a smoker with lung cancer might commit suicide because of depression caused by the disease. In both examples the result would be to bias the conclusions in favour of the supposed risk factor, so that it seems to have less effect on disease than it does actually have.

7. The basic design only allows one risk factor to be studied. When several risk factors are of interest a more sensible approach is to use a single baseline sample (Section 5.1.3).

### 5.1.3    Alternative designs

As well as the basic design, there are many alternative types of cohort study, any of which may be preferable in a given situation. Several of the alternatives have economic advantages.

1. Omission of the non-factor group. This is not recommended since without parallel study of a control group we cannot judge whether any effects seen are due to the factor, study effects or simply 'background' effects such as air pollution.

2. Use of an external comparison group rather than a non-factor group. This has the advantage of studies of type 1, that only one group has to be monitored, whilst maintaining a comparative aspect. The external group is often the national population. For example, in a study of workers exposed to styrene in the reinforced plastics and composites industry, Wong (1990) calculated cause-specific death rates for a cohort of workers and compared these with routine statistics for the USA. The major difficulty with this approach is the possibility of bias. Routine statistics may not be complete (even in the USA) and are unlikely to be as detailed as the information collected on the cohort. Study effects could also cause differential bias. One important difference with this design is that *rates*, rather than risks, are generally the basic unit of measurement. As such, it requires a special approach to analysis; we defer discussion of this until Section 5.6.

3. A single baseline sample is used to define the factor and non-factor groups. This is a very common design used, for example, in the Scottish Heart Health Study (SHHS). As explained in Section 2.2.1, at baseline a random sample of Scottish men and women were sampled and invited to complete a questionnaire and attend at a screening clinic. Consequently information on several possible risk factors for coronary heart disease was obtained which could then be used to subdivide the sample in several ways – for example by baseline smoking status (current smoker/non-smoker) and parental history of coronary heart disease (yes/no). When the cohort was followed up over time relative risks etc. were calculated for each individual risk factor (as well as combinations), as already seen in several examples in Chapter 4. More examples follow in this and later chapters. One extra advantage of this design is that, provided the sample is randomly selected, an estimate of the prevalence of the risk factor is also obtained (for example, the percentage of people who are current smokers at baseline). This is necessary in order to obtain a direct estimate of the attributable risk (Section 3.7).

4. Mortality, rather than morbidity, is the outcome recorded. As already mentioned, this was the method used by Wong (1990), whose major aim was to study the relationship between exposure to styrene and cancer. Death is a sensible outcome measure here, but would not be should diseases which rarely lead to death, such as skin disorders, be of major interest. The disadvantage of only recording deaths is that the number of positive

outcomes found is smaller (or at least, no bigger) than when episodes of sickness are used. This means that either a larger cohort or a longer time horizon needs to be used to identify the same number of positive outcomes. Clearly there could also be important differences between relationships of risk factors with morbidity and mortality, since the latter represents the extreme. The SHHS recorded both types of outcome.

5. Event notification arises from routine statistics, rather than special observation. As mentioned for studies of type 2, routine statistics (such as death registrations, hospital patient administration systems and disease registers) may be incomplete or insufficiently detailed. There may also be substantial loss to follow-up through migration. Even so, this is likely to be the only viable method of monitoring in a large study. Provided that the factor and non-factor groups experience equal problems, this method is sound. In the SHHS the cohort was monitored by having each member flagged by the Registrar General for Scotland. Whenever a member died the death certificate was copied and sent to the study team for analysis. The cohort was also followed up for coronary morbidity by linking hospital in-patient records for patients with chosen diagnoses to the SHHS database (linking by name, age, sex and address).

6. Retrospective cohort studies. Sometimes it is possible to trace the cohort backwards in time to ascertain risk factor status some years before. This method is attractive since it does not involve having to wait for years before the study is complete. It is, however, essential to have complete and accurate records for the method to give unbiased results. For example, it would not be sensible to study the hazards of smoking by asking a sample of people to recall their smoking habits 10 years ago and then comparing morbidity between people who were smokers and non-smokers at that time. Besides problems of accurate recall, we would expect that a greater proportion of those who smoked 10 years ago will already have died. Retrospective cohort studies are frequently used in studies of occupational mortality, including the study already cited by Wong (1990).

7. Comparison of several groups. Although we have only considered two groups so far, the cohort method is unrestricted in the number of groups involved. Hence in a study of smoking we could define three groups, 'current smoker', 'ex-smoker' and 'never-smoker'. Indeed the risk factor could be continuous, when recorded from a single baseline sample. Studies of type 3 allow different risk factors, in different formats, to be analysed.

We conclude this section with an example of a cohort study. This falls into category 3 above. Note the size, scope and longevity of this study, which is typical of cohort investigations based in the community.

*Example 5.1*   The Avon Longitudinal Study of Pregnancy and Childhood (ALSPAC) is a cohort study of all pregnancies amongst women resident in three English health districts, with expected delivery dates between 1 April 1991 and 31 December 1992. The study recruited 14 893 pregnancies, leading to 14 210 surviving children. This builds on previous national studies (of 1946, 1958 and 1970 birth cohorts) and is part of a European network of similar studies (ALSPAC, 1995).

The ALSPAC protocol requires collection of information from the subjects, on average, every 4 months, until the children reach the age of 7. Information is gathered from a number of sources, including self-completion questionnaires given to mothers and fathers, hospital and other health records and biological samples from mother and/or child (urine, blood, teeth, hair, nails and placenta). When the child is aged 7 he or she will be invited to a clinic where detailed assessments of growth, vision, hearing and other faculties will be made. Thereafter it is hoped to follow the child through to adulthood.

The study aims to investigate various factors that may be associated with the development of children and the well-being of parents and their offspring – for example, the physical and emotional effects of twin pregnancies (Thorpe *et al.*, 1995) and the effects of maternal smoking on birthweight (Passaro *et al.*, 1996).

## 5.2   Analytical considerations

### 5.2.1   Concurrent follow-up

If everyone in the cohort starts at the same time and is followed up for the same length of time (or, at least, until the event of interest occurs) then analysis may proceed as in Chapter 3, taking account of confounding and interaction as necessary, as explained in Chapter 4. This is the **fixed cohort** situation, and is relatively easy to deal with. Sections 5.2.2–5.2.5 will consider situations where the opposite, the **variable cohort** situation, occurs. This is where the set of individuals at risk changes during the study for reasons other than loss due to qualifying events.

Even with a fixed cohort, the simple analyses of risk based, for example, on relative risks have the disadvantage that they cannot differentiate between short- and long-term effects. This would be a problem, for instance, should a high blood pressure at age 50 be a risk factor for all-causes mortality (death from any cause) in the first few years, but not a noticeable risk in the review made after 30 years of follow-up. Of course everyone must die eventually, so that relative risks for death must inevitably tend to unity as follow-up time increases.

An alternative approach is to carry out a **survival analysis**, which is a simultaneous analysis of progress for different durations of follow-up: the times of events are analysed rather than the mere fact of the events. Survival analysis is ideal for the variable cohort situation. Note that the word 'survival' here does not necessarily relate to lack of death; it could mean failure to become diseased. In general, 'survival' means lack of experience of the event of interest. We shall develop the basic ideas of survival analysis in Section 5.3. A further alternative, based upon the person-years of experience of the cohort, is described in Section 5.6.

### 5.2.2   Moving baseline dates

Sometimes recruitment into a study is not simultaneous, but happens over a period of time. For instance, in the SHHS follow-up was recorded from the day the individual attended a clinic, where blood pressure, height, weight, etc. were recorded (Section 2.2.1). The nurses who administered these clinics had to travel to different parts of Scotland; hence subjects from different parts of the country had different baseline dates. Indeed, there were 35 months between the first and last clinic sessions.

The usual way to deal with this problem is simply to ignore it: follow-up is measured as elapsed time since baseline, using a different starting point for each subject. This assumes that any effects are homogeneous (unchanged) with respect to calendar time. Provided that the baseline dates do not vary greatly, this is usually a reasonable assumption: see Section 5.7 for further discussion.

### 5.2.3   Varying follow-up durations

As just noted, baseline calendar times may vary. Conversely, the calendar time at which evaluation of effects is made will generally be the same for each member of the cohort. There may, therefore, be varying lengths of follow-up. For example, the paper by Tunstall-Pedoe et al. (1997), which is the source of information about the follow-up in the SHHS used here, described coronary events (hospital diagnosis of myocardial infarction, coronary artery surgery or death) for every member of the SHHS cohort up to the last day of 1993. At this date, elapsed follow-up time since baseline varied from 9.1 years for the earliest recruits (November 1984 to December 1993) to 6.2 years for the last recruits (October 1987 to December 1993). The mean elapsed time was 7.7 years. Notice that elapsed time here is *potential* follow-up time: some individuals will have early termination due, for example, to coronary death.

There are three ways in which we could seek to use the simple risk analyses of Chapter 3 in this situation. In each case we seek to treat the study as that of a fixed cohort. The first is to analyse only those with complete (potential) follow-up. This is wasteful of information, and not acceptable unless the wastage is only marginal.

The second is to perform a simple risk analysis for all events up to, but not exceeding, the minimum elapsed time. In the SHHS this is 6.2 years. For ease of interpretation this might be rounded down to some convenient value. Thus Examples 3.13, 4.3 and 4.13 (and their extensions) all used the first 6 years of observation in the SHHS. This approach is fine for providing simple examples that are easy to interpret, but is unsatisfactory as a definitive analysis of risk. Again, this is because it wastes information. For instance, those people known to have had their first coronary event in their seventh, eighth or ninth year of study would, nevertheless, be counted as disease-free in the 6-year follow-up analysis.

The third method uses this extra information by simply ignoring the variation in follow-up durations. That is, we record each individual as either disease positive or negative during his or her follow-up, and proceed as in Chapter 3. Of course, this means that some people will have had rather longer to experience their event; thus, all else being equal, they have more chance of an event than those with shorter follow-ups. This should not cause a problem provided that the time homogeneity assumption is satisfied (which generally requires the variation in follow-up to be small) and that the length of follow-up is not related to the risk factor being studied.

As an example of where a problem could occur, consider the analysis of coronary risk by housing tenure status (owner-occupiers versus renters) in the SHHS. As explained in Section 5.2.2, the date of entry into the SHHS varies with the location of the local clinic. Consequently the elapsed follow-up time, up to the end of 1993, varies by the area of residence of the subject. Suppose that, by chance, early recruitment was made in areas where rented accommodation is far more common than is the norm in Scotland. Renters will then tend to have been observed for longer periods of follow-up, and thus have more chance of an event, all else being equal. The analysis, based upon the assumption of a fixed cohort, would then be biased against renters.

In fact no such problems of bias have been noted in the SHHS data. Consequently, analysis of varying follow-up periods will be used for these data as illustrations in Chapter 10, where statistical models for the situations of Chapter 3 are presented. Nevertheless, this is not the preferred method of dealing with varying follow-ups; survival analysis is better because it removes the chance of bias. Published accounts of the SHHS follow-up use survival analysis for this and other reasons.

Since survival analysis considers risk during successive duration intervals, it can easily deal with varying follow-ups. For instance, someone who joins a study only two years before its closure can provide information for risk calculation in the first and second but not in subsequent years. Separating out the years in this way makes it unimportant that the number at risk (the denominator in the risk calculation) varies by year.

Anyone who has not yet experienced an event but has a follow-up time that is less than the maximum possible is said to be **censored**; the data supplied by such a person are **censored data**. So in a study of the 20-year risk of working in the coal-mining industry that finishes today, someone who started work 10 years ago and is still in good health has been censored. Notice that censoring can only occur for people who have yet to experience an event. Even someone recruited only a few days before the study ends will be uncensored should he or she have had an event, such as the illness under study, in the few available days. When the study is effectively open-ended, so that there is no predetermined maximum follow-up time, all subjects who have no recorded event at the time of review are censored. This is so in the SHHS example; live subjects continued to be followed up after the review date of 31 December 1993 used in Tunstall-Pedoe *et al.* (1997) and here.

### 5.2.4    Withdrawals

As noted in Section 5.1.2, **withdrawals** are a possible complication. Withdrawals are people who are lost to follow-up before experiencing an event. Their duration of study (the length of time they were at risk of an event) will be less than the difference between the dates of the end of the study and their entry. We cannot know whether they would have had an event should they have lasted for their complete possible follow-up duration.

For example, in the SHHS withdrawals occur when a study member leaves the United Kingdom. Figure 5.2 illustrates the progress of SHHS subjects from their baseline (in 1984, 1985, 1986 or 1987) to the 'closing date' of 31 December 1993. For any year of entry, some individuals will experience an event before the closing date, some will still be event-free survivors at the closing date (censored) and some will have left the UK before the closing date (withdrawn). Each line represents a representative subject from a specific year of entry and, for simplicity, each representative is shown as entering in mid-year.

Let us suppose that the withdrawal happened for reasons not associated with the disease of interest – for instance, a subject who left the study environment in order to take up a promotion at work. If we choose to analyse the cohort data using simple risk analyses, as in Chapter 3, in the presence of withdrawals, we clearly cannot treat the withdrawals as event-positive. We have two choices: either we ignore the withdrawals altogether or we include them amongst those negative for the event. In the former case we will ignore the known information that they survived for some time without an event, and thus tend to

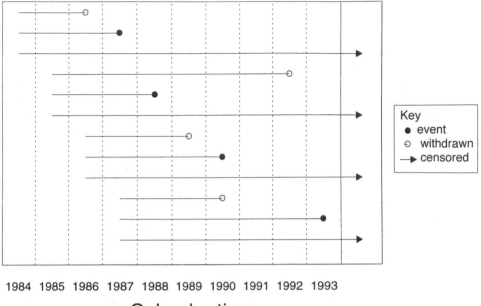

1984  1985  1986  1987  1988  1989  1990  1991  1992  1993

## Calendar time

**Figure 5.2**   Follow-up periods in the SHHS.

overestimate the risk. In the latter we ignore the fact that they could have gone on to experience an event had they been fully followed up, and thus tend to underestimate the risk. Thus neither choice is ideal. Simple risk analysis will only be acceptable if the number of withdrawals is small – for instance, in the SHHS where only 14 of the 11 629 subjects were withdrawals.

Assuming that the reason for withdrawal is unimportant, the problem of withdrawals is very similar to that of variable follow-up durations. Hence, withdrawals may be treated as censored subjects in a survival analysis, as we shall do for data from the SHHS. Should withdrawal occur for some reason connected with the outcome of interest, as in the bronchitis example in Section 5.1.2 (migration due to illness), then withdrawal should be counted as a positive event.

If withdrawal is related to the risk factor, but not the outcome variable, this does not invalidate the analysis, but may suggest that the outcome measure is insubstantial. For instance, if many people leave the coal-mining industry, but not other industries, due to heart disease, then the study of bronchitis introduced in Section 5.1, which treats such withdrawals as censored, would still be valid but might not be the most useful study of occupational risk for miners.

### 5.2.5   Competing causes of failure

Although the cohort study may be designed to study only one disease – for example, heart disease – follow-up may be terminated through death which is due to an alternative condition, for example cancer. In a sense, heart disease and cancer are then **competing risks**. The simplest way to deal with an alternative, competing cause is to treat those who 'fail' due to this cause as withdrawals. They would thus be treated like any other censored subjects. This only makes sense provided the competing cause is independent of the disease under study. We shall adopt this simple procedure when dealing with SHHS data in this and subsequent chapters. More complex procedures are possible, and have the advantage of allowing valid comparisons between the competing causes (for example, see Lunn and McNeil, 1995), but they are beyond our current scope.

## 5.3   Cohort life tables

A **cohort life table**, which will simply be called a life table here, is a tabular presentation of the progress of a cohort through time. To construct the life table, the first step is to divide the entire follow-up period into consecutive intervals of time. Then calculate the following quantities: $n_t$ the number of survivors at time $t$; $e_t$ the number of events in the study interval that begins at time $t$; $p_t$ the estimated probability of surviving the entire study interval that begins at $t$; $q_t$ the estimated probability of an event of interest (or **failure**) during the study interval that begins at $t$; and $s_t$ the estimated probability of surviving from baseline to the end of the study interval that begins at $t$. Taking baseline to be time 0, then $n_0$ will be the total number of subjects in the study. As explained in Section 5.2.1, 'survival' is a general term meaning absence of experience of the event of interest. In many instances the event of interest will be death, whence survival will have the most straightforward interpretation. Notice that the intervals of time need not be equal in length, although they will be in the next few examples.

All the $n$ and $e$ results come from observation. The $q$ values are risks and so, by (3.1) or simple logic,

$$q_t = e_t/n_t. \tag{5.1}$$

Since surviving is the complement to experiencing an event,

$$p_t = 1 - q_t. \tag{5.2}$$

Finally, since each $p$ value gives the estimated probability of survival during a particular interval (indexed by $t$) the estimated probability of complete, or **cumulative**, survival from baseline to the end of a given interval will be the product of all $p$ values up to and including that for the given interval. That is,

$$s_t = p_0 p_1 p_2 \cdots p_t. \tag{5.3}$$

When the event of interest is an attack of the disease that is not necessarily fatal, it will be possible for any one individual to suffer more than one event during follow-up. Then the word 'event' in all the above will be taken to refer to the first event. Once an individual has an event, he or she is immediately treated as a non-survivor. For example, when analysing coronary events in the SHHS, someone who has a hospital diagnosis of myocardial infarction after 26 months' follow-up, but dies of a subsequent heart attack some months later, would nevertheless have a completed survival time of 26 months.

*Example 5.2* A cohort of 1000 men at high risk of disease, but currently disease-free, is recruited. In the first year of study 5 of the men are newly diagnosed with the disease. In the second year a further 10; in the third year 20; in the fourth year 35; and in the fifth year 50 new cases are identified. The resultant life table, employing (5.1)–(5.3), is given in Table 5.1.
. From this table we see that the estimated probability of survival for five years is 0.88. This could well be the most useful single outcome measure for the study. Notice that we could get this in a straightforward manner from the $n$ column: 880 survivors at time 5 compared with 1000 at time 0 gives an estimated five-year survival probability of 880/1000 = 0.88.

Figure 5.3 shows the estimated cumulative survival probability, $s_t$, for the data in Table 5.1, plotted against time: a graph of the estimated **survival function**, or a **survival plot**. This is a **step function**; that is, it moves in discrete steps rather than in a smooth curve. As a consequence, the chance of survival to a point which is intermediate to those enumerated in the life table will be

**Table 5.1**  Life table for a hypothetical cohort

| Time (t) | No. free of disease (n) | No. of events (e) | Interval risk (q) | Interval survival (p) | Cumulative survival (s) |
|---|---|---|---|---|---|
| 0 | 1000 | 5 | 0.0050 | 0.9950 | 0.9950 |
| 1 | 995 | 10 | 0.0100 | 0.9899 | 0.9850 |
| 2 | 985 | 20 | 0.0203 | 0.9797 | 0.9650 |
| 3 | 965 | 35 | 0.0363 | 0.9637 | 0.9300 |
| 4 | 930 | 50 | 0.0538 | 0.9462 | 0.8800 |
| 5 | 880 | | | | |

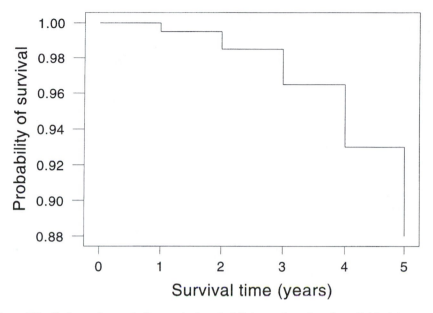

**Figure 5.3**  Estimated cumulative survival probabilities against time from Table 5.1.

estimated to be equal to that chance evaluated at the previous life table time cut-point. Thus the estimated chance of survival for 2.5 years is taken as equal to the estimated chance of survival for 2 years, 0.9850. The steps in a survival plot must always be in a downward direction since the chance of survival cannot increase with time.

Notice that $s_t$ is not plotted against $t$, but rather against the value of the next time cut-point. This is because $s_t$ is the estimated probability of survival up to the end of the interval beginning at time $t$. By definition, the probability of survival to time 0 is unity.

### 5.3.1   Allowing for sampling variation

We can estimate the standard error of the interval-specific risks by using (3.3):

$$\hat{se}(p_t) = \sqrt{p_t(1 - p_t)/n_t}.$$

Similarly,

$$\hat{se}(q_t) = \sqrt{q_t(1 - q_t)/n_t}.$$

Further inferences on these interval-specific probabilities follow from Section 2.5.2.

We can estimate the standard error of the cumulative survival probability (Greenwood, 1926) as

$$\hat{se}(s_t) = s_t \sqrt{\sum_{i=0}^{t} \frac{q_i}{n_i - e_i}}, \tag{5.4}$$

from which an approximate 95% confidence interval (using a normal approximation) for cumulative survival from baseline to the end of the interval that begins at time $t$ is

$$s_t \pm 1.96\hat{se}(s_t). \tag{5.5}$$

*Example 5.3*   The estimated standard error of the estimated 5-year survival probability in Example 5.2 is, from (5.4),

$$\hat{se}(s_4) = s_4 \sqrt{\sum_{i=0}^{4} \frac{q_i}{n_i - e_i}} = 0.88 \sqrt{\frac{0.0050}{995} + \frac{0.0100}{985} + \frac{0.0203}{965} + \frac{0.0363}{930} + \frac{0.0538}{880}}$$

$$= 0.01028.$$

Hence, from (5.5) and Table 5.1, the approximate 95% confidence interval for survival up to 5 years is

$$0.8800 \pm 1.96 \times 0.01028,$$

that is, $0.8800 \pm 0.0201$ or $(0.8599, 0.9001)$.

We are 95% sure that the interval from about 0.86 to 0.90 contains the true probability of surviving for 5 years.

An approximate test of the null hypothesis that the cumulative survival probability is $s$, where $s$ is some preconceived value, comes from comparing

$$\left\{\frac{s_t - s}{\hat{se}(s_t)}\right\}^2 \tag{5.6}$$

to chi-square with 1 d.f.

### 5.3.2   Allowing for censoring

As explained in Section 5.2, subjects may be lost to follow-up for various reasons. Here we shall not distinguish between these causes, but will take them all into the single category of censored individuals. For instance, Table 5.2 shows the results of follow-up for a selected subset of men in the SHHS. This subset consists of men who were free of coronary disease and had known category of housing tenure at baseline; housing tenure will be used to define subgroups in subsequent examples. Follow-up has been subdivided into whole-year intervals from baseline. As Figure 5.2 shows, the calendar date of baseline

**Table 5.2**  Number of men experiencing a CHD event or being censored by period of observation, SHHS selected subset

| Period of follow-up (years) | Censored | Events | Total |
|---|---|---|---|
| 0 but less than 1 | 7 | 17 | 24 |
| 1 but less than 2 | 12 | 22 | 34 |
| 2 but less than 3 | 24 | 26 | 50 |
| 3 but less than 4 | 19 | 23 | 42 |
| 4 but less than 5 | 21 | 37 | 58 |
| 5 but less than 6 | 15 | 38 | 53 |
| 6 but less than 7 | 501 | 31 | 532 |
| 7 but less than 8 | 2143 | 20 | 2163 |
| 8 but less than 9 | 1375 | 5 | 1380 |
| 9 but less than 10 | 66 | 0 | 66 |
| Total | 4183 | 219 | 4402 |

varies by individual and the maximum possible completed follow-up time, from baseline to study end at 31 December 1993, is less than 10 years.

There are several ways of adapting the basic life table approach to allow for withdrawals. Consider the first interval in Table 5.2. The 7 men censored before a single completed year of follow-up could all have been lost at the beginning. Since 4402 men were recruited in all, this would lead to an estimated failure probability of $17/(4402 - 7) = 0.003868$ in this year, using (5.1). If, instead, the 7 men all left at the end of the first year the appropriate estimated failure probability would be $17/4402 = 0.003862$. Clearly the truth lies somewhere in-between these two extremes. A reasonable approximation is to subtract only half the number censored from the raw denominator, 4402. That is, we take the estimated failure probability to be $17/(4402 - 3.5) = 0.003865$.

A general formula for this censoring-adjusted estimated failure probability is

$$q_t = e_t/n_t^*  \tag{5.7}$$

where

$$n_t^* = n_t - \tfrac{1}{2}c_t  \tag{5.8}$$

and $c_t$ is the number censored during the interval which begins at time $t$. When (5.8) is used, the life table method is called the **actuarial method** for survival data. Using (5.7), the procedures described by (5.2) and (5.3) are still valid for this new situation; (5.4) becomes

$$\hat{\mathrm{se}}(s_t) = s_t \sqrt{\sum_{i=0}^{t} \frac{q_t}{n_t^* - e_t}} \tag{5.9}$$

and (5.5) and (5.6) are still valid.

*Example 5.4*    Table 5.3 is the life table for SHHS men using the data in Table 5.2 and, consecutively, (5.8), (5.7), (5.2), (5.3) and (5.9). The $n_t^*$ values are given in the 'adjusted number' column. Figure 5.4 shows the estimated cumulative survival probabilities from Table 5.3, together with 95% confidence intervals calculated from (5.5).

As in Example 5.2, a useful summary measure for the life table is the longest possible survival probability: here the probability of survival for 9 years, estimated as 0.941081. Notice that this is not the same as the total number of men who have not experienced an event divided by the total number studied, $4183/4402 = 0.950250$, since the latter takes no account of loss to follow-up. Now the intermediate life table values *are* required to produce an appropriate measure of overall survival.

### 5.3.3    Comparison of two life tables

As discussed in Section 5.1, cohort studies are much more useful if they involve an element of comparison. Life tables can be constructed for each subgroup of

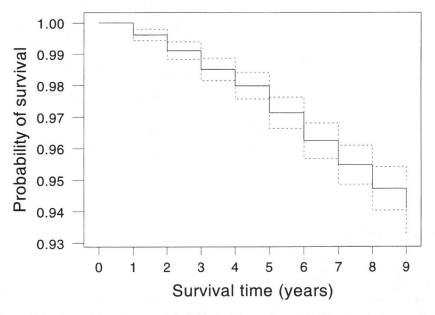

**Figure 5.4**    Actuarial estimates and 95% confidence intervals for cumulative survival probabilities of coronary events; selected subset of SHHS men.

**Table 5.3** Life table for coronary events, selected subset of SHHS men

| Time (years) | Number | Censored | Adjusted number | Events | Interval risk | Interval survival | Cumulative survival probability Estimate | Cumulative survival probability Standard error |
|---|---|---|---|---|---|---|---|---|
| 0 | 4402 | 7 | 4398.5 | 17 | 0.003 865 | 0.996 135 | 0.996 135 | 0.000 935 6 |
| 1 | 4378 | 12 | 4372.0 | 22 | 0.005 032 | 0.994 968 | 0.991 122 | 0.001 415 2 |
| 2 | 4344 | 24 | 4332.0 | 26 | 0.006 002 | 0.993 998 | 0.985 174 | 0.001 825 3 |
| 3 | 4294 | 19 | 4284.5 | 23 | 0.005 368 | 0.994 632 | 0.979 885 | 0.002 122 6 |
| 4 | 4252 | 21 | 4241.5 | 37 | 0.008 723 | 0.991 277 | 0.971 337 | 0.002 526 8 |
| 5 | 4194 | 15 | 4186.5 | 38 | 0.009 077 | 0.990 923 | 0.962 521 | 0.002 880 4 |
| 6 | 4141 | 501 | 3890.5 | 31 | 0.007 968 | 0.992 032 | 0.954 851 | 0.003 169 7 |
| 7 | 3609 | 2143 | 2537.5 | 20 | 0.007 882 | 0.992 118 | 0.947 325 | 0.003 563 6 |
| 8 | 1446 | 1375 | 758.5 | 5 | 0.006 592 | 0.993 408 | 0.941 081 | 0.004 503 3 |
| 9 | 66 | 66 | | 0 | | | | |

the cohort and the survival experiences compared by graphical, or more formal, methods. In Section 5.5 we shall develop a global test for the comparison of survival; here we shall restrict ourselves to comparing two specific survival probabilities, one from each of the two subgroups.

The standard error of the difference between two cumulative survival probabilities, $s_t^{(1)}$ and $s_t^{(2)}$, is estimated as

$$\hat{se}\left(s_t^{(1)} - s_t^{(2)}\right) = \sqrt{\hat{se}\left(s_t^{(1)}\right)^2 + \hat{se}\left(s_t^{(2)}\right)^2},\tag{5.10}$$

leading to an approximate 95% confidence interval for the true difference of

$$s_t^{(1)} - s_t^{(2)} \pm 1.96\hat{se}\left(s_t^{(1)} - s_t^{(2)}\right).\tag{5.11}$$

An approximate test of the null hypothesis that the two survival probabilities are equal is given by comparing

$$\left\{\frac{s_t^{(1)} - s_t^{(2)}}{\hat{se}(s_t^{(1)} - s_t^{(2)})}\right\}^2\tag{5.12}$$

to chi-square with 1 d.f.

*Example 5.5*  The data of Table 5.2 were disaggregated by housing tenure status, and separate life tables were constructed for owner-occupiers and renters. The essential results are shown in Table 5.4, from which Figure 5.5 was drawn to compare the two survival functions pictorially. The chance of survival without a coronary event is greatest in the owner-occupier group at all times. This agrees with, but adds to, the finding of Example 4.3: those who live in rented accommodation (predominantly those of lower social status in Scotland) are more likely to experience CHD.

We might wish to compare 9-year survival to see whether the observed difference is statistically significant. Using (5.10), the test statistic (5.12) becomes,

$$\frac{(0.949563 - 0.929946)^2}{0.0057661^2 + 0.0071534^2} = 4.56.$$

From Table B.3 this result is significant at the 5% level of significance ($0.05 > p > 0.025$). Hence there is evidence of a real difference.

Suppose that, for some reason, 5-year survival was of key interest. An approximate 95% confidence interval for the difference in the probability of survival for 5 years for owner-occupiers compared with renters is, from (5.10) and (5.11),

$$0.977287 - 0.963597 \pm 1.96\sqrt{0.0030006^2 + 0.0043024^2}$$

that is, $0.01369 \pm 0.01028$ or $(0.00341, 0.02397)$.

Figure 5.6 shows the difference in estimated survival probabilities up to each whole number of years of survival. In this instance 99% confidence intervals for this difference are shown. Recall that, as in other cases based upon the normal distribution, we can make the formula for a 95% confidence interval into one for an alternative percentage of confidence by

**Table 5.4**  Extract from life tables for SHHS men living in owner-occupied and rented accommodation

| Time (years) | Owner-occupiers | | | Cumulative survival probability | | Renters | | | Cumulative survival probability | |
| --- | --- | --- | --- | --- | --- | --- | --- | --- | --- | --- |
| | Number | Censored | Events | Estimate | Standard error | Number | Censored | Events | Estimate | Standard error |
| 0 | 2482 | 2 | 8 | 0.996 776 | 0.001 138 2 | 1920 | 5 | 9 | 0.995 306 | 0.001 560 9 |
| 1 | 2472 | 5 | 12 | 0.991 932 | 0.001 796 8 | 1906 | 7 | 10 | 0.990 075 | 0.002 265 7 |
| 2 | 2455 | 10 | 11 | 0.987 478 | 0.002 234 9 | 1889 | 14 | 15 | 0.982 184 | 0.003 028 2 |
| 3 | 2434 | 9 | 8 | 0.984 227 | 0.002 505 8 | 1860 | 10 | 15 | 0.974 241 | 0.003 632 3 |
| 4 | 2417 | 12 | 17 | 0.977 287 | 0.003 000 6 | 1835 | 9 | 20 | 0.963 597 | 0.004 302 4 |
| 5 | 2388 | 4 | 21 | 0.968 686 | 0.003 512 6 | 1806 | 11 | 17 | 0.954 499 | 0.004 794 3 |
| 6 | 2363 | 247 | 15 | 0.962 197 | 0.003 867 9 | 1778 | 254 | 16 | 0.945 249 | 0.005 276 2 |
| 7 | 2101 | 1286 | 9 | 0.956 258 | 0.004 321 2 | 1508 | 857 | 11 | 0.935 617 | 0.005 968 4 |
| 8 | 806 | 755 | 3 | 0.949 563 | 0.005 766 1 | 640 | 620 | 2 | 0.929 946 | 0.007 153 4 |
| 9 | 48 | 48 | 0 | | | 18 | 18 | 0 | | |

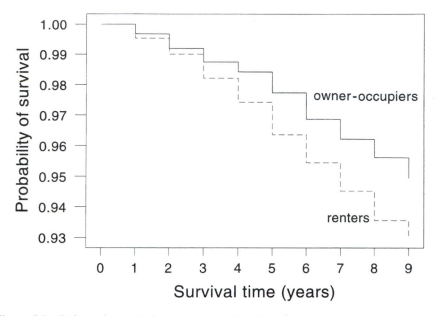

**Figure 5.5** Estimated cumulative survival probabilities for coronary events comparing owner-occupiers (solid line) and renters (dashed line), SHHS men.

replacing the two-sided 5% critical value, 1.96, with the appropriate alternative – here 2.5758, the 1% critical value (see Table B.2).

The difference in survival always favours owner-occupiers and tends to increase with time. Confidence limits also grow wider with time. Since there are few events and many censored at that time, we should expect the considerable lack of precision in the final year that the figure shows.

### 5.3.4    Limitations

We have already noted that the life table approach produces a step function, leading to consequent overestimation of survival probabilities at points intermediate to the cut-points that define the life table intervals. This suggests that it will be better to choose small intervals whenever several specific probabilities are likely to be of interest.

For each interval in the life table, the actuarial approach used to produce (5.7) assumes that the number of events amongst $n_t - c_t$ people who are at risk for the entire interval and $c_t$ people who are at risk for part of the interval is equal to the expected number of events from $n_t - \frac{1}{2}c_t$ people who are at risk for the entire interval. This will be accurate if the average time to censoring is half

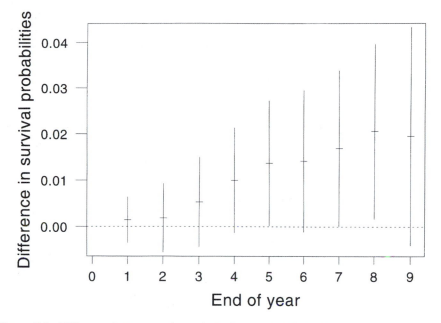

**Figure 5.6**   Difference between estimated survival probabilities for owner-occupiers and renters by year of follow-up; SHSS men.

the length of the interval, which would be true if censoring occurs uniformly within the interval, and if the risk of an event in any small time period is constant throughout the interval.

In some situations the approximation is not reasonable because either or both of these conditions are known to be violated. It may be that the average time to censoring is not half-way through the interval. Perhaps, for example, it is two-thirds of the way through. In this case we adjust (5.8) accordingly: here to

$$n_t^* = n_t - \tfrac{1}{3}c_t.$$

In general, we might prefer to use

$$n_t^* = n_t - (1 - a_t)c_t, \tag{5.13}$$

where $a_t$ is the average proportion of the interval that is survived before censoring occurs, for the interval that begins at time $t$. Sometimes $a_t$ will be unknown and a value of 0.5, leading to (5.8), will be the best 'guess'. If the interval length is small then the number censored, $c_t$, is unlikely to be large and hence the choice of value for $a_t$ in the general expression, (5.13), is unlikely to be important. Notice that this is certainly not the case in Examples 5.4 and 5.5 where there are hundreds censored in the seventh, eighth and ninth years of follow-up.

Alternatively, it may be that the risk of an event in, say, any single day increases (or decreases) as a person progresses through the interval defined by the life table. Consider a whole human life-span represented by 10-year intervals in a life table. During the first 10 years the instantaneous risk of death decreases rapidly, particularly during the first year as the baby develops in strength. During the last 10 years of life the instantaneous risk of death will increase as the elderly person becomes frailer with ageing. A child leaving the study, say, half-way through the 10-year interval will have already experienced the most vulnerable period. Using (5.7) with (5.8) will then overestimate the risk of death. Similarly, we can expect underestimates when censoring occurs in the final 10-year interval.

To avoid such problems, small intervals are recommended (again). Then the exact time at which withdrawals occur will not be crucial to the approximation, and instantaneous risk is unlikely to vary substantially within any of the intervals. Small intervals may only be required at survival durations where censoring is common or where risk is known to be changing rapidly.

## 5.4   Kaplan–Meier estimation

The **Kaplan–Meier** (KM) or **product-limit** approach to estimating the survival function (Kaplan and Meier, 1958) provides a response to the limitations of the standard life table identified in Section 5.3.4. In the KM approach the observed event times for the cohort being studied define the values of $t$ at which $s_t$ is evaluated; in the life table approach these values are usually set in advance of data collection. The KM approach leads to a life table with the smallest possible intervals. This uses the maximum amount of information in the data, ensuring that the steps in $s_t$ are as small as possible. Furthermore, the possible problems concerned with withdrawals are minimized. The only disadvantages are that the KM approach requires more (usually much more) computation and produces a less useful tabular display.

Essentially, KM estimation is life table estimation with the life table times (cut-points used to define the intervals) taken to be equal to the times of events in the cohort. Thus, with no censoring, (5.1)–(5.6) are still valid. However, in the presence of censoring (5.1) and (5.4) are used rather than (5.7) and (5.9) , or any other adjusted formula. As already mentioned, the choice of approximation used to deal with censoring is unlikely to be important when the intervals in the equivalent life table are small. The procedures for comparing cumulative survival probabilities given in Section 5.3.3 are also applicable, including (5.10)–(5.12).

Applying the KM methodology to the SHHS data analysed in Example 5.4 leads to a presentational problem: the resultant life table will be huge because there are hundreds of events. Instead we shall, for illustrative purposes, go through the calculations for the first year of follow-up (up to 365 days from a subject's baseline) only.

*Example 5.6*   During the first year of follow-up in the SHHS the completed survival times (in days) for the male subset defined in Section 5.3.2 were:

$$1, 46, 91^*, 101, 101, 103, 119, 133^*, 137, 145^*, 156, 186^*,$$
$$208, 215, 235, 242, 251, 294, 299, 300, 309^*, 312, 336^*, 357^*.$$

Here * denotes a censored observation (others are event times). A schematic representation of the loss to follow-up in year 1 is given by Figure 5.7. Note the double event at time 101.

The KM estimates of the survival function and their estimated standard errors are given in Table 5.5 (from Table 5.3 we already know that there were 4402 men at baseline). There were 17 coronary events during the year, two of which occurred on the same day of follow-up. Hence, excluding the start and end rows, there are 18 rows in Table 5.5. The seven censoring times do not define a row of the table, but the loss due to censoring must be accounted for when determining the number who survive to each specified time. Thus, for example, since 4401 survived to 46 days, then one man experienced a coronary event on this day, then another man was censored at 91 days, the number surviving to 101 days is $4401 - 1 - 1 = 4399$. At 365 days there were $4402 - 17 - 7 = 4378$ still under study and event-free. Conceptually each time in the KM life table is just *before* the time of the event (or events) occurring on that day. If censoring occurs on the same day, this is assumed not to occur before the same-day event(s).

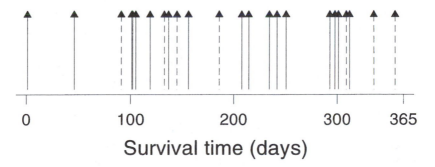

**Figure 5.7**   Loss to follow-up during the first year of study; selected subset of SHHS men. Solid arrows denote coronary events; dashed arrows denote censoring.

**Table 5.5**   Data and Kaplan–Meier estimation of the survival function, year 1 of follow-up for the selected subset of SHHS men

| Time (days) | Number | Events | Survival probability Estimate | Standard error |
|---|---|---|---|---|
| 0 | 4402 | | 1 | |
| 1 | 4402 | 1 | 0.999 773 | 0.000 227 1 |
| 46 | 4401 | 1 | 0.999 546 | 0.000 321 2 |
| 101 | 4399 | 2 | 0.999 091 | 0.000 454 2 |
| 103 | 4397 | 1 | 0.998 864 | 0.000 507 7 |
| 119 | 4396 | 1 | 0.998 637 | 0.000 556 1 |
| 137 | 4394 | 1 | 0.998 410 | 0.000 600 7 |
| 156 | 4392 | 1 | 0.998 182 | 0.000 642 1 |
| 208 | 4390 | 1 | 0.997 954 | 0.000 681 0 |
| 215 | 4389 | 1 | 0.997 727 | 0.000 717 8 |
| 235 | 4388 | 1 | 0.997 500 | 0.000 752 8 |
| 242 | 4387 | 1 | 0.997 273 | 0.000 786 2 |
| 251 | 4386 | 1 | 0.997 045 | 0.000 818 3 |
| 294 | 4385 | 1 | 0.996 818 | 0.000 849 1 |
| 299 | 4384 | 1 | 0.996 591 | 0.000 878 8 |
| 300 | 4383 | 1 | 0.996 363 | 0.000 907 5 |
| 312 | 4381 | 1 | 0.996 136 | 0.000 935 4 |
| 365 | 4378 | | | |

## 5.4.1   An empirical comparison

It is of interest to compare KM results with the actuarial results (from Section 5.3). The probability of survival to 1 year in Table 5.5 is 0.996136, compared to 0.996135 in Table 5.3. These are in excellent agreement; this magnitude of difference is no more than might be expected from rounding error.

In general, there will be differences due to the different methods of dealing with withdrawals. When KM estimation was used for the entire 9 years of SHHS data, the end-of-year estimates were as shown in Table 5.6, which also gives the actuarial results reproduced from Table 5.3 for ease of comparison. The agreement, in both the estimates of survival probabilities and their standard error, is very good until the last three years, when they begin to drift apart. This is not surprising since this is the period when there are several hundred censored and relatively few events. As noted already, the study described here could not be expected to produce accurate results for these latter years.

When there are many events, published tabular displays of KM analyses will generally be extracts from the whole life table, such as are given in Table 5.6. Graphical displays are more straightforward: Figure 5.8 gives KM estimates

**Table 5.6** Comparison of actuarial and Kaplan–Meier (KM) results for the survivor function, SHHS selected subset

| Time (years) | Estimate | | Standard error (× 10 000) | |
|---|---|---|---|---|
| | Actuarial | KM | Actuarial | KM |
| 1 | 0.996 135 | 0.996 136 | 9.356 | 9.354 |
| 2 | 0.991 122 | 0.991 125 | 14.152 | 14.148 |
| 3 | 0.985 174 | 0.985 177 | 18.253 | 18.249 |
| 4 | 0.979 885 | 0.979 885 | 21.226 | 21.226 |
| 5 | 0.971 337 | 0.971 339 | 25.268 | 25.267 |
| 6 | 0.962 521 | 0.962 525 | 28.804 | 28.800 |
| 7 | 0.954 851 | 0.954 982 | 31.697 | 31.607 |
| 8 | 0.947 325 | 0.947 144 | 35.636 | 36.308 |
| 9 | 0.941 081 | 0.936 608 | 45.033 | 70.003 |

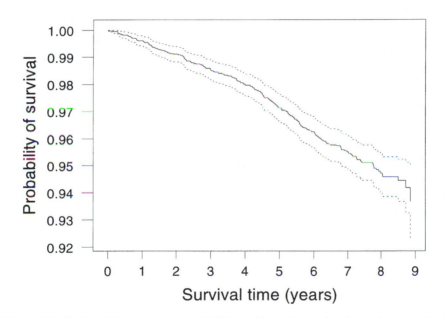

**Figure 5.8** Kaplan-Meier estimates and 95% confidence intervals of cumulative survival probabilities for coronary events; selected subset of SHHS men.

(and 95% confidence intervals) for the entire follow-up of the SHHS cohort. This is the direct equivalent of Figure 5.4; notice that the steps in the KM survival function are much less pronounced than in the actuarial function, leading to a smoother display.

## 5.5    Comparison of two sets of survival probabilities

In Section 5.3.3 we saw how to use Greenwood's formula (5.4) to construct a test for equality and confidence interval for the difference between two cumulative survival probabilities, one from each of two cohorts (or two subgroups of a single cohort). Here we consider the more general problem of comparing two complete sets of such probabilities; that is, we seek summary measures of comparative survival across the entire period of follow-up.

### 5.5.1    Mantel–Haenszel methods

Suppose that the follow-up times for both the cohorts to be compared are divided into the same consecutive intervals, just as in Table 5.4. Consider the number surviving to the start of each interval and the number of events in each interval, just as we have done before. Table 5.7 shows the relevant values extracted from Table 5.4.

Consider the first interval (0–1 years of follow-up). We can write the survival experience of the two groups during this interval as a $2 \times 2$ table (Table 5.8). We could then use the methods of Chapter 3 to compare the survival experiences within this first year, although this would take no account of those censored. Of more interest here is the fact that tables akin to Table 5.8 may be constructed for each interval in Table 5.7: nine tables in all. We seek a summary measure of the chance of an event, or conversely of survival, across the nine intervals: a situation analogous to that of Section 4.6, where Mantel–

**Table 5.7**    SHHS coronary survival data for men living in owner-occupied and rented accommodation

| Interval (years) | Owner-occupiers | | Renters | |
|---|---|---|---|---|
| | Number[a] | Events | Number[a] | Events |
| 0 but less than 1 | 2482 | 8 | 1920 | 9 |
| 1 but less than 2 | 2472 | 12 | 1906 | 10 |
| 2 but less than 3 | 2455 | 11 | 1889 | 15 |
| 3 but less than 4 | 2434 | 8 | 1860 | 15 |
| 4 but less than 5 | 2417 | 17 | 1835 | 20 |
| 5 but less than 6 | 2388 | 21 | 1806 | 17 |
| 6 but less than 7 | 2363 | 15 | 1778 | 16 |
| 7 but less than 8 | 2101 | 9 | 1508 | 11 |
| 8 but less than 9 | 806 | 3 | 640 | 2 |

[a]Number at the beginning of the interval.

**Table 5.8**  Survival experience by housing tenure status during the first year of follow-up, SHHS men

| Housing tenure | Event | No event | Total |
|---|---|---|---|
| Renters | 9 | 1911 | 1920 |
| Owner-occupiers | 8 | 2474 | 2482 |
| Total | 17 | 4385 | 4402 |

Haenszel methodology was used to produce summaries over strata defined by a confounding variable. Now the strata are the intervals of time, but otherwise the methodology transfers.

*Example 5.7*  Mantel–Haenszel methods will now be used to summarize survival in the SHHS example. Table 5.9 gives the set of $2 \times 2$ tables produced from Table 5.7 (the first of which is Table 5.8). Underneath each table $E(a_i)$ and $V(a_i)$ are given ($i = 1, 2, \ldots, 9$), the mean and variance of each top left-hand cell value (see Table 4.12). These are calculated from (4.19).

From (4.21), the continuity-corrected Cochran–Mantel–Haenszel test statistic for the null hypothesis of no overall difference in survival experience between the housing tenure groups is

**Table 5.9**  Survival experience by housing tenure status for each interval defined in Table 5.7 (see Table 5.8 for labels)

| 9  | 1911 | 1920 | | 10 | 1896 | 1906 | | 15 | 1874 | 1889 |
|----|------|------|--|----|------|------|--|----|------|------|
| 8  | 2474 | 2482 | | 12 | 2460 | 2472 | | 11 | 2444 | 2455 |
| 17 | 4385 | 4402 | | 22 | 4356 | 4378 | | 26 | 4318 | 4344 |

$E(a_1) = 7.415$
$V(a_1) = 4.166$
$\qquad$ $E(a_2) = 9.578$
$V(a_2) = 5.382$
$\qquad$ $E(a_3) = 11.306$
$V(a_3) = 6.353$

| 15 | 1845 | 1860 | | 20 | 1815 | 1835 | | 17 | 1789 | 1806 |
|----|------|------|--|----|------|------|--|----|------|------|
| 8  | 2426 | 2434 | | 17 | 2400 | 2417 | | 21 | 2367 | 2388 |
| 23 | 4271 | 4294 | | 37 | 4215 | 4252 | | 38 | 4156 | 4194 |

$E(a_4) = 9.963$
$V(a_4) = 5.618$
$\qquad$ $E(a_5) = 15.968$
$V(a_5) = 9.000$
$\qquad$ $E(a_6) = 16.364$
$V(a_6) = 9.235$

| 16 | 1762 | 1778 | | 11 | 1497 | 1508 | | 2 | 638  | 640  |
|----|------|------|--|----|------|------|--|---|------|------|
| 15 | 2348 | 2363 | | 9  | 2092 | 2101 | | 3 | 803  | 806  |
| 31 | 4110 | 4141 | | 20 | 3589 | 3609 | | 5 | 1441 | 1446 |

$E(a_7) = 13.310$
$V(a_7) = 7.540$
$\qquad$ $E(a_8) = 8.357$
$V(a_8) = 4.839$
$\qquad$ $E(a_9) = 2.213$
$V(a_9) = 1.230$

$$\frac{(|\sum a_i - \sum E(a_i)| - \frac{1}{2})^2}{\sum V(a_i)} = \frac{(|115 - 94.474| - 0.5)^2}{53.363} = 7.52.$$

From Table B.3, for 1 d.f., this is significant at the 0.1% level (the exact $p$ value is 0.006). Hence, there is evidence of a difference in the overall chance of survival. Since the sum of observed values ($\sum a_i$) is greater than the sum of expected ($\sum E(a_i)$) for those who experience an event amongst renters, we can conclude that renters are the more likely to have a coronary attack.

We can use (4.10) or (4.15) to estimate the common odds ratio or relative risk across the intervals. These both turn out to be 1.46. Hence we estimate that renters are almost half as likely again to experience a coronary event within any one year of the nine. This may be compared with Example 4.3, where the relative risk for an event within six years was found to be about 1.3, when no account was taken of those censored. The difference is explained by reference to Table 5.4: a disproportionate number of renters were censored (mainly due to death from other causes) in the earlier years of follow-up.

## 5.5.2  The log-rank test

In Section 5.5.1 the treatment of censored individuals was rather crude. For instance, it may be that one of the two cohorts (subgroups) loses several subjects during an interval whilst the other does not. The analysis would then be biased against the cohort with no censoring. As in Section 5.4, we can minimize the chance of such a problem by taking the intervals to be as small as possible. In this case we choose the intervals between successive events for the two subgroups *combined*.

When the Cochran–Mantel–Haenszel test of Section 4.6.2 is applied to survival data using KM intervals it is called the **log-rank test**. In Example 5.8 we apply this test to data from the first year of the SHHS. As with KM estimation, the log-rank test is computationally intensive and it would be impractical to provide a detailed example of its application to the entire nine years of the SHHS.

The name 'log-rank test' (or 'logrank test') is sometimes applied to other, similar, test procedures. These include the procedures given in Section 5.5.3 and the test used by Peto *et al.* (1977). This is unfortunate as it may lead to confusion. An alternative derivation of the log-rank test, as defined here, is given by Cox and Oakes (1984)

*Example 5.8*  During the first year of follow-up in the SHHS the completed survival times (in days) for the men in owner-occupied accommodation were:

$$46, 101, 103, 119, 208, 215, 235, 299, 309^*, 336^*.$$

For those in rented accommodation, they were:

$$1, 91^*, 101, 133^*, 137, 145^*, 156, 186^*, 242, 251, 294, 300, 312, 357^*.$$

Again * denotes a censored observation. We could proceed, as in Example 5.7, to list the set of sixteen $2 \times 2$ tables of tenure by survivorship (one for each interval between events). However, this is not necessary in order to apply (4.21), the continuity-corrected log-rank test statistic. A table in the format of Table 5.7 has all the necessary information, from which (4.21) can be applied repeatedly by interpreting the items in each row in terms of the $2 \times 2$ table that they define. This shorthand approach has been used in Table 5.10 (from Table 5.4 we already know that there were 2482 owner-occupiers and 1920 renters at baseline). The columns labelled $\overline{E}_i$ and $E_i$ are the number of survivors (after events and censoring have been accounted for) at the start of interval $i$ and $c_i$ and $a_i$ are the numbers of events within interval $i$, for owner-occupiers and renters respectively. This notation is derived from Table 4.12.

As an example of the calculations required to obtain the final two columns, consider the first row of Table 5.10. By reference to Table 4.12 and analogy with Example 5.7, (4.19) gives

$$E(a_1) = \frac{(1+0) \times 1920}{1920 + 2482} = 0.4362,$$

$$V(a_1) = \frac{(1+0)((1920-1) + (2482-0)) \times 1920 \times 2482}{(1920 + 2482)^2(1920 + 2482 - 1)} = 0.2459.$$

Notice that the expected number of events in the renters group, under the null hypothesis of no difference (in survival) between the groups, is equal to the risk of an event in the combined cohort times the number at risk in the renters group. This seems intuitively reasonable.

**Table 5.10**  SHHS coronary survival data during the first year of follow-up for men living in owner-occupied and rented accommodation

| Interval (days) | Owner-occupiers | | Renters | | Expectation $E(a_i)$ | Variance $V(a_i)$ |
|---|---|---|---|---|---|---|
| | $\overline{E}_i$ | $c_i$ | $E_i$ | $a_i$ | | |
| 1 to less than 46 | 2482 | 0 | 1920 | 1 | 0.4362 | 0.2459 |
| 46 to less than 101 | 2482 | 1 | 1919 | 0 | 0.4361 | 0.2459 |
| 101 to less than 103 | 2481 | 1 | 1918 | 1 | 0.8720 | 0.4917 |
| 103 to less than 119 | 2480 | 1 | 1917 | 0 | 0.4360 | 0.2459 |
| 119 to less than 137 | 2479 | 1 | 1917 | 0 | 0.4361 | 0.2459 |
| 137 to less than 156 | 2478 | 0 | 1916 | 1 | 0.4360 | 0.2459 |
| 156 to less than 208 | 2478 | 0 | 1914 | 1 | 0.4358 | 0.2459 |
| 208 to less than 215 | 2478 | 1 | 1912 | 0 | 0.4355 | 0.2458 |
| 215 to less than 235 | 2477 | 1 | 1912 | 0 | 0.4356 | 0.2459 |
| 235 to less than 242 | 2476 | 1 | 1912 | 0 | 0.4357 | 0.2459 |
| 242 to less than 251 | 2475 | 0 | 1912 | 1 | 0.4358 | 0.2459 |
| 251 to less than 294 | 2475 | 0 | 1911 | 1 | 0.4357 | 0.2459 |
| 294 to less than 299 | 2475 | 0 | 1910 | 1 | 0.4356 | 0.2459 |
| 299 to less than 300 | 2475 | 1 | 1909 | 0 | 0.4354 | 0.2458 |
| 300 to less than 312 | 2474 | 0 | 1909 | 1 | 0.4355 | 0.2458 |
| 312 to 365 | 2473 | 0 | 1908 | 1 | 0.4355 | 0.2458 |
| Total | | 8 | | 9 | 7.4086 | 4.1798 |

From (4.21), the continuity-corrected log-rank test statistic is

$$\frac{(|9 - 7.4086| - 0.5)^2}{4.1798} = 0.2850.$$

This is to be compared with $\chi_1^2$ but is clearly not significant at any reasonable significance level. We conclude that there is no evidence of a difference, between coronary survival probabilities, in the first year of follow-up.

Just as the choice of which group to place in the first row of Tables 5.8 and 5.9 is arbitrary, we could choose to swap the owner-occupiers and renters data, keeping the labels for $\bar{E}_i$ etc. fixed, in Table 5.10. We would then find that $\sum a_i - \sum E(a_i)$ has the same magnitude but opposite sign to that found above. $\sum V(a_i)$ would remain the same. As a consequence the value of the log-rank test statistic would stay the same.

### 5.5.3   Weighted log-rank tests

A class of alternative tests to the log-rank test are the **weighted log-rank tests**. These are generally derived from the log-rank statistic without continuity correction (4.20), which may be written as

$$L = E^2/V, \tag{5.14}$$

where

$$E = \sum(a_i - E(a_i)), \qquad V = \sum V(a_i), \tag{5.15}$$

and the summations run over all time intervals. Weighted log-rank test statistics are of the form

$$L_w = E_w^2/V_w, \tag{5.16}$$

where

$$E_w = \sum w_i(a_i - E(a_i)), \qquad V_w = \sum w_i^2 V(a_i) \tag{5.17}$$

and the $\{w_i\}$ are a set of weights, one for each time interval. The log-rank test itself is a special case where $w_i = 1$ for all $i$. Weighted log-rank test statistics are each compared to chi-square with 1 d.f.

The most common weighted log-rank test takes $w_i = n_i$, the number at risk at the start of time interval $i$. This test is variously known as the **Breslow, Gehan** or **(generalized) Wilcoxon test**. It gives greatest weight to the time intervals with the greatest number at risk; inevitably these are the earliest time intervals. Most other weighting schemes take $w_i$ to be some function of $n_i$; for example $w_i = \sqrt{n_i}$ leads to the **Tarone–Ware test**.

*Example 5.9*   Figure 5.9 shows the KM estimates of the survivor function for coronary events by housing tenure status for the entire 9 years of the SHHS data. Once more we see that owner-occupiers have the best outcomes at all times. The complete set of data (as used

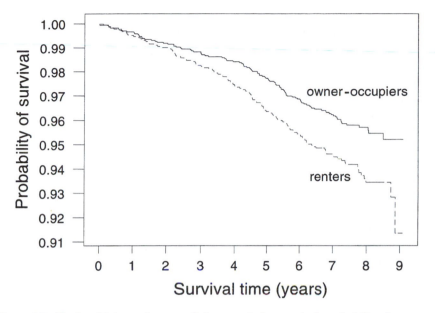

**Figure 5.9** Kaplan–Meier estimates of the cumulative survival probability for owner-occupiers (solid line) and renters (dashed line); SHHS men.

here in its entirety, and earlier in summary or extract) is available electronically: see Appendix C.

The application of the log-rank test to the entire data set is a straightforward extension of Example 5.8. It turns out that $E = 20.435$ and $V = 53.7180$, using (5.15). The continuity-corrected log-rank statistic is then, from (4.21) and (5.14),

$$(20.435 - 0.5)^2/53.7180 = 7.40$$

whilst the uncorrected form, (5.14), is

$$20.435/53.7180 = 7.77.$$

As we saw earlier, the SHHS results are unreliable in the final couple of years due to the large number censored and the small number of events. Hence there is a case for weighting the test procedure in favour of the earlier intervals. The generalized Wilcoxon test was applied to the data and gave $E_w = 78\,493$ and $V_w = 8.866 \times 10^8$ using (5.17). From (5.16), the test statistic is

$$78493^2/(8.866 \times 10^8) = 6.95.$$

Neither the continuity correction, nor the Wilcoxon weighting, has had a large effect upon the result in this example. When each of these three test statistics is compared to $\chi_1^2$ the $p$ value is below 0.01 (see Table B.3). Hence, we can conclude that there is evidence of a real difference; the benefit of being an owner-occupier does not seem to be simply due to chance. Contrast this conclusion with that of Example 5.8; Figure 5.9 shows that there is little difference between the tenure groups in the first year, but a widening gap thereafter.

In Section 4.6.3 we noted that the Cochran–Mantel–Haenszel test assumes that the comparative chance of an event does not vary by level of the confounding factor. Translated into the current application, the log-rank test assumes that the comparative chance of an event does not vary by the time intervals between events. This is widely known as the **proportional hazards** assumption. We shall consider this assumption more fully in Chapter 11. For now it is sufficient to note that it is an assumption of time homogeneity: the chance of an event in the two groups is assumed to be in constant proportion over time.

The null hypothesis for the log-rank test is that the constant proportion is unity (that is, no difference). The alternative hypothesis is that this constant proportion is something other than unity. Under conditions of proportional hazards, the log-rank test is the most powerful test available (see Section 8.2 for a formal definition of 'power'). Otherwise, a weighted test will be preferable. Hence, we require a method of testing for proportional hazards. This issue is discussed in Section 11.8. In most applications the log-rank test is used rather than any kind of weighted test unless the proportional hazards assumption is clearly false.

### 5.5.4    Allowing for confounding variables

The log-rank test may easily be extended to allow adjustment for confounding variables. We split the data into strata defined by the levels of the confounder. Then we find the $E$ and $V$ statistics of (5.15) for each stratum: call these $E_j$ and $V_j$ for the $j$th stratum. The **stratified log-rank test statistic** is then

$$L_s = \sum E_j^2 \Big/ \sum V_j,$$

where the summations run over all strata. This is, once more, compared against chi-square with 1 d.f.

Similar stratified tests may be constructed for weighted log-rank tests. An alternative way of dealing with confounding is through a statistical model for survival analysis: see Chapter 11.

### 5.5.5    Comparing three or more groups

The log-rank test, and its associates, may be extended to deal with the problem of comparing three or more sets of survival functions: see Collett (1994). In practice, such situations are more commonly dealt with using the statistical models of Chapter 11.

## 5.6    The person-years method

An alternative to the life table method of analysis for cohort data is the person-years method. The person-years incidence rate is estimated to be

$$\hat{\rho} = e/y, \tag{5.18}$$

where $e$ is the number of events (just as in earlier sections) and $y$ is the number of person-years of follow-up. To calculate $y$ we must sum all the follow-up periods of the study subjects. Once someone is censored, or has an event, that person's follow-up is terminated. This gives an alternative way of dealing with censoring. Sometimes (5.18) is called an **incidence density** to distinguish it from a rate when the denominator is a number of people, as in (3.28).

The only difference between (3.28) and (5.18) lies in the denominator. We develop inferential procedures for each rate assuming that its denominator is a fixed quantity; the only variable quantity is the numerator, which is the number of events in each case. Hence, the confidence intervals and tests given in Section 3.8 are applicable in the current context; we simply replace the number, $n$, by the person-years, $y$, in each formula (where necessary).

*Example 5.10*  Suppose that the eight male employees who work in a high-exposure (to potential toxic substances) department of a chemical company are investigated in an all-causes mortality study. Table 5.11 shows the dates when each man joined the study (that is, began employment in the high-exposure department) and the dates of leaving the study (through death, leaving for another job, retirement or end of study).

Notice that years studied have been calculated to the nearest month. It would be possible to calculate more accurately by counting individual days. If we further approximate 1 month = $1/12$ = 0.0833 years we get $y$ = 177.1667 years. From (5.18), the mortality rate is then $e/y = 4/177.1667 = 0.0226$ or 22.6 per thousand per year.

**Table 5.11**    Data from a hypothetical chemical company

| Individual no. | Date entered | Date left | Years studied | Death? |
|---|---|---|---|---|
| 1 | 5 Oct 1956 | 1 Dec 1993 | 37y 2m | yes |
| 2 | 10 Oct 1969 | 31 Dec 1997 | 28y 3m | no |
| 3 | 10 Jun 1979 | 31 Dec 1997 | 18y 7m | no |
| 4 | 30 Aug 1984 | 28 Sep 1994 | 10y 1m | no |
| 5 | 8 May 1962 | 8 Jul 1991 | 29y 2m | yes |
| 6 | 1 Nov 1966 | 10 May 1979 | 12y 6m | yes |
| 7 | 21 Mar 1954 | 30 Jun 1991 | 37y 3m | no |
| 8 | 8 Jun 1961 | 29 Jul 1965 | 4y 2m | yes |
| | | Total | 177y 2m | yes = 4 |
| | | | | no = 4 |

## 5.6.1  Age-specific rates

Since age is often a basic determinant of propensity for disease, person-years analyses usually take account of age. This is achieved by dividing the time spent in the study up into periods spent within distinct age groups, separately for each subject. Of course, during follow-up each individual could pass through several age groups. If $e_i$ is the number of events which occurred whilst subjects were in age group $i$ and $y_i$ is the number of years in total spent in the study whilst in age group $i$ (the person-years at age $i$) then the person-years incidence rate for age group $i$ is estimated, using (5.18), as

$$\hat{\rho}_i = e_i/y_i. \tag{5.19}$$

Calculation of the component of $y_i$ attributable to any particular individual is somewhat tricky, and would normally be done by computer for any large cohort. Figure 5.10 is a flow-chart specifying a general method for calculating $y_i$ for a single person within a single age interval denoted by $i$. The results from all individuals will be summed to give the value of $y_i$ in (5.19) for each $i$.

*Example 5.11*   Consider Example 5.10 again, but now include information on date of birth: see Table 5.12. This enables the total employment experience of each person to be divided up by the time spent at different ages. Three age groups are used here; notice that they do not have to span an equal number of years. All durations are rounded to the nearest month, as before.

  Age at start and end have been calculated using the start and end dates from Table 5.11. For example, consider individual number 1:

$$\text{age at entry} = (5\,\text{Oct}\,1956) - (31\,\text{Jul}\,1929) = 27\text{y}\,2\text{m},$$
$$\text{age at leaving} = (1\,\text{Dec}\,1993) - (31\,\text{Jul}\,1929) = 64\text{y}\,4\text{m}.$$

The components of $y_i$ for each $i$ ($i = 1, 2, 3$) were calculated using Figure 5.10. When $i = 1$, min $= 0$ and max $= 40$. When $i = 2$, min $= 40$ and max $= 55$. When $i = 3$, min $= 55$ and max $= \infty$. Consider, again, the first individual. For him, sage $= 27.167$ and fage $= 64.333$. Following the flow-chart through for age group 1 we obtain

$$y = \text{max} - \text{sage} = 40 - 27.167 = 12.667\,\text{years}\ (\text{or 12y 10m}).$$

For age group 2 we obtain

$$y = \text{max} - \text{min} = 55 - 40 = 15\,\text{years}.$$

For age group 3 we obtain

$$y = \text{fage} - \text{min} = 64.333 - 55 = 9.333\,\text{years}\ (\text{or 9y 4m}).$$

## 5.6.2  Summarization of rates

The set of age-specific estimated rates $\{\hat{\rho}_i\}$ is generally summarized using the standardized event ratio (SER), as defined by (4.4). This requires some suitable

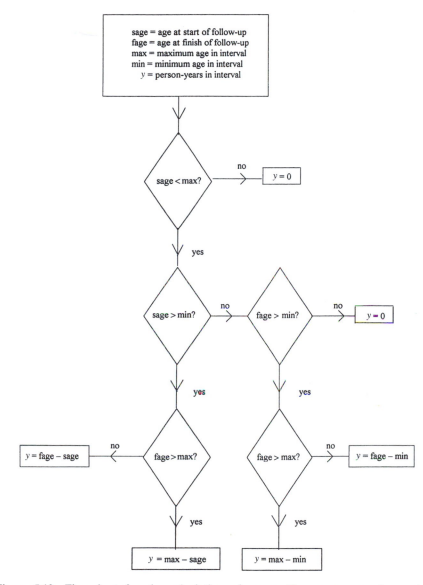

**Figure 5.10** Flow-chart for the calculation of age-specific person-years for a single individual and a single age group.

**Table 5.12**    Further data from a hypothetical chemical company ($+$ denotes a death)

| Individual no. | Date of birth | Age at start | Age at finish | Experience when aged (years) Below 40 | 40–54 | 55 and over |
|---|---|---|---|---|---|---|
| 1 | 21 Jul  1929 | 27y 2m | 64y 4m | 12y 10m | 15y 0m | 9y 4m+ |
| 2 | 1 Aug  1933 | 36y 2m | 64y 5m | 3y 10m | 15y 0m | 9y 5m |
| 3 | 8 Jun  1951 | 28y 0m | 46y 7m | 12y 0m | 6y 7m | – |
| 4 | 17 Jun  1944 | 40y 2m | 50y 3m | – | 10y 1m | – |
| 5 | 3 Jan  1931 | 31y 4m | 60y 6m | 8y 8m | 15y 0m | 5y 6m+ |
| 6 | 14 May  1936 | 30y 6m | 43y 0m | 9y 6m | 3y 0m+ | – |
| 7 | 30 Jun  1926 | 27y 9m | 65y 0m | 12y 3m | 15y 0m | 10y 0m |
| 8 | 10 Aug  1926 | 34y 10m | 39y 0m | 4y 2m+ | – | – |
| | | | Total | 63y 3m | 79y 8m | 34y 3m |
| | | | $e_i$ | 1 | 1 | 2 |
| | | | $y_i$ | 63.250 | 79.667 | 34.250 |
| | | | $\hat{\rho}_i$ | 0.01581 | 0.01255 | 0.05839 |

standard population as a basis for comparison. This will often be the national population of which the cohort followed is a subset.

*Example 5.12*    Suppose that the national statistical digest for the country from which data were collected in Examples 5.10 and 5.11 reported average annual male death rates (per thousand) of 1.8 for 25–39-year-olds, 9.0 for 40–54-year-olds and 19.2 for 55–64-year-olds. The expected number of deaths in the chemical company department, during the course of the cohort study, is then, from (4.3),

$$E = 1.8 \times 63.250 + 9.0 \times 79.667 + 19.2 \times 34.250 = 1488.453$$

per thousand. Hence we would expect to see 1.488 deaths if the chemical company employees had the same chance of death as all males in the country. From (4.4) the standardized mortality ratio (SMR: the SER when the events are all deaths) is $4/1.488 = 2.69$, or 269% . Hence the high-exposure department of the chemical factory is, apparently, a dangerous place to work, with a death rate that is 2.69 times the national average (age-standardized).

If the population from which the cohort was selected has the same chance of an event as does the standard population, after age adjustment, then observed and expected numbers of events should be very similar. We can test for equality (that is, study population SER $= 1$) by calculating

$$\frac{(|e - E| - \tfrac{1}{2})^2}{E}, \tag{5.20}$$

which is compared to chi-square with 1 d.f. Note that the $\tfrac{1}{2}$ is a continuity correction which is appropriate here because $e$ comes from a Poisson distribution and can only take integer values.

Approximate 95% confidence intervals for the SER may be obtained from the approximate result that $\sqrt{e}$ has a normal distribution with variance $\frac{1}{4}$ (Snedecor and Cochran, 1980). This leads to the limits for the study population SER of

$$\text{SER}\left(1 \pm \frac{1.96}{2\sqrt{e}}\right)^2. \tag{5.21}$$

Unfortunately both (5.20) and (5.21) are inaccurate when $e$ is small. When $e$ is below 20 exact procedures are recommended: see Breslow and Day (1987) and Gardner and Altman (1989). Neither (5.20) nor (5.21) would be suitable for the hypothetical data of Example 5.11. They could be used for each deprivation group in Example 4.7. The methods of this (and the next) section may be applied equally well to data from other types of study that are summarized as SERs or indirect standardized rates.

### 5.6.3   Comparison of two SERs

The methodology of Sections 5.6.1 and 5.6.2 would be applicable when a single cohort is followed. When two (or more) cohorts or sub-cohorts are observed we would normally seek to compare them. We can do this directly, using an extension of the Mantel–Haenszel procedure (see Section 5.6.4) or indirectly by comparing SERs. The latter comparison is indirect because an SER is already a comparative measure, where the 'base' is the standard population. If we take the same standard population for each SER then we have a logical framework for comparison.

By analogy with the idea of a relative risk, we can calculate the **relative SER**,

$$\omega_s = \frac{\text{SER}_2}{\text{SER}_1}, \tag{5.22}$$

to compare two standardized event rates, $\text{SER}_2$ relative to $\text{SER}_1$. Since, by (4.6), the indirect standardized rate is a constant times the SER, $\omega_s$ may also be called a **standardized relative rate**.

From Breslow and Day (1987), 95% confidence limits for $\omega_s$ are given by $(\omega_L, \omega_U)$, where

$$\omega_L = \frac{E_1 e_2}{E_2 F_L(e_1 + 1)}, \qquad \omega_U = \frac{E_1 F_U(e_2 + 1)}{E_2 e_1}. \tag{5.23}$$

Here $e_1$ and $E_1$ are, respectively, the observed and expected number of events in cohort 1; similarly for cohort 2. $F_L$ is the upper $2\frac{1}{2}\%$ point of the $F$ distribution with $(2e_1 + 2, 2e_2)$ d.f. and $F_U$ is the upper $2\frac{1}{2}\%$ point of the $F$ distribution with $(2e_2 + 2, 2e_1)$ d.f.: see Table B.5(c).

Breslow and Day (1987) also derive an approximate test of the null hypothesis that two SERs are equal. This requires calculation of the test statistic (with continuity correction),

$$\frac{(|e_1 - E_1^*| - \frac{1}{2})^2}{E_1^*} + \frac{(|e_2 - E_2^*| - \frac{1}{2})^2}{E_2^*}, \qquad (5.24)$$

which is to be compared to chi-square with 1 d.f. In (5.24),

$$E_i^* = (\text{SER})E_i, \qquad (5.25)$$

for $i = 1, 2$, where SER is the overall standardized event ratio for the two cohorts combined. Since (5.24) is only an approximation it will not necessarily agree with the result from (5.23). When the results are in conflict it will be better to base the test on inclusion (accept $H_0$) or exclusion (reject $H_0$) of unity within the confidence interval. Breslow and Day (1987) also give an exact test which requires evaluating probabilities from the binomial distribution.

*Example 5.13*  In addition to the chemical company that was the subject of the last three examples, another (much larger) chemical company in the same country has employees working in similar high-exposure conditions. In the period 1955–97 there were 43 deaths amongst this company's high-exposure work-force. This compares with 38.755 that were expected according to national statistics.

Clearly both work-forces have higher than expected numbers of deaths when compared with the experiences of the country as a whole. We shall now compare the second work-force with the first.

Letting subscript '1' denote the original chemical company, we have from the above and Examples 5.10 and 5.12,

$$e_1 = 4, \qquad e_2 = 43$$
$$E_1 = 1.488, \qquad E_2 = 38.755.$$

Hence the estimated relative SMR, from (4.4) and (5.22), is

$$\hat{\omega}_s = \frac{43/38.755}{4/1.488} = 0.413$$

So the second work-force has less than half the (indirectly standardized) rate of the first.

To obtain 95% confidence limits for $\omega_s$ we first find the upper $2\frac{1}{2}\%$ point of $F$ with $(2 \times 4 + 2, 2 \times 43) = (10, 86)$ and $(2 \times 43 + 2, 2 \times 4) = (88, 8)$ d.f. From a statistical computer package these were found to be 2.201 and 3.749, respectively. Using these, (5.23) gives the lower and upper confidence limits as

$$\frac{1.488 \times 43}{38.755 \times 2.201 \times (4 + 1)} = 0.150, \qquad \frac{1.488 \times 3.749 \times (43 + 1)}{38.755 \times 4} = 1.583.$$

Thus the 95% confidence limits are (0.150, 1.583): there is quite a wide range of error which includes a relative age-standardized mortality rate of unity.

We can go on (if we wish) to test the hypothesis that the relative SMR is unity using (5.24). First we find the overall SMR: this is, from (4.4),

$$\frac{4 + 43}{1.488 + 38.755} = 1.168.$$

Using this in (5.25) gives

$$E_1^* = 1.168 \times 1.488 = 1.738,$$
$$E_2^* = 1.168 \times 38.755 = 45.266.$$

Substituting into (5.24) gives the test statistic

$$\frac{(|4 - 1.738| - 0.5)^2}{1.738} + \frac{(|43 - 45.266| - 0.5)^2}{45.266} = 1.855.$$

This value is well below the 10% critical value from $\chi_1^2$, so that the null hypothesis fails to be rejected. We conclude that there is no conclusive evidence that either company is worse than the other, after allowing for age differentials.

### 5.6.4    Mantel–Haenszel methods

In Sections 5.6.2 and 5.6.3 we have seen how to use standardization to control for variation in age (the confounding variable) and then how to compare two cohorts (or subgroups of a single cohort) using the standard population as an intermediate reference. A more direct way of comparing two cohorts is to use a Mantel–Haenszel (MH) procedure.

As in Section 4.6, the MH approach requires the data for the two cohorts to be subdivided by the strata of the confounding variable(s). As in Sections 5.6.1–5.6.3, we will take age to be the sole confounder (although this is not necessary). Suppose that membership of one cohort denotes 'exposure', whilst membership of the other is 'no exposure': for example, smokers versus non-smokers. Then we record, $e_{1i}$ number of events in the $i$th age group of cohort 1 (unexposed), and $y_{1i}$ number of person-years in the $i$th age group of cohort 1. Here $i$ ranges over all the age groups used. Similar variables $e_{2i}$ and $y_{2i}$ are defined for cohort 2 (exposed).

It is useful to compare these definitions with those given by Table 4.12 for the fixed cohort problem (where no individual is censored). Two of the terms are identical: $a_i = e_{2i}$ and $c_i = e_{1i}$, but $y_{1i}$ takes the place of $\overline{E}_i$ whilst $y_{2i}$ takes the place of $E_i$. The latter two relationships are not equalities because whilst the $E$s are real numbers of people, the $y$s are accumulated durations. Nevertheless, the MH estimate of the age-adjusted **relative rate**, $\hat{\omega}_{MH}$, turns out to be remarkably similar to the MH estimate of the age-adjusted relative risk, $\hat{\lambda}_{MH}$, given by (4.15). The estimate is

$$\hat{\omega}_{MH} = \frac{\sum e_{2i} y_{1i} / y_i}{\sum e_{1i} y_{2i} / y_i}, \qquad (5.26)$$

where $y_i = y_{1i} + y_{2i}$ is the total number of person-years at age $i$ (which takes the place of $n_i$ in (4.15)) and the summations run over all age groups. Since person-years are used, (5.26) could also be called an age-adjusted **incidence density ratio**. Note that (5.26) compares the exposed to the unexposed. See Rothman and Boice (1979) for a derivation of this MH estimator, and Greenland and Robins (1985) for further comment. Breslow (1984) suggests the following estimate for the standard error of the log of the MH estimate:

$$\hat{se}(\log_e \hat{\omega}_{MH}) = \sqrt{\sum(y_{1i}y_{2i}e_i/y_i^2)} \Big/ \left( \sqrt{\hat{\omega}_{MH}} \right) \left( \sum (y_{1i}y_{2i}e_i/y_i(y_{1i} + \hat{\omega}y_{2i})) \right),$$

(5.27)

where $e_i = e_{1i} + e_{2i}$ is the total number of events at age $i$, and the summations run over all age groups.

From (5.27) we get approximate 95% confidence limits $(L_{\log}, U_{\log})$ for $\log_e \omega_{MH}$ of

$$L_{\log} = \log_e \hat{\omega}_{MH} - 1.96\hat{se}(\log_e \hat{\omega}_{MH})$$
$$U_{\log} = \log_e \hat{\omega}_{MH} + 1.96\hat{se}(\log_e \hat{\omega}_{MH}),$$

(5.28)

and hence approximate 95% confidence limits $(L, U)$ for $\omega_{MH}$ itself are

$$L = \exp(L_{\log}),$$
$$U = \exp(U_{\log}).$$

(5.29)

Breslow and Day (1987) provide the following test statistic of the null hypothesis $\omega_{MH} = 1$, that is, no association between exposure and disease after allowing for age differences:

$$\frac{(|e_2 - \sum(y_{2i}e_i/y_i)| - \frac{1}{2})^2}{\sum(y_{1i}y_{2i}e_i/y_i^2)}.$$

(5.30)

This is compared to chi-square with 1 d.f. Here $e_2 = \sum e_{2i}$ is the total number of events in the exposed group. Once again, the summations run over all age groups and the $\frac{1}{2}$ is a continuity correction.

Finally, recall that MH summarization is only appropriate if there is homogeneity of exposure–disease association across the age strata (Section 4.6.3). A test of the null hypothesis that the relative rate is homogeneous across age groups is given by comparing

$$\sum \frac{(e_{1i} - \hat{e}_{1i})^2}{\hat{e}_{1i}} + \sum \frac{(e_{2i} - \hat{e}_{2i})^2}{\hat{e}_{2i}}$$

(5.31)

to chi-square with $\ell - 1$ d.f., where $\ell$ is the number of age groups (the number of items in each summation) and

$$\hat{e}_{1i} = \frac{e_i y_{1i}}{y_{1i} + \hat{\omega}_{MH} y_{2i}},$$

$$\hat{e}_{2i} = \frac{e_i y_{2i} \hat{\omega}_{MH}}{y_{1i} + \hat{\omega}_{MH} y_{2i}}. \tag{5.32}$$

This result is derived by Breslow and Day (1987), although they also suggest an improved, but more complex, procedure which requires the use of an alternative estimator for $\omega$ to the MH estimator used in (5.32).

*Example 5.14*   We now return to the example from the SHHS used in earlier sections. Using the algorithm of Figure 5.10, the person-years of follow-up were calculated, by 5-year age group, both for men who rent and men who occupy their own houses. Further, all coronary events were also grouped by the same 5-year age groups. Results are given in Table 5.13. For completeness, age-specific coronary event rates and the relative rate (renters versus owner-occupiers), calculated from (5.18) and (3.31), are included. Since the SHHS studied 40–59-year-olds, and the maximum follow-up time is less than 10 years, there are no person-years of observation at ages above 69 years.

The age-specific relative rates range from 0.51 to 1.88. We can summarize these by the MH estimate (5.26),

$$\omega_{MH} = \frac{(2 \times 1619.328)/(1619.328 + 1107.447) + \cdots + (2 \times 356.394)/(356.394 + 351.710)}{(3 \times 1107.447)/(1619.328 + 1107.447) + \cdots + (4 \times 351.710)/(356.394 + 351.710)}$$

$$= \frac{64.584}{45.888} = 1.407,$$

**Table 5.13**   Number of coronary events and person-years by age group and housing tenure, SHHS men

| Age group (years) | Housing tenure | Coronary events | Person-years | Coronary rate (per thousand) | Relative rate |
|---|---|---|---|---|---|
| 40–44 | Renters | 2 | 1 107.447 | 1.806 | 0.97 |
|       | Owners  | 3 | 1 619.328 | 1.853 | |
| 45–49 | Renters | 24 | 3 058.986 | 7.846 | 1.88 |
|       | Owners  | 19 | 4 550.166 | 4.176 | |
| 50–54 | Renters | 31 | 3 506.530 | 8.841 | 1.72 |
|       | Owners  | 25 | 4 857.904 | 5.146 | |
| 55–59 | Renters | 28 | 3 756.650 | 7.453 | 1.25 |
|       | Owners  | 27 | 4 536.832 | 5.951 | |
| 60–64 | Renters | 28 | 2 419.622 | 11.572 | 1.19 |
|       | Owners  | 26 | 2 680.843 | 9.698 | |
| 65–69 | Renters | 2 | 351.710 | 5.687 | 0.51 |
|       | Owners  | 4 | 356.394 | 11.224 | |
| Total | Renters | 115 | 14 200.945 | 8.098 | 1.45 |
|       | Owners  | 104 | 18 601.467 | 5.591 | |

which is, as expected, different from the unadjusted relative rate, 1.45 (seen in the 'total' line in Table 5.13).

Notice that, since renters provide the numerator for the relative rate, they take the place of the 'exposed' group, with subscript 2 in (5.26)–(5.32). $\hat{\omega}_{\mathrm{MH}}$ can be used, in (5.32) and then (5.31), to test whether the relative rate is homogeneous across the age strata. First we require all six values of $\hat{e}_{1i}$ and $\hat{e}_{2i}$ from (5.32). For example, when $i = 1$ (age group 40–44 years),

$$\hat{e}_{11} = \frac{(3+2) \times 1619.328}{1619.328 + 1.407 \times 1107.447} = 2.548,$$

$$\hat{e}_{21} = \frac{(3+2) \times 1107.447 \times 1.407}{1619.328 + 1.407 \times 1107.447} = 2.452.$$

When all such terms are calculated, (5.31) becomes $1.981 + 1.699 = 3.68$. This is to be compared to chi-square with $(6 - 1) = 5$ d.f. and is not significant ($p > 0.5$). Hence we conclude that the difference in observed relative rates by age group was merely due to sampling variation.

We have now established that it is sensible to use a summary measure of the relative rate, and shall go on to consider the accuracy of our chosen measure, $\hat{\omega}_{\mathrm{MH}}$. From (5.27),

$\hat{\mathrm{se}}(\log \hat{\omega}_{\mathrm{MH}})$

$$= \frac{\sqrt{(1619.328 \times 1107.447 \times (3+2)/(1619.328 + 1107.447)^2 + \cdots)}}{\sqrt{1.407((1619.328 \times 1107.447 \times (3+2)/((1619.328 + 1107.447)(1619.328 + 1.407 \times 1107.447))) + \cdots)}}$$

$$= \frac{\sqrt{53.771}}{\sqrt{1.407} \times 45.599} = 0.1356.$$

This leads to 95% confidence limits for $\log_e \omega_{\mathrm{MH}}$ of $\log_e 1.407 \pm 1.96 \times 0.1356$, that is, $0.3415 \pm 0.2658$, using (5.28). Raising the two limits to the power e gives the 95% confidence interval for $\omega_{\mathrm{MH}}$ itself, $(1.08, 1.84)$, as specified by (5.29).

Finally we can test whether the common relative rate is significantly different from unity by computing (5.30), which turns out to be,

$$\frac{(|115 - 96.304| - 0.5)^2}{53.771} = 6.16.$$

This is compared to $\chi_1^2$: from Table B.3, $0.025 > p > 0.01$, and hence we conclude that there is evidence that renters have higher coronary rates than do owner-occupiers, after correcting for age.

## 5.6.5    Further comments

Although the person-years method has been described so that adjustment is made for age, it is frequently used to adjust simultaneously for calendar period. This means extending the algorithm of Figure 5.10 to subdivide follow-up by calendar time as well as age.

Sometimes the 'exposure' to the risk factor may alter during follow-up: for example, a smoker may quit smoking during the study. The individual person-years of follow-up for any exposure level only accumulate the years when the individual was at that particular exposure level. For example, if someone dies whilst exposed he or she will still have made a contribution to the person-years for non-exposure provided that his or her exposure started after the study began. More details of this specific point and of person-years methodology in general are given by Breslow and Day (1987). This includes extensions to the situation of only two exposure levels, although this generalization is often achieved in practice through the Poisson regression model described in Section 11.9.

As was seen directly in Example 5.14, the use of Mantel–Haenszel methods with person-years data provides an alternative to the survival analysis methods of Sections 5.3–5.5. Kahn and Sempos (1989) compare the two methods and conclude that there is little to choose between them in terms of the assumptions needed for validity; for example, both assume lack of bias caused by withdrawals. However, the person-years method often requires a considerable amount of work to produce the basic data, via Figure 5.10, for example. Also there is an advantage in observing how survival probability alters with follow-up duration, which is a direct result of survival analysis.

Person-years analysis will not, therefore, be the generally recommended method for analysing cohort data. There are two exceptions: first, when there is no control group, other than some standard population which has not been followed up for the purposes of the study; second, when exposure varies, as explained above. In the former case, the methods of Section 5.6.2 are ideal. In the latter, special regression models for survival data (Section 11.6.1) may be useful.

## 5.7    Period-cohort analysis

In this chapter we have assumed that any effects that are investigated are homogeneous over calendar time, so that subjects with different baseline times may be taken together (Section 5.2.2). In this final section we review, briefly, the case when this assumption is invalid.

We will expect lack of homogeneity (a **period-cohort effect**), due to such things as changes in general health care or natural fluctuations in disease, whenever baseline dates vary over several years. As an example, Table 5.14 shows some data from the Connecticut Tumor Registry which are presented and analysed by Campbell et al. (1994). The table shows breast cancer incidence data for the years 1938–82, by 5-year intervals.

The year-of-birth groups define birth cohorts (at least approximately, since there will have been migration into and out of Connecticut). The baseline dates (years of birth) range over more than 60 years, so we should consider the

**Table 5.14**  Breast cancer rates (cases per 100 000 woman-years) in 1938–82 by age group and year of birth, Connecticut, USA (data prepared by the National Cancer Institute)

| Year of birth | Age group (years) | | | | | | | | | | | | |
|---|---|---|---|---|---|---|---|---|---|---|---|---|---|
| | 20–24 | 25–29 | 30–34 | 35–39 | 40–44 | 45–49 | 50–54 | 55–59 | 60–64 | 65–69 | 70–74 | 75–79 | 80–84 |
| 1888–1892 | | | | | | | 106.8 | 152.7 | 174.5 | 193.9 | 228.1 | 263.0 | 302.2 |
| 1893–1897 | | | | | | 91.8 | 102.5 | 156.5 | 170.8 | 211.1 | 235.4 | 275.0 | 317.7 |
| 1898–1902 | | | | | 85.8 | 104.3 | 117.6 | 150.9 | 168.3 | 213.6 | 257.5 | 318.8 | 320.2 |
| 1903–1907 | | | | 39.8 | 84.8 | 126.9 | 129.1 | 170.2 | 189.7 | 237.8 | 285.8 | 321.7 | |
| 1908–1912 | | | 19.7 | 48.3 | 97.6 | 127.2 | 154.3 | 183.6 | 214.5 | 263.5 | 303.8 | | |
| 1913–1917 | | 5.9 | 15.8 | 53.4 | 100.0 | 138.6 | 147.6 | 184.5 | 229.0 | 271.8 | | | |
| 1918–1922 | 1.5 | 8.2 | 26.2 | 56.2 | 102.9 | 150.1 | 171.6 | 226.9 | 254.4 | | | | |
| 1923–1927 | 1.5 | 6.3 | 24.5 | 57.5 | 114.1 | 168.3 | 195.9 | 214.1 | | | | | |
| 1928–1932 | 3.5 | 9.0 | 27.5 | 59.5 | 127.4 | 183.9 | 174.4 | | | | | | |
| 1933–1937 | 0.4 | 9.6 | 25.0 | 55.6 | 106.9 | 160.8 | | | | | | | |
| 1938–1942 | 0.8 | 9.1 | 24.1 | 55.8 | 95.3 | | | | | | | | |
| 1943–1947 | 0.2 | 8.3 | 26.0 | 58.8 | | | | | | | | | |
| 1948–1952 | 1.8 | 8.0 | 25.9 | | | | | | | | | | |

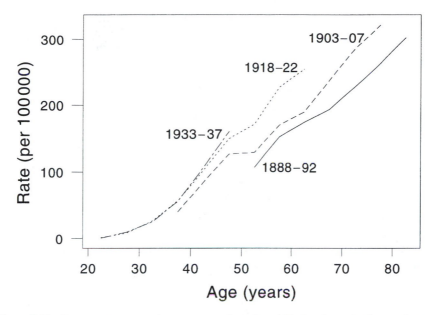

**Figure 5.11**    Breast cancer rates by age group for selected birth cohorts in Connecticut.

possibility of period-cohort effects. If there is time homogeneity the age-specific rates should be reasonably constant over the cohorts. They are clearly not, from inspection of any column in Table 5.14 or from Figure 5.11, which illustrates rates for selected cohorts from Table 5.14.

Another example where it will be advisable to consider time-specific cohorts is an occupational health study where there are known to have been important recent improvements in safety precautions.

The simplest analysis, when time homogeneity fails, will be to analyse the cohorts separately. However, this results in small numbers, incomplete estimation in most cohorts (see the gaps in Table 5.14) and may not ultimately be necessary if the sole object is to compare survival or person-years rates between levels of a risk factor. In the latter case, cohort amalgamation may still be acceptable if there is no *interaction* associated with the risk factor. For instance, the roughly parallel curves in Figure 5.11 suggest that the risk factor, age, may act in the same relative way throughout (see the comments in Section 4.7). Hence, for analyses of the effect of age the whole data set might still be considered as one. Campbell *et al.* (1994) fit a statistical model to the complete data set in Table 5.14, using both period and cohort information.

Methods for dealing with time-specific cohorts, allowing for interactions with age, are discussed by Kupper *et al.* (1985). A thorough treatment of the modelling issues is given by Clayton and Schifflers (1987a; 1987b).

### 5.7.1   Period-specific rates

Finally, we consider a topic which, although closely allied to the material of this chapter, is actually a technique for use with cross-sectional data. This is the use of rates calculated from data collected in a single time period (for instance, over the past year) to produce a view of how a population would be expected to progress if it always experienced these rates.

For example, the breast cancer rates by age group in Connecticut during 1978–82 (the most recent 5-year period covered by the data) may be extracted from Table 5.14 by considering how old each birth cohort would be once they reach the period 1978–82. It turns out that the appropriate rates are those along the bottom diagonal: that is, from 25.9 (for 35–39-year-olds) to 320.2 (for 80–84-year-olds), as plotted in Figure 5.12 (solid line).

Period-specific rates have the advantage of being relatively quick to calculate; to construct Figure 5.12 we only need data on population size and breast cancer incidence in 1978–82 rather than any protracted follow-up. They are also up to date; we would need to go back to the 1898–1902 cohort in Table 5.14 to obtain cohort-specific data on 80–84-year-olds, but then data from this cohort give an analysis of, say, 40–44-year-olds that is of considerable vintage. Often period-specific rates are calculated from readily available data such as national demographic publications which give mid-year population estimates and deaths in the past 12 months (such as appear in Table 3.15).

Unfortunately, period-specific rates are misleading whenever there is an important period-cohort effect. For example, Figure 5.12 (solid line) shows a slight fall in the rate of breast cancer at around age 80. This suggests that the oldest women alive may have some protection conferred by their age. This is seen to be misleading when we consider the first three birth cohorts (1888–1902) in Table 5.14. For each of these cohorts, the rates continue to increase with age. The dip in the solid line of Figure 5.12 arises because the 80–84-year-olds alive in 1978–82 lived through the time of least overall risk from breast cancer (over all the time studied): we can see this from the general tendency for rates to increase as we go down the columns of Table 5.14, starting at the third row. As a consequence they have accumulated less risk than the 75–79-year-olds alive in 1978–82. Two risk processes are influencing the results: an increase of risk with age and an increase of risk with calendar time (possibly caused by changes in lifestyle or environmental pollution).

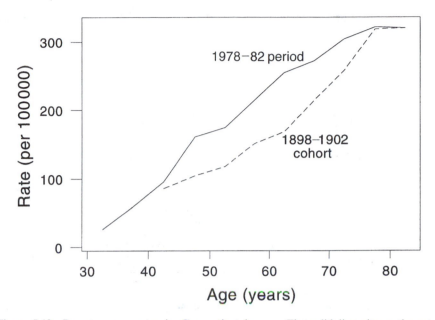

**Figure 5.12**  Breast cancer rates in Connecticut by age. The solid line shows the rates recorded during the most recent period of observation (1978–82). The dashed line shows the rates experienced by the 1898–1902 birth cohort as it passed through successive time periods from age 40 onwards.

The same phenomenon may lead to underestimation of relative rates by age group, which could be constructed from Figure 5.12 (solid line) or (more accurately) from the bottom diagonal of Table 5.14. For example, the relative rate comparing 75–79-year-olds to 50–54-year-olds using 1978–82 data (Table 5.14's diagonal) is $321.7/174.4 = 1.84$. For each of the four cohorts within which this calculation is possible in Table 5.14 (the 1888–1907 birth cohorts) the same relative rate varies between 2.46 and 2.71. To illustrate the underestimation of relative rates, the data from one of the birth cohorts (1898–1902) has been added to Figure 5.12 (as a dashed line). The dashed line gives much lower rates in the earlier years of life, producing a greater contrast with the later years than does the solid line. Such problems are always possible with cross-sectional data, but are not always acknowledged.

Period-specific rates by age may be used to construct a period-specific life table, usually called a **current life table**. This is the type of life table found in demographic yearbooks and publications of national statistical services. The layout of a current life table is similar to that of a cohort life table, although extra functions are often added. Several examples of their use are given by Pollard *et al.* (1990); fine details of their construction are given by Shryock *et al.* (1976).

## Exercises

5.1 Shaper *et al.* (1988) describe a cohort study of a random sample of 7729 middle-aged British men. Each man was asked, at baseline, his alcohol consumption (amongst other things). During the next 7.5 years death certificates were collected for any of the cohort who happened to die. The table given below was compiled.

|  | Alcohol consumption group | | | | |
|---|---|---|---|---|---|
|  | *None* | *Occasional* | *Light* | *Moderate* | *Heavy* |
| Number of subjects | 466 | 1845 | 2544 | 2042 | 832 |
| Number of deaths | 41 | 142 | 143 | 116 | 62 |

Note that occasional drinkers are defined to be those whose alcohol consumption is less than 1 unit per week; light drinkers consume 1–15 units per week; moderate drinkers 16–42 units per week; and heavy drinkers more than 42 units per week.

(i)  Calculate the risk and the relative risk (using the non-drinkers as the base group) of death for each alcohol consumption group. Calculate 95% confidence intervals for each risk and relative risk. Plot a graph of the relative risks, showing the confidence limits. What do the results appear to show about the health effects of drinking?

(ii) Why might the conclusions based on the above table alone be misleading? Given adequate funding, describe how you would go about answering the question of how alcohol consumption is related to middle-aged mortality. State the data collection method you would employ and which variables you would record.

5.2 Refer to the brain metastases data of Table C.4, treating anyone who did not die from a tumour as censored.

(i)  Construct a life table using intervals of 6 months (so that the cut-points are 0, 6, 12 etc.) using the actuarial method. Include 95% confidence intervals for the survival probabilities.

(ii) Find the Kaplan–Meier estimates of the survivor function, together with 95% confidence intervals.

(iii) Produce a diagram to compare your estimates in (i) and (ii).

(iv) Construct separate life tables with intervals of 6 months (using the actuarial method) for those who have and have not received prior treatment. Use these to compare survival probabilities at 12 months for those who have and have not received prior treatment, giving a 95% confidence interval for the difference.

(v)  Use the Mantel–Haenszel test on the life table results to compare survival experiences for those who have and have not received prior treatment.

(vi) Find Kaplan–Meier survival estimates for the two prior treatment groups. Then use the log-rank test to compare survival experiences for those who have and have not received prior treatment.

(vii) Use the generalised Wilcoxon test to repeat (vi). Compare the two results with that of (v).

5.3 Refer to the lung cancer data of Table C.1.

(i) Find the Kaplan–Meier estimates of survival function for literate and illiterate people separately.

(ii) Plot these estimates on a single graph.

(iii) Compare the two one-year survival probabilities, giving a 99% confidence interval for each and for their difference.

(iv) Use the log-rank test to compare survival experience between literate and illiterate people.

(Note: this question is very tedious without the help of a computer.)

5.4 An investigation has been carried out to explore the relationship between industrial exposure to hydrogen cyanide and coronary heart disease. The investigation studied men employed in a variety of factories, all of whom were regularly exposed to hydrogen cyanide at work. Over a 10-year period, 280 men died from coronary heart disease. In all, 15 000 man-years of follow-up were observed.

(i) If the national annual death rate from coronary heart disease amongst the male working population is 182 per 100 000, calculate the relative rate for those exposed to industrial hydrogen cyanide using the national working population as the base. Does this suggest that industrial exposure to hydrogen cyanide is an important risk factor for coronary heart disease?

(ii) Discuss the shortcomings of this investigation. Suggest ways in which the study design could be improved so as to provide better insight into the relationship of interest.

5.5 Liddell *et al.* (1977) describe an occupational cohort study of all 10 951 men born between 1891 and 1920 who worked for at least one month in the chrysotile mining and milling industry in Quebec. The paper, from which data are given below, describes 20 years' follow-up for each man until the end of 1973. From estimates of the concentration of airborne respirable dust, year by year, for each specific job within the industry and using full employment records, the investigators calculated the overall dust exposure for each man. The number of lung cancer deaths was presented within a number of dust

| Total dust exposure ($pf^{-3}y \times 10^{6}$) | Lung cancer deaths | |
| --- | --- | --- |
| | Observed | Expected |
| Less than 3 | 28 | 31.93 |
| 3–10 | 11 | 19.09 |
| 10–30 | 17 | 18.76 |
| 30–100 | 37 | 40.08 |
| 100–300 | 34 | 45.02 |
| 300–600 | 43 | 31.04 |
| 600 or greater | 28 | 12.13 |

exposure groups and compared to the expected number based on the complete cohort. Calculate the SMR for each dust exposure group, together with 95% confidence intervals. Plot the results as a graph and describe the effect of dust exposure in words.

5.6 Kitange *et al.* (1996) studied adult mortality in Tanzania, where no accurate death registration system exists. During the period from 1 June 1992 to 31 May 1995 adult deaths were recorded in three areas of the country through a system of field reports and 'verbal autopsies'. Censuses of population were also carried out for each area. The areas chosen were within the urban centre of Dar es Salaam and the rural areas of Hai and Morogoro. The table below gives observed and expected numbers of deaths for women in each area (expected numbers have been estimated from other statistics given in the source paper and cannot be accurately quoted with more significant digits). The standard population used by the authors was the female population of England and Wales in 1991.

| Deaths | Dar es Salaam | Hai | Morogoro |
|---|---|---|---|
| Observed | 615 | 693 | 1070 |
| Expected | 69.4 | 153 | 111 |

(i) Estimate the standardized mortality ratios (SMRs), together with 95% confidence intervals, within each area.
(ii) Compare the SMR for women in Hai to that in Dar es Salaam by calculating the relative SMR and its 95% confidence interval.
(iii) Repeat (ii) comparing Morogoro to Dar es Salaam.
(iv) Interpret your results.

5.7 In a cohort study of 34 387 menopausal women in Iowa, intakes of certain vitamins were assessed in 1986 (Kushi *et al.*, 1996). In the period up to the end of 1992, 879 of these women were newly diagnosed with breast cancer. The table below shows data for two vitamins, classified according to ranked categories of intake.

| Category of intake | Vitamin C | | Vitamin E | |
|---|---|---|---|---|
| | Events | $PY^a$ | Events | $PY^a$ |
| 1 (low) | 507 | 124 373 | 570 | 143 117 |
| 2 | 217 | 57 268 | 129 | 33 950 |
| 3 | 76 | 19 357 | 71 | 19 536 |
| 4 | 55 | 17 013 | 28 | 6 942 |
| 5 (high) | 24 | 7 711 | 81 | 22 176 |

$^a$PY = woman-years (as reported: note that their sum differs by one between vitamins).

For each vitamin, calculate the relative rates (with 95% confidence intervals) taking the low-consumption group as the base. Do your results suggest any beneficial (or otherwise) effect of additional vitamin C or E intake?

5.8 Refer to the data on smelter workers in Table C.5.

  (i)   Find the overall relative rate of death, high versus low arsenic exposure, together with a 95% confidence interval.

  (ii)  Find the Mantel–Haenszel relative rate corresponding to (i), adjusting for age group and calendar period simultaneously. Give the corresponding 95% confidence interval.

  (iii) Test whether exposure has an effect, adjusting for age group and calendar period.

  (iv)  Carry out a test of the assumption necessary for the application of the Mantel–Haenszel method.

# 6

# Case–control studies

## 6.1 Basic design concepts

The first step in a **case–control**, **case–referent** or **retrospective** study is to detect a number of people with the disease under study: the **cases**. We then select a number of people who are free of the disease: the **controls**. The cases and controls are then investigated to see which risk factors differ between them.

*Example 6.1* Autier *et al.* (1996) describe a study of cutaneous melanoma in which 420 adult cases (selected from five hospitals in Belgium, France and Germany) were compared to 447 adult controls (selected from the local communities served by the hospitals). Of the cases, 75% reported that they had not been protected against sunlight (for instance, by wearing a hat or applying sunblock) during their childhood. This exceeds the corresponding percentage, 69%, amongst controls. Hence being a case is more closely associated with lack of childhood protection than is being a control, and exposure to sunlight in childhood may thus be a risk factor for melanoma.

The clear difference between a case–control and a cohort study is that here we select by disease status and look back to see what, in the past, might have caused the disease. By contrast, in a cohort study we wait to see whether disease develops. Diagrammatically the comparison may be made between Figures 6.1 and 5.1.

### 6.1.1 Advantages

1. Case–control studies are quicker and cheaper than follow-up studies because there is no waiting time involved. This makes them particularly suitable for diseases with a long latency.
2. Many risk factors can be studied simultaneously. For example, the cases and controls may be asked a series of questions on aspects of their lifestyle.
3. Case–control studies are particularly well suited to investigations of risk factors for rare diseases, where otherwise there may well be problems in generating a sufficient number of diseased people to produce accurate results.

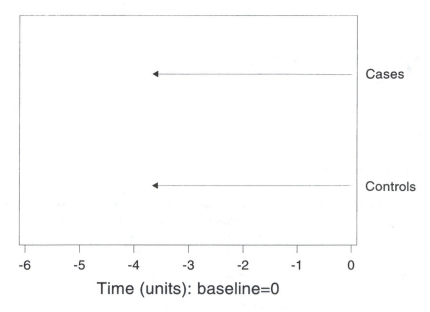

**Figure 6.1**    A representation of a case–control study.

4. Case–control studies usually require much smaller sample sizes than do equivalent cohort studies. Sample size calculation is the subject of Chapter 8; case–control and cohort study sample sizes are compared in Section 8.7.3.
5. Case–control studies are generally able to evaluate confounding and interaction rather more precisely for the same overall sample size than are cohort studies. This is because case–control studies are usually more equally balanced.

### 6.1.2   Disadvantages

1. Case–control studies do not involve a time sequence, and so are not able to demonstrate causality. For example, when more of the cases are heavy drinkers, how do we know that drinking preceded the disease? Perhaps the disease led to heavy drinking as a source of comfort. Sometimes it will be possible to question the time sequence of risk factor exposure and disease, but there are frequently problems with the accuracy of recall.
2. Being a case might reflect survival rather than morbidity. For instance, suppose that heavy smokers who have a heart attack tend to die immediately, before they reach hospital. A case–control study of heavy smoking and myocardial infarction (MI), which selects both cases and

controls from hospital, will then find that there are rather fewer heavy smokers amongst the cases than the controls. This may even appear to suggest that heavy smoking is protective against MI.

3. Case–control studies can investigate only one disease outcome. This is because sampling is carried out separately within the study groups (case and control), which are defined according to the disease outcome. Other diseases would produce different study groups.

4. Case–control studies cannot provide valid estimates of risk or odds, and can only provide approximate estimates of relative risk which are inaccurate in certain circumstances (Section 6.2).

5. Case–control studies are very likely to suffer from bias error. In many instances, problems arise from the way controls are sampled (Section 6.4). Another source of bias is differential quality of information. Cases, being more interesting in a medical sense, may be researched more thoroughly. The very fact that someone has a disease may mean that he or she has been subjected to a more rigorous investigation, perhaps X-ray screening, blood testing and the like. Also, when asked to provide information themselves, the cases may well be more likely to be accurate then the controls, simply because they have personal interest in the results of the research (see Example 6.2). In most such instances, a case is more likely to be correctly recorded as having been exposed to a particular risk factor. However, by contrast, in a comparison of recall of mothers from a case–control study of sudden infant death syndrome, Drews *et al.* (1990) found that mothers of cases were more likely to report false prior medical events. Either way there is bias against the misreported variable when it is considered as a risk factor.

Disadvantage 5 is the one most often quoted in the criticism of the case–control approach. Together with disadvantage 1, this places case–control studies below cohort studies in the hierarchy of study validity when the purpose is to investigate cause and effect. Since this is such a common goal in epidemiological investigations, this is a serious drawback.

Generally case–control studies are used for pragmatic reasons (for example, to save cost or time) rather than for considerations of validity. As a consequence, case–control studies need to be conducted very carefully, with full regard to possible sources of bias. To be persuasive, they need to be reported with evidence of avoidance or minimization of bias. Steps to avoid bias include blindness of the analyst to the case or control status of any one individual (Section 7.3.2) and careful selection of cases and controls (Sections 6.3 and 6.4).

Where possible, checks for bias should be carried out. For example, consider Example 1.1. Subsequent to their initial work, Doll and Hill (1952) were able to identify a number of lung cancer 'cases' who were wrongly diagnosed – that is, they were treated as cases in the analysis but should have been treated as controls (or, perhaps, ignored altogether). They found no difference between the smoking habits (as ascertained during the case–control study) of this misclassified set and the controls, although the true cases had much higher levels of tobacco consumption. Hence there was no evidence of a bias in risk factor assessment.

Although bias error might occur, it is unlikely fully to explain large estimates of association between risk factor and disease, such as odds ratios that exceed 3. Furthermore, we can be confident that bias has had no important effect whenever a dose-response effect (greater odds ratio, compared to the base level, at higher levels of the risk factor) is found.

*Example 6.2*  During January 1984 six cases of legionnaires' disease were reported to the health authority in Reading, UK, all of whom became ill between 15 and 19 December 1983 (Anderson *et al.*, 1985). This cluster suggested a point source outbreak. A local search was then conducted to discover whether there had been any other legionnaires' disease cases with onsets within the same 5 days. General practitioners and hospital physicians were asked to consider recent referrals and report any possible cases for further consideration, whilst hospital discharge and autopsy records were reviewed and outpatient X-rays were checked for possible cases, so far undiagnosed. The result was that 13 cases were detected in all. The cases had no obvious factor in common, such as all working in the same place, so that no clear source of the legionella bacterium (an aquatic organism) was apparent. However, all cases had visited Reading town centre just before their illness.

A case–control study was mounted to compare exposure between the cases and a selected set of 36 people without the disease (the controls). Cases and controls were compared by the number who had visited each of six designated parts of Reading town centre, just prior to the outbreak. Results are given in Table 6.1.

Frequency of visiting most parts of Reading was high amongst both groups, which is not surprising as the period covered was just before Christmas. However, most of the cases, but

**Table 6.1**  Number of people visiting parts of Reading town centre in the 2 weeks preceding the onset of legionnaires' disease

| Area of Reading | Cases | Controls |
| --- | --- | --- |
| Abbey Square | 9 | 19 |
| Butts Centre | 12 | 21 |
| Forbury Gardens | 3 | 6 |
| Minster Street | 9 | 21 |
| South Street | 4 | 9 |
| Railway Station | 3 | 9 |
| Overall | 13 | 36 |

rather fewer controls, visited the Butts Centre shopping mall. This suggests that the Butts Centre might be a source of the legionella bacterium. A formal analysis is given in Example 6.10.

Subsequently a water sample from a cooling tower in one of the buildings in the Butts Centre was found to have the legionella species, *Legionella pneumophila*. The contaminated tower had been drained, cleared and refilled 2 weeks before the outbreak occurred. It was concluded that the disease may have been spread by atmospheric drift of contaminated water droplets from this tower.

In this investigation the case–control approach is the only one possible. Speed of hypothesis testing was of paramount importance since further infections could lead to deaths. Cohort studies of legionnaires' disease will, in any case, be impractical because of the rare nature of the disease (only 558 cases were reported in England and Wales in the four years preceding the Reading outbreak), despite the common presence of the bacterium in many natural and human-made water supplies. Hence extremely large samples would be required.

One possible bias in this study is differential quality of reporting. Cases are likely to have given careful thought to what they did just before becoming ill. On the other hand, controls, with no personal interest in the disease, may well have been rather less precise in their recall. For example, some controls may have forgotten a trip that they made, several weeks before being questioned, to the shops in the Butts Centre. Hence the observed case–control differential may be due to bias error. This type of bias is sometimes called **anamnestic bias**.

### 6.1.3   Synthetic studies

A variant on the basic approach is a case–control study based upon a cohort. That is, the cases are identified as those in the cohort study who have developed disease and controls are selected from those without disease. Such studies are called **synthetic** case–control studies. Synthetic studies have the advantage over cohort studies in that they save resources (see Mantel, 1973). This includes situations where, after the cohort study has begun, it is decided that further risk factors or confounding variables should be measured. In the synthetic design only those chosen to be studied need be recalled for measurements of these 'new' variables.

For instance, in a cohort study of cancer risk factors, Lin *et al.* (1995) recruited 9775 men. Blood samples were taken and frozen at recruitment into the cohort study. Subsequently 29 cases of gastric cancer were identified from follow-up investigations, such as collection of cancer registrations. These 29 were compared to 220 healthy controls drawn from the same cohort. One hypothesis was that there was a link between *Helicobacter pylori* and subsequent gastric cancer. *H. pylori* prevalence was assessed by a test on the subject's blood. For the synthetic study the hypothesized relationship could be assessed by unfreezing and analysing only the blood samples from the cases and controls. This meant that laboratory work was much reduced compared with analysing the entire cohort, although notice that there is an underlying assumption that freezing has no effect on the results.

When the time at which subjects develop disease is known, this can be incorporated into the analysis. Controls may then be selected in a matched way (Section 6.5), taking time of disease as the matching variable: the result is called a **nested** case–control study (see Wacholder, 1991). Controls are selected from all those who are non-cases at the time concerned, including future cases (see Robins *et al.*, 1986a). Sometimes 'nested' is used in a less specific way to refer to any kind of synthetic case–control study.

Synthetic studies are generally less prone to bias error than ordinary case–control studies. For instance, the quality of information obtained on risk factor status is more likely to be the same for cases and controls when this information is captured before case or control status is determined.

## 6.2    Basic methods of analysis

### 6.2.1    Dichotomous exposure

Consider, first, the simple situation where exposure to the risk factor is dichotomous. Without loss of generality, we shall (as usual) refer to the two outcomes as 'yes' or 'no' to exposure. Data from the study then appear as a $2 \times 2$ table in the form of Table 3.1. For example, Table 6.2 gives the data reported by Autier *et al.* (1996), described in Example 6.1. No data were available for 43 subjects whose childhood protection against the sun could not be ascertained.

As in Example 6.1, it is straightforward to compare the proportion (or percentage) of cases and controls with (or without) sun protection. However, this is not the most useful comparison. The epidemiologist would really like to compare the chance of disease for those who have, and those who have not, been protected from the sun.

Since Table 6.2 is in the form of Table 3.1, the temptation is to calculate any of the summary estimates of association given in Chapter 3, including the risk

**Table 6.2**  Sun protection during childhood by case–control status for cutaneous melanoma in Belgium, France and Germany

| Sun protection? | Cases | Controls | Total |
|---|---|---|---|
| Yes | 99 | 132 | 231 |
| No | 303 | 290 | 593 |
| Total | 402 | 422 | 824 |

and relative risk. This would be incorrect, because we do not have a single random sample when a case–control study is undertaken. Instead we have a sample of cases and a separate sample of controls: a sample that is **stratified** by case–control status. This means that our overall sample would not necessarily contain anything like the same proportion of diseased subjects as are in the population within which the study is based. Since cases are generally rare and controls are plentiful, the proportion of diseased individuals in the sample will usually be much higher. For instance, the proportion of melanoma cases in the sample presented in Table 6.2 is $402/824 = 0.49$. Considerably fewer than 49% of adults have cutaneous melanoma: the annual incidence rate is approximately 1 per 10 000 and the lifetime risk is about 1 in 200 (Boyle *et al.*, 1995).

To understand what we can estimate using case–control data it is useful to consider the distribution of diseased and undiseased people by risk factor exposure status in the population: see Table 6.3(a). After Schlesselman (1982), let us suppose that the case–control study samples a fraction $f_1$ of those diseased and a fraction $f_2$ of those without the disease. That is, we sample from the *columns* of Table 6.3(a). The result is Table 6.3(b).

The risk in the population is, from (3.1), $A/(A + B)$ for those exposed to the risk factor and $C/(C + D)$ for those unexposed; whilst the relative risk is, from (3.2),

$$\frac{A(C + D)}{C(A + B)},$$

comparing the exposed to the unexposed. The expected values of these quantities in the case–control sample are, for those exposed to the risk factor,

$$f_1A/(f_1A + f_2B) \neq A/(A + B);$$

for those unexposed,

$$f_1C/(f_1C + f_2D) \neq C/(C + D);$$

and for the relative risk,

**Table 6.3**  Risk factor status by (a) disease status in the population and (b) case–control status in the sample (showing expected values)

| Risk factor status | (a) Population values | | | (b) Expected values in the sample | | |
|---|---|---|---|---|---|---|
| | Diseased | Not diseased | Total | Cases | Controls | Total |
| Exposed | $A$ | $B$ | $A + B$ | $f_1A$ | $f_2B$ | $f_1A + f_2B$ |
| Not exposed | $C$ | $D$ | $C + D$ | $f_1C$ | $f_2D$ | $f_1C + f_2D$ |
| Total | $A + C$ | $B + D$ | $N$ | $f_1(A + C)$ | $f_2(B + D)$ | $n$ |

$$\frac{f_1 A(f_1 C + f_2 D)}{f_1 C(f_1 A + f_2 B)} \neq \frac{A(C + D)}{C(A + B)}.$$

This demonstrates that the sample risk and the sample relative risk are not valid estimates of their population equivalents in a case–control study.

A similar problem arises for the odds. In the population the odds of disease are, from (3.8), $A/B$ for those exposed to the risk factor and $C/D$ for those unexposed. The expected values of the odds in the case–control sample are

$$f_1 A / f_2 B \neq A/B$$

for those exposed and

$$f_1 C / f_2 D \neq C/D$$

for those unexposed. However, for the odds ratio the sampling fractions $f_1$ and $f_2$ cancel out. That is, using (3.9), the expected sample value is

$$\frac{(f_1 A)(f_2 D)}{(f_2 B)(f_1 C)} = \frac{AD}{BC} = \psi,$$

where $\psi$ (as usual) is the odds of disease in the population. Hence we can use a case–control study to estimate the odds ratio, but not the risk, relative risk or odds.

The only exception to the above statement would be when $f_1 = f_2$. However, as already indicated, this is very unlikely in practice. The fraction of the diseased sampled, $f_1$, will tend to be much closer to 1 than will the fraction of the non-diseased sampled, $f_2$.

Lack of ability to estimate the relative risk directly is not too much of a disadvantage provided the disease is rare amongst both those with and without the risk factor, which is very often the situation when a case–control study is undertaken. In this situation the odds ratio is a good approximation to the relative risk (Section 3.3.1). Indeed many authors use the term relative risk to refer to the odds ratio from a case–control study. This is confusing, and the distinction will be maintained here.

Although there are restrictions on the range of estimation available from a case–control study, the chi-square test of Section 3.5 is applicable without modification. Similarly, Fisher's exact test (Section 3.5.4) may be used, where necessary.

Note that in a cohort study (with a fixed cohort) the estimation problems described above do not arise, even when stratified sampling is used. This is because the sampling will be from the rows of Table 6.3(a). Consequently sampling factions will always cancel out whatever measure of chance, or comparative chance, of disease is used in a cohort study.

*Example 6.3*    From the data in Table 6.2 we estimate the odds ratio for melanoma (sun protection versus no sun protection) to be

$$\frac{99 \times 290}{132 \times 303} = 0.72$$

using (3.9). The approximate standard error of the log of this odds ratio is calculated from (3.10) to be

$$\sqrt{\frac{1}{99} + \frac{1}{132} + \frac{1}{303} + \frac{1}{290}} = 0.1563.$$

From (3.11) and (3.12), approximate 95% confidence limits for the odds ratio are thus

$$\exp\{\log_e 0.72 \pm 1.96 \times 0.1563\}$$

that is, (0.53, 0.98). Hence sun protection in childhood reduces the risk of melanoma by a factor of around 0.72 (those protected have 72% of the risk of the unprotected). We are 95% sure that the interval from 0.53 to 0.98 contains the true odds ratio (approximate relative risk). If we prefer to write conclusions in terms of the elevated risk of lack of protection, we could say that the relative risk (95% confidence interval) for lack of protection versus protection is $1/0.72$ ($1/0.98$, $1/0.53$) that is, 1.39 (1.02, 1.89).

To test the null hypothesis of no association between exposure and case–control status, we use (3.16). The observed value of this is

$$\frac{824\{|99 \times 290 - 132 \times 303| - 824/2\}^2}{231 \times 593 \times 402 \times 422} = 4.19.$$

From Table B.3, this is significant at the 5% level (the exact *p* value is 0.04). Hence there is real evidence that lack of sun protection in childhood is associated with melanoma in adulthood. Note that this conclusion is consistent with unity lying just outside the 95% confidence interval.

## 6.2.2    *Polytomous exposure*

When exposure to the risk factor is measured at several levels we proceed as in Section 3.6. That is, we choose a base level and compare all other levels to this base.

*Example 6.4*    Table 6.4 gives results from a case–control study of *Escherichia coli* by Fihn *et al.* (1996). Cases were women aged 18–40 selected from the records of a health maintenance organization in Washington State, USA. Controls were randomly sampled from the same database, chosen from those women without *E. coli* infections within the same age structure as the cases. Table 6.4 gives odds ratios for ethnicity relative to the chosen base group. Caucasians were chosen as the base because they are the largest group in number, and thus most accurately measured.

There is some evidence of a relationship between ethnicity and case–control status: the chi-square statistic, (2.1), is 11.10 ($p = 0.03$). Those with *E. coli* seem more likely to be Hispanics and Asians, and less likely to be 'Others'. However, only 'Others' seem to be significantly different from the Caucasians at the 5% level, since unity is inside all the other 95% confidence intervals for the odds ratio.

**Table 6.4**   Ethnicity by case–control status in a study of *E. coli* in Washington State

| Ethnicity | Cases | Controls | Odds ratio (95% CI) |
|---|---|---|---|
| Caucasian | 514 | 541 | 1 |
| African American | 25 | 25 | 1.05 (0.60, 1.86) |
| Hispanic | 13 | 5 | 2.74 (0.97, 7.73) |
| Asian | 32 | 21 | 1.60 (0.91, 2.82) |
| Other | 20 | 37 | 0.57 (0.33, 0.99) |
| Total | 604 | 629 | |

When the levels are ordinal we would normally wish to consider a trend in the odds ratios. This cannot be achieved by the method of Section 3.6.2, since that uses risks which are non-estimable here. A method for analysing trend in odds ratios is given in Section 10.4.4.

### 6.2.3   Confounding and interaction

Just as with any kind of epidemiological study, the results obtained for a single risk factor may be compromised by confounding or interaction with other variables. The Mantel–Haenszel method of Section 4.6 may be applied to deal with confounding. Indeed, the source paper (Mantel and Haenszel, 1959) analysed a case–control study: see Example 4.12. Unfortunately, confounding may arise through the selection process in a case–control study; we should then only adjust if the confounder has a known association with disease in the parent population (see Day *et al.*, 1980). Interaction in case–control studies may be analysed as described in Section 4.8.2. Alternatively, virtually all of Chapter 10 is appropriate to case–control studies; there statistical models are used to adjust for confounding or to deal with interaction.

### 6.2.4   Attributable risk

In Section 3.7 attributable risk, $\theta$, was defined as the proportion of cases of disease that were, apparently, due to the risk factor. We can estimate $\theta$ from a case–control study provided that:
1. the odds ratio is a good approximation to the relative risk;
2. the prevalence of the risk factor amongst controls is a good approximation to the prevalence in the entire population.

The rare disease assumption, previously used only to justify proposition 1, makes these reasonable propositions provided that controls are sampled randomly from amongst those without the disease (see Cole and MacMahon, 1971).

In symbols, using the notation of Section 3.7,

1. $ad/bc$ is an approximate estimate of $\lambda$,
2. $b/(b + d)$ is an approximate estimate of $p_E$.

Hence (3.27) gives, after some algebraic manipulation,

$$\tilde{\theta} = \frac{ad - bc}{d(a + c)}, \tag{6.1}$$

where $\tilde{\theta}$ is the estimated attributable risk from a case–control study.

Assuming that the disease is rare, we can obtain approximate 95% confidence limits for the attributable risk in a case–control study as

$$\left\{ 1 + \frac{1 - \tilde{\theta}}{\tilde{\theta}} \exp(\pm u) \right\}^{-1}, \tag{6.2}$$

where

$$u = \frac{1.96d(b + d)}{a(b + d) - b(a + c)} \sqrt{\frac{a}{c(a + c)} + \frac{b}{d(b + d)}}. \tag{6.3}$$

These limits were suggested by Leung and Kupper (1981), using the same method that gave rise to (3.24). A logistic regression modelling approach to adjust the attributable risk for confounders is described by Benichou and Gail (1990); a SAS macro to carry out their computations is given by Mezzetti *et al.* (1996). Other methods are reviewed by Coughlin *et al.* (1994) and Benichou (1991).

*Example 6.5*   In a case–control study of paternal smoking and birth defects in Shanghai, China, 1012 cases with non-smoking mothers were identified during the period from 1 October 1986 to 30 September 1987. An equal number of controls with non-smoking mothers were selected from problem-free births during the same period (Zhang *et al.*, 1992). Results are given in Table 6.5.

From Table 6.5 we can estimate the odds ratio for a birth defect, comparing babies whose father smokes to those whose father does not, to be

**Table 6.5**   Paternal smoking by case–control status for birth defects in Shanghai

| Paternal smoking? | Cases | Controls |
|---|---|---|
| Yes | 639 | 593 |
| No | 373 | 419 |
| Total | 1012 | 1012 |

$$\hat{\psi} = \frac{639 \times 419}{593 \times 373} = 1.21.$$

To be able to go on to calculate attributable risk we need to ascertain that birth defects are rare and that the controls are a fair sample from the population of babies. During the year of monitoring of births in this study, 75 756 new-born were recorded, of whom 1013 (less than 2% ) had defects. Note that only one of these had to be excluded from the case definition used for Table 6.5 due to maternal smoking. Although case and control selection was based on hospital records, the controls should be a random selection from the community at large because all deliveries in Shanghai are made in hospital. Hence we can estimate attributable risk from these data.

From Table 6.5 the prevalence of paternal smoking amongst controls is

$$\frac{593}{1012} = 0.58597.$$

Hence, from (6.1), the estimated attributable risk is

$$\hat{\theta} = \frac{639 \times 419 - 593 \times 373}{419 \times 1012} = 0.10979.$$

To calculate the corresponding 95% confidence interval, we first use (6.3) to find

$$u = \frac{1.96 \times 419 \times 1012}{639 \times 1012 - 593 \times 1012} \sqrt{\frac{639}{373 \times 1012} + \frac{593}{419 \times 1012}} = 0.99262.$$

Then, from (6.2), the 95% confidence limits are

$$\left\{ 1 + \frac{1 - 0.10979}{0.10979} \exp(\pm 0.99262) \right\}^{-1} = (0.0437, 0.2497).$$

Hence we estimate that 11.0% of birth defects are attributable to paternal smoking, and we are 95% sure that the interval from 4.4% to 25.0% contains the true attributable percentage.

## 6.3    Selection of cases

Thus far the issues of subject selection have been deliberately skimmed over, so as to provide a simplified introductory account. This complex issue in the design of a case–control study will now be addressed. Case selection is considered here; control selection, and its relation with case selection, is the subject of Section 6.4.

### 6.3.1    Definition

Before cases can be selected, a precise definition of the disease to be studied must be formulated. If this is not precise there will be a danger of misclassification of potential cases and controls. If the definition is too broad then the case–control study may be futile. For instance, the definition 'mental illness' will encompass a range of conditions with very different aetiology. Even if certain clinical conditions are strongly associated with specific risk factors, the complete set of cases may have no, or only a minimal, excess of these risk factors compared with controls.

When the disease is very rare there is always a temptation to broaden the definition so as to capture extra cases. Thus in some analyses of the legionnaires' disease study (Example 6.2), people diagnosed with primary pneumonia were included together with proven legionnaires' disease sufferers because the two are difficult to distinguish. The danger is that this dilutes the true effect of exposure on the real disease. The legionnaires' disease study considered several different definitions, and thus had several different, but overlapping, case series. However, this type of approach might lead to bias if only the best results are presented.

### 6.3.2   Inclusion and exclusion criteria

Sometimes subjects with the disease are only considered eligible to be cases if they satisfy certain inclusion and exclusion criteria. These may be chosen so as to improve the validity of the study; for example, when subjects with co-existing diseases or well-established risk factors are excluded. Thus, babies with mothers who smoke were excluded from the cases in Example 6.5. It may be desirable to restrict selection to those cases with an onset of disease within a limited time period, and in a specific place. This is so whenever a **point source** of disease (in time and space) is sought; for example, during an outbreak of food poisoning and in the legionnaires' disease study of Example 6.2. Some restrictions on time and place are, in any case, necessary for practical reasons in all case–control studies.

Sometimes diseased people are excluded from the case series because they have no, or very little, chance of exposure to the risk factor. Thus in a study of oral contraceptives as a risk factor for breast cancer we should exclude post-menopausal women. Including them would be a waste of resources. Exclusions on grounds of efficiency often utilize age and sex criteria.

### 6.3.3   Incident or prevalent?

Incident disease is a better criterion for case selection. Prevalent cases introduce a greater element of ambiguity in the time sequence, as discussed in Sections 1.4.1 and 3.4. For instance, alcohol consumption may be associated with the absence of angina simply because many of those with angina have been told to stop drinking by their doctor.

The great advantage with prevalent cases is their ready availability in large numbers for certain conditions. This would represent a distinct saving in time and effort when studying a rare, but non-fatal, chronic condition. When prevalent cases are used, steps should be taken to minimize the chance of error. For example, the reasons for, and not just the fact of, use of medication or clinical procedures should be questioned.

### 6.3.4   Source

Cases are usually selected from medical information systems. The most common source is hospital admission records, but operating theatre or pathology department records, sickness absence forms and disease registers are other potential sources. Further possibilities are given in Example 6.2. As in the study described there, several sources may be utilized so as to broaden the search, where necessary.

### 6.3.5   Consideration of bias

Case selection will be biased if the chance of having the risk factor is different for those from whom the cases are drawn, and for all of those who have the disease (that is, in the parent population). If we let $p_{case}$ be the probability of exposure (assumed, for simplicity, to be dichotomous) amongst cases and $p_{disease}$ be the corresponding probability for all those with the disease, then we have bias if

$$p_{case} \neq p_{disease}.$$

Such bias will occur whenever the chance of becoming as case depends, in some way, on the fact of exposure to the risk factor.

An example arises where hormone replacement therapy (HRT) is considered as a risk factor for cervical cancer. Women patients registered with a particular health centre who take HRT daily are required to attend at an annual HRT clinic, held at the health centre, as a condition of renewal of their prescription. At the clinic they undergo a cervical smear. Although other female patients will routinely be given notice that they are due for a smear, this is only done at intervals of several years and many will not attend for the screening test. Hence undetected cervical cancer is more likely amongst those who are not receiving HRT and

$$p_{case} > p_{disease}.$$

In this example the potential problem might be removed if only advanced stages of the disease are considered. Then it may well be that all the diseased will have been detected, whatever the subject's history.

A second example shows bias in the opposite direction. Pearl (1929) studied data from autopsies and found that cancer and tuberculosis (TB) were rarely found together. He thus suggested that cancer patients might be treated with tuberculin (the protein of the TB bacterium). Hence (lack of) TB is supposed to be a risk factor for cancer. However, not all deaths were equally likely to be autopsied. It happened that people who died from cancer and TB were less likely to be autopsied than those who died from cancer alone. Hence

$$p_{case} < p_{disease}$$

In this case the bias arises specifically because of the source (autopsies) used. This type of bias is known as **Berkson's bias**, as reviewed by Walter (1980a) and Feinstein *et al.* (1986). More examples appear in Section 6.4.

Although we should be concerned whenever the case selection is biased, this may not, in itself, invalidate the case–control analysis. As seen in Section 6.2, the analysis will be based on a comparison of cases and controls. Consequently the result (that is, the odds ratio for exposure versus no exposure) will only be biased if there is *differential* bias in case and control selection. Further details appear in Section 6.4.2.

## 6.4    Selection of controls

Controls should be a representative subgroup of those members of the same base group that gave rise to cases, who have the particular characteristic that they have not (yet) developed the disease. With all else equal (specifically, exposure to the risk factor of interest), a case and a control should have had the same chance as becoming classified as a case, had they become diseased.

In practice such comparability is often difficult to achieve, making this the most challenging aspect of case–control study design. A thorough exposition of principles and practice is given by Wacholder *et al.* (1992) and several numerical examples are given by Sackett (1979). A more concise account is provided in this section.

### 6.4.1    General principles

Four general principles involved in control selection may be identified. The first two of these derive from the general requirement of comparability given above.

The other two are concerned with efficiency and validity of attribution of effect of the particular risk factor.

1. Controls should be drawn from amongst those who are free of the disease being studied. Usually we would exempt anyone who, although disease-free now, has had the disease in the past.

2. Controls should be drawn from the same general population as gave rise to the cases. This is necessary to protect (as far as possible) against the possible distorting effects of unknown, or unmeasured, confounders and effect modifiers. The same inclusion/exclusion criteria as used for cases (Section 6.3.2) should be applied, as far as is appropriate, without introducing any new criteria. Thus, in Example 6.5 controls were drawn from non-smoking mothers since the decision had been made to exclude cases whose mother smoked.

3. The source from which controls are selected should not give rise to bias error. By analogy with Section 6.3.5, bias in inferences drawn specifically about controls arises when

$$p_{\text{control}} \neq p_{\text{undiseased}}$$

where $p$ denotes the chance of exposure. We shall see examples of this problem in Section 6.4.2.

4. Controls should have some potential for the disease. For instance women who have had their womb removed should not be considered as controls in a study of endometrial cancer. If they were, some of those without a womb but with the risk factor would be expected to have become cases had they retained their womb. Consequently the comparison between cases and controls would underestimate the effect of the risk factor, assuming that there is no equal (or greater) bias associated with the cases.

Notice that there is not, as sometimes stated, any reason to exclude a control purely because he or she has no potential for exposure to the risk factor. Besides the issues raised in 1–4 above, we are interested in comparing all those who have no exposure. See Poole (1986) for a discussion of this issue.

Controls are either drawn from the same source (such as the same hospital) as were cases, or from the community served by the same medical services. Hospital controls are considered in Section 6.4.2, community controls in Section 6.4.3 and other types of control in Section 6.4.4. Where possible, more than one type of control group might be used. In this situation, comparison of the control groups may highlight problems. If the groups are the same (in terms of risk factor profiles) then no particular problem is found and the control groups should be combined. This does not rule out bias caused by selection of controls, but makes it less likely. If the control groups are different in some important way there may well be bias associated with at least one of them, and further investigation is necessary. This may result in ignoring one (or more) of the control groups subsequently. Drawbacks are that it may not be easy to reconcile differences, and the whole process will be demanding in resources. When the disease is particularly rare, the make-up of the control group may be checked against the make-up (say by age, sex and race) of the national population as a whole.

*Example 6.6*   Moritz *et al.* (1997) describe a comparison of hospital and community controls when female cases of hip fracture aged 45 years or more were selected from hospitals in New York City and Philadelphia, USA. They found that the estimates of effect for some risk factors differed greatly when the different control groups were used separately in the analysis. Table 6.6 shows a selection of their results.

When community controls (a sample of women living in the communities where the cases lived) were used, then falling during the past 6 months, smoking and stroke were much more important risk factors than when hospital controls (sampled from the same hospitals as the cases) were used. On the other hand, the use of hospital controls (women sampled from surgical, orthopaedic or medical wards) suggested a stronger effect of poor vision on the risk of a hip fracture. For all these four risk factors there is a significant ($p < 0.05$) effect when one source of controls is used, but not when the alternative is used.

The explanation for the difference is likely to be that hospital controls tend to be less healthy in a general sense (although apparently not in terms of eyesight). The authors of the source paper suggest that community controls may be better for studying frail, elderly individuals.

## 6.4.2   Hospital controls

Hospitals are a convenient and cheap source of controls, especially in situations where a clinical procedure, such as a blood sample, is required to measure the risk factor. They have the advantage that their medical data are likely to be of comparable quality to those from the cases, and may have been collected prior to classification as controls (removing the possibility of observer bias). There is a good chance that their quality of recall will also be similar to

**Table 6.6**   Odds ratios (with 95% confidence intervals)[a] in a study of hip fracture using two different control groups

| Risk factor | Hospital controls | Community controls |
| --- | --- | --- |
| Fall in past 6 months | 1.08 (0.71, 1.53) | 1.70 (1.22, 2.35) |
| Current (versus never) smoking | 1.30 (0.85, 1.98) | 2.49 (1.61, 3.83) |
| Stroke | 1.36 (0.87, 2.11) | 2.51 (1.60, 3.94) |
| Poor vision | 2.62 (1.27, 5.37) | 1.42 (0.81, 2.48) |

[a]Adjusted for several potential confounding variables.

that for cases (reducing the chance of anamnestic bias), since they are in the same environment. As with the cases, they are likely to be thinking about the antecedents of their disease and they are likely to be co-operative, especially as they have time to spare.

One disadvantage is that the risk factor for the study disease may also be a risk factor for the condition that a particular control has, this condition being the cause of his or her hospitalization. For example, in the study of lung cancer and smoking by Doll and Hill (Example 1.1) the controls were to be non-cancer patients selected from the same hospitals as the cases. As mentioned in Section 1.2, several of the controls had been hospitalized for diseases that we now know to be related to smoking. Hence

$$p_{\text{control}} > p_{\text{undiseased}},$$

and there was thus a bias in favour of the risk factor in the analysis that compares lung cancer cases and controls. Exactly the same kind of bias appears to have operated when hospital controls were used in the study reported in Example 6.6 (no significant effect of smoking was found, despite the contrary conclusion when community controls were used).

The reverse situation could occur if we studied aspirin and MI. We would expect lack of aspirin taking to be likely to lead to hospitalization for MI because of aspirin's platelet-inhibiting property. However, if our controls contain, for example, large numbers who suffer from arthritis then we should expect many of these to be taking aspirin to alleviate pain. Hence when we consider lack of aspirin as the risk factor for MI,

$$p_{\text{control}} < p_{\text{undiseased}}$$

and we have bias in the direction contrary to the risk factor – that is, we have a reduced estimate of the benefit of aspirin for avoiding a heart attack.

To reduce such problems it is best to choose controls from a range of conditions, exempting any disease that is likely to be related to exposure (as discussed by Wacholder and Silverman, 1990). In order to ensure comparability with cases, conditions for which the hospital (of the cases) is a regional specialty might be excluded. Otherwise the controls may have, for example, a much wider socio-economic profile since they are drawn from a wider catchment population. If the hospital is a regional specialty for the disease under study (that is, the condition suffered by the cases) then a number of local hospitals might be used to provide controls.

The second major disadvantage is the possibility of Berkson's bias – differential rates of hospitalization. To see how this arises, consider the distribution of exposure and disease in the population, Table 6.3(a), once

**Table 6.7** Risk factor by disease status for hospital patients (disease refers to the specific disease being studied)

| | Disease status | |
|---|---|---|
| Risk factor status | Disease | No disease |
| Exposed | $f_1 A$ | $f_2 B$ |
| Unexposed | $f_3 C$ | $f_4 D$ |

again. Suppose that fractions $f_1$ of those exposed and diseased, $f_2$ of those exposed and not diseased, $f_3$ of those unexposed and diseased and $f_4$ of those unexposed and not diseased are hospitalized. The result is Table 6.7, showing the hospital population distribution. If all those hospitalised were studied in the case–control study then the odds ratio is

$$\psi_H = \frac{f_1 A f_4 D}{f_2 B f_3 C} = \left(\frac{f_1 f_4}{f_2 f_3}\right)\frac{AD}{BC} = \left(\frac{f_1 f_4}{f_2 f_3}\right)\psi. \tag{6.4}$$

If the hospitalization fractions (the *f*s) are different then $\psi_H \neq \psi$, the true odds ratio for the entire population. When a random sample is drawn from amongst those in hospital with the study disease and/or (more likely) those in hospital without this disease, $\psi_H$ is the expected value, and the same problem arises. Differential hospitalization rates might be caused by the influence of a second disease.

*Example 6.7*  Sackett (1979) reports a study of 2784 individuals sampled from the community. Of these 257 had been hospitalized during the previous six months. Data from the whole and for the hospitalized subset only are given in Table 6.8. Both data displays show the presence or absence of respiratory disease and the presence or absence of diseases of the bones and organs of movement (labelled 'bone disease').

**Table 6.8**  Bone disease by respiratory disease status in (a) the general population and (b) in hospitalized subjects

| | Respiratory disease in | | | |
|---|---|---|---|---|
| | (a) Population | | (b) Hospital | |
| Bone disease? | Yes | No | Yes | No |
| Yes | 17 | 184 | 5 | 18 |
| No | 207 | 2376 | 15 | 219 |
| % Yes | 8% | 7% | 25% | 8% |

If we were to consider bone disease as a risk factor for respiratory disease we would find a large effect should we draw our case–control sample from hospital (25% versus 8%). However, there is really almost no effect (8% versus 7% in the entire population).

More particularly,

$$\hat{\psi}_H = \frac{5 \times 219}{18 \times 15} = 4.06,$$

whereas

$$\hat{\psi} = \frac{17 \times 2376}{1840 \times 207} = 1.06.$$

Hence hospital subjects would give a misleading picture of risk. Comparing the two parts of Table 6.8, we can see that hospitalization rates are much higher when someone has both diseases ($f_1 = 5/17 = 0.29$) than when he or she has only one disease ($f_2 = 0.10$, $f_3 = 0.07$) or neither disease ($f_4 = 0.09$). This causes the bias in the hospitalized odds ratio.

In general we might expect higher hospitalization rates when someone has multiple illnesses (as in Example 6.7), since then they are rather more ill than when they have only one condition. This can cause a bias even when the 'second' condition is not a subject of study, because the risk factors for this second condition will then be over-represented amongst cases of the condition of interest. For instance, suppose lack of vitamin K is a risk factor for bone disease. Hospital cases of respiratory disease will, on the basis of Example 6.7, be more likely to have low levels of vitamin K than the controls, even though vitamin K consumption has no effect on respiratory disease.

One point to emphasize about Berkson's bias is that (in this context) it requires *differential* hospitalization rates between cases and controls. For instance, we would not expect this kind of bias should there be (as often happens) lower rates of hospitalization amongst those of lower social class or amongst ethnic minority groups, provided that the effect of class or ethnicity is the same for those diseased and undiseased.

We can see this from (6.4). Suppose that exposure to the risk factor multiplies the chance of hospitalization by a factor of $e$, regardless of the health problem. For example, the most deprived members of society might have 80% of the chance of hospitalization that others have, whenever they become sick (that is, $e = 0.8$). Then,

$$f_1 = f_3 e \quad \text{and} \quad f_2 = f_4 e$$

so that (6.4) becomes

$$\psi_H = \frac{(f_3 e) f_4}{(f_4 e) f_3} \psi = \psi.$$

For this and other potential sources of bias, we will not have bias in the overall measure of comparison, $\psi$, when there is equal bias in case and control selection. Of course, in practice, we may often suspect that bias occurs, without having the means to quantify it and thereby see whether it is equally distributed.

### 6.4.3  Community controls

Controls drawn from the community have the great advantage of being drawn directly from the true population of those without the disease. Assuming that they are drawn randomly, they provide a valid basis for the estimation of the attributable risk when the disease is rare (Section 6.2.4). They would almost certainly be the ideal source when cases are also identified in the community because of the complete generalizability in this situation. Even when cases are detected in hospital, community controls do not have the problem of selection bias that is due to their exposure status.

The disadvantages with random community controls are that they are inconvenient to capture and their data are often of inferior quality. Random sampling requires a sampling frame, such as a list of all adults in a town, which may be difficult to obtain. Interviews will often need to be carried out, and medical investigations may be required, which will necessitate personal contact being made. Locating and visiting selected controls at home may be expensive and time-consuming. Subjects may be unwilling to co-operate, especially when asked to attend a clinic and/or to submit to invasive procedures. Convenient sampling frames, such as telephone directories, may introduce a selection bias (for example, socio-economic bias). Indeed, all the types of bias generally associated with sample surveys, such as bias caused by non-response and poor-quality fieldwork, may occur. Such problems may not arise for cases, especially when they are drawn from hospitals, and hence there could be an important differential bias.

Another possible problem is that there may be bias in case selection which might well 'cancel' out if hospital controls were used and only becomes important when community controls are employed. For instance, those with the disease might be more likely to be hospitalized if they are of high socio-economic status, particularly if the disease is not generally fatal (for example, conditions related to fertility). Controls (for instance, parents identified from school records) will presumably have a complete social mix. The effect of factors associated with social status will then be judged in a biased way. Thus, if the well-off eat a diet that is relatively high in protein, then

$$p_{case} > p_{disease}$$

where $p$ is the probability of a high-protein diet. Assuming controls are sampled randomly, no equivalent bias occurs in controls. The study might thus find an erroneous link between dietary protein and infertility.

### 6.4.4  Other sources

Other sources for controls are medical systems other than hospitals (as in Example 6.4) and special groups in the community who have some relation to the cases (such as friends, neighbours and relatives). Relative controls should be particularly useful when genetic factors are possible confounders.

Usually the medical systems used to locate controls are those that give rise to the cases (as in Example 6.4). The issues will be similar to those discussed in Section 6.4.2.

Special community controls are generally only used in **matched** case–control studies. In the simplest kind of matched study each case is individually paired with a control who is (say) a near neighbour. The idea is that this should ensure that such factors as exposure to air pollution, socio-economic status and access to medical care are balanced between cases and controls, thus removing any confounding effect. A full description of matched studies appears in Sections 6.5 and 6.6: the question of whether or not to match is a further issue in the selection of controls.

Special community controls have the advantage of not requiring a sampling frame, although neighbourhood controls may be difficult to obtain due to non-response within a limited population. For example, the legionnaires' disease study of Example 6.2 used neighbourhood controls and this led to many revisions of the control selection, due to failure to locate co-operative neighbours who satisfied other inclusion criteria (see Example 6.10).

Friends and relatives are unlikely to refuse to co-operate, and so are easy and cheap both to identify and to obtain. However, other types of bias are often a problem, particularly since the sample is necessarily non-random. For instance, lonely people will be missed out of friend control groups and small households are relatively unlikely to yield neighbourhood controls, if only because there is more chance of an empty house when a call is made. In both cases there might be a consequent bias against social activities, such as smoking and drinking, in the final analysis. An example is given by Siemiatycki (1989). On the other hand, special controls are often too similar to the cases, meaning that the risk factor tends to be rather more common in controls than it would otherwise be, leading to bias in the other direction. This problem is known as **overmatching** (discussed further in Section 6.5.2).

### 6.4.5   How many?

Sometimes the number of cases is fixed, because we can detect no more. This was certainly true in the legionnaires' disease outbreak in Reading (Example 6.2) where case searching was intense and thus probably all-inclusive. On the other hand, the number of available controls is usually very large, indeed virtually unlimited in some situations. A naive approach would be to choose just as many controls as there are cases, but where it is possible to choose more, should we do so?

Almost certainly the answer to this question is 'yes', because there will then be greater precision in estimates and tests. Economic and time considerations may also come into play, especially as the extra precision will be subject to the 'law of diminishing returns'. Rarely will it be worth having a case : control ratio of above 1 : 4.

One measurement of precision is the power of the test for no exposure–disease relationship (see Section 8.2 for a definition of 'power'). Figure 6.2 shows how power increases as the number of controls increases, when the number of cases is fixed. The points on this figure correspond to situations

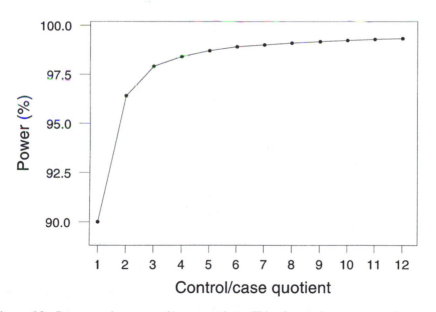

**Figure 6.2** Power against control/case quotient. This shows the power to detect an approximate relative risk of 2 when the risk factor has a prevalence of 30%, a two-sided 5% significance test is to be used and 188 cases are available.

where the number of controls is an integer multiple of the number of cases (between 1 and 12). Of course this multiple could be fractional; consideration of fractional multiples would produce a smooth curve for the figure.

Notice how much better a 1 : 2 study is than a 1 : 1 study, showing that it is worthwhile to double the number of controls. The extra power soon becomes less important as the control/case quotient increases; above 4 (a case : control ratio of 1 : 4) there is little improvement when the control/case quotient is increased.

The theory required to produce Figure 6.2 is given in Section 8.7; in particular, (8.22) defines the power. Figure 6.2 illustrates a special situation suggested by Example 8.18, but the concept it illustrates is a general one.

## 6.5   Matching

In Chapter 4 we have seen how to adjust for confounding during the analysis stage of an epidemiological investigation. Such adjustment may, instead, be made at the design stage by the process of **matching**. The simplest type of matching is where each case is matched with a single control (**1 : 1 matching** or **pair matching**), so that the control has identical (or, at least, very similar) values of the confounding variables. In this design the case and control groups are identically balanced, and so any difference between them cannot be due to the confounders.

Common matching variables are age and sex. In particular circumstances, race, marital status, hospital, time of admission to hospital, neighbourhood, parity, blood group and social class (amongst others) may be sensible matching criteria. Continuous variables, such as age, are matched within a pre-specified range. Sometimes this is done by grouping the variables; for example, age might be categorized into 5-year age groups and the control must be within the same 5-year age group as the case. A better technique is to insist that the control is aged within so many years either side of the case's age – for example, no more than $2\frac{1}{2}$ years younger or older. The finer the groupings the more effective the matching.

### 6.5.1   Advantages

1. There is direct control of the confounders. This means that the 'adjustment' of the relationship between risk factor and disease is achieved automatically and intuitively, leading to a clear interpretation. This is the most common reason for matching.

2. It ensures that adjustment is possible. In exceptional circumstances there might be no overlap between the cases and a randomly sampled set of controls. For instance, all the cases may be elderly, but the controls include no elderly people. Adjusting for age, using the Mantel–Haenszel (Section 4.6) or some other procedure, would not then be possible.

3. Under certain conditions, matching improves the efficiency of the investigation. For instance, a smaller sample size could be used, or the effect of the risk factor could be estimated with a shorter confidence interval. Many studies of relative efficiency of matched and unmatched case–control studies have been carried out: for example, McKinlay (1977), Kupper et al. (1981), Thompson et al. (1982) and Thomas and Greenland (1983). The comparison is complex because relative efficiency depends upon several factors, many of which may be difficult to quantify in advance of data collection. In summary, the matched design is only more efficient if the matching variable is a true confounder (that is, related both to the disease and to the risk factor), and if there are only a moderate number of rejected controls (controls which cannot be matched to a case).

### 6.5.2   Disadvantages

1. Data collection is more complex. It may be difficult to find a suitable match, especially when there are several matching variables. For example, we may have to locate a disease-free Afro-Caribbean woman in her fifth pregnancy from a neighbourhood that is predominantly Caucasian. This may make the investigation more expensive than the corresponding unmatched study, especially when the potential controls have to be questioned before a decision can be reached as to whether they should be accepted or discarded (see McKinlay, 1977). Of course we can always relax the matching criteria, perhaps by eliminating a matching factor or widening the groups for a continuous variable, but this inevitably reduces the fundamental benefit of matching.

2. Data analysis must take account of the matching. A matched study requires a matched analysis, which is often considerably more complex both to understand and compute (Section 6.6).

3. The effect (on disease) of the matching variable cannot be estimated. By design we know that the probability of being a case, given a certain level of exposure to the matching variable, in a paired study is $\frac{1}{2}$. So we cannot take account of the matching variable as a risk factor in its own right. We can, however, estimate the interaction of the risk factor and the matching variable (see Thomas and Greenland, 1985).

4. Adjustment cannot be removed. We cannot estimate the effect of the risk factor without adjustment for the matching variable. Sometimes the contrast between unadjusted and adjusted odds ratios is an important component of the interpretation of the epidemiological data.
5. There may be overmatching. This is where the matching has been done incorrectly or unnecessarily. That is, the matching variable has some relationship with the risk factor or disease, but it is either not a true confounder or is so highly correlated with other matching variables as to be superfluous. This may simply result in loss of efficiency, but may also cause biased results. MacMahon and Trichopoulos (1996) suggest an example of overmatching where the consequent odds ratio is correct, but the procedure is inefficient because many data items are redundant. This is where matching is done on religion in a study of oral contraceptive risk. Assuming religion is unrelated to disease, matching on religion may well produce many case–control pairs who have no chance of exposure to oral contraceptives because of their religious beliefs. They can provide no information about risk.

Whether or not to match is not an easy question to answer. As discussed already, when the matching variable is not a true confounder matching is probably less efficient; when it is a true confounder it is probably more efficient, unless the cost of matching is high. The precise comparison between the efficiency of matched and unmatched designs depends upon several factors, including the strengths of relationships, the way confounding is addressed in the analysis of the unmatched design and the type of matching used. When there is a large pool of controls, from which information on risk factor and confounder exposure may be obtained cheaply, it is unlikely that a pair-matched study, with many rejected controls, will be a worthwhile alternative to the unmatched design. See Thompson *et al.* (1982) and Thomas and Greenland (1983) for detailed discussions.

### 6.5.3   One-to-many matching

Since it is highly likely that there are many more controls available than there are cases, we can often contemplate matching each case with several controls, so as to improve efficiency (for example, precision of estimates). We shall refer to this as $1 : c$ matching, meaning that one case is matched to $c$ controls. As $c$ increases more and more of the 'spare' controls will be used up, provided they can be matched with cases. This increases overall sample size, and hence gives more precise estimation.

The relative precision of matching, say, $r$, rather than $s$ controls to each case was studied by Ury (1975). He shows that the relative efficiency is

**Table 6.9**   Relative efficiencies (using the criteria of Ury, 1975) for the number of matched controls per case

| Number of controls | Relative efficiency compared to one less | Relative efficiency compared to pairing |
|---|---|---|
| 2 | 1.333 | 1.333 |
| 3 | 1.125 | 1.500 |
| 4 | 1.067 | 1.600 |
| 5 | 1.042 | 1.667 |
| 6 | 1.029 | 1.714 |
| 7 | 1.021 | 1.750 |
| 8 | 1.016 | 1.778 |
| 9 | 1.013 | 1.800 |
| 10 | 1.010 | 1.818 |

$r(s+1)/s(r+1)$. Using this formula, Table 6.9 has been constructed to show the relative efficiency for a range of numbers of controls compared both to pairing and to one less control (for each case). Clearly pairing is inefficient: even 1 : 2 matching is a third again as efficient. In agreement with the comments for unmatched studies (in Section 6.4.5), there is little gain from having more than four matched controls per case (for example using five controls is only 4% more efficient than using four).

### 6.5.4   Frequency and category matching

A similar procedure to individual matching, as presented above, is to ensure that the control sample has a similar overall make-up to the case sample. Hence, if the cases consist of 100 young men, 50 old men, 25 young women and 25 old women then the control sample will be made the same. This will be referred to as **frequency matching**, although this term sometimes has other connotations. In practice, frequency matching may be only approximately achieved due to drop-outs or failure to locate the total number required. It requires the distribution of cases to be known, which is not possible if cases are identified sequentially as the study progresses.

Frequency matching has a great advantage over pair matching in that the loss of a case (or control) does not imply the automatic loss of the corresponding control (or case). As McKinlay (1977) and Kleinbaum *et al.* (1982) point out, pairing is often arbitrary in that a case could have been matched with another case's control when two or more cases have common matching variable outcomes. Frequency matching effectively combines in a single group cases which match with each other and their corresponding controls. Intuitively this seems preferable.

As with individual matching, frequency matching does not have to seek groups of equal size: the controls could be chosen to have a similar *proportional* make-up, in terms of the confounding variables, to the cases. In general, we could sample an arbitrary number of cases and an arbitrary number of controls from within each category defined by the cross-classification of the matching variables. This is known as **category matching**; frequency matching is the most efficient version of category matching. See also Section 6.6.4.

### 6.5.5   *Matching in other study designs*

Although matching is given here as a methodology for case–control studies, it could also be applied to cohort or intervention studies. There we would match risk factor status, rather than disease status. For example, we might match a smoker to a non-smoker of the same sex and age in a cohort study of lung cancer. As Kleinbaum *et al.* (1982) show, matching has theoretical attractions for such follow-up designs.

## 6.6   The analysis of matched studies

When a case–control study (or, indeed, any other type of study) is matched the analysis *must* take account of the matching. If, instead, the standard unmatched analysis is used the odds ratio will tend to be closer to unity; hence we are liable to miss detecting the effect of a true risk factor. This is because the cases and controls will be more similar to each other than they should be, if independent sampling had taken place.

The appropriate analysis for matched studies turns out to be very simple for 1 : 1 matching (Section 6.6.1) but more complex in the general case (Sections 6.6.2–6.6.4). In this section we restrict to analyses based on $2 \times 2$ tables, or combinations of such tables. An alternative, more general approach, through statistical modelling is given in Section 10.11.2. There, again, the 1 : 1 situation turns out to be a simple special case.

### 6.6.1   *1 : 1 matching*

The results of a paired study, with subjects classified by exposure/no exposure to the risk factor of interest, should be presented in terms of the study pairs. In particular, the format of Table 6.10 is appropriate to display the data, rather

**Table 6.10**    Display of results from a paired case–control study

| Case exposed to the risk factor? | Control exposed to the risk factor? Yes | No |
|---|---|---|
| Yes | $c_1$ | $d_1$ |
| No | $d_2$ | $c_2$ |

than Table 3.1. Table 6.10 displays information about the case–control pairs observed. Each member of the pair is either exposed or unexposed to the risk factor, and is (of course) either a case or a control, giving the four possible outcomes shown in the table.

Pairs with the same exposure status for both case and control are called **concordant** pairs; the total number of concordant pairs is $c_1 + c_2$. Pairs with different exposures are called **discordant**; there are $d_1 + d_2 = d$ discordant pairs.

Let $\phi$ be the probability that a discordant pair has an exposed case. Then, from Table 6.10, $\phi$ is estimated by the proportion,

$$\hat{\phi} = d_1/(d_1 + d_2) = d_1/d. \tag{6.5}$$

Under the usual null hypothesis that there is no association between the risk factor and disease, each discordant pair is just as likely to have the case exposed as to have the control exposed. Thus the null hypothesis can be written as

$$H_0 : \phi = \tfrac{1}{2}.$$

This is a test of the value of a proportion. Adopting a normal approximation, the general case of this is considered in Section 2.5.2. From (2.4), a test of no association in a paired study has the test statistic

$$\frac{\hat{\phi} - 0.5}{\sqrt{0.5(1 - 0.5)/d}} = \frac{2d_1 - d}{\sqrt{d}}. \tag{6.6}$$

We compare (6.6) to the standard normal distribution (Table B.1 or B.2). Alternatively, we could square (6.6) to give

$$\frac{(2d_1 - d)^2}{d}, \tag{6.7}$$

which we compare to chi-square with 1 d.f. (Table B.3). As usual (Section 3.5.3), a continuity correction might be applied to either (6.6) or (6.7). For instance, (6.8) is the continuity-corrected chi-square statistic

$$\frac{(|2d_1 - d| - 1)^2}{d}. \tag{6.8}$$

The test based on any of (6.6)–(6.8) is referred to as **McNemar's test**, the test for no association in a paired study of proportions. It is a direct analogue of the paired $t$ test for quantitative data (Section 2.7.4).

To obtain an estimate of the odds ratio, $\psi$, we may use the following relationship between $\phi$ and $\psi$,

$$\psi = \phi/(1 - \phi), \tag{6.9}$$

which is easy to prove from basic rules of probability (see Cox, 1958). Taking (6.5) and (6.9) together gives an estimate for $\psi$ of

$$\hat{\psi} = d_1/d_2. \tag{6.10}$$

Note that (6.9) shows that when $\phi = \frac{1}{2}$ the value of the odds ratio $\psi$ is 1. Hence (6.6)–(6.8) give tests of $\psi = 1$, as we would anticipate.

When $d$ is large we can use (2.2) to get 95% confidence limits for $\phi$ by a normal approximation, thus leading to confidence limits for $\psi$ using (6.9). However, $d$ is often fairly small in paired case–control studies and it is then necessary to use exact limits for $\psi$. Breslow and Day (1980) give these limits as $(\psi_L, \psi_U)$, where

$$\psi_L = d_1/\{(d_2 + 1)F_L\}, \qquad \psi_U = (d_1 + 1)F_U/d_2, \tag{6.11}$$

in which $F_L$ and $F_U$ are the upper $2\frac{1}{2}$% points of $F$ with $(2(d_2 + 1), 2d_1)$ and $(2(d_1 + 1), 2d_2)$ d.f., respectively.

Since McNemar's test is an approximate one, when $n$ is small a preferable testing procedure (for $H_0 : \psi = 1$) at the 5% level is to calculate the 95% confidence interval for $\psi$ from (6.11) and reject $H_0$ if unity is outside it. A more direct method is given by Liddell (1980).

*Example 6.8*  A case–control study of presenile dementia by Forster *et al.* (1995) identified 109 clinically diagnosed patients aged below 65 years from hospital records. Each case was individually paired with a community control of the same sex and age, having taken steps to ascertain that the control did not suffer from dementia.

Table 6.11 shows the status of the 109 pairs for one of the risk factors explored in the study: family history of dementia. Information on the relationship between family history of

**Table 6.11**  Family history of dementia and case–control status in a paired study of presenile dementia

| Case has a relative with dementia? | Control has a relative with dementia? | |
| --- | --- | --- |
| | Yes | No |
| Yes | 6 | 25 |
| No | 12 | 66 |

dementia and disease comes from the 37 discordant pairs, 25 of which had an exposed case. The 66 pairs where neither person had a relative with dementia and 6 pairs where both had a relative with dementia yield no information about this relationship.

Using (6.8), McNemar's continuity-corrected test statistic is

$$\frac{(|2 \times 25 - 37| - 1)^2}{37} = 3.89.$$

Compared to $\chi_1^2$, using Table B.3, this is just significant at the 5% level. Hence there is evidence of an effect of family history on dementia.

From (6.10) the odds ratio is estimated to be

$$25/12 = 2.08,$$

so that a family history of dementia roughly doubles an individual's chance of presenile dementia.

The 95% confidence limits for the odds ratio are, from (6.11),

$$\psi_L = 25/13F_L, \qquad \psi_U = 26F_U/12$$

where $F_L$ and $F_U$ are the upper $2\frac{1}{2}$% points of F on $(2 \times 13, 2 \times 25) = (26, 50)$ and $(2 \times 26, 2 \times 12) = (52, 24)$ d.f., respectively. From a computer package these were found to be 1.9066 and 2.1006, respectively. Hence the 95% confidence interval for the odds ratio is

$$(25/(13 \times 1.9066), 26 \times 2.1066/12) = (1.01, 4.55).$$

## 6.6.2    1 : c matching

When each case is matched to $c$ controls a test statistic which generalizes McNemar's test may be derived using the same methodology as that used in Section 6.6.1. Alternatively, the Mantel–Haenszel (MH) approach may be used. Both approaches give the same results, as shown by Pike and Morrow (1970). We will consider the MH derivation only. Derivations of formulae will be provided, using the results of Section 4.6. Details may be omitted without loss of ability to use the consequent formulae.

In order to apply the MH methodology we must first define the strata. In Section 4.6 the strata were the groups defined by the confounding variable; here each case–control matched set is a distinct stratum.

### 1 : 1 Matching revisited

To fix ideas consider, again, 1 : 1 matching, where each set (stratum) is of size 2. Given $n$ case–control pairs we have $n$ strata, but the strata can only be of four types. Table 6.12 shows these four possibilities. Each of the constituent tables is of the form of Table 3.1; notice that it is correct to consider the data *within* a matched set in this form. For convenience, Table 6.12 is divided into three sections, each classified by the number exposed within the pair. When there is one exposure there are two possible tables (case exposed or control exposed). Each table naturally has an overall total of 2, since all sets are of this size.

**Table 6.12**  Types of table (showing risk factor exposure status by case–control status) possible for each pair in a paired case–control study

**No exposures**

|  | Cases | Controls | Total |
|---|---|---|---|
| Exposed | 0 | 0 | 0 |
| Unexposed | 1 | 1 | 2 |
| Total | 1 | 1 | 2 |

**One exposure**

|  | Cases | Controls | Total |  | Cases | Controls | Total |
|---|---|---|---|---|---|---|---|
| Exposed | 1 | 0 | 1 | Exposed | 0 | 1 | 1 |
| Unexposed | 0 | 1 | 1 | Unexposed | 1 | 0 | 1 |
| Total | 1 | 1 | 2 | Total | 1 | 1 | 2 |

**Two exposures**

|  | Cases | Controls | Total |
|---|---|---|---|
| Exposed | 1 | 1 | 2 |
| Unexposed | 0 | 0 | 0 |
| Total | 1 | 1 | 2 |

The Cochran–Mantel–Haenszel (CMH) test statistic, (4.21), requires calculation of the expectation and variance of the top left-hand cell of each table.

The expectation, from (4.19), is the product of the 'cases' total and the 'exposed' total divided by $n$, the grand total (which is always 2). For a 'no exposures' table this is $1 \times 0/2 = 0$, for a 'one exposure' table it is $1 \times 1/2 = \frac{1}{2}$ and for a 'two exposures' table it is $1 \times 2/2 = 1$.

The variance, from (4.19), is the product of the four marginal totals divided by $n^2(n-1) = 2 \times 2 \times 1 = 4$. For a 'no exposures' table this is $1 \times 1 \times 0 \times 1/4 = 0$, for a 'one exposure' table it is $1 \times 1 \times 1 \times 1/4 = \frac{1}{4}$ and for a 'two exposures' table it is $1 \times 1 \times 2 \times 0/4 = 0$. Notice that the 'no exposures' and 'two exposures' tables have no variance and thus provide no information. We can exclude them from further consideration on these grounds, but we shall retain them for now to see what happens.

In order to compute the CMH test statistic we need to sum the elements in the top left-hand cell of each table making up the whole data set, to sum the expectations and sum the variances. Hence we need to know how many there are of each kind of table. As usual, let $a$ denote the observed number in this top left-hand cell for some arbitrary case–control set. Also, let $t_i$ be the number of sets with $i$ exposures, and $m_i$ the number of the $t_i$ in which the case is exposed. Then the four $2 \times 2$ tables making up Table 6.12 have, reading downwards and left to right, $t_0, m_1, t_1 - m_1$ and $t_2$ occurrences respectively in the observed data. These tables have, respectively, $a = 0$, $a = 1$, $a = 0$ and $a = 1$ and thus

$$\sum a = t_0 \times 0 + m_1 \times 1 + (t_1 - m_1) \times 0 + t_2 \times 1 = m_1 + t_2.$$

Using $E$ and $V$ to denote the corresponding expectations and variances gives

$$\sum E = t_0 \times 0 + t_1 \times \tfrac{1}{2} + t_2 \times 1 = \tfrac{1}{2}t_1 + t_2,$$
$$\sum V = t_0 \times 0 + t_1 \times \tfrac{1}{4} + t_2 \times 0 = \tfrac{1}{4}t_1.$$

Notice that, when calculating $\sum E$ and $\sum V$ (but not $\sum a$) we do not need to distinguish the two types of table with one exposure. Note also that $m_0 = 0$ and $m_2 = t_2$.

The continuity-corrected CMH test statistic, (4.21), is

$$\frac{\left( |\sum a - \sum E| - \tfrac{1}{2} \right)^2}{\sum V} = \frac{\left( |(m_1 + t_2) - (\tfrac{1}{2}t_1 + t_2)| - \tfrac{1}{2} \right)^2}{\tfrac{1}{4}t_1} = \frac{\left( |2m_1 - t_1| - 1 \right)^2}{t_1}.$$
$$(6.12)$$

Now $t_1$ is the number of pairs with one exposure – that is, the number of discordant pairs. In Section 6.6.1 we called this quantity $d$. Similarly $m_1 = d_1$ in the notation of Section 6.6.1. With these substitutions (6.12) reduces to the McNemar test statistic, (6.8).

Thinking, once more, of each case–control set (pair, in the 1 : 1 situation) as a stratum, a MH estimate of the odds ratio, $\hat{\psi}_{\text{MH}}$, may be obtained similarly from (4.10). There is a simplification here that $n = 2$ in every stratum. The odds ratio turns out to be the sum of the products of diagonals in each stratum's $2 \times 2$ table, divided by the sum of the products of the off-diagonals. For each of the tables making up Table 6.12 the diagonal products are, respectively, $0 \times 1, 1 \times 1, 0 \times 0$ and $1 \times 0$. Hence the numerator for $\hat{\psi}_{\text{MH}}$ is

$$t_0 \times 0 + m_1 \times 1 + (t_1 - m_1) \times 0 + t_2 \times 0 = m_1.$$

The corresponding off-diagonal products are $0 \times 1, 0 \times 0, 1 \times 1$ and $1 \times 0$, giving a denominator for $\hat{\psi}_{\text{MH}}$ of

$$t_0 \times 0 + m_1 \times 0 + (t_1 - m_1) \times 1 + t_2 \times 0 = t_1 - m_1.$$

Thus

$$\hat{\psi}_{\text{MH}} = m_1/(t_1 - m_1), \qquad (6.13)$$

which reduces to the estimate of the odds ratio given in Section 6.6.1, (6.10), when we substitute $d = t_1$ and $d_1 = m_1$.

Notice, finally, that neither (6.12) nor (6.13) contains any contribution from the 'no exposures' or 'two exposures' tables. The terms from either type of concordant pair have either been zero or have cancelled out. In general, it does no harm to include concordant sets in calculations since they will make no overall contribution. However, excluding them simplifies the arithmetic.

*1 : 2 matching*
So far the MH approach has provided no new results, but the notation and methodology for $c = 1$ is easily extended to $c > 1$. Now there will be $2(c + 1)$ different types of $2 \times 2$ table to consider, each table representing a type of matched set. One further example will be given before the general results are stated. This is the situation where $c = 2$; all strata now are of size 3 (one case and two controls in each set). The $2(c + 1) = 6$ different $2 \times 2$ tables and appropriate calculations for each type of table are given in Table 6.13.

Using Table 6.13, with (4.21) , the CMH test statistic is thus

$$\frac{(|\sum a - \sum E| - \frac{1}{2})^2}{\sum V} = \frac{(|m_1 + m_2 - \frac{1}{3}t_1 - \frac{2}{3}t_2| - \frac{1}{2})^2}{\frac{2}{9}(t_1 + t_2)}. \tag{6.14}$$

Also, from (4.10),

$$\hat{\psi}_{MH} = \frac{2m_1 + m_2}{(t_1 - m_1) + 2(t_2 - m_2)}, \tag{6.15}$$

thus we have the appropriate calculations for a 1 : 2 matched study. Note, again, that concordant sets provide no contribution in the final equations (that is, none of $m_0, t_0, m_3$ or $t_3$ appear in (6.14) or (6.15)).

*General 1 : c matching*
General results for 1 : $c$ matching are obtained from the same approach. The CMH test statistic for testing the null hypothesis of no association between case–control status and exposure status is

$$\left( \left| \sum_{i=1}^{c} m_i - \sum_{i=1}^{c} \left( \frac{i}{c+1} \right) t_i \right| - \frac{1}{2} \right)^2 \Bigg/ \sum_{i=1}^{c} \left\{ \frac{i(c+1-i)}{(c+1)^2} \right\} t_i.$$

This may be rewritten as

$$\left( \left| (c+1) \sum_{i=1}^{c} m_i - \sum_{i=1}^{c} i t_i \right| - (c+1)/2 \right)^2 \Bigg/ \sum_{i=1}^{c} i(c+1-i) t_i. \tag{6.16}$$

We compare (6.16) to chi-square with 1 d.f.

**Table 6.13** Types of table (showing risk factor exposure status by case–control status) possible for each set in a 1 : 2 case–control study (DP = diagonal product, OP = off-diagonal product)

---

**No exposures**

| 0 | 0 | 0 |
|---|---|---|
| 1 | 2 | 3 |
| 1 | 2 | 3 |

$$E = \frac{1 \times 0}{3} = 0$$

$$V = \frac{1 \times 2 \times 0 \times 3}{3^2 \times 2} = 0$$

No. of tables: $t_0$
$a = 0, DP = 0, OP = 0$

**One exposure**

| 1 | 0 | 1 |
|---|---|---|
| 0 | 2 | 2 |
| 1 | 2 | 3 |

| 0 | 1 | 1 |
|---|---|---|
| 1 | 1 | 2 |
| 1 | 2 | 3 |

$$E = \frac{1 \times 1}{3} = \frac{1}{3}$$

$$V = \frac{1 \times 2 \times 1 \times 2}{3^2 \times 2} = \frac{2}{9}$$

No. of tables: $m_1$    No. of tables: $t_1 - m_1$
$a = 1, DP = 2, OP = 0$    $a = 0, DP = 0, OP = 1$

**Two exposures**

| 1 | 1 | 2 |
|---|---|---|
| 0 | 1 | 1 |
| 1 | 2 | 3 |

| 0 | 2 | 2 |
|---|---|---|
| 1 | 0 | 1 |
| 1 | 2 | 3 |

$$E = \frac{1 \times 2}{3} = \frac{2}{3}$$

$$V = \frac{1 \times 2 \times 2 \times 1}{3^2 \times 2} = \frac{2}{9}$$

No. of tables: $m_2$    No. of tables: $t_2 - m_2$
$a = 1, DP = 1, OP = 0$    $a = 0, DP = 0, OP = 2$

**Three exposures**

| 1 | 2 | 3 |
|---|---|---|
| 0 | 0 | 0 |
| 1 | 2 | 3 |

$$E = \frac{1 \times 3}{3} = 1$$

$$V = \frac{1 \times 2 \times 3 \times 0}{3^2 \times 2} = 0$$

No. of tables: $t_3$
$a = 1, DP = 0, OP = 0$

---

The MH estimate of the odds ratio is

$$\hat{\psi}_{MH} = \frac{\sum_{i=1}^{c} (c + 1 - i)m_i}{\sum_{i=1}^{c} i(t_i - m_i)}. \tag{6.17}$$

When $c = 1$ (6.16) and (6.17) reduce to (6.12) and (6.13), respectively; when $c = 2$ they reduce to (6.14) and (6.15).

Miettinen (1970) gives an approximate formula for the standard error of $\log_e \hat{\psi}$:

$$\text{se}(\log_e \hat{\psi}) = \left[ \psi \sum_{i=1}^{c} \frac{i(c+1-i)t_i}{(i\psi + c + 1 - i)^2} \right]^{-0.5}. \tag{6.18}$$

We can substitute $\hat{\psi}_{MH}$ for $\psi$ in (6.18) to obtain an estimated result, $\hat{\text{se}}(\log_e \hat{\psi})$. An approximate 95% confidence interval for $\log_e \psi$ is then $(L_{\log}, U_{\log})$, given by

$$\log_e \hat{\psi}_{MH} \pm 1.96 \hat{\text{se}}(\log_e \hat{\psi}), \tag{6.19}$$

leading to approximate 95% confidence limits for $\psi$ of

$$(\exp(L_{\log}), \exp(U_{\log})). \tag{6.20}$$

Alternatively, the method of Robins *et al.* (1986b) given by (4.11)–(4.14) could be applied to the individual case–control sets.

*Example 6.9* Rodrigues *et al.* (1991) describe a study of the protection against tuberculosis conferred by BCG vaccination amongst children of Asian ethnic origin born in England. Cases were selected from lists of notifications of the disease, picking out names associated with the Indian subcontinent. Controls were selected from district child health registry or school health records, again picking out Asian names only.

Five controls were matched to each case on the basis of sex and date of birth. BCG vaccination history was determined from historical records, for both cases and controls. Results are given in Table 6.14, which is in a compact form, suitable for publication. Using the notation introduced earlier, the first three columns of Table 6.15 re-express the data. The remaining columns of Table 6.15 give the components of (6.16) and (6.17) which are then summed. Notice that $c + 1 = 6$ here.

For example, Table 6.14 shows that there are three matched sets with the case and three controls exposed, and seven matched sets with the case unexposed but four controls exposed. There are thus 10 sets with four exposures, of which three have the case exposed (shown in row four of Table 6.15). The $t_i$ values come from adding successive diagonals across Table 6.14 (i.e. $1 + 15, 5 + 11, 1 + 5$, etc.), and the $m_i$ values are the numbers in the 'Yes' row of Table 6.14. Concordant sets (the bottom left-hand and top right-hand cells of Table 6.14) do

**Table 6.14** Exposure amongst matched sets showing the number of cases and matched controls who had a history of BCG vaccination

| Case with BCG? | Number of controls with BCG | | | | | | Total no. of sets |
|---|---|---|---|---|---|---|---|
| | 0 | 1 | 2 | 3 | 4 | 5 | |
| Yes | 1 | 5 | 1 | 3 | 20 | 27 | 57 |
| No | 11 | 15 | 11 | 5 | 7 | 5 | 54 |

**Table 6.15**  Calculations for Example 6.9, where $i$ is the number of exposures, $t_i$ the total number of sets with $i$ exposures and $m_i$ the number of the $t_i$ in which the case is exposed

| $i$ | $m_i$ | $t_i$ | $it_i$ | $i(6-i)t_i$ | $(6-i)m_i$ | $i(t_i - m_i)$ |
|---|---|---|---|---|---|---|
| 1 | 1 | 16 | 16 | 80 | 5 | 15 |
| 2 | 5 | 16 | 32 | 128 | 20 | 22 |
| 3 | 1 | 6 | 18 | 54 | 3 | 15 |
| 4 | 3 | 10 | 40 | 80 | 6 | 28 |
| 5 | 20 | 25 | 125 | 125 | 20 | 25 |
| Total | 30 | | 231 | 467 | 54 | 105 |

not contribute to inferences and hence are ignored in Table 6.15. If they were included in the table, results would stay the same.

From (6.16) and the first three totals in Table 6.15, we have the test statistic

$$(|6 \times 30 - 231| - 6/2)^2 \big/ 467 = 4.93.$$

Compared to $\chi_1^2$ this is significant at the 5% level: from Table B.3, $0.05 > p > 0.025$.

From (6.17) and the final two totals in Table 6.15, the odds ratio for BCG versus no BCG is estimated to be $54/105 = 0.51$. Hence BCG vaccination seems to approximately halve the chance of tuberculosis amongst Asian children born in England.

In order to estimate $\text{se}(\log_e \hat{\psi})$, Table 6.16 was constructed. Here the first three columns are all copied from Table 6.15. $\psi$ is estimated as $54/105$, the MH estimate just derived. When the total given in Table 6.16 is substituted into (6.18), we obtain

$$\hat{\text{se}}(\log_e \hat{\psi}) = \left[\frac{54}{105} \times 24.9696\right]^{-0.5} = 1 \big/ \sqrt{12.8415} = 0.2791.$$

From (6.19), approximate 95% confidence limits for $\log_e \psi$ are

$$\log_e\left(\frac{54}{105}\right) \pm 1.96 \times 0.2791$$

that is, $(-1.2120, -0.1179)$. Exponentiating both limits gives approximate 95% confidence limits for $\psi$ of $(0.30, 0.89)$ as stated by (6.20).

**Table 6.16**  Extra calculations (for a confidence interval) for Example 6.9, notation as in Table 6.15

| $i$ | $t_i$ | $H = i(6-i)t_i$ | $J = (i\psi + 6 - i)^2$ | $H/J$ |
|---|---|---|---|---|
| 1 | 16 | 80 | 30.4073 | 2.6309 |
| 2 | 16 | 128 | 25.2865 | 5.0620 |
| 3 | 6 | 54 | 20.6376 | 2.6166 |
| 4 | 10 | 80 | 16.4604 | 4.8601 |
| 5 | 25 | 125 | 12.7551 | 9.8000 |
| | | | Total | 24.9696 |

### 6.6.3    1 : variable matching

On occasions a study may plan to match each case with $c$ controls (where $c > 1$), but the data that eventually arrive for analysis have some incomplete sets. This may be because of failure to locate $c$ controls with all the matching criteria, due to drop-outs or as a consequence of missing values (failure to ascertain the exposure status of some controls). In such situations we have a 1 : variable matched study. Although conceptually more difficult, these studies are straightforward to deal with using the methodology of Section 6.6.2.

Suppose that we let $j$ denote the number of controls that are matched with any one case, where $j = 1, 2, \ldots, c$. We can derive a test of $H_0 : \psi = 1$ by calculating the $E$s and $V$s according to (4.19) for each value of $i$ within each value of $j$ in the observed data.

Using a superscript $(j)$ to denote the matching ratio we obtain

$$E_i^{(j)} = \left(\frac{i}{j+1}\right)t_i^{(j)}, \qquad V_i^{(j)} = \left\{\frac{i(j+1-i)}{(j+1)^2}\right\}t_i^{(j)}, \tag{6.21}$$

for $i = 1, 2, \ldots, j$ within each value of $j$. Substituting into (4.21) gives the CMH test statistic

$$\left(\left|\sum_{j=1}^{c}\sum_{i=1}^{j} m_i^{(j)} - \sum_{j=1}^{c}\sum_{i=1}^{j} E_i^{(j)}\right| - \tfrac{1}{2}\right)^2 \bigg/ \left(\sum_{j=1}^{c}\sum_{i=1}^{j} V_i^{(j)}\right), \tag{6.22}$$

which is to be compared with $\chi_1^2$.

A similar method gives rise to an estimate of the odds ratio,

$$\hat{\psi}_{\mathrm{MH}} = \sum_{j=1}^{c}\sum_{i=1}^{j} T_i^{(j)} \bigg/ \sum_{j=1}^{c}\sum_{i=1}^{j} B_i^{(j)}, \tag{6.23}$$

where

$$\begin{aligned} T_i^{(j)} &= (j+1-i)m_i^{(j)}/(j+1) \\ B_i^{(j)} &= i(t_i^{(j)} - m_i^{(j)})/(j+1). \end{aligned} \tag{6.24}$$

Similarly, (6.18) may be generalized to give a standard error for $\log_e \hat{\psi}$ of

$$\left[\psi \sum_{j=1}^{c}\sum_{i=1}^{j} \frac{i(j+1-i)t_i^{(j)}}{(i\psi + j + 1 - i)^2}\right]^{-0.5},$$

from which a 95% confidence interval for $\psi$ follows using (6.19) and (6.20).

**Table 6.17**   Exposure amongst matched sets, showing the number of cases and matched controls visiting Reading's Butts Centre in the 2 weeks preceding the case's onset of illness

| Matching ratio | Case visited the Butts Centre? | Number of controls visiting the Butts Centre | | | |
|---|---|---|---|---|---|
| | | 0 | 1 | 2 | 3 |
| 1:1 | Yes | 0 | 1 | | |
| | No | 0 | 0 | | |
| 1:2 | Yes | 0 | 1 | 0 | |
| | No | 0 | 0 | 0 | |
| 1:3 | Yes | 2 | 2 | 2 | 4 |
| | No | 0 | 1 | 0 | 0 |

Note: discordant sets are marked in bold.

*Example 6.10*   In the study of legionnaires' disease in Reading (Example 6.2) each person with the disease was supposed to be matched by three controls. The matching criteria were age (within 10 years), sex, neighbourhood of residence and mobility (ability to move around). Due to the combination of the factors, only one control could be found for one of the cases and only two controls for one of the others. The remaining 11 cases all received three matched controls.

Tables of exposure status against case–control status were drawn up for each designated area in Reading. Table 6.17 gives the table for 'exposure' to the Butts Centre.

Calculation of the test statistic and estimate of the odds ratio is illustrated by Table 6.18. Substituting the totals from this table into (6.22) gives the test statistic

$$\frac{(|7 - 3.9167| - 0.5)^2}{1.6597} = 4.02,$$

which is significant at the 5% level (see Table B.3). Also, the odds ratio for visiting the Butts Centre compared to not is, from (6.23),

$$\frac{3.3333}{0.2500} = 13.33.$$

**Table 6.18**   Calculations for Example 6.10, where $j$ is the number of controls matched to a case, $i$ the number of exposures, $t_i^{(j)}$ the total number of sets of size $j + 1$ with $i$ exposures, $m_i^{(j)}$ the number of the $t_i^{(j)}$ in which the case is exposed, $E_i^{(j)}$ and $V_i^{(j)}$ are defined by (6.21) and $T_i^{(j)}$ and $B_i^{(j)}$ are defined by (6.24)

| $j$ | $i$ | $m_i^{(j)}$ | $t_i^{(j)}$ | $E_i^{(j)}$ | $V_i^{(j)}$ | $T_i^{(j)}$ | $B_i^{(j)}$ |
|---|---|---|---|---|---|---|---|
| 2 | 2 | 1 | 1 | 0.6667 | 0.2222 | 0.3333 | 0 |
| 3 | 1 | 2 | 3 | 0.7500 | 0.5625 | 1.5000 | 0.2500 |
| | 2 | 2 | 2 | 1.0000 | 0.5000 | 1.0000 | 0 |
| | 3 | 2 | 2 | 1.5000 | 0.3750 | 0.5000 | 0 |
| Total | | | 7 | 3.9167 | 1.6597 | 3.3333 | 0.2500 |

Hence there is a strong indication that the Butts Centre was a source of the legionella bacterium.

### 6.6.4    Many : many matching

A major disadvantage with 1 : 1 matching is that, should the matched control be 'lost' (for example, due to a failed blood analysis) then the corresponding case is inevitably also lost. This not only reduces accuracy in the final results, but also means that time and resources (for example, in laboratory testing of this case's blood) will have been wasted. The adoption of a 1 : many scheme, with the fall-back of a 1 : variable scheme if necessary, protects against this problem. With this scheme, however, should the *case* be lost, the corresponding matched controls will also be lost. To protect against this (opposite) problem a many : many matched scheme may be possible in special circumstances. This is the category matching situation introduced in Section 6.5.4.

The MH methodology of Section 4.6 can often be easily applied directly to the matched sets. However, if there are many sets this may require extensive computation. Alternatively (and completely equivalently) the approach of Sections 6.6.2 and 6.6.3 may be extended to the many : many situation. Practical situations generally will have variable numbers of both cases and controls (that is, variable : variable ratios) and consequently this is the situation which we will consider. Of course, this is the most general situation, from which the fixed ratio situation may be derived as a special case.

Suppose that $m_{ik}^{(rs)}$ is the number of matched sets with $r$ cases and $s$ controls in which there are $i$ exposures to the risk factor, $k$ of which are exposed cases. The test statistic for testing no association ($\psi = 1$) is

$$\left( \left| \sum km_{ik}^{(rs)} - \sum E_{ik}^{(rs)} \right| - \tfrac{1}{2} \right)^2 \bigg/ \left( \sum V_{ik}^{(rs)} \right), \qquad (6.25)$$

where

$$E_{ik}^{(rs)} = \left( \frac{ir}{r+s} \right) m_{ik}^{(rs)},$$

$$V_{ik}^{(rs)} = \left\{ \frac{i(r+s-i)rs}{(r+s)^2(r+s-1)} \right\} m_{ik}^{(rs)}. \qquad (6.26)$$

The estimated odds ratio (exposure versus no exposure) is

$$\hat{\psi}_{\text{MH}} = \left( \sum T_{ik}^{(rs)} \right) \bigg/ \left( \sum B_{ik}^{(rs)} \right), \qquad (6.27)$$

where

$$T_{ik}^{(rs)} = k(s - i + k)m_{ik}^{(rs)}/(r + s),$$
$$B_{ik}^{(rs)} = (i - k)(r - k)m_{ik}^{(rs)}/(r + s).$$

(6.28)

In (6.25) and (6.27) the summations are quadruple summations over $r$, $s$, $i$ and $k$. The procedure required is to calculate the value $km_{ik}^{(rs)}$ and the four quantities in (6.26) and (6.28), for each observed combination of $r$, $s$, $i$ and $k$. Each of the five sets of quantities is then summed and the sums are substituted into (6.25) and (6.27). To save unnecessary work, all concordant sets may be discarded at the outset (as usual).

*Example 6.11*    In a synthetic case–control study of D-dimer and MI carried out by Professor G.D.O. Lowe at the University of Glasgow, cases and controls were identified from the Scottish Heart Health Study cohort, there being insufficient funds to measure D-dimer on all subjects. Cases were cohort members who developed MI during the period of follow-up to December 1993. Controls were matched to cases by baseline coronary disease status, 5-year age group, sex, district of residence and time of recruitment to the cohort study.

Since D-dimer was to be measured on frozen blood samples that had been stored for several years, problems with quality were anticipated – for example, through degeneration of blood samples and disattached labels. Hence there was a good chance that some cases or controls would have no D-dimer result. In order to protect against losing matched subjects whenever this happened, a many : many scheme was adopted. All subjects, whether case or control, who shared the same values of each combination of matching criteria were taken as a single matched set (on condition that there had to be at least one case and one control in each set). The result was 384 cases and 1304 controls, making up 277 matched sets.

So as to provide a tractable example, 20 of the 277 sets were randomly sampled and their data are presented in Table 6.19. Here we take 'exposure' to D-dimer to be a high value of D-dimer, itself defined to be a value above the median of the entire 1688 subjects. Table 6.19 has data for 28 cases and 107 controls. Two of the sets (2 and 4), involving 2 cases and 6 controls, are concordant and can be discarded. Calculations, using (6.26) and (6.28), on the remaining 18 sets are presented in Table 6.20. In order to clarify the calculations, each set is taken separately in Table 6.20, rather than grouping together sets with common values of $r$, $s$, $i$ and $k$ (that is, sets 5, 6 and 7 and sets 10 and 11). As a consequence $m_{ik}^{(rs)} = 1$ in each row of the table, and so we can use each of (6.25), (6.26) and (6.28) with the $m_{ik}^{(rs)}$ term deleted.

From substituting the totals from Table 6.20 into (6.25), the test statistic is

$$(|14 - 12.8047| - 0.5)^2/5.2230 = 0.09,$$

which is clearly not significant at any reasonable significance level. The estimated odds ratio is, from (6.27) and the totals of the final two columns in Table 6.26,

$$\hat{\psi}_{\text{MH}} = 5.7111/4.5158 = 1.26.$$

Hence those with high D-dimer have approximately 1.26 times the risk of MI compared to those with low D-dimer, but this contrast is not significant. A confidence interval for $\psi_{\text{MH}}$ may be found from (4.11)–(4.14) using the 20 sets as 20 strata. This gives a 95% confidence

**Table 6.19**    Results from a matched case–control study of D-dimer and myocardial infarction (exposure = high D-dimer)

| Set number | Matching ratio | Number of exposed | |
|---|---|---|---|
| | | Cases | Controls |
| 1 | 1 : 2 | 0 | 1 |
| 2 | 1 : 3 | 0 | 0 |
| 3 | 1 : 3 | 1 | 1 |
| 4 | 1 : 3 | 1 | 3 |
| 5 | 1 : 4 | 0 | 1 |
| 6 | 1 : 4 | 0 | 1 |
| 7 | 1 : 4 | 0 | 1 |
| 8 | 1 : 4 | 0 | 2 |
| 9 | 1 : 4 | 0 | 3 |
| 10 | 1 : 4 | 1 | 1 |
| 11 | 1 : 4 | 1 | 1 |
| 12 | 1 : 4 | 1 | 2 |
| 13 | 1 : 4 | 1 | 3 |
| 14 | 1 : 7 | 1 | 3 |
| 15 | 2 : 7 | 1 | 2 |
| 16 | 2 : 7 | 1 | 5 |
| 17 | 2 : 8 | 1 | 7 |
| 18 | 2 : 8 | 2 | 3 |
| 19 | 3 : 11 | 1 | 4 |
| 20 | 3 : 12 | 2 | 8 |

Note: discordant sets are marked in bold.

interval of (0.53, 3.02). Applying (4.10) and (4.21) to the same 20 strata gives the same results as above for the test statistic and estimate, as it must.

### 6.6.5    A modelling approach

An alternative method for analysing matched case–control studies is through a conditional logistic regression model (Section 10.11.2). This approach can conveniently extend the range of analyses presented here to deal with multiple exposure levels, confounding variables not included in the matching criteria and interaction.

**Table 6.20** Calculations for Example 6.11 on a set-by-set basis, so that $m_{ik}^{(rs)} = 1$: the $E$, $V$, $T$ and $B$ variables are defined by (6.26) and (6.28)

| Set no. $r$ | Cases $r$ | Controls $s$ | Exposures $i$ | Cases exp. $k$ | $E_{ik}^{(rs)}$ | $V_{ik}^{(rs)}$ | $T_{ik}^{(rs)}$ | $B_{ik}^{(rs)}$ |
|---|---|---|---|---|---|---|---|---|
| 1 | 1 | 2 | 1 | 0 | 0.3333 | 0.2222 | 0 | 0.3333 |
| 3 | 1 | 3 | 2 | 1 | 0.5000 | 0.2500 | 0.5000 | 0 |
| 5 | 1 | 4 | 1 | 0 | 0.2000 | 0.1600 | 0 | 0.2000 |
| 6 | 1 | 4 | 1 | 0 | 0.2000 | 0.1600 | 0 | 0.2000 |
| 7 | 1 | 4 | 1 | 0 | 0.2000 | 0.1600 | 0 | 0.2000 |
| 8 | 1 | 4 | 2 | 0 | 0.4000 | 0.2400 | 0 | 0.4000 |
| 9 | 1 | 4 | 3 | 0 | 0.6000 | 0.2400 | 0 | 0.6000 |
| 10 | 1 | 4 | 2 | 1 | 0.4000 | 0.2400 | 0.6000 | 0 |
| 11 | 1 | 4 | 2 | 1 | 0.4000 | 0.2400 | 0.6000 | 0 |
| 12 | 1 | 4 | 3 | 1 | 0.6000 | 0.2400 | 0.4000 | 0 |
| 13 | 1 | 4 | 4 | 1 | 0.8000 | 0.1600 | 0.2000 | 0 |
| 14 | 1 | 7 | 4 | 1 | 0.5000 | 0.2500 | 0.5000 | 0 |
| 15 | 2 | 7 | 3 | 1 | 0.6667 | 0.3889 | 0.5556 | 0.2222 |
| 16 | 2 | 7 | 6 | 1 | 1.3333 | 0.3889 | 0.2222 | 0.5556 |
| 17 | 2 | 8 | 8 | 1 | 1.6000 | 0.2844 | 0.1000 | 0.7000 |
| 18 | 2 | 8 | 5 | 2 | 1.0000 | 0.4444 | 1.0000 | 0 |
| 19 | 3 | 11 | 5 | 1 | 1.0714 | 0.5828 | 0.5000 | 0.5714 |
| 20 | 3 | 12 | 10 | 2 | 2.0000 | 0.5714 | 0.5333 | 0.5333 |
| Total | | | | 14 | 12.8047 | 5.2230 | 5.7111 | 4.5158 |

## Exercises

6.1   In a case–control study of use of oral contraceptives (OCs) and breast cancer in New Zealand, Paul et al. (1986) identified cases over a 2-year period from the National Cancer Registry and controls by random selection from electoral rolls. The data shown below were compiled.

| Used OCs? | Cases | Controls |
|---|---|---|
| Yes | 310 | 708 |
| No | 123 | 189 |
| Total | 433 | 897 |

(i)   Estimate the odds ratio for breast cancer, OC users versus non-users. Specify a 95% confidence interval for the true odds ratio.

(ii)  Test whether OC use appears to be associated with breast cancer.

6.2   Morrison (1992) carried out a case–control study of risk factors for prostatic hypertrophy in Rhode Island. Cases were all men who had a first experience of prostatic surgery, but who did not have prostatic or bladder cancer, during the period from November 1985 to October 1987. Random population controls were selected from administrative lists, filtering out those with a history of prostatic surgery or prostatic or bladder cancer by telephone interview. Of 873 cases, 48 reported that they were Jewish. Of 1934 controls, 64 were Jewish.

    (i)  Calculate the odds ratio (with a 95% confidence interval) for prostatic surgery for Jews compared to non-Jews.

    (ii)  Test for the significance of a relationship between being of the Jewish religion and undergoing prostatic surgery.

6.3    In September 1993 only the second outbreak of *Salmonella enteritidis* phage type 4 (SE) occurred in the USA (Boyce *et al.*, 1996). As with the first, the infection occurred amongst people who had eaten at a certain Chinese fast-food restaurant in El Paso, Texas. To investigate the second outbreak, a case–control study was instigated. Cases were people with diarrhoea or culture-confirmed SE that occurred after the patient ate at the restaurant between 27 August and 15 September 1995. Controls were either well meal companions of the cases or persons subsequently identified as having eaten at the restaurant, without undue effects, during the outbreak. The table below shows the number of cases and controls who reported eating each of four menu items from the restaurant.

| Food item | Cases ($n = 19$) | Controls ($n = 17$) |
|---|---|---|
| Breaded chicken | 14 | 11 |
| Any chicken | 16 | 16 |
| Egg rolls | 14 | 3 |
| Fried rice | 14 | 9 |

    Which food item do you suspect is the source of SE? Provide suitable analytical evidence to support your assertion.

6.4    Scragg *et al.* (1993) report a study of bed sharing and sudden infant death syndrome (SIDS). Cases of SIDS were compared to a random sample of controls selected from lists of births. Of the 393 cases, 248 usually shared a bed, whereas of the 1591 controls, 708 usually shared a bed. Estimate the attributable risk of SIDS for bed sharing, together with a 95% confidence interval.

6.5    Horwitz and Feinstein (1978) report that a side-effect of exogenous oestrogen use is vaginal bleeding. Vaginal bleeding is itself a potential sign of endometrial cancer amongst post-menopausal women. Consider the implications of these observations in the design of a case–control study of oestrogen intake and endometrial cancer.

6.6    In a case–control study of risk factors for dental caries, McMahon *et al.* (1993) present data relating to age of child, age of mother and whether or not the child has dental caries, as shown below. Caries is defined here as a minimum of four decayed, missing or filled teeth.

| Age of mother (years) | Age of child (months) | | | | | |
|---|---|---|---|---|---|---|
| | < 36 | | 36–47 | | ≥48 | |
| | Caries | Control | Caries | Control | Caries | Control |
| < 25 | 1 | 1 | 1 | 5 | 8 | 9 |
| 25–34 | 4 | 16 | 18 | 67 | 46 | 113 |
| ≥35 | 1 | 2 | 3 | 14 | 10 | 35 |

Find (i) unadjusted (raw) and (ii) Mantel–Haenszel adjusted (for child age) odds ratios for dental caries by age of mother, taking the oldest women as the reference group. Give 95% confidence intervals in each case. (iii) Interpret your results.

6.7 For each of Examples 6.8, 6.9 and 6.10 find the odds ratio *ignoring* matching. What effect has ignoring matching had on each odds ratio?

6.8 A case–control study of acute lymphoblastic leukaemia amongst Spanish children found 128 cases aged below 15 years from hospital records (Infante-Rivard *et al.*, 1991). Each case was matched by year of birth, sex and municipality to a single control. Community controls were randomly selected using Census lists.

The table below shows an analysis of the mothers' exposure to dust from cotton, wool or synthetic fibres during pregnancy. Exposure was established by personal interview, either at home or in hospital. Some of the cases had already died by the time of the interview.

| Case exposed to dust? | Control exposed to dust? | |
|---|---|---|
| | Yes | No |
| Yes | 1 | 11 |
| No | 2 | 114 |

(i) Find the estimated odds ratio for exposure compared to non-exposure, together with an estimated 95% confidence interval.

(ii) Test the null hypothesis that exposure to dust is not associated with the leukaemia.

6.9 In a study of the relationship between criminality and injury, cases were selected from English-speaking men with acute traumatic spinal cord injuries admitted to hospital in Louisiana between 1 January, 1965 and 31 December 1984 who were still alive at the time of study and could be contacted by telephone (Mawson *et al.*, 1996). Controls were selected from holders of Louisiana drivers' licenses, matched with individual cases on age, sex, race, Zip code of residence and educational attainment. Subjects were asked if they had ever been arrested, convicted of a crime or placed in a correctional institution before the date of their spinal injury. Controls were asked the same questions, with the relevant date being that of the spinal injury of the case to whom they had been matched. Results for arrests before the age of 17 years for case–control pairs are given below:

| Case arrested? | Control arrested? | |
|---|---|---|
| | Yes | No |
| Yes | 7 | 33 |
| No | 16 | 83 |

(i)   Calculate the odds ratio for spinal cord injury, comparing those with a history of criminal arrests to those without. Give a 95% confidence interval for your estimate.

(ii)  Test the null hypothesis that criminality is not associated with spinal injury.

(iii) Given the same problem to research, are there any changes that you would consider making to the study design or analysis as presented here?

6.10  Miller *et al.* (1978) identified 136 cases of bladder cancer at Ottowa Civic Hospital in Canada. Each case was matched by two controls for sex and 10-year age group, controls being largely recruited from the same hospital as the cases. The table shown below gives a classification of the number of heavy smokers (20 or more cigarettes per day) within each of the case–control triples.

| Number of exposures in the triple | Number of triples | Number of triples with an exposed case |
|---|---|---|
| 0 | 12 | 0 |
| 1 | 40 | 17 |
| 2 | 53 | 42 |
| 3 | 31 | 31 |

(i)  Estimate the odds ratio for bladder cancer, heavy smokers versus not. Give a 95% confidence interval for the true odds ratio.

(ii) Test whether heavy smoking is associated with bladder cancer.

6.11  Pike *et al.* (1970) give the results of a matched case–control study of children with microscopically proven Burkitt's lymphoma at Mulago Hospital, Uganda. Patients were individually matched with one or two unrelated persons of the same age, sex, tribe and place of residence. The method used was to visit homes near the home of the patient until one or two suitable subjects were found. Individuals were then characterized as

| Burkitt's tumour patient | Matched controls | | | | |
|---|---|---|---|---|---|
| | Single controls | | Two controls | | |
| | AA | AS | AA, AA | AA, AS | AS, AS |
| AA | 13 | 6 | 7 | 3 | 1 |
| AS | 2 | 1 | 1 | 2 | 0 |

either haemoglobin AA or AS to test the hypothesis that haemoglobin AA is a risk factor for Burkitt's lymphoma. The table above reproduces the way in which results are given in the paper.

(i) Test the hypothesis of no association against the one-sided alternative that children with haemoglobin AA are more susceptible to the lymphoma.

(ii) Estimate the corresponding odds ratio together with a 99% confidence interval.

(iii) Interpret your results.

6.12 For the venous thromboembolism matched case–control data of Table C.6, confirm the summary table given below.

| | Case uses | Number of controls using HRT | | |
|---|---|---|---|---|
| Matching ratio | HRT? | 0 | 1 | 2 |
| 1 : 1 | Yes | 7 | 3 | |
| | No | 17 | 1 | |
| 1 : 2 | Yes | 15 | 15 | 4 |
| | No | 27 | 11 | 3 |

Using this summary table, answer the following questions:

(i) Test for no association between hormone replacement therapy use and venous thromboembolism.

(ii) Estimate the odds ratio, together with a 95% confidence interval, for users versus non-users.

6.13 A medical investigator plans to carry out a case–control study of risk factors for asthma amongst infants. Cases are to be identified from referrals to the Paediatric Department of a certain hospital. Each case will be matched by two controls selected from the hospital records, matching being on the basis of whether or not the baby was born in a high-level care department of a hospital (such as an intensive care unit). Is this a sensible matching criterion? Suggest other possible matching criteria and identify how you would select your controls.

# 7

# Intervention studies

## 7.1 Introduction

An intervention study is an experiment which is applied either to existing patients, in order to decide upon an appropriate therapy, or to those presently free of symptoms, in order to decide upon an appropriate preventive strategy. Two types of intervention study may be identified. **Clinical trials** are where treatments are allocated to individual people; **community trials** are where treatments are allocated to groups – for example, when fluoride is added to a town's water supply with the aim of reducing dental caries. Community trials are relatively rare and supply rather less precise information. For instance, we could not be sure that any particular person living in a town with a fluoridated water supply would habitually drink that water. For these reasons the remainder of this chapter will address clinical trials. Community trials will normally be analysed as outlined in Section 7.4.

The term 'clinical trial' is most often associated with experiments undertaken by pharmaceutical companies – for example, to test the efficacy of a novel drug formulation in the treatment of a specific disease. The term is also used to include issues such as a comparison of hospital procedures (day care against overnight stay, or medical against surgical treatment for patients with similar complaints), field trials of vaccines and evaluation of contraceptive practices. The essential feature is that the allocation of patient to treatment is *planned* – that is, the investigators decide who should receive which treatment (usually using some probabilistic mechanism). Contrast this with cross-sectional surveys, cohort and case–control studies, where there is no control over who is and who is not, for example, a cigarette smoker.

*Example 7.1* Crombie *et al.* (1990) describe a clinical trial of vitamin and mineral supplementation to improve verbal and non-verbal reasoning of schoolchildren which was carried out in Dundee, Scotland. To begin with, various reasoning (IQ) tests were applied to two groups of schoolchildren aged between 11 and 13 years. One group (of size 42) then received vitamin and mineral supplements. The other group (of size 44) received a **placebo** treatment, inactive tablets which were indistinguishable from the active tablets. The tablets were taken for 7 months, after which time the IQ tests were repeated. Table 7.1 gives the baseline and final values for two of the tests administered.

**Table 7.1**   Initial and final values of IQ scores for 86 children in Dundee

| *Placebo group* (*n* = 44) | | | | *Active group* (*n* = 42) | | | |
| --- | --- | --- | --- | --- | --- | --- | --- |
| *Non-verbal test* | | *Verbal test* | | *Non-verbal test* | | *Verbal test* | |
| *Initial* | *Final* | *Initial* | *Final* | *Initial* | *Final* | *Initial* | *Final* |
| 89 | 83 | 87 | 84 | 70 | 87 | 57 | 63 |
| 82 | 97 | 73 | 87 | 91 | 91 | 68 | 75 |
| 107 | 107 | 59 | 72 | 106 | 104 | 78 | 89 |
| 95 | 101 | 105 | 108 | 92 | 87 | 86 | 84 |
| 110 | 100 | 97 | 105 | 103 | 114 | 81 | 93 |
| 106 | 97 | 75 | 84 | 105 | 115 | 85 | 89 |
| 114 | 112 | 113 | 118 | 106 | 106 | 85 | 86 |
| 97 | 96 | 86 | 89 | 82 | 78 | 80 | 82 |
| 103 | 103 | 95 | 97 | 101 | 98 | 86 | 84 |
| 109 | 122 | 101 | 94 | 86 | 106 | 76 | 86 |
| 97 | 80 | 84 | 89 | 101 | 102 | 99 | 97 |
| 93 | 103 | 93 | 93 | 97 | 97 | 100 | 93 |
| 107 | 110 | 96 | 94 | 84 | 85 | 76 | 85 |
| 84 | 102 | 73 | 86 | 90 | 100 | 87 | 97 |
| 69 | 79 | 70 | 80 | 88 | 90 | 77 | 85 |
| 109 | 100 | 97 | 95 | 121 | 106 | 95 | 92 |
| 98 | 101 | 77 | 76 | 101 | 110 | 82 | 89 |
| 72 | 78 | 86 | 87 | 100 | 97 | 91 | 89 |
| 70 | 78 | 82 | 87 | 116 | 126 | 108 | 110 |
| 99 | 122 | 79 | 79 | 108 | 121 | 98 | 111 |
| 105 | 118 | 96 | 104 | 127 | 125 | 94 | 98 |
| 133 | 133 | 130 | 126 | 95 | 100 | 88 | 88 |
| 87 | 93 | 84 | 82 | 90 | 91 | 83 | 92 |
| 104 | 120 | 101 | 89 | 112 | 117 | 101 | 93 |
| 118 | 112 | 98 | 95 | 115 | 119 | 98 | 109 |
| 113 | 121 | 105 | 118 | 112 | 111 | 80 | 87 |
| 89 | 99 | 90 | 92 | 104 | 108 | 99 | 107 |
| 101 | 97 | 76 | 79 | 107 | 98 | 88 | 88 |
| 95 | 95 | 82 | 83 | 137 | 131 | 109 | 109 |
| 103 | 101 | 98 | 100 | 109 | 115 | 91 | 99 |
| 99 | 107 | 90 | 96 | 99 | 116 | 82 | 85 |
| 101 | 111 | 89 | 89 | 80 | 82 | 84 | 90 |
| 118 | 104 | 106 | 104 | 105 | 112 | 90 | 99 |
| 114 | 115 | 103 | 100 | 99 | 104 | 82 | 84 |
| 111 | 105 | 87 | 89 | 78 | 85 | 70 | 77 |

**Table 7.1** *cont.*

| Placebo group ($n=44$) | | | | Active group ($n=42$) | | | |
|---|---|---|---|---|---|---|---|
| Non-verbal test | | Verbal test | | Non-verbal test | | Verbal test | |
| Initial | Final | Initial | Final | Initial | Final | Initial | Final |
| 81 | 75 | 78 | 64 | 70 | 98 | 92 | 89 |
| 90 | 74 | 89 | 77 | 135 | 135 | 117 | 116 |
| 104 | 87 | 75 | 74 | 117 | 129 | 108 | 104 |
| 83 | 91 | 69 | 79 | 84 | 88 | 91 | 80 |
| 101 | 98 | 79 | 86 | 103 | 104 | 87 | 88 |
| 113 | 98 | 78 | 98 | 108 | 112 | 85 | 87 |
| 97 | 101 | 83 | 92 | 130 | 128 | 102 | 100 |
| 93 | 92 | 84 | 89 | | | | |
| 119 | 130 | 121 | 126 | | | | |

Note: These data are available electronically; see Appendix C.

Simple analyses of these data are given by $t$ tests (Section 2.7.3). Since there could be important differences between the two groups before treatment began, it is more meaningful to compare the differences in IQ scores – that is, final minus initial score – for each test. Summary statistics and the results of $t$ tests, using (2.14)–(2.16), are given in Table 7.2. Although those on active treatment show the greatest improvement (on average), there is no significant difference between the supplement and placebo groups for either test. We conclude that there is no evidence of an effect upon IQ of supplementation. More complete analyses are given in the source paper.

## 7.1.1   Advantages

1.  Clinical trials are most efficient for investigating causality, because we can ensure that the 'cause' precedes the 'effect'. This makes them an attractive proposition for epidemiological investigations into possible causal relationships between risk factors and disease.
2.  We can ensure that possible confounding factors do not confuse the results. This is because we can allocate patients to treatment in any way we choose. For instance, consider a comparative trial of two treatments for a chronic

**Table 7.2**   Mean differences (with standard errors in parentheses) in IQ scores, together with tests of no difference between treatments

| IQ test | Placebo group | Active group | $t$ test | |
|---|---|---|---|---|
| | | | Statistic | p value |
| Non-verbal | 1.50 (1.49) | 3.90 (1.24) | 1.24 | 0.22 |
| Verbal | 2.64 (1.06) | 3.14 (0.90) | 0.36 | 0.72 |

condition which inevitably worsens with age. We can ensure that age does not affect the evaluation of the treatments by allocating each treatment to patient groups with the same (or very similar) age make-up.

3.  We can ensure that treatments are compared efficiently. This means using our control over allocation to spread the sample over the treatment groups so as to achieve maximum power in statistical tests. such as the $t$ test of Example 7.1. This may simply require allocating an equal number of patients to each treatment group (Section 8.4.3). We may also wish to look for effects of combinations of treatments, or interactions between treatments and personal characteristics. Then we can arrange to obtain sufficient numbers of observations of each distinct type, in order to evaluate such effects efficiently.

### 7.1.2   Disadvantages

1.  Since clinical trials involve the prospective collection of data they may share many of the disadvantages of cohort studies listed in Section 5.1.2.
2.  There are ethical problems concerned with giving experimental treatments. These are considered in more detail in Section 7.2, but note that such considerations often rule out the use of clinical trials in epidemiological investigations. For example, it is unethical to force chosen individuals to drink heavily merely for experimental purposes, since heavy drinking has known undesirable effects.
3.  In many instances intervention studies screen out 'problem' subjects, such as the very young, the elderly and pregnant women, who may have a special (possibly adverse) reaction to treatment. This may restrict the generalizability of results.

## 7.2   Ethical considerations

Most medical researchers accept the need for clinical trials to evaluate new therapies scientifically. There is, however, an inevitable load for the clinical trial participant to bare, be it the risk of unknown side-effects or simply the inconvenience of recording data and attending for frequent clinic visits. Ethical considerations must, therefore, be taken into account before a trial is begun, as considered at length by Pocock (1983). Of course such issues are relevant to all epidemiological investigations, but they are particularly important in this context. The most important condition to satisfy is that the trial itself is conducted ethically, which includes taking steps to avoid bias in the results (Section 7.3) and using an adequate sample size (Chapter 8). Each patient should receive an explanation of the trial, and his or her consent should be obtained before treatment.

The ethical requirements of clinical trials throughout the world are defined by the Declaration of Helsinki issued by the World Medical Association in 1960 and revised at the meeting in Tokyo in 1975. One of its principles is that the trial should have a **protocol** (see Section 7.2.2) which is submitted to an independent committee for approval. In the United Kingdom protocols must be submitted to local ethical committees and the Committee on Safety of Medicines must also be approached before any new drug is tested. Regulatory bodies exist to ensure that any new drug has been properly tested before a marketing licence is issued. In the UK this is the Committee on Safety of Medicines, once again; in the USA it is the Food and Drug Administration. Similar bodies exist in many countries.

### 7.2.1  Stages of experimentation

To reduce the problem of side-effects, new pharmaceuticals are subjected to several stages of experimentation before first being given to humans. This would often involve *in vitro* and animal experimentation, although the latter provokes further ethical deliberation. Even once human experimentation begins, a cautious stepwise approach is adopted for new treatments.

The clinical trials carried out by the pharmaceutical industry are generally grouped into four stages or 'phases' which reflect successive experimentation on human subjects:

- **Phase one trials**. These are concerned with the basic safety of the drug, rather than its efficacy. Volunteers are often used; sometimes these are healthy people, such as employees of the pharmaceutical company involved.
- **Phase two trials**. As with subsequent phases, these are always applied to patients – that is, people with the illness that the drug is to treat. Phase two trials try to identify a suitable formulation of the drug, possibly the dosage which is most effective without causing unpleasant side-effects. This requires careful monitoring, often associated with a wide range of measurements. Consequently the numbers involved are relatively small, although possibly slightly higher than in phase one trials.
- **Phase three trials**. These are large-scale comparative clinical investigations which seek to evaluate the efficacy of a treatment, or treatments. This is the most substantial and formal of the phases, and is what many researchers mean when they use the term 'clinical trial'. A drug which 'passes' phase three will subsequently be referred to the regulatory body for a product

licence to be issued, enabling the drug to be marketed. The sample size would often be determined using preliminary information derived from the earlier-phase trials.

- **Phase four trials**. These are studies which are undertaken after the drug has been marketed. They study long-term effects of the treatment in question, in terms of both efficacy and side-effects. Since side-effects may be felt by only very small percentages or very particular types of patients, phase four trials often involve several hundred (or even thousand) subjects. In fact, although phase four studies are spoken of as clinical trials, they are most often sample surveys rather than experiments. Information is sought from those patients who have received the treatment under investigation, and these patients will not generally have been allocated treatment for the purpose of the study.

Epidemiological investigations will rarely have such a multi-phase aspect. However, they will sometimes use evidence from pharmaceutical trials at the stage of study design and when seeking to interpret results. Hence it is relevant for the epidemiologist to understand the terminology introduced here.

### 7.2.2    The protocol

The protocol serves two main purposes. First, it is a justification for the clinical trial which will be scrutinized by ethical committees (and, possibly, funding agencies). Second, it is a reference manual for use by all those involved in the administration and analysis of the trial. Although no list can possibly cover the needs of all protocols, the following is a specimen list of section headings. This should serve as a framework for the construction of a protocol. Although some of the items are clearly specific to intervention studies, several will be appropriate for protocols in observational studies also. Further details on protocol design are provided by Sylvester *et al.* (1982).

1. Rationale: The background to the study, explanation of how the novel treatment is thought to work against the disease in question, why it might be an improvement on existing treatment and references to previous literature on the subject.
2. Aims of study: What, exactly, does the trial seek to discover? For instance the aims may be to compare efficacy (suitably defined) and side-effects of a new against an existing treatment.
3. Design of study: A specification of the basic design used (Sections 7.4–7.6) and how the measures to avoid bias (Section 7.3) will be implemented.

4.  Selection of patients: This should include the number to be assigned to each treatment group, as well as inclusion and exclusion criteria. Inclusion criteria usually contain the precise definition of disease to be used (for example, the symptoms which must be exhibited) and appropriate age limits (if any) for entry to the trial. Exclusion criteria often include other medical conditions which may cause complications, including pregnancy. Patients may also be excluded because they have received treatment, such as steroid therapy, which may affect their responses in the current investigation.

5.  Drugs and dosages: A list of the medications (or alternatives) to be taken by the subjects, the dosage(s) to be used and the form of the medication (tablets, injections, inhalers etc.). The drug supplier is mentioned here if not specified elsewhere.

6.  Assessments: What will be measured during the trial. This is likely to include measures of efficacy (blood pressure, lung function etc.), records of adverse events (headaches, nausea etc.) plus records of compliance (how many tablets were actually taken each day) and concurrent medication (or other form of treatment) received. Compliance is recorded because we would normally exclude from the analysis any patient who has deviated importantly from the rules of the protocol. Records of concurrent medication may be used in two main ways. If this medication is something which alleviates the symptoms of the very disease that is being studied then its consumption is evidence of lack of efficacy of the treatment allocated. If the medication is normally taken for other complaints then its consumption might indicate a side-effect of the treatment allocated. Furthermore, in the event that many subjects take the same concurrent medication, we may wish to look at the effect of taking a combination of the study treatment and the concurrent medication.

7.  Documentation: A list of the forms for recording information. This may include physicians' record cards to be completed during clinic visits and daily record cards to be completed by the patient. The latter would typically record compliance and side-effects plus self-assessments of well-being (particularly in trials concerning chronic conditions).

8.  Procedure: This is usually the longest part of the protocol, and specifies what should be done, and by whom, at each stage of the trial. Many clinical trials involve several clinic visits, and here we should state, for example, what measurements will be taken at each particular visit, including the precise methodology to use (for example, 'diastolic blood pressure by sphygmomanometer taking the fifth Korotkoff sound'). Instructions for the doctor to give to his or her patients would also be

included (such as how many tablets should be taken per day, and how the daily record card should be completed).

9. Withdrawals: Patients may withdraw themselves or be removed from the study by the investigating physician (or others), possibly for medical reasons or because of serious protocol deviations. This section of the protocol specifies how the reasons for withdrawal should be recorded (often on a special form) and describes any other consequent administrative procedures. Reasons for withdrawal may, of course, provide evidence of side-effects.

10. Adverse events: As for withdrawals. Severe adverse events would usually lead to withdrawal in any case.

11. Patient consent: A statement that patient consent will be sought and, if appropriate, what rules will be followed.

12. Ethics: A statement that the appropriate ethical committee will be, or has already been, consulted. A copy of the ethical guidelines to be adopted, such as the Declaration of Helsinki, is often included as an appendix.

13. Analysis: Outline details (at least) of the statistical methods to be used upon the subsequent data set. If there are special features of the required analysis, such as omission of certain data when assessing efficacy or separate subgroup analyses (for example, by age), these should be given here.

14. Data discharge: Details of data confidentiality and the rules governing disclosure.

15. Investigators' statement: A declaration that the protocol will be followed, which the principal investigators (and others) will sign.

## 7.3   Avoidance of bias

Just as in any other exercise in data collection, clinical trials may suffer from bias error if not conducted in an appropriate fashion. In this section we will consider four principles which should be followed in order to reduce the chance of a biased conclusion. See also Section 7.4 for some examples of the application of these principles.

### 7.3.1   Use of a control group

Just as for cohort studies, epidemiological intervention studies should be *comparative* – that is, a control group should be researched alongside a treated group. Here we assume, as we will subsequently in this chapter, that only two groups are involved, but in general there could be several treatment groups. The control group may be treated with a placebo (as in Example 7.1) or another active treatment, such as the existing standard therapy.

If there had been no placebo group in the Dundee vitamin study the only data would be the right-hand portion of Table 7.1. Then the appropriate procedure (for each IQ test) would be to use a paired $t$ test (Section 2.7.4). The $t$ statistics are 3.16 and 3.50, leading to $p$ values of 0.003 and 0.001, for non-verbal and verbal tests, respectively. Thus, without the control group, we would conclude that vitamin supplementation *does* improve IQ, the opposite to the conclusion in Example 7.1. One contributory factor to the result here is likely to be the increased experience of the children between testing dates; some improvement in certain aspects of IQ might be expected regardless of treatment.

If we fail to use a control group then we can never be sure that our results are not, at least in part, due to 'background' causes. One possible 'background' influence is the psychological boost of treatment which may cause an improvement in patient health all by itself. This is demonstrated in the following example, which is described in greater detail by Miao (1977) and Freedman *et al.* (1978).

*Example 7.2* In 1962 gastric freezing was introduced as an innovative treatment for duodenal ulcers on the evidence of an uncontrolled trial (that is, with no control group) of 24 patients, all of whom had relief of symptoms when the trial concluded after 6 weeks (Wangensteen *et al.*, 1962). Since the standard treatment in non-severe cases was not curative, and in severe cases involved surgery which sometimes failed and sometimes was fatal, this new treatment soon became popular. Seven years later a controlled trial of gastric freezing was published using 82 patients in the treated (gastric freeze) group and 78 in the control (pretend freeze) group. When the trial was evaluated after 6 weeks both groups tended to show an improvement; after 2 years, however, both groups tended to become clinically worse. There was no significant difference between the two groups at any time. This is suggestive of a short-term psychological boost after treatment, which disappeared in the long term. Gastric freezing appears to have no real effect. Partially as a result of the second, properly conducted, trial, gastric freezing was abandoned as a treatment for duodenal ulcers.

## 7.3.2 Blindness

Blindness is the policy of keeping someone unaware of which treatment has been given. Trials are said to be **single-blind** if the patient does not know which treatment he or she has received. This is desirable to avoid psychological boosts which may affect the results. For instance, those who know that they have received a placebo are unlikely to receive the same lift as those who know their treatment is active. For this reason, the controlled gastric freezing trial

(Example 7.2) used a pretend freeze, identical to the actual freeze in all observable aspects, for the control group.

Trials are **double-blind** if both the doctor, nurse or whoever is assessing the outcomes (patient response, physical measurements, laboratory tests etc.) and the patient are unaware of the treatment received. This avoids **observer bias** – that is, situations where the observer 'sees' an imaginary benefit (such as an improved state of health or fewer side-effects) for those patients treated with the observer's preferred treatment. However subconscious the observer's prejudice may be, the results would be biased in favour of his or her preconceived preference. Sometimes the person interpreting the set of results, possibly a statistician, is also kept blind for similar reasons. The trial would then be **triple-blind**.

Although blindness is desirable, it is not always possible. An obvious example is where a radiation treatment is compared with a surgical treatment of breast cancer. In drug trials blindness is usually easy to achieve by the use of dummy tablets, such as used in the Dundee vitamin study (Example 7.1). On the other hand, it is essential that the treatment allocation is coded and that there is always someone available to break the code in times of medical problems during the trial and, of course, at the end of the study.

### 7.3.3   Randomization

Subjects should be allocated to treatment group according to some chance mechanism. When this is done the trial is called a **randomized controlled trial** (RCT). Randomization is necessary to avoid systematic bias. Further details are given in Section 7.7, but the following example provides a cautionary tale of what can happen without randomization.

*Example 7.3*   Gore and Altman (1982) describe a controlled trial of free milk supplementation to improve growth amongst schoolchildren in Lanarkshire, Scotland, in 1930. Ten thousand children were allocated to the treated group, those who received the milk, and a similar number to the control group, who received no supplementation. Well-intentioned teachers decided that the poorest children should be given priority for free milk, rather than using strictly randomized allocation. The consequence was that the effects of milk supplementation were indistinguishable from (that is, confounded with) the effects of poverty. Since the poorer children were lighter at baseline this could bias in favour of milk 'treatment' because the lightest children had more potential to grow. Furthermore, the study began in winter and ended in summer, and at both times the children were weighed fully clothed. This unfortunate procedure is likely to have led to an underestimation of weight gain in both groups, but less so in the poorer (milk 'treatment') group because their warm winter clothes were sure to have been lighter. Again, there is a bias towards better results in the group given extra milk. There are, of course, other potential effects associated with poverty.

Quite how much, and even in what direction overall, the non-randomized allocation procedure affected the results is unclear. Firm conclusions about the benefit or otherwise of milk supplementation cannot be drawn from this trial.

### 7.3.4  Consent before randomization

To avoid bias in the eventual composition of the treatment groups, patients should be checked for consent (and eligibility) for each treatment before being randomly allocated to a treatment group. It is usually more attractive to a physician to randomize first, since then he or she will only have to explain one treatment to any one patient. As well as being easier, this avoids possible loss of the patient's trust when his or her doctor has to admit uncertainty about which of the treatments is best in this individual case. However tempting it may be, allocation before consent should be avoided because there is always the chance that a specific treatment will be rejected by a specific type of person, leading to potential bias. For example, in a comparison of drug and homeopathic treatments for a severe chronic condition it may well be that those who agree to participate after being allocated to homeopathic treatment are predominantly people who have been failed by 'normal' treatments and hence, are, inherently, rather more sick. Bias is then against the homeopathic treatment. Further discussion of the general problem is given by Kramer and Shapiro (1984).

## 7.4   Parallel group studies

All of the intervention studies described so far are of the simplest design where subjects are allocated into two (or more) treatment groups and everyone within a group receives the same treatment, which is different from the treatment given to other group(s). Furthermore, the number of subjects to be allocated to each group (notwithstanding withdrawals) is fixed in advance. Such studies are called **parallel group studies**; Sections 7.5 and 7.6 consider two alternative study designs for clinical trials.

Although the design is very different, the analysis of a parallel group intervention study proceeds exactly as for an equivalent cohort study. Here we shall look at two further examples of simple parallel group studies, so as to reinforce the basic ideas and provide illustrations of how the principles of Section 7.3 are put into practice. More complex examples may involve issues such as censoring, and thus require the analytical methods introduced in Chapter 5.

*Example 7.4*    Several accounts have been given of the large-scale field trial of the Salk polio vaccine carried out in the USA in 1954, including those by Snedecor and Cochran (1980) and Pocock (1983). The description here draws mainly on the account by Freedman *et al.* (1978).

Although the first outbreak of poliomyelitis did not happen until 1916, by 1954 hundreds of thousands of Americans, particularly children, had contracted the disease. The vaccine of Jonas Salk was just one of many proposed, but had already proved successful at generating antibodies to polio during laboratory tests. A field trial of the vaccine amongst children was deemed appropriate. Since the annual incidence rate of polio was, thankfully, only about 1 in 2000, several thousand subjects were needed (Chapter 8).

There were ethical objections to the use of a placebo control group in the field trial, given the nature of the disease, but this was overruled because polio tends to occur in epidemics. The number of cases in the USA in 1953, for instance, was about half of that in 1952, so that a drop during 1954 might have been attributable to a natural lull in the disease had an uncontrolled experiment been used.

Two different approaches to allocating children to treatment (vaccination or control) group were used. The National Foundation for Infantile Paralysis (NFIP) suggested vaccinating all children in the second grade whose parents gave consent. First- and third-grade children were to act as controls (without seeking parental consent). There are two serious flaws in this approach. First, it is likely that a greater proportion of consenting parents would be from advantaged social classes than we would expect to find in the general population. This is primarily because the more advantaged are usually better educated. Schoolchildren from high social class families are more likely to contract polio since they live in more hygienic accommodation and so are less likely to have already contracted a mild form of the disease in early life, when protected by maternal antibodies. Hence, to confine vaccination to children whose parents gave consent is to bias against the vaccine. The error is, of course, akin to that of seeking consent before allocation (Section 7.3.4). The second problem with the NFIP method is that, because of the contagious nature of polio, a clustering effect is highly likely. Hence, just by chance, there could have been a relatively high (or low) incidence amongst second-grade children in 1954, even if the trial had never occurred.

The second design used was an RCT which included all children whose parents consented to their entering the trial. These children were subsequently randomly assigned to either the vaccinated or control group within each participating school. Randomization was carried out within schools so as to balance out any geographic variations (for example, some schools may have been in particularly high-risk areas).

The RCT was double-blind. Children and their families were kept blind to treatment allocation by the use of saline fluid injections for the control group which mimicked the active vaccinations. The evaluating physicians were also kept blind because some forms of polio were difficult to diagnose, and it was thought likely that a sick child who was known to be unvaccinated was more likely to receive a positive diagnosis for polio than a child known to be vaccinated. Since the merits of the Salk vaccine were still being debated, subconscious bias during evaluation was very possible.

Some schools used the NFIP method whilst others adopted the RCT. Table 7.3 gives rounded figures to summarize the results. In this table results from those children without parental consent have been omitted, but these were also recorded.

There is a clear benefit of vaccine in both trials, with either 29 or 43 fewer cases of polio per 100 000 children after vaccination. Formal significance tests could be carried out for each

**Table 7.3**  Polio incidence rates per hundred thousand (with sample size in parentheses) in the two Salk vaccine trials

| Group | NFIP | RCT |
|---|---|---|
| Vaccinated | 25 (225 000) | 28 (200 000) |
| Control | 54 (725 000) | 71 (200 000) |
| Difference | −29 | −43 |

trial using the methods of Section 3.5 to compare two proportions on the exact source data. In fact it is clear, even from the rounded figures, that both trials produced extremely significant results (given the enormous sample sizes). However, Table 7.3 also shows a clear difference between the two trials, with the RCT predicting a much greater effect of vaccination. This demonstrates the bias, as expected, from the NFIP method; in fact it underestimates the effect of the vaccine by $43 - 29 = 14$ cases per 100 000. Due to the evidence of this RCT, the Salk vaccine was subsequently put into widespread use.

*Example 7.5*  The study of Crowther *et al.* (1990), already met in Example 3.9, was a parallel group study of the benefits of hospitalization for bed rest (from 28–30 weeks' gestation until delivery) in twin pregnancies. Subjects were women attending a special multiple pregnancy antenatal clinic. Women with cervical sutures, hypertension, a Caesarean section scar, an anteparteum haemorrhage or uncertain gestational age were excluded. Subjects were randomly allocated to either the treated (hospitalized bed rest) group or the control (no hospitalization, normal routine) group. Consent was obtained before randomization and ethical approval was granted by the local University Research Board. Although it was clearly not possible to make the subjects blind, the neonatalogist who made gestational age assessments was unaware of the treatment given.

Randomization achieved two groups of women that were fairly similar in all important aspects (average height, weight, gestational age etc.). There were no withdrawals or loss to follow-up. However, of the 58 women in the treated group, four did not attend for hospitalization and a further 11 required leave of absence from hospital for domestic reasons. Of the 60 women in the control group, 22 required antenatal admission to hospital because complications developed. Rather than being treated as protocol deviations to be excluded, they were retained in the analysis. Crowther *et al.* (1990) conclude that the study is thus truly a comparison of a policy of recommended routine hospitalization in uncomplicated twin pregnancy against a policy of advising hospitalization only if complications supervened.

Various end-points of the trial were analysed. Mean values (for example, mean gestational age at delivery) were compared using $t$ tests, and proportions (for example, the proportion who underwent a Caesarean section) were compared by using odds ratios (Section 3.2). In Example 7.1 we saw an example of the analysis of means. To illustrate an analysis of data in the form of proportions, consider Table 7.4, which gives data on delivery time from the study of Crowther *et al.* (1990). From this it is easy to calculate the odds ratio for bed rest versus no bed rest, from (3.9), as

$$\hat{\psi} = \frac{36 \times 20}{22 \times 40} = 0.82.$$

**Table 7.4**  Treatment group by gestational age for the bed rest study

| Treatment group | Gestational age (weeks) | | |
| --- | --- | --- | --- |
| | Below 37 | 37 or more | Total |
| Best rest | 36 | 22 | 58 |
| Control | 40 | 20 | 60 |
| Total | 76 | 42 | 118 |

The 95% confidence limits for this odds ratio are easily derived from (3.12) to be (0.39, 1.74). Since unity lies within this interval, we conclude that there is no significant effect of hospitalization for bed rest upon the odds of a delivery before 37 weeks. A chi-square test (with and without a continuity correction, as explained in Section 3.5.3) gives a $p$ value of 0.60. Notice that the analysis of Table 7.4 could equally well have been based on the relative risk rather than the odds ratio (Section 3.3.1).

No significant differences were found in any measure of pregnancy outcome, but twins in the treated group were significantly heavier and less likely to be either small for gestational age or stillbirths (although the analysis used ignores any correlation between siblings). Hence the study suggests that recommended bed rest may enhance fetal growth but provides no evidence of any effect on aspects of the pregnancy itself.

## 7.5  Cross-over studies

The most important drawback of a parallel group study is that any differences between the two (or more) treatment groups will affect the results. Although randomization will prevent any systematic differences occurring, chance imbalances in such variables as age, sex, height and weight between groups are possible, especially if the size of the study is fairly small. Even if the between-group differences in these so-called **prognostic factors** (which would be called confounding variables at the analysis stage) are not significant, such person-to-person differences cause extra variation in the measurements obtained, which decreases the precision of the results (for example, it increases the width of the confidence intervals).

An alternative is the **cross-over study** in which each treatment is given, at different times, to each subject. An introduction to cross-over studies is given by Senn (1993). The simplest example, and the only one we will consider here, is the two-period, two-treatment (or $2 \times 2$) cross-over. More complex designs are discussed in the comprehensive text by Jones and Kenward (1989).

In the $2 \times 2$ design subjects are (randomly) assigned to one of two groups; call them groups A and B. Subjects in group A receive treatment 1 for a suitable length of time and then receive treatment 2. Subjects in group B receive the two treatments in the opposite order (2 followed by 1). Usually the treatment periods are of equal length, typically a few weeks. Single blindness may be achieved by the **double-dummy** technique where each subject always receives a combination of two treatments, the appropriate active treatment plus a placebo which is indistinguishable from the other active treatment.

In a cross-over study the effect of (say) treatment 1 compared with treatment 2 may be assessed for each individual subject. Such **within-subject differences** are then summarized to obtain an overall evaluation of efficacy. Since within-subject variation is almost certainly less than between-subject variation, a cross-over should produce more precise results than a parallel group study of the same size. Alternatively, this advantage of cross-overs could be viewed as a saving in sample size: a cross-over should obtain the same precision as a parallel group study without using as many subjects. This saving of resources is the most common justification for using a cross-over design.

Unfortunately, there are several disadvantages to cross-overs which restrict their application. These are:

1.  Justification: The advantage of more precision, or fewer subjects, is only valid when within-subject variation *is* less than between-subject variation. Although this does generally happen in practice there is no theoretical reason why it should always.
2.  Suitability: Cross-over studies are only suitable for long-term conditions for which treatment only provides short-term relief (and certainly not a cure). Otherwise there could be no justification for the second treatment period. Examples of use include studies of bronchitis, angina, hypertension, migraine, 'jet lag', colostomy appliances and contraceptive devices.
3.  Duration: Each subject has to spend a long time in the trial, possibly twice as long as in the comparable parallel group study. This may lead to several withdrawals and non-compliance because of fatigue. Sample size (at analysis) may then be reduced so much that the consequent precision of results is unacceptably low. With extremely long trials, problems of cost and changes in the condition of the illness may also occur.
4.  Carry-over effects: There is a possibility that one treatment has, when given first, a residual effect in the second period, called a **carry-over effect**. An obvious case where this is likely is when treatment 1 is active and treatment 2 is a placebo. Subjects in group A may still have some benefit from treatment 1 even after they have crossed over to the placebo. A straightforward comparison of within-subjects differences would then be biased against the active treatment, since some (group A) placebo results are better than they should be. To protect against carry-overs, many cross-

over trials include a **wash-out** period between the two treatment periods. Sometimes a placebo is applied during this period, or sometimes the second period treatment is applied 'early' – that is, before the start of the second treatment period proper. Some trials have a **run-in** period before the first treatment period proper begins, so as to wash out any residual effects of any previous medications (as well as to acclimatize subjects to trial conditions).

A differential carry-over effect is one of several possible causes of a **treatment by period interaction** – that is, a differential effect of treatment in different periods. A test for the presence of such an interaction may be constructed (as we shall see later), but unfortunately this test usually has low power, by which we mean that there is a good chance of failing to detect an interaction (caused by carry-over or otherwise) even when it is medically important (see Section 8.2 for technical details). The reason for this is that this particular test is based upon between-subject differences, and the sample size is usually small. Note that the treatment by period interaction is indistinguishable from (aliased with) an effect of treatment group in a two-treatment two-period cross-over.

5. Complexity: Cross-overs are more complex to analyse than parallel group studies.

### 7.5.1   Graphical analysis

As in many other situations, the first step in analysing cross-over data should be to plot the data. Various different plots have their use in 2 × 2 cross-overs (as discussed by Hills and Armitage, 1979). Consider, first, graphs of mean response against period, labelled by treatment received. Figure 7.1 illustrates six of the possible forms for such a graph for a trial of treatments R and S. In each case the responses under the same treatment have been joined by a line. This should not be interpreted as subjects' progress through the trial: remember that someone who takes R in period 1 will take S in period 2 and vice versa. The lines emphasize treatment by period interactions, when they occur, since these are manifested as non-parallel lines. In extreme cases of interaction (Section 4.7) the lines will cross. A case-study example of the type of plot given in Figure 7.1 is included as Figure 7.2.

For other useful plots, see the figures associated with Example 7.6. Figure 7.3 shows response against period for each subject separately for each treatment group. Here the lines *do* represent subjects' progress (the left-hand side marks the response in period 1 and the right the response in period 2, for a

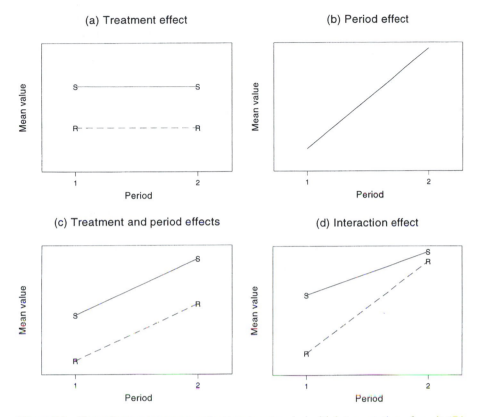

**Figure 7.1**   Plots of mean response against treatment period with interpretation of result: 'R' denotes that treatment R was used, 'S' denotes that treatment S was used (points are co-incident in (b)).

given subject). These plots are able to show up atypical subjects, such as those whose trial progress goes in the opposite direction to that of others, or who have very small or very large effects. Such subjects require further scrutiny, in order to decide whether to report them separately; for instance, they may be protocol violations. **Scatterplots** may also be useful in this respect. Figure 7.4 shows a scatterplot of results in period 2 against results in period 1, labelled by treatment group. A treatment effect would show as a clustering of symbols either side of the diagonal line. A similar scatterplot, but showing results when using the different treatments, rather than in different periods, could be used to detect period effects. Period effects are probably not of direct interest; the study aims to explore treatment effects. They may, however, be of secondary interest. For instance, Figures 7.1(b) and 7.1(c) are cases where response has increased over time for each treatment group (that is, regardless of order), which suggests a benefit of longer-term treatment. Figure 7.1(a) suggests no such effect.

### 7.5.2  Comparing means

The plots of Figure 7.1 are somewhat idealized, since exactly parallel lines are unlikely in practice. Furthermore, we would like to be able to quantify what is a small and a large difference. Hence we continue by assessing the statistical significance of the various possible effects.

Before we can test for a treatment (or period) effect we should first test for a treatment by period interaction. If there is no evidence for such an interaction, then we may go ahead and test for treatment (and period) effects using the cross-over data (see below). However, if there is an interaction, then we cannot use the information from the second period to assess the treatment effect since this would introduce bias. Instead we would be forced to use only the data from the first period of treatment and analyse as a parallel group study.

To develop the tests we need some basic notation. Let $x_{A1}$ denote an observation from group A in period 1, and $x_{A2}$ denote an observation from group A in period 2; similarly for group B. Then let $t_A$ denote the total of the two observations for a subject in group A, and $d_A$ denote the difference between first and second period observations for subjects in group A; similarly for group B. Hence,

$$t_A = x_{A1} + x_{A2}, \qquad d_A = x_{A1} - x_{A2};$$
$$t_B = x_{B1} + x_{B2}, \qquad d_B = x_{B1} - x_{B2}.$$

Also let $n_A$ be the number of subjects in group A, $\bar{t}_A$ and $s(t)_A$ be the mean and standard deviation of the $t_A$, and $\bar{d}_A$ and $s(d)_A$ be the mean and standard deviation of the $d_A$; and similarly for group B.

Analysis will be based upon these sums and differences across periods. We shall assume that the data obtained approximate to a normal distribution reasonably well, so that $t$ tests may be used. Otherwise transformations (Section 2.8.1) should be tried and if these fail to 'induce' normality, non-parametric alternatives may be used (Section 2.8.2). We shall also assume that the pooled estimate of variance, (2.16), is appropriate to use. In the case of totals this will be

$$s(t)_p^2 = \frac{(n_A - 1)s(t)_A^2 + (n_B - 1)s(t)_B^2}{n_A + n_B - 2}; \qquad (7.1)$$

and, in the case of differences,

$$s(d)_p^2 = \frac{(n_A - 1)s(d)_A^2 + (n_B - 1)s(d)_B^2}{n_A + n_B - 2}. \tag{7.2}$$

Three tests are possible, for the effects now listed.

1. **Treatment by period interaction** If there were no such interaction then the means of the two totals ($t_A$ and $t_B$) should be equal. This is tested formally by applying (2.14) to the data on totals for the separate groups; that is, we compare

$$\frac{\bar{t}_A - \bar{t}_B}{\sqrt{s(t)_p^2 \left[\frac{1}{n_A} + \frac{1}{n_B}\right]}} \tag{7.3}$$

with $t_{n_A + n_B - 2}$ using some appropriate significance level. As has been mentioned, this test has low power. To protect against this, it is a good idea to use a higher significance level than that planned for the test of treatment difference. For instance, we might use a 5% test to compare treatments, but a 10% test here. If this test is significant then, unless we have some way of accounting for the interaction from other data, we should abandon the cross-over analysis, as already explained.

2. **Treatment difference** Cross-over data are paired data, and hence the paired $t$ test (Section 2.7.4) could be applied to the entire set of differences (that is, the $d_A$ and $d_B$ combined), which would be compared with zero. The weakness of this test is that it ignores the period effect, and in the presence of an important period effect it may give misleading results. A rather safer procedure, which is not affected by period differences, is the two-sample $t$ test to compare the means of the $d_A$ and $d_B$. Here $\bar{d}_A$ estimates $\mu_R - \mu_S$ where $\mu_R$ and $\mu_S$ are the true mean effects of treatments R and S respectively, where R is the treatment taken in the first period by subjects in group A, and S the other treatment. $\bar{d}_B$ will estimate $\mu_S - \mu_R$. Hence a test of $\mu_R - \mu_S = 0$ (no treatment effect) can be made by comparing $\bar{d}_A - \bar{d}_B$ with zero. Hence the test statistic

$$\frac{\bar{d}_A - \bar{d}_B}{\sqrt{s(d)_p^2 \left[\frac{1}{n_A} + \frac{1}{n_B}\right]}} \tag{7.4}$$

is compared with $t_{n_A + n_B - 2}$. An unbiased estimate for $\mu_R - \mu_S$ is given by $\frac{1}{2}(\bar{d}_A - \bar{d}_B)$. The associated confidence interval, derived from (2.18), also includes the factor $\frac{1}{2}$. It is

$$\frac{1}{2}(\bar{d}_A - \bar{d}_B) \pm \frac{1}{2}(t_{n_A+n_B-2})\sqrt{s(d)_p^2 \left[\frac{1}{n_A} + \frac{1}{n_B}\right]}. \qquad (7.5)$$

3. **Period difference** If it is interesting, this may be tested (regardless of any treatment effect) by comparing the average of the $d_A$ against the average of the *negative* values of $d_B$. This follows from the method used to compare treatments. In the calculations the only change now is that we must replace $-\bar{d}_B$ by $+\bar{d}_B$ in (7.4) and (7.5).

The procedures given here may easily be implemented using standard software that applies the pooled $t$ test and associated confidence interval. Generalizations of the approach, using statistical modelling, are given by Barker *et al.* (1982) and Jones and Kenward (1989).

*Example 7.6* Hill *et al.* (1990) describe a $2 \times 2$ cross-over trial to compare lysine acetyl salicylate (Aspergesic) with ibuprofen in the treatment of rheumatoid arthritis. Here ibuprofen was the usual prescribed treatment; there was interest in whether a cheap, over-the-counter medicine might work equally well. Thirty-six patients were randomly assigned to the two treatment order groups at entry (half to each). After two weeks on their first treatment,

**Table 7.5** Average pain scores from the rheumatoid arthritis study, showing sums and differences across treatment periods

| Ibuprofen–Aspergesic group ($n = 15$) | | | | Aspergesic–ibuprofen group ($n = 14$) | | | |
|---|---|---|---|---|---|---|---|
| Period 1 | Period 2 | Sum | Diff. | Period 1 | Period 2 | Sum | Diff. |
| 3.143 | 3.286 | 6.429 | −0.143 | 1.286 | 2.214 | 3.500 | −0.928 |
| 3.000 | 2.429 | 5.429 | 0.571 | 4.100 | 4.444 | 8.544 | −0.344 |
| 3.071 | 2.357 | 5.428 | 0.714 | 3.357 | 3.267 | 6.624 | 0.090 |
| 3.286 | 2.929 | 6.215 | 0.357 | 3.214 | 2.929 | 6.143 | 0.285 |
| 2.846 | 2.200 | 5.046 | 0.646 | 3.286 | 3.714 | 7.000 | −0.428 |
| 2.571 | 2.071 | 4.642 | 0.500 | 3.800 | 3.231 | 7.031 | 0.569 |
| 3.214 | 3.143 | 6.357 | 0.071 | 3.143 | 2.214 | 5.357 | 0.929 |
| 3.929 | 3.571 | 7.500 | 0.358 | 3.467 | 3.615 | 7.082 | −0.148 |
| 3.909 | 3.000 | 6.909 | 0.909 | 2.714 | 2.154 | 4.868 | 0.560 |
| 2.615 | 2.692 | 5.307 | −0.077 | 1.786 | 1.929 | 3.715 | −0.143 |
| 1.786 | 2.214 | 4.000 | −0.428 | 2.714 | 2.857 | 5.571 | −0.143 |
| 1.429 | 1.286 | 2.715 | 0.143 | 2.930 | 3.710 | 6.640 | −0.780 |
| 3.000 | 2.929 | 5.929 | 0.071 | 2.143 | 2.071 | 4.214 | 0.072 |
| 3.250 | 4.000 | 7.250 | −0.750 | 2.860 | 2.430 | 5.290 | 0.430 |
| 2.500 | 1.214 | 3.714 | 1.286 | | | | |
| | Total | 82.87 | 4.228 | | Total | 81.58 | 0.021 |
| | Mean | 5.52 | 0.282 | | Mean | 5.83 | 0.0015 |
| | Std dev. | 1.35 | 0.524 | | Std dev. | 1.45 | 0.527 |

patients crossed over to the opposite treatment. A further two weeks later the trial ended. There was no run-in or wash-out period, but the trial was double-blind (including use of the double-dummy procedure).

At baseline a general medical examination was carried out, and the recorded baseline values of the two treatment groups were found to be similar (in summary terms). At the two subsequent clinic visits (at half-way and the end) patient and investigator assessments of progress were recorded and several measurements (grip strength, blood pressure, haematology etc.) were taken. Between the clinic visits (that is, whilst on treatment) diary cards were completed each day by the patients. The data recorded included a pain assessment score on a 1–5 scale (1 = no pain, 2 = mild pain, 3 = moderate pain, 4 = severe pain, 5 = unbearable pain). These data are summarized in Table 7.5, which shows the average (mean) pain score for each patient in each treatment period (plus derived values). Table 7.5 only represents 29 of the original 36 patients. Five withdrew from the trial, one was considered non-compliant because of the vast quantities of study medication that he returned unused, and one patient failed to return his second diary card.

Graphical analyses of these data are given in Figures 7.2–7.4. Figures 7.3 and 7.4 suggest that there is little treatment effect, because several of the lines on each side of Figure 7.3 go up and several go down, and the points in Figure 7.4 are both near to the diagonal and not separated by type of symbol (representing group membership). Figure 7.2 suggests that there could be a treatment by period interaction since the lines (just) cross. Mean pain scores are virtually identical, except when Aspergesic is taken in the second period in which case they are lower. This agrees with Figure 7.3 and Table 7.5 where we note that 11/15 do better with

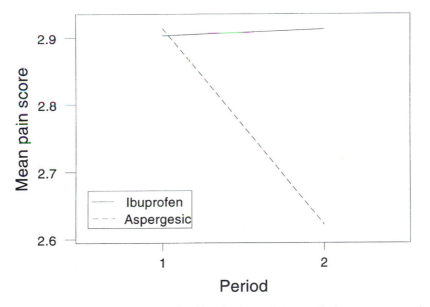

**Figure 7.2** Mean pain score (over all subjects) when using a particular treatment against treatment period, arthritis study.

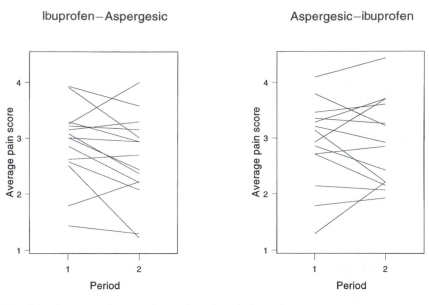

**Figure 7.3**  Average pain score (over a 2-week period) against treatment period classified by treatment group, arthritis study.

Aspergesic when it is used in the second period compared with half (7/14) when it is used first. So, perhaps Aspergesic works better when taken *after* ibuprofen, which would imply a treatment by period interaction, perhaps caused by a differential carry-over of ibuprofen (although there could be other explanations). Other diagrams (boxplots and histograms not shown here) suggest that the pain scores in Table 7.5 have a distribution reasonably close to the normal distribution (for instance, no severe skew). Hence $t$ tests are acceptable.

A test for treatment by period interaction involves computing

$$s(t)_{\mathrm{p}}^2 = \frac{14 \times 1.35^2 + 13 \times 1.45^2}{15 + 14 - 2} = 1.96$$

from (7.1). Substituting this into (7.3) gives

$$\frac{5.52 - 5.83}{\sqrt{1.96\left(\frac{1}{15} + \frac{1}{14}\right)}} = -0.60,$$

which is not significant when compared to $t$ with 27 d.f. ($p > 0.5$ from Table B.4). Despite our earlier concern, there is no evidence of an interaction and hence the lack of parallel lines seen in Figure 7.2 is attributable to chance variation. We can thus go on to use the full cross-over to test for treatment and period effects. We need to calculate first:

$$s(d)_{\mathrm{p}}^2 = \frac{14 \times 0.524^2 + 13 \times 0.527^2}{15 + 14 - 2} = 0.276$$

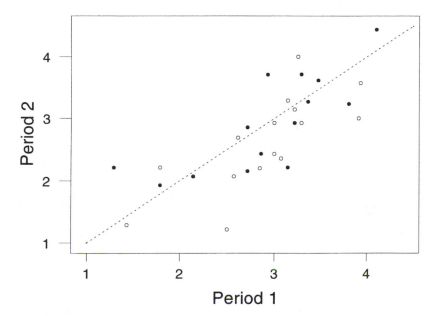

**Figure 7.4** Average pain score (over a 2-week period) in the second period against the same quantity (for the same subject) in the first period of treatment, arthritis study. Open circles represent the ibuprofen–Aspergesic group; closed circles represent the Aspergesic–ibuprofen group.

from (7.2). Substituting this into (7.4) gives

$$\frac{0.282 - 0.0015}{\sqrt{0.276\left(\frac{1}{15} + \frac{1}{14}\right)}} = 1.44$$

which is not significant when compared against $t$ with 27 d.f. ($p > 0.2$ from Table B.2). A similar test for a period effect requires comparison of

$$\frac{0.282 + 0.0015}{\sqrt{0.276\left(\frac{1}{15} + \frac{1}{14}\right)}} = 1.45$$

with the same $t$ value. Again, this is not significant. Hence we conclude that there is no significant effect of either treatment or period of treatment. Aspergesic is as good as, but no better or worse than, ibuprofen.

Using (7.5), we can quantify the difference in pain score when taking Aspergesic. This gives the 95% confidence interval as

$$\frac{1}{2}(0.282 - 0.0015) \pm \frac{1}{2} \times 2.052 \times \sqrt{0.276\left(\frac{1}{15} + \frac{1}{14}\right)},$$

that is, $0.14 \pm 0.20$. In this calculation 2.052 is $t_{27}$ at the two-sided 5% level, obtained from a computer package. As the hypothesis test has already shown it must, the interval contains 0. We expect Aspergesic to produce an average of 0.14 more 'units of pain' than ibuprofen, but this is not significantly different from 'no difference' in mean pain score. The 95% confidence interval for period difference is unlikely to be required here, but for completeness it is

$$\frac{1}{2}(0.282 + 0.0015) \pm 0.20,$$

or $0.14 \pm 0.20$. This is the extra mean pain score in period 1 compared to period 2. Notice that, to two decimal places, it is the same as the treatment difference. This is not, of course, generally so. This has happened here because $\bar{d}_B$ is so small.

One final point about the analysis is that Figure 7.3 shows the possible existence of an outlier. One patient in the ibuprofen–Aspergesic group has a very large decrease in pain between periods 1 and 2 (this is the last patient in this group in Table 7.5). Reference to this patient's other data from the trial gave no reason to suspect an error in these reports. To be safe, the data were reanalysed omitting this patient; the conclusions from the hypothesis tests were not altered.

### 7.5.3   *Analysing preferences*

At the end of a cross-over trial subjects are sometimes asked to state which treatment period they preferred. This may be a general question such as 'During which period did you feel better?' or a more particular question such as 'In which period did you experience the fewest problems?'. Sometimes the investigating physician may also be asked to state the treatment period in which he or she thought the subject's health was better. We wish to analyse such data to discover which (if any) treatment is preferred. This can be achieved using **Prescott's test** (Prescott, 1981), which is a test for linear trend in a contingency table of treatment group against preference stated. The general layout of such a table is shown as Table 7.6.

Prescott's test statistic may be derived directly from (3.19). However, since the numbers in cross-over trials are usually quite small, it is advisable to use a continuity correction. This means subtracting $\frac{1}{2}n$ from the numerator of (3.19). The result is

$$\frac{n(n(n_{A3} - n_{A1}) - n_A(n_3 - n_1) - \frac{1}{2}n)^2}{n_A n_B(n(n_3 + n_1) - (n_3 - n_1)^2)} \tag{7.6}$$

which should be compared to chi-square with 1 d.f.

The drawback with this procedure is that the approximation to chi-square will be in doubt if some of the expected frequencies are very small. In this event we would be forced to use the exact form of Prescott's test, which is akin to Fisher's exact test (Section 3.5.4) but computationally more demanding An alternative, but less sensitive test, which is easier to compute in the exact form

**Table 7.6**   Display of preference data

| Treatment group | Prefer 1st period treatment | No preference | Prefer 2nd period treatment | Total |
|---|---|---|---|---|
| A | $n_{A1}$ | $n_{A2}$ | $n_{A3}$ | $n_A$ |
| B | $n_{B1}$ | $n_{B2}$ | $n_{B3}$ | $n_B$ |
| Total | $n_1$ | $n_2$ | $n_3$ | $n$ |

is **Gart's test** (Gart, 1969), sometimes known as the **Mainland–Gart** test. This is based upon the $2 \times 2$ contingency table formed by deleting the 'no preference' column from Table 7.6. Now Fisher's exact test may be applied, if necessary.

Treatment effect is usually estimated by the odds ratio,

$$\hat{\psi} = \frac{n_{A1}/n_{A3}}{n_{B1}/n_{B3}}, \tag{7.7}$$

which gives the relative odds in favour of a preference for treatment R, *given that a preference is stated*. As in Section 7.5.2, R is the treatment given in period 1 to subjects in group A.

The procedures described so far are all for treatment effects. Just as in Section 7.5.2, we can also look at period effects, and as before this is achieved by a minor change to the equations for treatment effects. Here we simply interchange $n_{B1}$ and $n_{B3}$ in Table 7.6. This causes changes in $n_1$ and $n_3$ (and the corresponding headings should now be 'Prefer treatment R' and 'Prefer treatment S', where S is the treatment given in period 2 to patients in group A), but all else is unchanged. We can then apply Prescott's (or Gart's) test to this new table or, equivalently, simply make the necessary changes to (7.6) and (7.7). The latter becomes the odds in favour of a preference for period 1, given that a preference is stated.

*Example 7.7*   In the trial described in Example 7.6 one of the questions at the end of the trial was 'Compared to the last visit [to the clinic], is your pain worse/the same/better?'. In our terminology these translate to: worse = treatment given in period 1 preferred, same = no preference, better = treatment given in period 2 preferred. There were 30 responses to this question (no missing values). The results are given in Table 7.7.

The numbers here are quite small, but we would expect the chi-square test with a continuity correction to be reasonably accurate. Using (7.6), the test statistic is

$$\frac{30(30(8-6) - 17(11-13) - 15)^2}{17 \times 13(30(11+13) + (11-13)^2)} = 1.18.$$

By Table B.3, this is not significant ($p > 0.1$).

**Table 7.7**  Preference data relating to pain assessment from the Aspergesic trial

| Treatment group | Prefer 1st period treatment | No preference | Prefer 2nd period treatment | Total |
|---|---|---|---|---|
| Ibuprofen–Aspergesic | 6 | 3 | 8 | 17 |
| Aspergesic–ibuprofen | 7 | 3 | 3 | 13 |
| Total | 13 | 6 | 11 | 30 |

To test for a period effect using the $\chi_1^2$ statistic for Prescott's test, we apply (7.6) to the table

$$
\begin{array}{ccc|c}
6 & 3 & 8 & 17 \\
3 & 3 & 7 & 13 \\
\hline
9 & 6 & 15 & 30
\end{array}
$$

which, from (7.6), results in the test statistic

$$
\frac{30(30(8-6) - 17(15-9) - 15)^2}{17 \times 13(30(15+9) - (15-9)^2)} = 0.64,
$$

which is clearly not significant at any reasonable significance level.

### 7.5.4   Analysing binary data

Another type of data that may arise from a cross-over study is the binary form – for example, the answer to the question 'Did you feel any chest pain since the last clinic visit?' in an angina study. In many clinical trials we would wish to compare the treatments for presence of side-effects, and this is another example of a success/failure variable.

Binary data may be analysed in exactly the same fashion as preference data. This is achieved by taking a subject who has success in period 1 but failure in period 2 as a 'period 1 preference', and similarly a patient who has success in period 2 but failure in period 1 is a 'period 2 preference'; all others have 'no preference'. We would then analyse as in Section 7.5.3.

## 7.6   Sequential studies

In many intervention studies, particularly those involving the allocation of treatments to patients, subjects are recruited at different times. For instance, a general practitioner may enter each new patient who arrives for consultation with a specific disorder into the study; unless the disorder is particularly common, this may require recruitment over several weeks, or even months. Consequently, results for particular patients, such as response to a 2-week exposure to treatment, may well be available serially in time. Suppose, then, that the benefits of one treatment over another are clear from the early results. Is there any point in continuing the experiment under these circumstances? Indeed, is it ethically acceptable to continue to allocate a treatment even when it is known to be inferior?

To avoid this ethical dilemma, some intervention studies use a **sequential** design. This means that the number of subjects studied is not fixed in advance, but is allowed to vary depending upon the clarity of the information received. Hence, if early observations show an obvious treatment difference, then the study will stop early. If not, it continues. Such a design is only suitable when data do arrive serially in time. As well as the ethical consideration, a sequential study (suitably designed and analysed) can be expected to finish before the conventional fixed-sample parallel group study would do so. This not only reduces costs for the current study, but also should be of benefit to future subjects, since the results will be available rather earlier than they would otherwise have been. The practical disadvantages are that the required quantities of the treatment, human resources and equipment are unknown in advance, and that data must be compiled and calculations made at regular intervals (these are sometimes called **interim analyses**). Sequential data are also more difficult to analyse, although specialist software is available (see Emerson, 1996). There is insufficient space to describe the methods of analysis here: see Whitehead (1997) for a thorough exposition. A simple picture will describe the essential idea (Figure 7.5). This shows the stopping boundaries for a particular sequential test called the **triangular test**. A suitable test statistic, the formula for which is determined by statistical theory, is calculated at each interim analysis, assumed here to happen when each single new result is obtained (this assumption is not necessary and may well be inconvenient in practice). Progress during the study, as results accumulate, is shown as a 'walk' across the plot from left to right. The walk begins within the 'No decision yet' zone and continues until either the 'Reject null hypothesis' or the 'Fail to reject' boundary is crossed. In the hypothetical example illustrated the rejection boundary was crossed, and the study terminated, once the 20th subject's result was available. The conclusion was that the null hypothesis should be rejected.

In many situations it is appropriate to plot some function of the accumulated sample size, rather than the sample size itself, on the horizontal axis. The

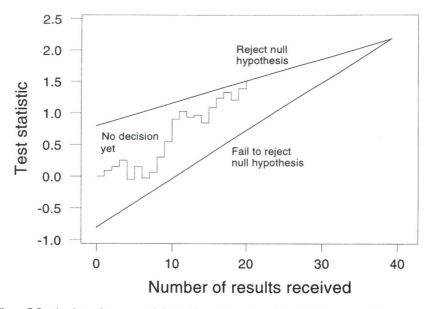

**Figure 7.5**    A triangular sequential test: the null hypothesis is that the mean subject response takes some predetermined value, against a one-sided alternative.

triangular test is only one of a number of sequential test designs available: see Whitehead (1997) for a general discussion and Jennison and Turnbull (1990) for a comparison of some of the more popular designs.

An example of a sequential intervention study is that described by Moss *et al.* (1996). This was a comparison of prophylactic therapy with an implanted cardioverter-defibrillator and conventional medicine in the treatment of subjects with specific severe coronary symptoms. The end-point recorded was death from any cause. A two-sided sequential triangular test was adopted; the test statistic used to formulate the stopping boundaries was the log-rank test (Section 5.5.2). Data were analysed weekly from the point when 10 deaths had been reported. By the time the study was terminated, the first of the 192 patients recruited had been followed up for 61 months and the last for 1 month (the average duration of follow-up was 27 months). The conclusion reached was that the treatments had a different effect ($p = 0.009$); the implant appeared to reduce mortality. Early stopping, compared with a fixed-sample design, meant that the results could be published, and acted upon, more quickly.

## 7.7    Allocation to treatment group

Whatever the design, any comparative clinical trial should have a set of rules for allocating subjects to treatment groups. Earlier we saw the benefit of randomization, which is to protect against systematic bias, so we will certainly want rules which involve a chance mechanism. We will assume that subjects will be allocated to either of two treatment groups, call them A and B – and that an equal number are required in each. Generalizations from these restrictions are not difficult. We will also assume that subjects arrive one at a time for recruitment by the investigator (assumed to be a physician, perhaps at a GP clinic or hospital). Consent should have been obtained before allocation begins (Section 7.3.4).

The allocation schemes described fall into two types: those which use global (unstratified) randomization (Section 7.7.1) and those which stratify randomization so as to achieve balance between the groups in terms of the prognostic factors (such as age and sex) which are thought to have an important effect on the outcome of the trial (Section 7.7.2).

In the examples that follow we shall use a random number table, Table B.6. To make things easier to follow we will always begin drawing random numbers at the top left-hand position and move left to right across the table. In general, a random starting point should be chosen as well, perhaps, as a random direction.

### 7.7.1    Global randomization

Here patients will be allocated to treatment groups A or B using randomization rules which are unrestricted with regard to prognostic factors. We shall look at four alternative schemes.

In **complete randomization**, each patient is allocated to group A or B using a fair coin (for example, heads = A; tails = B) or some equivalent mechanism, such as Table B.6. To use a random number table we assign an equal number of random digits to each group; for example, we could allocate 0–4 to A and 5–9 to B. Then, since the first ten random numbers in Table B.6 are

$$1, 4, 7, 2, 6, 0, 9, 2, 7, 2,$$

the allocations for the first ten subjects are

$$A, A, B, A, B, A, B, A, B, A.$$

There are two drawbacks to this simple scheme: overall imbalance between the groups is fairly likely (in the example there are six As and only four Bs) and prognostic factors may not be balanced (for example, all the As could, by chance, be men and all the Bs could be women). These problems are unlikely to be important for very large studies, in which case this is the preferred allocation scheme because of its simplicity.

In the **alternation** scheme, the first patient is allocated as above, and thereafter the assignments alternate. Hence, using Table B.6, we draw the first random number, 1, which corresponds to allocation A (by the rules used above). The sequence of allocations thus is

$$A, B, A, B, A, B, A, B, A, B, \ldots.$$

This scheme ensures equal allocation (obviously this is only exactly true if the overall sample size is even). It still does not guarantee balance in prognostic factors and, furthermore, has the disadvantage of predictability. Once the investigating physician has discovered the pattern he or she may defer or refuse recruitment because the next allocation is known in advance. This will lead to bias in many cases. Clearly the problem is not as bad in double-blind studies, but it is not impossible for a few subjects' codes to be broken, inadvertently or due to medical necessity. The investigator may then be able to guess the pattern.

An improvement on alternation is a block allocation scheme, **random permuted blocks**, which is much less predictable. We will look at the specific example of blocks of size 4. Consider all the different possible sequences of allocations of four successive subjects containing two As and two Bs. These are the permuted blocks:

1. A, A, B, B
2. A, B, A, B
3. A, B, B, A
4. B, A, A, B
5. B, A, B, A
6. B, B, A, A.

Blocks are then chosen at random by selecting random numbers between 1 and 6. This could be done (for example) with a fair die or by using Table B.6 (ignoring the numbers 7, 8, 9 and 0). Hence the first five numbers obtained from Table B.6 are

$$1, 4, 2, 6, 2$$

Referring back to the numbering scheme above gives the allocation of the first 20 subjects as

$$A, A, B, B, B, A, A, B, A, B, A, B, B, B, A, A, A, B, A, B$$

(split the letters into groups of four to see the relationship with the list of permuted blocks).

This scheme may not be entirely unpredictable, since in single-blind studies an investigator who discovers the block size will then know at least every last assignment in the block in advance, assuming that he or she is devious enough to keep a record of past assignments. This problem is unlikely to occur when the block size is large (say 10 or more), but it may be worthwhile varying the block size as allocation proceeds. Prognostic factors are likely to be unbalanced.

The **biased coin method** is akin to complete randomization except that, at each allocation, we evaluate the correspondence in treatment group size up to that point, and allocate to the group currently undersized with a probability of more than 1/2. The probabilities used are commonly 3/5, 2/3 or 3/4. We will take 2/3 as an example. To apply the scheme we will take the random numbers 1, 2, 3, 4, 5, 6 for the smallest group, and 7, 8, 9 for the largest group. In the case of a tie in sample size we simply allocate to each group with probability 1/2, exactly as for the complete randomization scheme (0–4 = A, 5–9 = B).

The first 10 numbers obtained from Table B.6 are now written with the consequent allocation according to the above rules; the lower-case letters in-between describe the relative sample sizes *before* the present allocation is made (a = A larger, b = B larger, t = tie):

| 1, | 4, | 7, | 2, | 6, | 0, | 9, | 2, | 7, | 2, | 9 |
|----|----|----|----|----|----|----|----|----|----|---|
| t | a | t | b | t | b | b | b | b | b | b |
| A, | B, | B, | A, | B, | | B, | A, | B, | A, | B |

Note that the zero has been rejected.

This scheme is not guaranteed to provide a balance in numbers (indeed the sample sizes are 6 : 4 in favour of B in the example), but the degree of inequality is unlikely to be important except in very small trials. Prognostic factors may be unbalanced.

### 7.7.2   Stratified randomization

Here we shall assume that a number of prognostic factors are known to have an influence on the outcome of the study. We shall look at two allocation schemes which seek to remove the differential effect of such prognostic factors by balancing their contribution to the two treatment groups. For example, we might wish to allocate as many men to group A as to group B, thus achieving balance with regard to sex.

Such balancing is not essential. For one thing, randomization itself should achieve at least an approximate balance in the long run (that is, big samples) since it is a 'fair' allocation scheme. The problem here is that trials are often fairly small in relation to the number of prognostic factors and the degree of balance that is required. Lack of balance may be allowed for at the analysis stage using methods designed to control for confounding (Chapter 4). Balance is, however, desirable on the grounds that the results are then more 'obvious' and more likely to be convincing. It is also statistically more efficient. Hence, provided that important prognostic factors are known and that the sample size overall is not big, restricted randomization is to be preferred. On the other hand, there is no point in trying to balance for a factor unless we are very confident that it has a real effect. Restricted randomization is more complex and more prone to error in application. Rarely will it be worthwhile balancing on more than three prognostic factors.

In what follows, as an example, we shall assume that we wish to balance on three factors: age, sex and severity of illness. Age is to be balanced at three levels (below 30, 30–49 and 50 years or more) and severity at two levels (severe, not severe).

In the **stratified random permuted blocks** scheme, subjects are grouped into cross-classified strata defined by the prognostic factors. In our example there are 12 such strata ($3 \times 2 \times 2$). A random permuted block scheme is used within each stratum using random numbers, just as in the unstratified scheme. The only difference now is that we shall have several (12 in the example) parallel sequences of random numbers, and thus blocks. With such a process there is little chance of predictability by the investigator, and blocks of size 2 (A, B and B, A only) may well be acceptable.

The drawback with this scheme is that it does not guarantee equality either in total group size or in the relative numbers for individual prognostic factors, between treatment groups. Either or both may have serious discrepancies. For our example, suppose that 100 patients are recruited to the trial and that the

**Table 7.8**  Cross-classification of 100 subjects by sex, severity of illness and age group

| Sex | Severity of illness | Below 30 | 30–49 | 50 and over |
|-----|---------------------|----------|-------|-------------|
| Men | Severe | 5 | 11 | 9 |
|     | Not severe | 9 | 13 | 0 |
| Women | Severe | 3 | 13 | 15 |
|     | Not severe | 7 | 15 | 0 |

*Age (years)* spans the last three columns (Below 30, 30–49, 50 and over).

**Table 7.9**   Result of stratified random permuted block (of size 2) allocation for the data in Table 7.8

| Allocation to A | | | Allocation to B | | |
|---|---|---|---|---|---|
| 2 | 5 | 4 | 3 | 6 | 5 |
| 4 | 7 | 0 | 5 | 6 | 0 |
| 2 | 7 | 8 | 1 | 6 | 7 |
| 4 | 8 | 0 | 3 | 7 | 0 |

Note: labels as in Table 7.8 for each treatment group.

number in each cross-class is as shown in Table 7.8. Suppose that random permuted blocks of size 2 are used within each stratum, and the resulting allocation is as shown in Table 7.9. This splits each individual number in Table 7.8 into two components and, because blocks of size 2 are used, there is never a difference of more than 1 between the left and right halves of Table 7.9. However, the sex ratio in group A is 29 : 22 in favour of women but in group B it is 25 : 24 in favour of men. Should the disease affect women more seriously than men, this imbalance would lead to bias (against the treatment given to group A in a parallel group trial), unless the analysis takes it into account. In this example there are also slight imbalances in overall sample size (51 : 49 in favour of A), age and severity of illness. Examples with serious imbalances in any of these are not difficult to construct. So, whilst the cross-classes are almost exactly balanced, the totals for any individual prognostic factor may be quite dissimilar.

In general, the problems illustrated by the example will tend to worsen as overall sample size decreases, block size increases and the number of cross-classes (that is, the number of prognostic factors or levels used within factors) increases. Hence small block sizes are preferable, but even then if subjects or resources are scarce, and there are several important prognostic factors, the scheme may not be suitable.

**Minimization** is a generalization of the biased coin method, by means of which we seek to balance the individual (marginal) totals of the prognostic factors. The basic idea is that when a new subject arrives for allocation we should calculate a score, for each treatment group, which reflects how similar the current allocation outcome is, in overall terms, to the characteristics of this new subject. The subject is then allocated to the group with lowest score using a probability greater than 1/2. As with the simple biased coin method, the probability taken is often 3/5, 2/3 or 3/4. Tied scores require the use of a probability of 1/2.

**Table 7.10**    Result of current allocations (within each sex, age and severity group separately) when the next patient arrives

| Factor | Level | A | B |
|--------|-------|---|---|
| Sex | Men | 27 | 25 |
|  | Women | 22 | 25 |
| Age | Below 30 | 12 | 11 |
| (years) | 30–49 | 25 | 27 |
|  | 50 and over | 12 | 12 |
| Severity | Severe | 28 | 28 |
| of illness | Not severe | 21 | 22 |

The simplest method of scoring is to count the number with each individual prognostic factor in common with the new subject, and sum over all the factors. For example, suppose the result of current allocations is given by Table 7.10. The next patient is a woman aged 26 without a severe case of the illness. To decide which treatment group she should go into we add up the numbers for the levels of Table 7.10 which have matching characteristics. These are: for A, $22 + 12 + 21 = 55$; for B : $25 + 11 + 22 = 58$. Hence we allocate her to group A with a probability of, say, 2/3. Notice that this particular outcome would be expected to improve the balance for overall group sizes, sex and severity of illness but actually increase the imbalance for age.

This scheme is not guaranteed to produce exactly equal numbers (as is clear from the example), but the degree of imbalance is unlikely to be important except in very small studies. Notice that minimization does not even try to balance out numbers in the cross-classes, such as those shown in Table 7.8. There may be perfect balance for each prognostic factor when taken alone, but serious imbalance across some cross-classes. For instance, groups A and B may have the same number of men and women and the same number of severe and non-severe cases, yet all the men in group A might be severe and all the men in B non-severe cases. This, of course, is the opposite problem to that encountered with stratified random permuted blocks. If we really would like balance across cross-classes with the minimization scheme we should take each cross-class as a separate classification, contributing to the score. However, this is likely to be tedious to implement.

Sometimes minimization is applied using an allocation probability of unity for the group with the smallest score. This is undesirable, since the process is now no longer random, but may be justifiable on pragmatic grounds in multi-centre trials and where there are several prognostic factors. Other rules for scoring, to be contrasted with the simple totalling method suggested here, are described by Whitehead (1997).

### 7.7.3 Implementation

Rather than having an investigator spin a coin, toss a die, use random number tables or some equivalent device for randomization during subject contact, randomization lists are normally prepared in advance. Often this list is transferred to a sequence of cards which are then placed in numbered, opaque, sealed envelopes. As each subject arrives the next envelope is then opened to reveal the allocation, A or B. Pocock (1983) cautions that doctors have been known to open and then reseal envelopes to discover forthcoming allocations in advance. Subjects may be rejected or deferred because the particular treatment is thought to be unsuitable for them, giving rise to bias. Often the randomization list is kept elsewhere and the investigator has to telephone for an allocation at the time of treatment.

Biased coin and minimization schemes require three sets of sealed envelopes, one for the situation where A is in the ascendancy (for example, with cards in the ratio 2 : 1 in favour of A), one for a tie (1 : 1) and one for B in the ascendancy (1 : 2). They also require that a careful check on past allocations be maintained. The stratified random permuted block scheme requires a set of envelopes for each stratum.

Double-blind studies introduce extra complexity. The indistinguishable A and B study medicines might be simply given (with labels) to the investigator in bulk. When A is allocated the medicine labelled A is given out. The problem with this is that when the code is broken for one subject it is automatically broken for all future subjects, thus violating the blindness. With the sealed envelope method this might be overcome by placing the medication, rather than a card, in the envelope. Otherwise the drugs might be issued by a third party.

Further details about allocation of subjects to treatment are given by Pocock (1979). Similar material is included in Pocock (1983). Modern methods of allocation use computer systems to simulate much of the above.

## Exercises

7.1 In the Lifestyle Heart Trial subjects with angiographically documented coronary heart disease were randomly assigned to an experimental or a usual-care group (Ornish *et al.*, 1990). Experimental subjects were prescribed a low-fat vegetarian diet, moderate aerobic exercise, stress management training, stopping smoking and group support. The usual-care subjects were not asked to change their lifestyle. Progression or regression of coronary artery lesions was assessed in both groups by angiography at baseline and after about a year.

Regression was observed in 18 of the 22 experimental subjects and 10 of the 19 control subjects.

    (i) Is this evidence of a significant effect of the lifestyle change regimen? Calculate suitable summary statistics to represent the effect.

    (ii) Discuss the potential problems of this intervention study and suggest moves that might be made to control these problems in similar studies.

7.2 In a study of four treatments for eradication of *H. pylori*, Tham *et al.* (1996) report the following eradication results (expressed as ratios of eradications to number treated):

Omeprazole + amoxycillin + metronidazole 6/20;

Ranitidine + amoxycillin + metronidazole 8/20;

Omeprazole + placebo 0/20;

Omeprazole + clarithromycin 4/20.

Test whether there is a significant difference between:

    (i) the first two treatments in this list.

    (ii) the third treatment (the only one not involving an antibiotic) and all the rest combined.

7.3 Refer to the cerebral palsy data of Table C.7.

    (i) Test whether the addition of rhizotomy has a significant effect on motor function.

    (ii) Summarize the effect of adding rhizotomy, giving a 95% confidence interval for your summary statistic.

7.4 Dorman *et al.* (1997) describe a randomized controlled comparison of a brief and a long questionnaire to ascertain quality of life for stroke survivors. Although the short questionnaire solicits less information it may be worth adopting, in future, if it leads to a higher response rate. The study involved 2253 survivors from the UK centres of the International Stroke Trial: 1125 received the short form and 1128 the long form, both sent out by post. After two mailings, 905 short and 849 long questionnaires had been returned.

    (i) Carry out a suitable test to ascertain whether the short questionnaire is worth considering further.

    (ii) Find a 99% confidence interval for the difference in response rates.

    (iii) If the short questionnaire were to be used, rather than the long one, in a study of 25 000 stroke survivors, how many extra respondents would you expect? Give a 99% confidence interval for this result.

7.5 Refer to the Norwegian Multicentre Study data of Table C.8.

    (i) Construct a separate actuarial life table for each treatment group. Include a standard error for each cumulative survival probability using Greenwood's formula.

    (ii) Plot the estimates of cumulative survival probability on a graph and interpret the presentation.

    (iii) Use a Cochran–Mantel–Haenszel test to compare overall survival between the Blocadren and placebo groups.

7.6 The following gives a series of objectives that have arisen, each of which suggests the use of an intervention study. State which kind of study design – parallel group, cross-over or sequential – you would suggest.

    (i) Comparison of two types of inhaler that are to be used to provide fixed amounts of salbutamol to patients with asthma. Lung function before and immediately after inhaler use will be compared.

    (ii) Comparison of the use and absence of use of antiarrhythmic drugs as an adjunct to electric shock treatment during episodes of ventricular fibrillation. The outcome measured will be survival for 1 hour.

(iii) Comparison of two diets that may cause reductions in blood cholesterol. Subjects to be healthy volunteers and the outcome measure to be change in serum total cholesterol after 4 weeks on the diet.

(iv) Comparison of a new and an existing treatment for a rare, fatal disease. Outcome to be survival time.

(v) Investigation of dental hygiene practices and blood coagulation. Volunteer subjects to be asked either to brush teeth twice a day or to refrain from tooth brushing. Changes in blood coagulation measures to be assessed after 2 weeks.

7.7 For the rheumatoid arthritis data of Table C.9, draw suitable diagrams to assess the treatment and period effects. Test for (i) a treatment by period interaction, (ii) a treatment effect and (iii) a period effect. Interpret your results.

7.8 Whitehead (1997) describes a sequential test, called a sequential probability ratio test, for the comparison of two proportions. This requires plotting $Z$ against $V$ at each time of observation, where

$$Z = \frac{nS - mT}{m + n}$$
$$V = \frac{mn(S + T)[(m - S) + (n - T)]}{(m + n)^3}.$$

Here $m$ and $n$ are, respectively, the number of patients in groups 1 and 2; and $S$ and $T$ are, respectively, the number of treatment successes in groups 1 and 2.

Du Mond (1992) describes a sequential study where this test is used to compare ganciclovir against placebo in the prevention of pneumonia following bone marrow transplantation. The upper and lower stopping boundaries for this test, for which results appear in Table C.10, turn out to be $Z = 2.58 + 0.675V$ and $Z - -2.58 + 0.675V$, respectively. Taking the ganciclovir group as group 1 and the placebo group as group 2, we conclude that ganciclovir is effective if we hit the upper boundary and we conclude 'no difference' if we hit the lower boundary.

(i) Using the data given in Table C.10, mark the boundaries given above and the results on a plot of $Z$ against $V$. What decision is made at the termination of the study?

(ii) Compare the boundaries for this test with those for the triangular test shown in Figure 7.5. Is there any particular disadvantage with the boundaries used in this test?

7.9 A study is planned to assess the desirability, and overall impact on the health services, of day surgery (hospital patients sent home after surgery without overnight stay). Several hospitals agree to take part in the study. At each hospital some surgical patients will be given day surgery and others will be kept as in-patients for at least one night. The two groups will be compared using various subjective criteria (including self-assessed health during the weeks following surgery) and factual criteria (such as the number of calls made to community and primary health care services during the weeks following surgery).

Describe a suitable method for allocating hospital patients to intervention groups. You may assume that a list of suitable surgical procedures for day surgery has already been established. Consider how you would put your allocation scheme into practice.

# 8

# Sample size determination

## 8.1 Introduction

Whenever an epidemiological study is being planned there is always the question of how many subjects to include – that is, what sample size to use. This is clearly a vital question and would constitute a crucial part of any research proposal. Too large a sample means wasted resources: the result may be statistically significant but have no practical significance, as when a very small relative risk, say below 1.05, turns out to be statistically significant – rarely will such a small increase in risk be biologically or medically important. This issue was discussed in Section 3.5.5, and is most likely found in large-scale cohort or cross-sectional studies. On the other hand, too small a sample leads to lack of precision in the results. This may render the entire study worthless: a result which would have medical significance has little chance of being found statistically significant when it is true. For instance, Gore and Altman (1982) report an investigation by Freiman *et al.* (1978) into 71 supposedly negative clinical trials. It transpired that two-thirds of these trials had a chance of 10% or more of missing a true improvement of 50% when comparing a 'new' against a 'standard' treatment. Seldom would a 50% improvement be of no medical importance, and hence such trials can be of little use.

The essential problem is to decide upon a value for the sample size, $n$, which is just sufficient to provide the required precision of results. The first consideration in calculating $n$ is the method of analysis which will subsequently be used on the data after collection. As we have seen in earlier chapters, this may well depend upon the type of data involved. Each different method of analysis will have an associated method for calculating sample size. This makes the entire subject too extensive, and often too complex, to cover fully here. Instead we shall restrict our description to the situation most commonly assumed when determining sample size in epidemiological research. This is when we wish to carry out a hypothesis test using a normal assumption or approximation. We shall look at four particular cases: tests for a single mean;

comparison of two means; a single proportion; and comparison of two proportions.

The approach of calculating $n$ for hypothesis tests is sometimes called the **power calculation method**. The application of this method in epidemiological research is generally straightforward provided that the sampling scheme to be used is simple random sampling. Case–control studies, however, require a slightly different approach to determining $n$, and hence they are considered separately in Section 8.7. More complex sampling methods are beyond our scope (see Cochran, 1977).

An alternative approach to the power calculation method is to determine $n$ so as to ensure that the resultant 95% (or other) confidence interval is of a specified maximum width. This method, which has much to commend it, is described by Bristol (1989). Sample size requirements when a more complex statistical analysis is planned, such as many : many matched case–control studies and survival analysis, tend to be covered in technical articles in statistical journals. For example, Freedman (1982) gives tables of sample sizes for use with the log-rank test, Hsieh (1989) gives sample sizes for use in logistic regression analysis (Chapter 10), whilst Schoenfield (1983) considers sample size for the proportional hazards model (Chapter 11). An extensive set of references is given by Lemeshow et al. (1990), a review is given by Donner (1984) and a useful set of tables for use in medical research is given by Machin and Campbell (1997).

Sometimes it may be useful to look at the sample size problem the other way around, that is to ask, given a particular value of $n$ (perhaps the most that can be afforded), what precision might be expected in the results. Here 'precision' might be the power (defined in the next section) or, say, the minimum relative risk that we can expect to find. This important problem will be addressed here along with the more usual direct computations of $n$. Such 'what if' questions can result in tedious calculation, especially as the formulae involved are quite complex. Consequently a computer package with sample size calculations is a real advantage in this situation; see Woodward (1989) for an example.

## 8.2   Power

The **power** of a hypothesis test is the probability that the null hypothesis is rejected when it is false. Often this is represented as a percentage rather than a probability. The distinction will not be crucial in our account, since it will be made clear which definition is being used.

In this section we shall consider, through examples, what determines the power of a hypothesis test. To simplify the explanation we shall consider one particular hypothesis test, the test for a mean value, as outlined in Section 2.7.2. Suppose that we wish to carry out a one-sided test, so that the two hypotheses under consideration are

$$H_0 \; : \; \mu = \mu_0,$$
$$H_1 \; : \; \mu > \mu_0.$$

Further, suppose that we plan to use a 5% significance test. For this test we know that we should reject $H_0$ whenever $T$ is greater than the upper 5% (one-sided) $t$ value with $n - 1$ d.f., where $T$ is the test statistic, (2.12),

$$T = \frac{\bar{x} - \mu_0}{s/\sqrt{n}}$$

for sample size $n$. The trouble with using this formula in any discussion of sample size is that the standard deviation, $s$, will be unknown before the sample is drawn. To simplify matters we will assume that the population standard deviation, denoted $\sigma$, is known. In this situation we replace (2.12) by

$$T = \frac{\bar{x} - \mu_0}{\sigma/\sqrt{n}}$$

and compare $T$ with the standard normal, rather than Student's $t$, distribution. Then we should reject $H_0$ in favour of $H_1$ whenever $T > 1.6449$. Note that 1.6449 is the critical value for a two-sided 10% test and thus a one-sided 5% test (see Table B.2). Hence by definition,

$$\text{Power} = p(T > 1.6449 \,|\, H_1 \text{ true}),$$

where the vertical line denotes 'given that'. In words, the power is the probability that the test statistic, $T$, exceeds 1.6449 given that the alternative hypothesis, $H_1$, is true.

It will be of interest to evaluate this equation for specific outcomes under the alternative hypothesis, $H_1$. That is, suppose we rewrite $H_1$ as

$$H_1 \; : \; \mu = \mu_1,$$

where $\mu_1 > \mu_0$. Then the power for the alternative $\mu = \mu_1$ becomes

$$\text{Power} = p(T > 1.6449 | \mu = \mu_1).$$

When $\mu = \mu_1$ the standardization process of taking away the mean and dividing by the standard error (Section 2.7) changes this to

$$\text{Power} = p\left(Z > 1.6449 + \frac{\mu_0 - \mu_1}{\sigma/\sqrt{n}}\right),$$

where $Z$ is a standard normal random variable (as tabulated in Tables B.1 and B.2). By the symmetry of the normal distribution, for any value $z$, $p(Z > z) = p(Z < -z)$. Hence,

$$\text{Power} = p\left(Z < \frac{\mu_1 - \mu_0}{\sigma/\sqrt{n}} - 1.6449\right). \tag{8.1}$$

We can evaluate the right-hand side of (8.1) and find an answer (at least approximately) from Table B.1. Alternatively, as noted in earlier chapters, values can be obtained from computer packages. We shall quote exact figures from the latter method here; the reader can check the results approximately with Table B.1.

*Example 8.1*   The male population of an area within a developing country is known to have had a mean serum total cholesterol value of 5.5 mmol/l 10 years ago. In recent years many Western foodstuffs have been imported into the country as part of a rapid move towards a Western-style market economy. It is believed that this will have caused an increase in cholesterol levels. A sample survey involving 50 men is planned to test the hypothesis that the mean cholesterol value is still 5.5 against the alternative that it has increased, at the 5% level of significance. From the evidence of several studies it may be assumed that the standard deviation of serum total cholesterol is 1.4 mmol/l. The epidemiologist in charge of the project considers that an increase in cholesterol up to 6.0 mmol/l would be extremely important in a medical sense. What is the chance that the planned test will detect such an increase when it really has occurred?

Here $\mu_0 = 5.5, \mu_1 = 6.0, \sigma = 1.4$ and $n = 50$. Substituting these into (8.1) gives the result,

$$\text{Power} = p\left(Z < \frac{6.0 - 5.5}{1.4/\sqrt{50}} - 1.6449\right)$$

$$= p(Z < 0.8805) = 0.8107.$$

Hence the chance of finding a significant result when the mean really is 6.0 is about 81%.

The determination of power for Example 8.1 is shown diagrammatically in Figure 8.1. The **rejection region** (or **critical region**) for the test is the area to the right of $T = 1.6449$. This is determined so as to contain 5% of the distribution of $T$ when the null hypothesis $\mu = 5.5$ is true (shaded). When the alternative hypothesis $\mu = 6.0$ is true the test statistic, $T$, no longer has mean zero; its mean is now

$$\frac{\mu_1 - \mu_0}{\sigma/\sqrt{n}} = \frac{6.0 - 5.5}{1.4/\sqrt{50}} = 2.5254$$

This causes the entire distribution of $T$ to be shifted 2.5254 units to the right. The area to the right of 1.6449 is now well over 5%; indeed it is clearly over 50% of the whole. As we have seen, it is actually 81%.

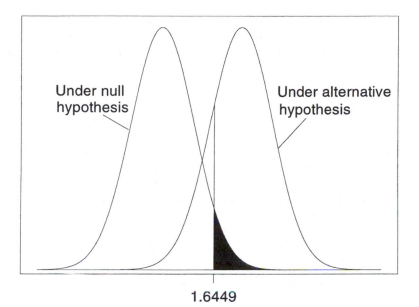

1.6449

**Figure 8.1**  Distribution of the test statistic, T, when $H_0$ is true and when $H_1$ is true for Example 8.1.

In Example 8.1 a difference of 0.5 mmol/l in mean cholesterol was thought to be medically important. Suppose that this was reconsidered and, instead, a difference of 0.6 was sought; that is $\mu_1 = 6.1$. Using this new value for $\mu_1$ in (8.1) gives the result,

$$\text{Power} = p(Z < 1.3856) = 0.9171.$$

That is, the power has increased from a little over 81% when seeking to detect a true mean of 6.0 to a little under 92% for a true mean of 6.1 mmol/l. We can see that an increase should be expected from Figure 8.1, because the right-hand normal curve would be moved further to the right if the mean under the alternative hypothesis was increased. There would then be a larger area to the right of the 1.6449 cut-point under the right-hand curve.

It may be useful to consider the power for a whole range of values for $\mu_1$. For Example 8.1 this simply means substituting repeatedly for $\mu_1$ in the equation,

$$\text{Power} = p\left( Z < \frac{\mu_1 - 5.5}{1.4/\sqrt{50}} - 1.6449 \right)$$

which is derived from (8.1). The results may be displayed in a graph called a
**power curve**. A power curve for Example 8.1 is given in Figure 8.2. Notice that
power increases, up to its maximum of 100%, as the value for the alternative
hypothesis, $H_1$, moves away from the $H_0$ value (5.5 mmol/l). This makes
intuitive sense: bigger differences should be far more obvious, and thus more
likely to be detected. Notice that the significance level of the test (5% in
Example 8.1) is obtained as the 'power' when $\mu_1 = \mu_0 = 5.5$ in Figure 8.2.

The power and significance level, when expressed as probabilities, are
(respectively) analogous to the specificity and $(1 - \text{sensitivity})$ for diagnostic
tests (Section 2.10). Instead of the power, some analysts prefer to consider the
complementary probability, $(1 - \text{power})$. This is known as the probability of
**type II** error, the error of failing to reject $H_0$ when it is false. This is generally
given the symbol $\beta$. Contrast this with type I error, $\alpha$, the error of rejecting $H_0$
when it is true (defined in Section 2.5.1), which is just the significance level
expressed as a probability. In Example 8.1, $\alpha = 0.05$ and $\beta = 1 - 0.8107 = 0.1893$.

In (8.1) we assumed that a 5% test was to be used. This will not always be
true. In general, if we plan to carry out a test at the $100\alpha\%$ level then we simply
need to replace 1.6449 with $z_\alpha$ in (8.1), where

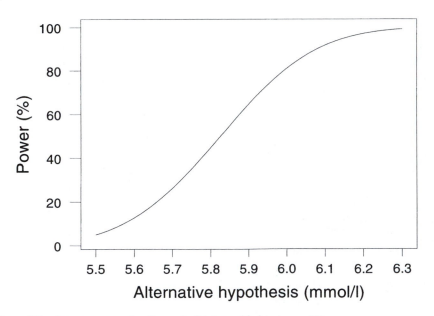

**Figure 8.2**    A power curve for Example 8.1 (one-sided test, $n = 50$).

$$p(Z < z_\alpha) = 1 - \alpha.$$

For some specific values of $\alpha$ we can find $z_\alpha$ directly from Table B.1 or indirectly from Table B.2. The equation for power, for a $100\alpha\%$ test then becomes,

$$\text{Power} = p\left(Z < \frac{\mu_1 - \mu_0}{\sigma/\sqrt{n}} - z_\alpha\right). \tag{8.2}$$

We are now in a position to specify what determines the power of a test. From (8.2), we can see that power will increase as

$$\frac{\mu_1 - \mu_0}{\sigma/\sqrt{n}} - z_\alpha$$

increases. In particular, therefore, power increases as
- $\sigma$ decreases,
- $\mu_1$ moves away from $\mu_0$,
- $z_\alpha$ decreases, i.e. $\alpha$ increases (becomes less extreme),
- $n$ increases.

Generally there is nothing that we can do to change $\sigma$ since it is an inherent property of the material at our disposal (in Example 8.1 we cannot change the person-to-person variability in cholesterol). We can alter the value of $\mu_1$ at which we evaluate power, but this will not change the essential characteristics of the test. We can alter $\alpha$, but an increased $\alpha$ means a greater chance of type I error. We can, however, increase $n$ so as to improve the test globally (albeit at extra cost). Intuitively this makes perfect sense: the larger the value of $n$ the more information we have available, and so the more precise our results (notwithstanding possible bias error). Hence the decision for the value of $n$ is crucial in any epidemiological study.

Figure 8.3 shows the power curves for the situation of Example 8.1, but where $n = 100$ and $n = 200$, superimposed on Figure 8.2 (where $n = 50$). When $n = 200$ the power reaches 100% (to three decimal places) for any alternative hypothesis value of 6.047 mmol/l or greater. This shows the pivotal role of sample size in hypothesis testing, tying in with the material of Section 3.5.5.

### 8.2.1    Choice of alternative hypothesis

Up to now we have only considered one-sided 'greater than' alternatives. In Example 8.1 we expect cholesterol to increase because of a move towards a Western diet. Suppose that a similar survey were planned in the United States, where we might expect cholesterol to have decreased over the last 10 years due to greater public awareness of the risks associated with elevated cholesterol

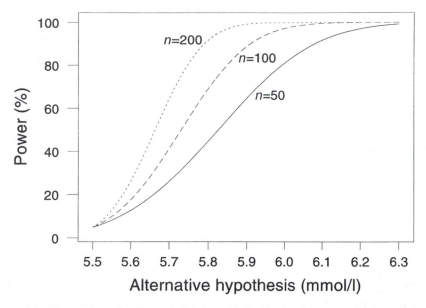

**Figure 8.3**    Power curves for Example 8.1 (one-sided test) when $n = 50$ (solid line), $n = 100$ (dashed line) and $n = 200$ (dotted line).

levels. In this situation we might decide that a one-sided test with a 'less than' alternative is appropriate. Due to the symmetry of the normal distribution, the only change to what went before is that we now reject $H_0$ whenever $T$ is less than $-1.6449$, rather than greater than $1.6449$, for a 5% test. The equation for power now becomes

$$\text{Power} = p\left( Z < \frac{\mu_0 - \mu_1}{\sigma/\sqrt{n}} - 1.6449 \right) \tag{8.3}$$

when $\mu = \mu_1$. This is exactly the same as (8.1) except that $\mu_0 - \mu_1$ has replaced $\mu_1 - \mu_0$. Consequently the new power curve is simply the mirror image of the old. For example, there must be an 81% chance of detecting a *reduction* of 0.5 mmol/l in mean serum total cholesterol according to the result of Example 8.1 (assuming $n = 50$, $\mu_0 = 5.5$ and $\sigma = 1.4$, as before) when a test against a 'less than' alternative is used.

When the alternative hypothesis is two-sided (as is most normal in practice) the hypotheses become

$$H_0 : \mu = \mu_0$$
$$H_1 : \mu = \mu_1,$$

where $\mu_1 \neq \mu_0$, such that $\mu_1$ can lie either side of $\mu_0$. The test statistic, $T$, is the same as for the one-sided case, but the critical value is now 1.96 because 5% of the standard normal distribution is either less than $-1.9600$ or greater than $1.9600$ (see Table B.2). Proceeding as in the one-sided situation, we can show that an approximate result for a 5% significance test is

$$\text{Power} = \begin{cases} p\left(Z < \dfrac{\mu_1 - \mu_0}{\sigma/\sqrt{n}} - 1.96\right) & \text{for } \mu_1 > \mu_0 \\[3mm] p\left(Z < \dfrac{\mu_0 - \mu_1}{\sigma/\sqrt{n}} - 1.96\right) & \text{for } \mu_1 < \mu_0. \end{cases} \tag{8.4}$$

*Example 8.2*   Consider a situation similar to Example 8.1, but where we wish to test for a cholesterol difference in either direction, so that a two-sided test is to be used. What is the chance of detecting a significant difference when the true mean is 6.0 mmol/l, and when the true mean is 5.0 mmol/l?
  When the true mean is 6.0, $\mu_1 > \mu_0$ and, by (8.4),

$$\text{Power} = p\left(Z < \frac{\mu_1 - \mu_0}{\sigma/\sqrt{n}} - 1.96\right)$$

$$= p\left(Z < \frac{6.0 - 5.5}{1.4/\sqrt{50}} - 1.96\right)$$

$$= p(Z < 0.5654) = 0.7141.$$

When the true mean is 5.0, $\mu_1 < \mu_0$ and, by (8.4), or by symmetry, the result is the same, 0.7141. Hence there is about a 71% chance of detecting an increase or decrease of 0.5 mmol/l using a two-sided test.

  The general formula for power with a $100\alpha\%$ two-sided test is

$$\text{Power} = \begin{cases} p\left(Z < \dfrac{\mu_1 - \mu_0}{\sigma/\sqrt{n}} - z_{\alpha/2}\right) & \text{for } \mu_1 > \mu_0 \\[3mm] p\left(Z < \dfrac{\mu_0 - \mu_1}{\sigma/\sqrt{n}} - z_{\alpha/2}\right) & \text{for } \mu_1 < \mu_0, \end{cases} \tag{8.5}$$

where $p(Z < z_{\alpha/2}) = 1 - (\alpha/2)$. For some values of $\alpha$, $z_{\alpha/2}$ can be read directly from Table B.2 where (using notation in this table) $P = 100\alpha\%$. With all else equal, the power is always lower using a two-sided test because $z_{\alpha/2}$ replaces $z_\alpha$ in the basic formulae: see also Examples 8.1 and 8.2. Just as before, power increases as $n$ increases, $\sigma$ decreases, $\alpha$ increases or $\mu_1$ moves away from $\mu_0$. The latter is illustrated by Figure 8.4, a power curve for the situation of Example 8.2. Notice the symmetry of such a two-sided power curve. As in Figures 8.2 and 8.3, the significance level of the test is given by the 'power' in the case where the null hypothesis ($\mu_1 = \mu_2$) is true.

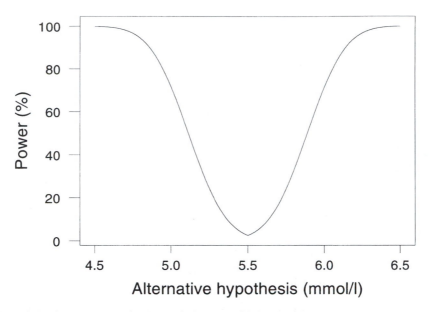

**Figure 8.4**    A power curve for Example 8.2 (two-sided test when $n = 50$).

## 8.3    Testing a mean value

The theory of Section 8.2 is directly applicable to the problem of determining
the size of a sample when the subsequent data will be used to test a hypothesis
about the mean of the parent population. This problem often arises in cross-
sectional epidemiological sample surveys. We will develop the methodology by
changing the terms of reference in our earlier example.

*Example 8.3*    Consider the problem of Example 8.1 again. The epidemiologist decides that
an increase in mean serum total cholesterol up to 6.0 mmol/l from the known previous value
of 5.5 mmol/l is so important that he would wish to be 90% sure of detecting it. Assuming
that a one-sided 5% test is to be carried out and that the standard deviation, $\sigma$, is known to
be 1.4 mmol/l, as before, what sample size should be used?

  Notice that the problem of Example 8.1 has now been turned around: power is known to
be 0.90, but $n$ is now to be determined. The problem is solved by turning (8.1) around in a
similar fashion. When the numerical values are substituted, (8.1) becomes

$$0.90 = p\left(Z < \frac{6.0 - 5.5}{1.4/\sqrt{n}} - 1.6449\right).$$

Now from Table B.2, $p(Z < 1.2816) = 0.90$ because the table shows us that 10% of the
standard normal is above 1.2816. Hence,

$$\frac{6.0 - 5.5}{1.4/\sqrt{n}} - 1.6449 = 1.2816;$$

when rearranged, this gives the formula,

$$n = \frac{(1.6449 + 1.2816)^2 1.4^2}{(6.0 - 5.5)^2} = 67.14.$$

In practice this will need to be rounded upwards, to be safe, so that 68 subjects should be sampled. In Example 8.1 we saw that the suggested sample size of 50 would give a test with 81% power, thus leaving a chance of almost 1 in 5 that the important difference would fail to be detected. This example shows that 18 further subjects are needed to increase power to the more acceptable level of 90%.

Consideration of Example 8.3 shows that the general formula for sample size for a one-sided test may be obtained from (8.2) as

$$n = \frac{(z_\alpha + z_\beta)^2 \sigma^2}{(\mu_1 - \mu_0)^2}, \tag{8.6}$$

where $100\alpha\%$ is the significance level for the test and $100(1 - \beta)\%$ is the predetermined power of detecting when the true mean is $\mu_1$ and, as usual,

$$p(Z < z_\alpha) = 1 - \alpha$$

and also, by analogy,

$$p(Z < z_\beta) = 1 - \beta.$$

*Example 8.4*   Consider Example 8.3 again, but suppose that the epidemiologist has decided to change his requirements. He now wishes to be 95% sure of detecting when the true mean is 6.1 mmol/l (with all else as before).
   This time, $1 - \beta = 0.95$, and from Table B.2, as seen already,

$$p(Z < 1.6449) = 0.95$$

so that $z_\beta = 1.6449$. If $\alpha = 0.05$ (as before), then $z_\alpha$ is also 1.6449. Substituting the numerical values into (8.6) gives

$$n = \frac{(1.6449 + 1.6449)^2 1.4^2}{(6.1 - 5.5)^2} = 58.92,$$

so that 59 subjects will be needed.

Next, we should consider other alternative hypotheses. As we have seen in Section 8.2.1, one-sided 'less than' alternatives simply involve swapping $\mu_1 - \mu_0$ for $\mu_0 - \mu_1$ in the formula for power, as with (8.1) and (8.3). Since $\mu_1 - \mu_0$ is squared in the formula for $n$, this formula, (8.6), is valid for both types of one-sided alternatives. Two-sided alternatives are, by a similar argument that led to (8.4), dealt with simply by substituting $\alpha/2$ for $\alpha$ in (8.6); that is,

$$n = \frac{(z_{\alpha/2} + z_\beta)^2 \sigma^2}{(\mu_1 - \mu_0)^2} \qquad (8.7)$$

for a two-sided test with significance level $100\alpha\%$.

Inspection of (8.6) and (8.7) shows that the sample size requirement increases as

- $\sigma$ increases,
- $\mu_1$ moves towards $\mu_0$,
- $z_\alpha$ or $z_{\alpha/2}$ increases, i.e. $\alpha$ decreases,
- $z_\beta$ increases, i.e. $\beta$ decreases, i.e. power increases.

As discussed in Section 8.2, the standard deviation, $\sigma$, is a property of the material being sampled and is not ours to vary. Intuitively it makes sense that a larger sample would be needed when the person-to-person variability is greater, since then we would expect to have to sample more widely to obtain an accurate overall picture. Sample size requirement should increase as $\mu_1$ moves towards $\mu_0$ because then we are trying to differentiate between hypotheses which are more similar, which inevitably requires more information. Since $\alpha$ and $\beta$ are each probabilities of error it seems reasonable that more information is required to reduce either of them.

### 8.3.1    Common choices for power and significance level

As we saw in Section 2.5.1, the significance level for a test is generally chosen to be either 5%, 1% or 0.1% (that is, $\alpha = 0.05$, 0.01 or 0.001). Power (as a percentage) is often chosen to be either 90% or 95% (that is, $\beta = 0.01$ or 0.05). For easy reference, Table 8.1 shows the values of $z_\alpha$ (or $z_{\alpha/2}$) and $z_\beta$ which correspond to these common choices (derived from Table B.2).

Other values for the significance level and percentage power are perfectly acceptable, and may well be more appropriate in certain circumstances (Table B.1 or a computer package would then need to be used). Usually the power and

**Table 8.1**    Values of $z_\alpha$ or $z_{\alpha/2}$ for common values of the significance level and of $z_\beta$ (in **bold**) for common values of power

| Significance level | | | | | | Power | |
|---|---|---|---|---|---|---|---|
| One-sided | | | Two-sided | | | | |
| 5% | 1% | 0.1% | 5% | 1% | 0.1% | 90% | 95% |
| 1.6449 | 2.3263 | 3.0902 | 1.9600 | 2.5758 | 3.2905 | **1.2816** | **1.6449** |

alternative hypothesis are chosen jointly, since $1 - \beta$ is the probability of detecting when the true mean really is $\mu_1$.

### 8.3.2  Using a table of sample sizes

Table 8.1 merely provides values of $z_\alpha$ (or $z_{\alpha/2}$) and $z_\beta$ for substitution into (8.6) or (8.7). Table B.7 in Appendix B goes further and gives the values of $n$. However, to make Table B.7 of manageable size it is necessary to introduce a new parameter, $S$, which is the standardized difference between the two hypothesized values for the mean, using the standard deviation as the standardizing factor. That is,

$$S = \frac{\mu_1 - \mu_0}{\sigma}. \tag{8.8}$$

When $\mu_1$ is less than $\mu_0$ (the 'less than' alternative hypothesis) the negative sign for $S$ should be ignored.

The values in Table B.7 have been calculated using six decimal places for the standard normal percentage points and have been rounded up to avoid trailing decimals. Consequently the answers given might disagree slightly with values calculated from (8.6) or (8.7) using Table 8.1, due to rounding error. Table B.7 gives values for $n$ appropriate to one-sided tests directly. For two-sided tests we should use the column of the table corresponding to half the significance level required (equivalent to using $z_{\alpha/2}$ rather than $z_\alpha$). Similar comments hold for Tables B.8–B.10.

*Example 8.5*  An intervention study is planned to compare drug treatment with alternative medicine in the treatment of a specific medical condition. The drug is to be stockpiled in health centres ready for distribution. The drug is supplied in sachets which are supposed to contain exactly 2 mg of the drug. It is thought that supplies may have been over-full, which could compromise the results of the study (although posing no danger to the subjects treated). Consequently, a number of sachets will be sampled, and their mean content tested against the null hypothesis that the mean really is 2.0. A 1% significance test will be used, since the health centre wishes to be very sure that the sachets are overweight before making a complaint to the supplier. The standard deviation of sachet contents is known, from past experience, to be 0.2 mg. The health centre decides that it is important to be 95% sure of detecting when the true mean content is 2.1 mg. How many sachets should be sampled?

Since the concern here is about over-filling, a one-sided test will be used. Now $\mu_0 = 2.0$, $\mu_1 = 2.1$, $\sigma = 0.2$ and, from Table 8.1, $z_\alpha = 2.3263$ and $z_\beta = 1.6449$. Using (8.6), we obtain

$$n = \frac{(2.3263 + 1.6449)^2 0.2^2}{(2.1 - 2.0)^2} = 63.08,$$

which would be rounded up to 64. Alternatively we could use Table B.7. Then we only need to calculate $S$ from (8.8),

$$S = \frac{2.1 - 2.0}{0.2} = 0.5$$

When $S = 0.5$, the significance level is 1% and power 95%, Table B.7 gives the answer 64, just as before.

*Example 8.6*    Take the situation of Example 8.5 again, but now suppose that there is also concern in case the sachets are underweight. This, too, is a potential source of bias in the study. A two-sided test would now be appropriate.

Assuming all else is unchanged, Table 8.1 gives $z_{\alpha/2} = 2.5758$ and $z_\beta = 1.6449$ and thus, by (8.7),

$$n = \frac{(2.5758 + 1.6449)^2 0.2^2}{(2.1 - 2.0)^2} = 71.26,$$

which rounds up to 72. Alternatively, to use Table B.7 we must look up the significance level of 0.5%, since our test is two-sided. As before, $S = 0.5$ and power is 95%. Table B.7 also gives the answer 72. Notice that a larger sample size is needed for this two-sided test compared to the one-sided equivalent in Example 8.5. This reflects the power differential between these two types of test, commented upon earlier.

Table B.7 cannot possibly include every possible value of $S$ (or significance level, or power). Thus the value of $S$ in Example 8.3 is $6.0 - 5.5/\,1.4 = 0.3571$, which does not appear in Table B.7. In these situations we can get a rough idea of sample size by taking the nearest figure for $S$. In the example, the nearest tabulated figure is 0.35 which has $n = 70$ (for one-sided 5% significance and 90% power). This is only slightly above the true value of 68 for $S = 0.3571$, given in Example 8.3. However, this process can lead to considerable error when $S$ is small. Since we have the complete formula here, (8.6), we should use this in preference.

### 8.3.3    The minimum detectable difference

Sometimes we have budgetary or other restrictions which cause the maximum possible value for $n$ to be determined by other than statistical considerations. In this case we may use (8.2) or (8.5) to determine the power with which we can expect to detect when the alternative hypothesis is true.

Alternatively, we might like to consider what is the difference from the null hypothesis, $d = \mu_1 - \mu_0$, which we can just expect to be able to detect with specified power. This is called the **minimum detectable difference**: we will be able to detect this, or any larger difference, with the given $n$ and specified power. By inverting (8.6) we get the result that

$$d = \frac{\sigma}{\sqrt{n}}(z_\alpha + z_\beta) \tag{8.9}$$

for a one-sided test. Replace $z_\alpha$ by $z_{\alpha/2}$ for a two-sided test, as usual.

*Example 8.7*  Suppose that, in the problem of Example 8.3, only one nurse is presently available to take the necessary blood samples. Due to time constraints, it is estimated that she will only be able to take blood from 50 patients. How small an increase in cholesterol from the known value of 5.5 mmol/l of 10 years ago can we expect to detect now, using a 5% test with 90% power?

Substituting the numerical values from Example 8.3 into (8.9) gives

$$d = \frac{1.4}{\sqrt{50}}(1.6449 + 1.2816) = 0.579\,\text{mmol/l}.$$

So we expect to be 90% certain of detecting when the true mean cholesterol is 5.5 + 0.579 = 6.079 mmol/l. The investigators now have to decide whether this is good enough (the minimum detectable difference of 0.579 is bigger than the difference of 0.5 which is considered medically important – see Example 8.3), or whether a second nurse should be employed so as to enable $n$ to be increased.

### 8.3.4  The assumption of known standard deviation

Notice that we have assumed throughout that the standard deviation, $\sigma$, is known. In practice, this is rarely true and we will, instead, have to rely upon an estimate, usually obtained from past experience. An alternative approach based on Student's $t$ distribution, which does not assume that $\sigma$ is known, is suggested by Snedecor and Cochran (1980). Theoretically this is preferable, but for good estimates of $\sigma$ and moderately large $n$ the results should be similar to those obtained from the equations given here.

## 8.4  Testing a difference between means

So far we have been concerned solely with one-sample situations where we wish to test a hypothesis about a mean. This is the simplest situation from which to introduce the methodology. Most often epidemiological investigations are comparative, and in this section we will extend our discussion to the problem of testing for the equality of two means. This situation is most likely to arise in a cross-sectional or intervention study. A similar problem could also arise in a cohort study with a fixed cohort, but in these studies the usual end-point of interest is a disease incidence, which is a proportion rather than a mean (Section 8.6).

Our new problem is a two-sample one; that is, we are to collect two samples and we wish to know how many subjects we should select altogether. There is, now, an extra factor to consider: how to distribute the sample between the two groups. Often equal sample sizes are used, but in some situations it may be sensible to allocate more to one or other of the groups. Thus in an experimental study of a new procedure against an existing standard, it might be worthwhile giving the new treatment to more than half of the patients simply in order to obtain more information about its performance (presumably the performance of the standard procedure is already well known). In a cross-sectional study we might prefer to sample proportionately to the population distribution of the grouping factor (if known). If we take a single random sample (rather than a separate one from each of the two groups) we certainly expect the sample distribution (say, by sex) to be as in the parent population, and thus not necessarily $1:1$ (Example 8.14). Economic considerations may also have an effect. For instance, one of the two treatments in an intervention study may be extremely expensive and this might cause us to prefer to allocate fewer to this treatment. In a case–control study the number of cases might be necessarily fixed, but the number of controls practically unlimited (Section 6.4.5).

We will assume, for simplicity, that the standard deviations are the same in each group. As before, we will assume that this common standard deviation, $\sigma$, is known. Let the sample sizes (to be determined) in the two groups be $n_1$ and $n_2$. Define the allocation ratio $r$ to be $n_1/n_2$ and let the overall sample size be $n$. That is,

$$n = n_1 + n_2 = (r+1)n_2.$$

Consider a test of the null hypothesis that the group means are equal against the alternative that their difference is $\delta$. Using the notation $\mu_1$ and $\mu_2$ for the two population means, the hypotheses are thus

$$H_0 : \mu_1 = \mu_2$$
$$H_1 : \mu_1 - \mu_2 = \delta,$$

where $\delta < 0$ or $\delta > 0$ for the two possible one-sided tests and $\delta \neq 0$ for a two-sided test. Sample size is to be determined so as to achieve a power of $1 - \beta$ of detecting when the true difference is $\delta$. The theory outlined in Sections 8.2 and 8.3 may be extended to show that

$$n = \frac{(r+1)^2(z_\alpha + z_\beta)^2\sigma^2}{\delta^2 r} \tag{8.10}$$

for a one-sided test (of either type). For a two-sided test the same formula is used except that $z_\alpha$ is replaced by $z_{\alpha/2}$.

*Example 8.8*  In Example 8.1, and its extensions, we assumed that the mean value of serum total cholesterol 10 years ago was known, and only the present-day value needed to be tested. Consider, now, the problem of deciding how many to sample in both of two surveys, separated in time by 10 years. Suppose that we wish to test, at the 5% level of significance, the hypothesis that the cholesterol means are equal in the two years against the one-sided alternative that the mean is higher in the second of the two years. Suppose that equal-sized samples are to be taken in each year, but that these will not necessarily be the same individuals – that is, the two samples are drawn independently (see Example 8.11 for the paired situation). Our test is to have a power of 95% for detecting when the later mean exceeds the earlier mean by 0.5 mmol/l. The standard deviation is assumed to be 1.4 mmol/l each time.

Here $\sigma = 1.4$, $\delta = 0.5$, $r = 1$ (since $n_1 = n_2$) and $z_\alpha = z_\beta = 1.6449$ (from Table 8.1). Hence, by (8.10),

$$n = \frac{(1+1)^2(1.6449 + 1.6449)^2 1.4^2}{0.5^2 \times 1} = 339.40.$$

To satisfy the set conditions this would need to be rounded up to the next highest *even* number, here 340. Hence we should sample 170 individuals in the first year and a further 170 in the second year.

### 8.4.1   Using a table of sample sizes

Notice that (8.10) is closely related to (8.6). If we consider that both $\delta$ and $\mu_1 - \mu_0$ are a difference between two means, then the relationship between the two equations is that (8.6) must be multiplied by $(r+1)^2/r$ to arrive at (8.10). Hence Table B.7 may be used in the two-sample situation. All that is necessary is to multiply each entry in the table by $(r+1)^2/r$. When $r = 1$ ( i.e. $1:1$ allocation) this multiplier becomes 4. Hence, for Example 8.8 we get the standardized difference, $S = 0.5/1.4 = 0.3571$. As we have seen already, the nearest tabulated value to this is 0.35. With 5% significance and 95% power, Table B.7 gives $n = 89$. Multiplying by 4 gives a value of 356 when $S = 0.35$, which is roughly comparable with the true answer of 340 when $S = 0.3571$.

*Example 8.9*   Undernourished women taking oral contraceptives sometimes experience anaemia due to increased iron absorption. A study is planned to compare regular intake of iron tablets against a course of placebos. Oral contraceptive users are to be randomly allocated to the two treatment groups and the mean serum iron concentrations compared after 6 months. It is thought, from earlier studies, that the standard deviation of the increase in serum iron concentration is $4\,\mu g\%$ over a 6-month period. The average increase in serum iron concentration without iron supplements is also $4\,\mu g\%$. The investigators wish to be 90% sure of detecting when the iron supplement doubles the serum iron concentration using a two-sided 5% significance test. It has been decided that four times as many women should be allocated to the iron tablet treatment since there is little chance of any side-effects, and this treatment is very cheap.

Here the difference to be detected is $8 - 4 = 4\,\mu g\%$ and, since $\sigma = 4\,\mu g\%$, we have that $S = 1$. Table B.7 gives a starting value for $n$ of 11, which needs to be multiplied by $(r+1)^2/r = (4+1)^2/4 = 6.25$. Hence the overall sample size required is 68.75, which needs to be rounded up to the nearest multiple of 5, that is, 70. We should allocate $70/5 = 14$

women to the placebo treatment and four times as many (56) to the iron tablet treatment. The reader might like to check that (8.10) gives exactly the same answer after rounding up.

Due to rounding error, Table B.7 can give different results to (8.10), but the difference is only likely to be important in extreme cases (very large or very small values for $r$).

Figure 8.5 shows how the sample size requirement decreases as the standardized difference, $S$ increases from 0.5 to 2.0 for Example 8.9. This emphasizes what should already be apparent from the use of $S$ in Table B.7: the sample size depends on the size of the difference to be tested *relative to* the standard deviation of the material in question. Figure 8.5 is a typical sample size curve, and shows that we should be prepared for very large samples if we wish to detect, with a high probability, a difference between means which is less than the standard deviation ($S < 1$). Note that Figure 8.5 gives results straight from (8.10) – that is, without rounding up to the nearest multiple of five.

### 8.4.2 Power and minimum detectable difference

It is a simple matter to turn (8.10) around to obtain expressions for the power given the sample size (and the difference to be detected) and for the minimum detectable difference given the sample size (and the power). These are, respectively,

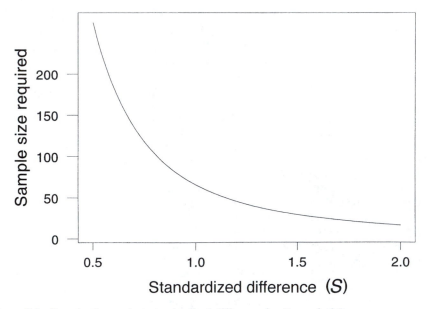

**Figure 8.5**  Sample size against standardized difference for Example 8.9.

$$z_\beta = \frac{\delta\sqrt{nr}}{(r+1)\sigma} - z_\alpha \qquad (8.11)$$

and

$$\delta = \frac{(r+1)(z_\alpha + z_\beta)\sigma}{\sqrt{nr}} \qquad (8.12)$$

In fact, (8.11) gives an expression for $z_\beta$ which would need to be converted into an expression for power $(1 - \beta)$ using the usual equation,

$$p(Z < z_\beta) = 1 - \beta.$$

As always, replace $z_\alpha$ by $z_{\alpha/2}$ in (8.11) and (8.12) for a two-sided test.

*Example 8.10*    Consider Example 8.8 again. Suppose that, because of human resources constraints, only 50 people may be sampled for blood in the first year, whilst it is anticipated that it will be possible to sample 100 in the second year. What is the minimum increase in cholesterol that can be detected with 95% power when a 5% significance test is used?

Here $n = n_1 + n_2 = 150$ and $r = n_1/n_2 = 2$. From Example 8.8, $\sigma = 1.4$ and $z_\alpha = z_\beta = 1.6449$. Hence, from (8.12),

$$\delta = \frac{(2+1)(1.6449 + 1.6449)1.4}{\sqrt{150 \times 2}} = 0.80 \text{ mmol/l}.$$

So, with the human resources available, the investigators can expect to find, with 95% power, an average increase of as little as 0.80 mmol/l of cholesterol.

Notice that Example 8.10 takes sample 2 to be the sample in the earlier year. If, instead, sample 1 were taken as the earlier sample we would have $r = n_1/n_2 = 0.5$. When substituted into (8.12) this gives exactly the same answer as before, but now we would interpret $\delta$ as a decrease over time. Strictly speaking, (8.12) gives a result for $\pm\delta$, but we can always choose to take sample 1 to be that with the highest mean and so force $\delta$ to be positive.

### 8.4.3    Optimum allocation of the sample

Given a fixed overall sample size, $n$, the optimum allocation of this between the two groups is an equal allocation. That is $n_1 = n_2$ or $r = 1$. This can be proven from (8.11) using differential calculus. Hence, if there are no strong reasons to do otherwise, we should allocate the sample equally between the two groups.

### 8.4.4    Paired data

So far we have assumed that the two samples are independent. If they are, instead, paired (for example, measurements before and after some medical intervention) then (8.10) is inappropriate. We should then apply (8.6) or (8.7) to the differenced data, where $\delta$ takes the place of $\mu_1 - \mu_0$. We now have to be careful that the variance, $\sigma^2$, is correct for the differenced data.

*Example 8.11*    Take the situation of Example 8.8 again, but this time suppose that the *same* individuals are to be sampled in the two years. The data are now paired and we should apply (8.6). Suppose that the standard deviation of the *increase* in cholesterol is known to be 1.0 mmol/l. Then taking all else as in Example 8.8, (8.6) gives

$$n = \frac{(1.6449 + 1.6449)^2 1.0^2}{0.5^2} = 43.29,$$

which is rounded up to 44. Here $S = 0.5/1.0 = 0.5$ and the answer may be obtained more directly from Table B.7.

Notice that the sample size requirement of 44 above is well below that of 169 (per sample) in the unpaired case (Example 8.8). Provided that the correlation between the 'before' and 'after' measurements is high and positive (as is likely in practice) pairing will give a considerable saving in sample numbers. There may, however, be costs elsewhere. In Example 8.11 it may be difficult to keep track of the 44 individuals over the 10-year period. Furthermore, there may also be bias error since the individuals concerned may be more health-conscious simply by virtue of being studied, which may lead them to (say) consume dietary cholesterol at a lower rate than other members of the population.

In the paired situation, (8.2) or (8.9) may be used to find power or minimum detectable difference, correcting for two-sided tests (when necessary), as usual.

## 8.5  Testing a proportion

All of our discussion about sample size requirements so far has been concerned with mean values. Similar formulae may be derived to deal with hypothesis tests for proportions by using a normal approximation to the binomial distribution which naturally arises, assuming independent outcomes. In this section we will consider one-sample problems.

Here the problem is to test the hypotheses

$$H_0 : \pi = \pi_0$$
$$H_1 : \pi = \pi_1 = \pi_0 + d,$$

where $\pi$ is the true proportion, $\pi_0$ is some specified value for this proportion which we wish to test for, and $\pi_1$ (which differs from $\pi_0$ by an amount $d$) is the alternative value which we would like to identify correctly with a probability (power) of $1 - \beta$. For one-sided tests $\pi_1 < \pi_0$ or $\pi_1 > \pi_0$ ($d < 0$ or $d > 0$) and for two-sided tests $\pi_1 \neq \pi_0$ ($d \neq 0$). Applying the power calculation method outlined in Sections 8.2 and 8.3 gives the result (assuming a $100\alpha\%$ significance test is used)

$$n = \frac{1}{d^2}\left[z_\alpha\sqrt{\pi_0(1-\pi_0)} + z_\beta\sqrt{\pi_1(1-\pi_1)}\right]^2 \tag{8.13}$$

for a one-sided test. Replace $z_\alpha$ by $z_{\alpha/2}$ for a two-sided test.

*Example 8.12*    Suppose that, over the last few years, a government target for health has been to reduce the prevalence of male smoking to, at most, 30%. A sample survey is planned to test, at the 5% level, the hypothesis that the proportion of male smokers in the population is 0.3 against the one-sided alternative that it is greater. The test should be able to find a prevalence of 32%, when it is true, with 90% power.

In this problem $\pi_0 = 0.30$ and $\pi_1 = 0.32$, and hence $d = 0.02$. For 5% significance (in a one-sided test) and 90% power, $z_\alpha = 1.6449$ and $z_\beta = 1.2816$ from Table 8.1. Hence, by (8.13),

$$n = \frac{1}{0.02^2}\left[1.6449\sqrt{0.3\times0.7} + 1.2816\sqrt{0.32\times0.68}\right]^2 = 4567.2$$

Thus, with rounding, 4568 should be sampled.

Notice that the sample size required in the last example is in the thousands. This is not uncommon in problems concerned with proportions.

### 8.5.1  Using a table of sample sizes

Example 8.12 could also be solved using Table B.8(a). In this table the answer 4567 appears in the fourth column of the second row. The difference (of one) is due to rounding error. Notice, from this table, that the values for $n$ increase as $\pi_0$ (the null hypothesis value) approaches 0.5 from either side. Also, as in Table B.7, $n$ increases as the difference to be detected, $d$, decreases.

### 8.5.2  Power and minimum detectable difference

Formulae for $z_\beta$ (which gives the power) and the least detectable difference, $d$, are easily obtained from (8.13) as

$$z_\beta = \frac{d\sqrt{n} - z_\alpha\sqrt{\pi_0(1-\pi_0)}}{\sqrt{\pi_1(1-\pi_1)}}$$

and

$$d = \frac{1}{\sqrt{n}}\left[z_\alpha\sqrt{\pi_0(1-\pi_0)} + z_\beta\sqrt{\pi_1(1-\pi_1)}\right].$$

## 8.6    Testing a relative risk

Consider, now, a two-sample problem in which the outcomes to be compared are proportions. The hypotheses to be tested may be written as

$$H_0 : \pi_1 = \pi_2$$
$$H_1 : \pi_1 - \pi_2 = \delta,$$

for some specified $\delta$, where $\pi_1$ and $\pi_2$ are the two population proportions. As in Section 3.1, it is usually more convenient to consider the relative risk, the ratio of $\pi_1$ to $\pi_2$, rather than the difference $\pi_1 - \pi_2$. Hence we will consider, instead,

$$H_0 : \pi_1 = \pi_2$$
$$H_1 : \pi_1/\pi_2 = \lambda.$$

Here group 2 will be the reference group since it is the denominator for the relative risk. For one-sided tests $\lambda < 1$ or $\lambda > 1$ and for two-sided tests $\lambda \neq 1$. Notice that, should we prefer to formulate the alternative hypothesis as a difference rather than a ratio (Section 3.3.2), we can easily calculate $\lambda$ as $\lambda = 1 + (\delta/\pi_2)$ and then proceed as below.

Problems of comparing proportions may arise in cohort studies, cross-sectional surveys and intervention studies. The methods discussed in this section are applicable in all such studies. Although a case–control study would also normally seek to compare two proportions, the equations given in this section would not be appropriate because of the special sampling design used (Section 8.7).

Using the power calculation method and adopting the notation of previous sections (including $r = n_1/n_2$) the total sample size requirement $(n_1 + n_2)$ for a one-sided test turns out to be

$$n = \frac{r+1}{r(\lambda-1)^2\pi^2}\left[z_\alpha\sqrt{(r+1)p_c(1-p_c)} + z_\beta\sqrt{\lambda\pi(1-\lambda\pi) + r\pi(1-\pi)}\right]^2,$$

$$(8.14)$$

where $\pi = \pi_2$ is the proportion in the reference group and $p_c$ is the common proportion over the two groups, which is estimated, from (2.7), as

$$p_c = \frac{\pi(r\lambda+1)}{r+1}. \qquad (8.15)$$

When $r = 1$ (equal-sized groups), (8.15) reduces to

$$p_c = \frac{\pi(\lambda+1)}{2} = \frac{\pi_1 + \pi_2}{2},$$

the arithmetic mean of the two separate proportions (under $H_1$). Replace $z_\alpha$ by $z_{\alpha/2}$ for a two-sided test.

Notice that $n$ depends upon $\pi = \pi_2$, the true proportion in the reference group. In general this will not be known, but will have to be estimated from past experience, or otherwise.

*Example 8.13*  A cohort study of smoking and coronary heart disease (CHD) amongst middle-aged men is planned. A sample of men will be selected at random from the population and asked to complete a questionnaire. Subsequently they will be monitored to record ill health and death. The investigators wish to submit their results for publication after 5 years, at which point they would like to be 90% sure of being able to detect when the relative risk for smoking is 1.4, using a one-sided 5% significance test. Previous evidence (Doll and Peto, 1976) suggests that non-smokers have an annual death rate from CHD of about 413 per 100 000 per year. Assuming that equal numbers of smokers and non-smokers are to be sampled, how many should be sampled overall?

Over a 5-year period the estimated chance of death is $5 \times 413/100000 = 0.02065$. This gives the value for $\pi$. The relative risk to be detected, $\lambda$, is 1.4, $z_\alpha = 1.6449$ and $z_\beta = 1.2816$ (from Table 8.1). We are assuming that the sample ratio, $r$, is unity. Then we must first use (8.15) to obtain

$$p_c = \frac{0.02065 \times 2.4}{2} = 0.02478.$$

Notice here that $\lambda\pi = 0.02891$ and that $p_c$ is the arithmetic mean of $\pi$ and $\lambda\pi$ as it should be, since $r = 1$. Then, by (8.14),

$$n = \frac{2}{0.4^2 \times 0.02065^2} \left[ 1.6449\sqrt{2 \times 0.02478 \times 0.97522} \right.$$
$$\left. + 1.2816\sqrt{0.02891 \times 0.97109 + 0.02065 \times 0.97935} \right]^2 = 12130.16.$$

So, rounding up to the next highest even number, 12 132 men should be sampled (6066 smokers and 6066 non-smokers).

In practice, the procedure assumed in the last example would be difficult to follow precisely because we have no way of knowing, in advance, whether a prospective sample recruit is a smoker or non-smoker. If, for example, one-third of all men in the population smoke, then we would expect to have to sample $6066 \times 3 = 18198$ men before arriving at a sample containing 6066 smokers. The excess number of non-smokers could simply be rejected, although it may be more sensible to retain them in the sample, once questioned. A better approach is to allow for the expected imbalance through the parameter $r$, as the next example shows.

*Example 8.14*  If the proportion of men smoking is one-third, then in a random sample we would expect to find $n_2 = n/3$. Hence $n_1 = 2n/3$ and thus $r = n_1/n_2 = 0.5$. Using this new value for $r$ in (8.14) and (8.15) for Example 8.13 gives

$$p_c = \frac{0.02065(0.5 \times 1.4 + 1)}{1.5} = 0.02340$$

$$n = \frac{1.5}{0.5 \times 0.4^2 \times 0.02065^2} \left[ 1.6449\sqrt{1.5 \times 0.02340 \times 0.97660} \right.$$

$$\left. + 1.2816\sqrt{0.02891 \times 0.97109 + 0.5 \times 0.02065 \times 0.97935} \right]^2 = 13543.30.$$

Rounding up gives a total sample size requirement of 13 544. We would expect that, after sampling, about a third of these would be smokers. Notice that 13 544 is not exactly divisible by 3, but any further rounding up would not be justifiable since we cannot guarantee the exact proportion of smokers.

### 8.6.1    Using a table of sample sizes

Table B.9 gives values for the overall sample size when equal numbers are allocated to each group ($r = 1$). Although unequal allocation is not uncommon, equal allocation is by far the most usual, especially in intervention studies.

*Example 8.15*    At a smoking cessation clinic the failure rate for the standard method of 'therapy' used is 20%. Trials of a new method of helping smokers to quit are to be carried out, and the investigator concerned has specified that he wishes to detect when the new method has 40% of the chance of failure that the standard method has with a probability of 0.90. If a two-sided 5% significance test is used with equal allocation to 'standard' and 'new' methods, what sample size is required?

Here $\pi = 0.20$ and $\lambda = 0.40$. This relative risk is to be detected with 90% power using a two-sided 5% test, so that Table B.9(c) is appropriate (treating this as a one-sided $2\frac{1}{2}$% test). The sample size required is 342 (171 in each treatment group). Approximately the same result comes from (8.14).

Figure 8.6 shows how $n$ varies when the relative risk that is to be detected with 90% power varies between 0.6 and 0.9 in the context of the above example. The shape of the curve is similar to that of Figure 8.5, but with two differences. First, the curve here looks like the mirror-image of the previous one because now we are considering alternative hypotheses which specify reductions, rather than increases, compared to the null. Second, the values for $n$ are considerably bigger. As with single-sample tests for proportions, large numbers are required to detect small differences between proportions (that is, relative risks close to unity). This is also obvious from study of Table B.9. As in Figure 8.5, the values for $n$ in Figure 8.6 have not been rounded up to produce integer answers.

In the literature there are several alternatives to (8.14). These include the different approximations given by Pocock (1983) and Altman (1991). Other variations include Fleiss (1981), who uses a continuity correction and Casagrande *et al.* (1978), who use Fisher's exact test. See Woodward (1992) for a review.

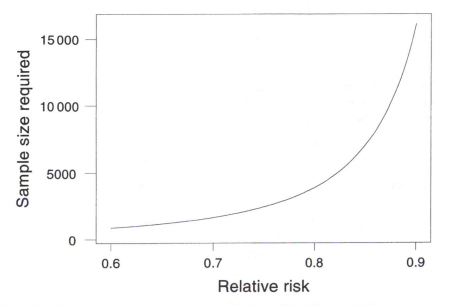

**Figure 8.6**  Sample size against relative risk to be detected for Example 8.15.

### 8.6.2  Power and minimum detectable relative risk

A formula for $z_\beta$ (and hence power) is easily derived from (8.14) to be

$$z_\beta = \frac{\pi(\lambda - 1)\sqrt{nr} - z_\alpha(r + 1)\sqrt{p_c(1 - p_c)}}{\sqrt{(r + 1)(\lambda\pi(1 - \lambda\pi) + r\pi(1 - \pi))}}$$

if $\lambda > 1$. If $\lambda < 1$ simply replace $\lambda - 1$ by $1 - \lambda$ in the leading term in the numerator. We cannot, however, invert (8.14) to provide a formula for the minimum detectable relative risk, $\lambda$. Instead we can use an approximate method. This derives from the approximation to (8.14) suggested by Pocock (1983). The approximate value for $\lambda$ turns out to be

$$\lambda \simeq \frac{1}{2a}\left[b \pm \sqrt{b^2 - 4ac}\right], \tag{8.16}$$

where

$$a = Y + \pi Z,$$
$$b = 2Y + Z,$$
$$c = Y - r(1 - \pi)Z,$$

in which

$$Y = rn\pi^2,$$

$$Z = (r+1)\pi(z_\alpha + z_\beta)^2.$$

This formula should be reasonably accurate when $r = 1$, but may be in considerable error when $r$ is very high or very low. A more accurate, but more complex, method is suggested in Woodward (1992).

*Example 8.16*    Consider the cohort study of Example 8.13. Suppose that the investigators decide that they can afford a sample size of 12 132 but no more. What is the minimum relative risk that they can expect to be able to detect with 90% power (all else as before)?

We know from Example 8.13 that the answer should be about 1.4. Using (8.16), we indeed get $\lambda = 1.4$. This arises from

$$Y = 12132 \times 0.02065^2 = 5.1734,$$

$$Z = 2 \times 0.02065(1.6449 + 1.2816)^2 = 0.35371,$$

$$a = 5.1734 + 0.02065 \times 0.35371 = 5.1807,$$

$$b = 2 \times 5.1734 + 0.35371 = 10.7005,$$

$$c = 5.1734 - (1 - 0.02065)0.35371 = 4.8270$$

$$\lambda \simeq \frac{10.7005 \pm \sqrt{10.7005^2 - 4 \times 5.1807 \times 4.8270}}{2 \times 5.1734}$$

$$= 1.40 \text{ (taking the positive root)}.$$

Note that the negative root gives a value below unity. If we were dealing with a protective factor this would be the result of interest.

## 8.7    Case–control studies

A case–control study typically aims to compare the disease incidence or prevalence between two groups: those exposed to some risk factor of interest and those not exposed. Hence the aim will be to test the hypotheses

$$H_0 : \pi_1 = \pi_2$$

$$H_1 : \pi_1/\pi_2 = \lambda,$$

where the probabilities $\pi_1$ and $\pi_2$ are explicitly

$$\pi_1 = p(\text{Disease}|\text{Exposed})$$

$$\pi_2 = p(\text{Disease}|\text{Not exposed}),$$

and $\lambda$ is, as usual, the relative risk; as in Section 8.2, the vertical bar is read as 'given', so that $\pi_1$ is 'the probability of disease given exposure'.

This is exactly the same formulation of hypotheses as in Section 8.6. There is, however, one crucial difference: here we cannot test $H_0$ directly because we have no means of estimating either $\pi_1$ or $\pi_2$. This is due to the design of the case–control study, which does not allow for such estimation (Section 6.2.1). Instead, what we can do is to test the hypotheses

$$H_0^* : \pi_1^* = \pi_2^*$$
$$H_1^* : \pi_1^*/\pi_2^* = \lambda^*,$$

where

$$\pi_1^* = p(\text{Exposed}|\text{Disease}) = p(\text{Exposed}|\text{Case}),$$
$$\pi_2^* = p(\text{Exposed}|\text{No Disease}) = p(\text{Exposed}|\text{Control})$$

(assuming no bias) since the case–control study samples from the populations of those diseased and those not diseased. The outcome of the analysis is now exposure rather than disease.

We are not interested in the items involved in $H_0^*$ and $H_1^*$, but luckily $\pi_1^*$ and $\pi_2^*$ turn out to have simple expressions in terms of $\lambda$ (which is what we *are* interested in) and $P = p(\text{Exposure})$, the prevalence of the risk factor. Using a theorem of probability known as Bayes' theorem (see Clarke and Cooke, 1992), we obtain

$$\pi_1^* = \frac{\lambda P}{1 + (\lambda - 1)P}$$

and

$$\pi_2^* \simeq P. \tag{8.17}$$

Thus we have

$$\lambda^* \simeq \frac{\lambda}{1 + (\lambda - 1)P} \tag{8.18}$$

The approximation (8.17) will be good if the disease is rare amongst those exposed to the risk factor (and amongst the population in general). It is an exact result if the null hypothesis ($H_0 : \pi_1 = \pi_2$) is true. See Schlesselman (1974) or Woodward (1992) for details.

Using (8.17) and (8.18) in (8.14) and (8.15), for the test of $H_0^*$ against $H_1^*$, gives

$$n = \frac{(r+1)(1 + (\lambda-1)P)^2}{rP^2(P-1)^2(\lambda-1)^2} \left[ z_\alpha \sqrt{(r+1)p_c^*(1-p_c^*)} \right.$$
$$\left. + z_\beta \sqrt{\frac{\lambda P(1-P)}{[1+(\lambda-1)P]^2} + rP(1-P)} \right]^2, \tag{8.19}$$

where

$$p_c^* = \frac{P}{r+1}\left(\frac{r\lambda}{1+(\lambda-1)P}+1\right) \tag{8.20}$$

for a one-sided test. As usual, replace $z_\alpha$ by $z_{\alpha/2}$ for a two-sided test. Notice that the sample size depends upon $P$, the population exposure prevalence, $\lambda$, the relative risk which it is important to detect, and $r$, the case : control ratio. As we have seen (in Section 6.2.1), a case–control study can only estimate the odds ratio. The approximation used in (8.17) ensures that the odds ratio is a good approximation to the relative risk. Hence, strictly we are considering the sample size needed to detect an *approximate* relative risk in a case–control study.

*Example 8.17*    A case-control study of the relationship between smoking and coronary heart disease is planned. A sample of men with newly diagnosed coronary disease will be compared for smoking status (smoker/non-smoker) with a sample of controls. Assuming an equal number of cases and controls, how many are needed to detect an approximate relative risk of 2.0 with 90% power using a two-sided 5% test? Government surveys have estimated that 30% of the male population are smokers.

Here $P = 0.3$, $r = 1$, $\lambda = 2$, $z_{\alpha/2} = 1.96$ and $z_\beta = 1.2816$ (see Table 8.1). Substituting into (8.20) gives

$$p_c^* = \frac{0.3}{2}\left(\frac{2}{1+0.3}+1\right) = 0.3808.$$

Then, by (8.19),

$$n = \frac{2\times 1.3^2}{0.3^2(-0.7)^2}\left[1.96\sqrt{2\times 0.3808 \times 0.6192}\right.$$
$$\left. + 1.2816\sqrt{\frac{2\times 0.3 \times 0.7}{1.3^2}+0.3\times 0.7}\right]^2 = 375.6.$$

So we should take 188 cases and 188 controls, that is, 376 individuals in all.

## 8.7.1    Using a table of sample sizes

The result of the last example may be obtained more easily from Table B.10. Here we need Table B.10(c), 5th column and 17th row to obtain the result. Schlesselman (1982) gives a comprehensive collection of tables for use in calculating sample size for case–control studies.

## 8.7.2    Power and minimum detectable relative risk

A formula for $z_\beta$ is easily derived from (8.19). First calculate

$$M = \left|\frac{(\lambda-1)(P-1)}{1+(\lambda-1)P}\right|. \tag{8.21}$$

Then

$$z_\beta = \frac{\dfrac{MP\sqrt{nr}}{\sqrt{r+1}} - z_\alpha\sqrt{(r+1)p_c^*(1-p_c^*)}}{\sqrt{\dfrac{\lambda P(1-P)}{[1+(\lambda-1)P]^2} + rP(1-P)}}, \tag{8.22}$$

from which we may calculate the power. As in Section 8.6, we cannot invert (8.19) directly to obtain an expression for $\lambda$. Instead, we can use a similar argument to that which gave rise to (8.16) and thus obtain an approximate result,

$$\lambda \simeq 1 + \frac{-b \pm \sqrt{b^2 - 4a(r+1)}}{2a},$$

where

$$a = rP^2 - \frac{nrP(1-P)}{(z_\alpha + z_\beta)^2(r+1)},$$

$$b = 1 + 2rP.$$

*Example 8.18*  In the situation of Example 8.17, suppose that we wish to find the power to detect an approximate relative risk of 2 using a two-sided 5% test when there are 188 cases and 940 controls available (a 1 : 5 case : control ratio). Assume a 30% prevalence of smoking once more.

Here $P = 0.3$, $\lambda = 2$, $z_{\alpha/2} = 1.96$, $z_\beta = 1.2816$, $n = 188 + 940 = 1128$ and $r = 188/940 = 0.2$. Substituting into (8.21),

$$M = \left|\frac{(2-1)(0.3-1)}{1+(2-1)0.3}\right| = |-0.5385| = 0.5385.$$

Also, from (8.20),

$$p_c^* = \frac{0.3}{(0.2+1)}\left(\frac{0.2 \times 2}{1+(2-1)0.3} + 1\right) = 0.3269.$$

With these results, (8.22) becomes

$$z_\beta = \frac{\dfrac{0.5385 \times 0.3\sqrt{1128 \times 0.2}}{\sqrt{0.2+1}} - 1.96\sqrt{(0.2+1)0.3269 \times 0.6731}}{\sqrt{\dfrac{2 \times 0.3 \times 0.7}{[1+(2-1)0.3]^2} + 0.2 \times 0.3 \times 0.7}} = 2.24.$$

From Table B.1 we see that the probability of a standard normal value below 2.24 is about 0.987. Hence the power of the test, with the given sample size allocation, is approximately 99%.

The result of Example 8.18 is included in Figure 6.2. We saw there that the power increases, but with a diminishing rate of return, as the number of controls increases, given a fixed number of cases.

To complete the interpretation, consider varying the allocation ratio, $r$, keeping the *overall* sample size fixed. This is the situation where we anticipate only being able to afford to interview so many people, but we wish to consider how many of these should be taken from the available cases (assuming a large supply). Figure 8.7 shows the result within the context of Example 8.17, taking the overall sample size to be fixed at 376. Note that $r$ is the reciprocal of the control/case quotient shown in Figure 8.7 (which is used for compatibility with Figure 6.2). Figure 8.7 illustrates situations where either the number of cases is an integer multiple of the number of controls (very unlikely in practice) or where the number of controls is an integer multiple of the number of cases. The integers used are from 1 to 12.

As suggested in Section 8.4.3, Figure 8.7 shows that optimum allocation (maximum power) occurs where $r = 1$ (equal allocation). When the number of cases is fixed we can always do better by recruiting more controls, but when the overall number of cases plus controls is fixed we cannot do better than to use equal allocation (compare Figures 6.2 and 8.7).

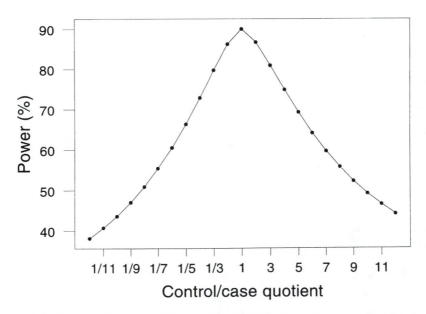

**Figure 8.7** Power against control/case quotient. This shows the power to detect an approximate relative risk of 2 when the risk factor has a prevalence of 30%, a two-sided 5% significance test is to be used and the overall sample size (cases plus controls) is fixed at 376.

### 8.7.3 Comparison with cohort studies

In most practical situations a case–control study requires a much smaller sample size than does a cohort study for the same problem. Consider, for example, a cohort study for the smoking and coronary disease problem of Example 8.17, such as that described in Example 8.13. To be able to calculate an equivalent value for $n$ in a cohort study we need an estimate of $\pi$, the chance of a coronary event (morbid or mortal) amongst non-smokers. Let us suppose that the cohort study is to last 10 years, and for this period $\pi$ is estimated (for example, from Example 3.1) to be 0.09. Notice that $P$, the prevalence of smoking, does not affect the value for $n$ in a cohort study. Conversely, $\pi$ does not affect the value for $n$ in a case–control study.

Table 8.2 compares $n$ for the two study designs over a range of values for the relative risk (or at least its approximate value from a case–control study). This illustrates the great advantage, in terms of sample size requirements, of a case–control study when the relative risk to be detected is small. In fact, coronary disease is not as rare as many diseases that are the subject of case–control studies. As Schlesselman (1974) shows, there are even greater savings with very rare diseases.

### 8.7.4 Matched studies

As discussed in Section 6.5, matching can improve the efficiency of a case–control study; in other words, we can detect the same approximate relative risk with the same power using rather fewer subjects. In this case, the sample size for an unmatched study acts as an upper limit for the matched sample size. However, this is not always true because the matched study must discard any

**Table 8.2** Sample size requirements to detect a given relative risk with 90% power using two-sided 5% significance tests for cohort and case–control studies

| Relative risk | Cohort study[a] | Case–control study[b] |
| --- | --- | --- |
| 1.1 | 44 398 | 21 632 |
| 1.2 | 11 568 | 5 820 |
| 1.3 | 5 346 | 2 774 |
| 1.4 | 3 122 | 1 668 |
| 1.5 | 2 070 | 1 138 |
| 2.0 | 602 | 376 |
| 3.0 | 188 | 146 |

[a] Using (8.14), assuming an incidence of 0.09 for the non-factor group.
[b] Using (8.19), assuming a prevalence of 0.3 for the risk factor.

concordant sets (Section 6.6). In a matched study where the number of concordant sets is very large we could even find a larger sample size requirement under matching. In addition, matching may require several potential controls to be rejected due to lack of matching properties. This is, in a sense, a component of sample size, although we shall not consider it further here.

For simplicity, we shall only look at 1 : 1 matched studies: see Walter (1980b) for formulae for sample size and power in 1 : variable case–control studies. In the paired situation we saw, in Section 6.6.1, that the test of the null hypothesis $\psi = 1$ is the same as the test of $\phi = 0.5$, where $\phi$ is the proportion of discordant pairs which have an exposed case. It will be simple to deal with $\phi$ because this is a single proportion, as already analysed in Section 8.5. The relationship between $\psi$ and $\phi$ is given by (6.9), $\psi = \phi/(1 - \phi)$. Let the alternative hypothesis be that the approximate relative risk is $\lambda$. Taking the odds ratio as this approximate relative risk, and using (6.9), we have that, under $H_1, \phi = \lambda/(1 + \lambda)$. Hence to test for the usual null hypothesis of no effect against the alternative that the approximate relative risk is $\lambda$ we, instead, can test $H_0 : \phi = 0.5$ versus $H_1 : \phi = \lambda/(1 + \lambda)$. This is the form of hypotheses assumed in Section 8.5 where $\pi_0 = 0.5$ and $\pi_1 = \lambda/(1 + \lambda)$, and hence

$$d = \pi_0 - \pi_1 = \frac{\lambda}{1 + \lambda} - \frac{1}{2} = \frac{\lambda - 1}{2(\lambda + 1)}.$$

Substituting these results into (8.13) gives

$$d = \frac{\left[z_\alpha(\lambda + 1) + 2z_\beta\sqrt{\lambda}\right]^2}{(\lambda - 1)^2}. \tag{8.23}$$

This result is labelled $d$ for consistency with Section 6.6.1, since it tells us the number of discordant pairs required. When sampling for the case–control study we shall also include concordant pairs. Let the probability of a discordant pair be $\pi_d$ and let $n_p$ be the total number of pairs sampled. Then $\pi_d = d/n_p$ and thus $n_p = d/\pi_d$. The total sample size is hence

$$n = 2d/\pi_d. \tag{8.24}$$

We can substitute (8.23) into (8.24) to arrive at the required sample size, provided we know $\pi_d$, or can at least find a reasonable estimate of it. The problem is that the chance of a discordant pair is rarely known, to any reasonable degree of approximation, before the study begins. The exception is where the results of a similar paired study are available. Contrast this with the situation in an unmatched study where we only need an estimate of the prevalence of the risk factor which is often easily obtained, perhaps from publications of the national statistics office.

Several approaches to this problem have been suggested (see Fleiss and Levin, 1988), all of which require estimation of some unknown parameter concerned with matching. Donner and Li (1990) give a formulation which depends upon the value of Cohen's kappa (Section 2.9.2) for the members of matched pairs.

*Example 8.19*  Consider Example 8.17 again, but this time suppose that a matched 1 : 1 case–control study is envisaged. A previous study has suggested that the chance of a discordant pair is about 0.5. Assuming that, as before, an approximate relative risk of 2 is to be found with 90% power using a two-sided 5% test, (8.23) gives

$$d = \frac{\left[1.96(2+1) + 2 \times 1.2816\sqrt{2}\right]^2}{(2-1)^2} = 90.34.$$

Substituting this into (8.24) gives

$$n = 2 \times 90.34/0.5 = 361.4.$$

Hence, after rounding up, 362 individuals are required; that is, 181 matched pairs. This gives a saving of seven pairs compared with the unmatched version of Example 8.17.

## 8.8   Concluding remarks

This chapter provides a set of equations which give the sample size requirements in the most straightforward situations that arise in epidemiological research. The one common requirement in each section of this chapter is for the epidemiologist to specify the difference, or sometimes the relative risk, that he or she wishes to be able to detect with some high probability (usually 0.90 or 0.95). This requires careful thought. Often the researcher will begin by being over-optimistic, specifying a difference which is so small that it requires an enormous sample to have a good chance of detecting it. Usually the value ultimately decided upon is some compromise between various objectives, including conserving resources. The ultimate decision may only be obtained after a few trial calculations. In this context the 'inverse' formulae for power and minimum detectable difference (relative risk) included in this chapter may well be useful. It is quite possible that the value for $n$ which is needed to be able to detect the difference we would really like to find with high probability is beyond our resources. There is no easy solution to this problem: we must either find more resources or accept reduced power.

Throughout we have assumed that sample size may be determined by considering only one variable of interest. Frequently the subsequent data set will include several variables; for instance, we might be planning a lifestyle survey which will measure height, weight, blood pressure, cholesterol, daily cigarette consumption and several other things. We might well find that the optimal value of $n$ for analysing height, say, is considerably different than that for analysing cholesterol. Similarly, there could be several end-points of interest in the subsequent data set; for example, the cohort phase of the Scottish Heart Health Study recorded both coronary events and deaths from all causes (Tunstall-Pedoe *et al.*, 1997). If there are multiple criteria, the value for $n$ might be calculated for each criterion. The maximum of all these gives the value for $n$ which satisfies all requirements. This will often be far more than is needed for some of the criteria, and hence may be considered to be too wasteful. An alternative approach is to pick the most important criterion and use this alone. So, if the effect of cholesterol on coronary death is considered to be the most crucial question in the lifestyle survey we would determine $n$ from considering this relationship alone. In practice, a strategy somewhere between these two may be preferred.

We should remember that the equations for sample size are based upon probabilities (through the power). There can be no absolute guarantee that the important difference will be detected, when it does exist, even with a very high power specification. All we can say is that we will run very little risk of missing it when we specify a high value for the power. The higher the power, the less the risk. Sample size evaluation is not an exact science, especially as some of the assumptions (such as normal distributions) may be violated by the data that ultimately are collected. Often we can only regard the sample size computed as a reasonable guide. Furthermore, if there is a strong possibility that some individuals will drop out before the end of the study, a common occurrence in cohort and intervention studies, then it would be wise to increase the nominal study size accordingly.

## Exercises

8.1 Vitamin A supplementation is known to confer resistance to infectious diseases in developing countries, although the precise mechanism is unclear. To seek to explain the mechanism, a group of healthy children will be given vitamin A supplement for a long period. At baseline, and at the end of the supplementation period, urine samples will be taken from all the children and neopterin excretion measured. The current level of neopterin is estimated as 600 mmol per millimole of creatinine, and the standard deviation of change due to supplementation has been estimated (from a small pilot sample) to be 200 mmol/mmol creatinine.

   (i) Suppose that a drop of 10% in neopterin is considered a meaningful difference, which it is wished to find with 95% power using a two-sided 1% test. How many children should be recruited?

(ii) Suppose that resources allow only 150 children to be given the supplements. What is the chance of detecting a drop of 10% in neopterin with a 1% two-sided test?

(iii) If 150 children are recruited, what is the smallest percentage reduction in neopterin that we can expect to detect with 95% power using a 1% two-sided test?

8.2 Various epidemiological studies compare smokers to non-smokers. One of the possible confounding variables in any such study is body mass index (BMI), since smokers have frequently been found to have lower BMIs.

Suppose that you decided to instigate a study to compare the mean BMIs of smokers and non-smokers. You plan to use a one-sided 5% significance test of the null hypothesis of no difference against the alternative that smokers have a lower BMI. From past experience the standard deviation of human BMI values is known to be about 4 kg/m$^2$.

(i) What sample size would you use to be 95% sure of detecting when smokers have a BMI that is 1 kg/m$^2$ lower (assuming an equal number of smokers and non-smokers is recruited)?

(ii) If resources only allow 600 subjects to be recruited, what is the anticipated power for detecting a difference of 1 kg/m$^2$ (assuming an equal number of smokers and non-smokers)?

(iii) If 200 smokers and 400 non-smokers were recruited, what would be the anticipated power for detecting a difference of 1 kg/m$^2$?

(iv) Suppose, now, that an alternative type of study is envisaged. Subjects who intend to give up smoking are to be recruited and their BMI will be recorded before and several years after giving up. If the conditions of the test to be applied to the subsequent data are as in (i) (that is, a difference of 1 kg/m$^2$ is to be detected with 95% power using a 5% one-sided test), under what condition does this design require fewer BMI recordings to be made than does the design used in (i)? You should assume that no subjects are 'lost' over time.

8.3 In Examples 8.13 and 8.14 one-sided tests were used, rather than the more usual two-sided. How do the sample size requirements change if a two-sided test is used in each case?

8.4 Basnayake et al. (1983) proposed an intervention study to test the hypothesis that Sri Lankan women are more suited to low-dose oral contraceptives (OCs). Women were to be randomly allocated to use either Norinyl (a standard-dose OC) or Brevicon (a low-dose OC). The aim is to determine the percentage of women continuing to use their allocated OC 12 months after entering the study.

(i) Suggest suitable inclusion and exclusion criteria for entering the study.

(ii) Suppose that the investigators wish to be 90% sure of detecting when the percentage of women continuing with the contraceptive after 12 months is 10% higher in the Brevicon group than in the Norinyl group. The 12-month continuation percentage amongst Norinyl users in previous studies was found to be 55%. In this study a two-sided 5% significance test will be used, with an equal number in each treatment group. How many women should be entered into the study (assuming no loss during follow-up)? How many should be entered if 5% can be expected to be lost to follow-up within 12 months?

(iii) Do you have any criticisms of using only the 12-month continuation percentage to compare the properties of the two OCs? State any other measures that you would wish to consider.

8.5 Researchers at a health promotions unit plan a study of the relationship between taking
diuretics and falling for old people. They believe that diuretics may be a risk factor for
falling because these reduce blood pressure. In their study the researchers plan to get
pharmacists, in chemist shops, to ask old people whether they have fallen in the past year
at the time that they issue them with prescribed medication. They will record two
variables for each elderly customer: whether they have received diuretics and whether
they have experienced a serious fall in the past year, both with yes/no responses.
Altogether 2000 subjects will be recruited.
  (i)  The researchers estimate that one-third of elderly people not taking diuretics will
       have experienced a serious fall within the previous year. Estimate the power of the
       test, assuming equal numbers in each group, to detect when the chance of a serious
       fall is 1.2 times as high amongst those who have received diuretics, using a two-sided
       5% significance test.
  (ii) Discuss any problems that you foresee for the proposed study.
8.6 To investigate the health effects of coffee drinking, a research team plans to carry out an
epidemiological study. Since coronary heart disease (CHD) is the leading cause of death
within the population to be studied, this is chosen as the basis for the sample size
calculation. It is known that the CHD incidence amongst non-coffee drinkers is 2.3 per
100 and that 40% of the population drink coffee (here taken as regular consumption of
four or more cups per day).
  What sample size is required (assuming equal-sized groups) to carry out a two-sided
5% significance test of the null hypothesis of no association between coffee drinking and
CHD, given that the team wishes to be 95% sure of detecting whenever coffee drinking
(at least approximately) doubles the risk of CHD, using:
  (i)  a cohort study?
  (ii) an unmatched case–control study?
It is also known that the risk of a specific type of cancer amongst non-coffee drinkers is 8
per 1000.
  (iii) How does the sample size requirement change in (i) and (ii) if the cancer is chosen as
        the basis for the sample size calculation instead of CHD (all else kept unchanged)?
8.7 An unmatched case–control study is to be carried out to ascertain the effect of occupation
on the chance of testicular cancer. Cases are to be new referrals to a hospital in a
particular area; controls will be recruited from amongst patients in the same hospitals
with any one of a number of pre-specified acceptable diagnoses. Each subject will be
interviewed, or his records will be consulted, to discover his current or last employment.
The various types of employment recorded will subsequently be grouped into a number of
mutually exclusive groups. Odds ratios will be calculated to compare each occupation
group (in turn) with all the rest combined. An odds ratio (approximate relative risk) of 2 is
considered so important that it should not be missed when a two-sided 1% significance
test is used. For the time available the investigators anticipate recruiting 400 cases. If
necessary, they estimate that they could recruit up to 1600 controls.
  What is the power for detecting an odds ratio of 2 for occupation groups that (i) 5%,
(ii) 10% and (iii) 20% of the national male adult population belong to, when equal
numbers of cases and controls (400 of each) are used?
  What are the equivalent results for occupation groups that (iv) 5%, (v) 10% and (vi)
20% belong to when all 1600 controls are used (together with the 400 cases)?

(vii) From your results, what recommendations would you make for the design of the study?

8.8 Schlesselman (1974) describes an unmatched case–control study of cono-truncal malformations in the baby and use of oral contraceptives by the mother. He assumes that 30% of all women use oral contraceptives, and that a 5% two-sided test is to be used with equal numbers in the two groups. Since the values of the parameters are all the same as here, Example 8.17 shows that 376 subjects (188 cases and 188 controls) are needed to detect an odds ratio (approximate relative risk) of 2 with 90% power.

(i) What is the smallest odds ratio greater than unity that one can expect to detect with 90% power using four times as many subjects (that is, 1504 subjects)?

(ii) Keeping the total number of subjects as 1504, produce a plot of the power against the smallest detectable odds ratio, varying the latter between 1.30 and 1.50. Interpret your graph.

# 9

# Modelling quantitative outcome variables

## 9.1  Statistical models

A statistical model has, at its root, a mathematical representation of the relationship between one variable, called the **outcome** or **y variable**, and one or more **explanatory** or **x variables**. For example, in the problem of finding a relationship between a smoker's daily cigarette consumption and the blood nicotine of his or her non-smoking spouse, $y$ is the blood nicotine and $x$ is the cigarette consumption.

Many models have the simple form

$$y = \frac{\text{systematic}}{\text{component}} + \frac{\text{random}}{\text{error}},$$

where the systematic component (but not the random error) is a mathematical function of the explanatory variables. The first aim of a modelling procedure will be to estimate the systematic component. This is achieved by analysing data from several subjects (smokers and their spouses in our example). We then obtain **fitted** or **predicted values**, expressed (as with other estimates) using the 'hat' notation:

$$\hat{y} = \frac{\text{systematic}}{\text{component}}.$$

Fitted values can be used to make epidemiological statements about the apparent relationship between $y$ and the other variable(s). For example, a prediction of the amount of blood nicotine is derived, on average, from the number of cigarettes smoked by the spouse. These predictions will clearly be incorrect by the amount of random error. For example, passive smoking may take place at a different rate for different people, even when each is exposed to the same basic conditions, if only due to physiological differences.

It is crucial that the model fitting ensures that the 'left-over' random component really is random, and does not contain any further systematic component which could be removed and incorporated within $\hat{y}$. For accurate predictions we also require the random error to be small; to reduce it we may need to take account of further explanatory variables in the systematic ('explained') part of the model. For example, blood nicotine may also depend upon the strength of the cigarette smoked. Consequently post-fitting model checking is advised (Section 9.8).

In this chapter we shall consider models for a quantitative outcome variable (such as the blood nicotine example). We shall assume, virtually throughout the chapter, that the random error has a normal probability distribution with zero mean and constant variance (Section 2.7). Some alternatives, where normality is not assumed, are discussed briefly in Section 9.10.

The models are generally classified into two types: analysis of variance (ANOVA) models, for which the explanatory variables are categorical; and regression models, for which the explanatory variables are quantitative. A common approach will be used, leading to the general linear model which allows explanatory variables of either type (Section 9.6).

## 9.2   One categorical explanatory variable

Models with a solitary explanatory variable are called **one-way ANOVA** models. It will be convenient to introduce them here in terms of hypothesis testing, although the estimation procedures which follow are generally more useful in practice.

### 9.2.1   The hypotheses to be tested

In Section 2.7.3 we saw how to use the $t$ test to compare two means, where the null hypothesis is that the two population means are equal. The one-way ANOVA extends this to provide a test of the null hypothesis that $\ell$ means are equal (for $\ell \geq 2$). As with the pooled $t$ test, the one-way ANOVA will assume that there is equal variance in each of the $\ell$ groups. A simple hypothetical example will be used to introduce the underlying concepts of the methodology.

*Example 9.1*   Suppose that a study of the effects of a diet that is lacking in meat has recruited six vegans, six lacto-vegetarians and six people with an unrestricted diet (omnivores). The data are presented in Table 9.1. There are three groups; the null hypothesis is

$$\mu_1 = \mu_2 = \mu_3$$

where the subscript 1 is for omnivores, 2 for vegetarians and 3 for vegans and each $\mu$ denotes a population mean for cholesterol. The alternative hypothesis is that at least one of the means is different from the others. In general, we write the hypotheses as

**Table 9.1**  Data from a hypothetical study of the effect of diet, showing total serum cholesterol (mmol/l) by type of diet for 18 different people

| Subject no. (within group) | Diet group | | | Total |
|---|---|---|---|---|
| | Omnivores | Vegetarians | Vegans | |
| 1 | 6.35 | 5.92 | 6.01 | |
| 2 | 6.47 | 6.03 | 5.42 | |
| 3 | 6.09 | 5.81 | 5.44 | |
| 4 | 6.37 | 6.07 | 5.82 | |
| 5 | 6.11 | 5.73 | 5.73 | |
| 6 | 6.50 | 6.11 | 5.62 | |
| Total | 37.89 | 35.67 | 34.04 | 107.60 |
| Mean | 6.32 | 5.95 | 5.67 | 5.98 |

$$H_0 : \mu_1 = \mu_2 = \cdots = \mu_\ell$$
$$H_1 : \mu_i \neq \mu_k \quad \text{for some } i \text{ and } k.$$

### 9.2.2  Construction of the ANOVA table

In order to provide formulae for the one-way ANOVA we shall need to introduce some mathematical notation. Even when the arithmetic will be done by a computer package, interpretation of the methodology and the results requires some insight into the underlying mathematical formulation.

Let $y_{ij}$ be the outcome for the $j$th subject in the $i$th group. For instance, in Example 9.1 the cholesterol reading for the 4th subject in the vegan group (group 3) is $y_{34} = 5.82$, from Table 9.1. If we let $\bar{y}$ be the overall sample mean and $\bar{y}_i$ be the sample mean in group $i$, then we can equate each $y_{ij}$ to a combination of $\bar{y}$ and $\bar{y}_i$ through

$$y_{ij} = \bar{y} + (\bar{y}_i - \bar{y}) + (y_{ij} - \bar{y}_i) \tag{9.1}$$

In words, (9.1) says

$$\text{observation} = \frac{\text{overall}}{\text{mean}} + \frac{\text{difference between}}{\text{specific and overall mean}} \quad \cdot$$

$$+ \frac{\text{difference between}}{\text{observation and specific mean}}$$

Removing the brackets and cancelling terms which are both added and subtracted on the right-hand side makes the truth of (9.1) obvious. Applied to an example from Table 9.1 we have, for the first subject in the omnivore group,

$$6.35 = 5.98 + (6.32 - 5.98) + (6.35 - 6.32)$$
$$= 5.98 + 0.34 + 0.03.$$

Subtracting $\bar{y}$ from both sides of (9.1) gives

$$(y_{ij} - \bar{y}) = (\bar{y}_i - \bar{y}) + (y_{ij} - \bar{y}_i).$$

When both sides of this expression are squared and then summed over the $i$ and $j$ subscripts it turns out (after some algebraic manipulation) that

$$\sum_i \sum_j (y_{ij} - \bar{y})^2 = \sum_i \sum_j (\bar{y}_i - \bar{y})^2 + \sum_i \sum_j (y_{ij} - \bar{y}_i)^2,$$

which can also be written as

$$\sum_i \sum_j (y_{ij} - \bar{y})^2 = \sum_i n_i(\bar{y}_i - \bar{y})^2 + \sum_i \sum_j (y_{ij} - \bar{y}_i)^2, \qquad (9.2)$$

where $n_i$ is the number of observations in group $i$ ($n_i = 6$ for each value of $i$ in Example 9.1). Often $n_i$ is called the number of **replicates** in group $i$. In words, (9.2) is represented as

$$\begin{array}{ccc} \text{total sum} & = & \text{group sum} \\ \text{of squares} & & \text{of squares} \end{array} + \begin{array}{c} \text{error sum} \\ \text{of squares} \end{array}.$$

This is the fundamental breakdown provided in the one-way ANOVA. The **total sum of squares** is the sum of squares (SS) of all deviations from the overall mean, sometimes called the **corrected sum of squares**. This is a measure of the overall variation in cholesterol from person-to-person, in the context of Example 9.1. The **group sum of squares** (often called the **treatment sum of squares** in an experimental situation) measures variation between the group-specific sample means, since it is based upon the $\bar{y}_i - \bar{y}$ differences. If $H_0$ is true we should expect this to be relatively small. The **error** (or **residual**) **sum of squares** simply measures the variation remaining after accounting for the variation between group means. This is sometimes called a **within-group sum of squares** because it is based upon the $y_{ij} - \bar{y}_i$ differences, which are differences between the observations and their mean within group $i$.

In speaking of the individual sums of squares as measures of variation based on squared differences, we are led into consideration of average measures. Just as in the definition of the variance, (2.9), we should divide the SS by the appropriate degrees of freedom if we are to define an average measure. As in (2.9), the appropriate d.f. for the total SS is $n - 1$ (the number of observations less one, equal to 17 in Example 9.1). Similarly, the group SS has $\ell - 1$ d.f., where $\ell$ is the number of groups ($\ell - 1 = 2$ in Example 9.1). This follows from the fact that when we know $\ell - 1$ of the group-specific means, assuming that the overall mean is known, we can calculate the final mean by subtraction (Section 2.6.3). For the error SS, each within-group measure of variation has $n_i - 1$ d.f., leading to $\sum (n_i - 1) = n - \ell$ d.f. overall. In Example 9.1 there are $18 - 3 = 15$ d.f. for error.

When the SS is divided by its d.f. the result is called a **mean square** (MS). We shall use the symbol $s_e^2$ to represent the error MS; this emphasizes the fact that this is a measure of variation, just like the overall sample variance, $s^2$. The error MS is the residual variation in the $y$ variable after the variation due to the group differences has been accounted for. Finally, the ratio of the group to the error mean squares is called the **F ratio** or **variance ratio**.

The general algebraic form of the ANOVA table is given by Table 9.2. By convention, the total MS (which is the variance for the $y$ variable) is omitted from the ANOVA table. Table 9.2. is arithmetically demanding to prepare and a far easier construction for hand calculation is given by Table 9.3. In this, equivalent expressions for the group and total SS are given, and the error SS and d.f. are found by subtracting the group component from the total. Table 9.3 requires the following additional definitions:

$$T_i = \sum_j y_{ij},$$

$$T = \sum_i T_i.$$

Hence $T_i$ is the total of the observations obtained from group $i$ and $T$ is the overall grand total of the sample values of the outcome variable, $y$. The term $T^2/n$, which is subtracted in both the group and total SS in Table 9.3, is called the **correction factor**.

*Example 9.2*   We shall now apply the formulae given in Table 9.3 to the data of Table 9.1. Note that summary averages and totals already appear in Table 9.1. Here $\ell = 3$ and $n_i = 6$ for each of the three values for $i$. The correction factor is

$$T^2/n = 107.60^2/18 = 643.209.$$

**Table 9.2**   The one-way ANOVA table for $\ell$ groups when $n_i$ observations are taken from the $i$th group: basic algebraic form

| Source of variation | Sum of squares | Degrees of freedom | Mean square | F ratio |
|---|---|---|---|---|
| Groups | $\sum n_i (\bar{y}_i - \bar{y})^2$ | $\ell - 1$ | $s_g^2 = \text{SS/d.f.}$ | $s_g^2/s_e^2$ |
| Error | $\sum\sum (y_{ij} - \bar{y}_i)^2$ | $n - \ell$ | $s_e^2 = \text{SS/d.f.}$ | |
| Total | $\sum\sum (y_{ij} - \bar{y})^2$ | $n - 1$ | | |

**Table 9.3**   The one-way ANOVA table for $\ell$ groups when $n_i$ observations are taken from the $i$th group: computational form

| Source of variation | Sum of squares | Degrees of freedom | Mean square | F ratio |
|---|---|---|---|---|
| Groups | $\sum \dfrac{T_i^2}{n_i} - \dfrac{T^2}{n}$ | $\ell - 1$ | $s_g^2 = \text{SS/d.f.}$ | $s_g^2/s_e^2$ |
| Error | By subtraction | By subtraction | $s_e^2 = \text{SS/d.f.}$ | |
| Total | $\sum\sum y_{ij}^2 - \dfrac{T^2}{n}$ | $n - 1$ | | |

The group SS is

$$\frac{37.89^2}{6} + \frac{35.67^2}{6} + \frac{34.04^2}{6} - 643.209 = 1.245.$$

The total SS requires calculation of $\sum\sum y_{ij}^2$. This is found by squaring each data item in Table 9.1 and summing the 18 squares. The total SS is thus

$$644.984 - 643.209 = 1.775.$$

Then, by subtraction, the error SS is

$$1.775 - 1.245 = 0.530.$$

The group d.f. is $3 - 1 = 2$, the total d.f. is $18 - 1 = 17$ and hence the error d.f. is $17 - 2 = 15$ (as noted earlier).

The group MS is thus $1.245/2 = 0.623$ and the error MS is $0.530/15 = 0.035$. The $F$ ratio is $0.623/0.035 = 17.8$. The formal ANOVA table is given in Table 9.4.

### 9.2.3   How the ANOVA table is used

To construct a test of significance for the null hypothesis that all means are equal we need to consider the average sums of squares, that is the mean squares. The error MS is an average of the individual variances within groups, and is essentially a generalization of the pooled estimate of variance in a two-sample $t$ test: see (2.16). It provides an estimate of the 'background variation' against which other components of variance can be compared. Here the only other component is that due to groups.

**Table 9.4**   ANOVA table for cholesterol in Examples 9.1 and 9.2

| Source of variation | Sum of squares | Degrees of freedom | Mean square | F ratio |
|---|---|---|---|---|
| Diets | 1.245 | 2 | 0.623 | 17.8 |
| Error | 0.530 | 15 | 0.035 | |
| Total | 1.775 | 17 | | |

The $F$ ratio compares the size of the group MS to the error MS. This should be small when $H_0$ is true (all population means are equal); large values are evidence against $H_0$. Precisely, we need to compare the $F$ ratio against the $F$ distribution with first d.f. given by the group d.f. and second d.f. given by the error d.f. This test requires one-sided critical values, such as are given in Table B.5. Hence we can read off values directly from this table in ANOVA problems.

From Table 9.4 we test the hypothesis of no difference in mean cholesterol between diet groups by comparing 17.8 with $F_{2,15}$. Table B.5(e) shows that the 0.1% critical value of $F_{2,15}$ is 11.3. Hence the test is significant for $p < 0.001$; there is a real difference in mean cholesterol by diet. Often the $p$ value is added as an extra column to the ANOVA table, as we shall do subsequently.

### 9.2.4    Estimation of group means

As we have seen, the ANOVA provides an overall test of equality of several means. Usually we shall also be interested in the size of the specific means.

The sample mean for group $i$, $\bar{y}_i$, is a straightforward estimate of the population mean for group $i$. To obtain a confidence interval for this mean we could apply (2.11) to that subset of the entire data which originates from group $i$. However, provided that the ANOVA assumption of equal variance in each group is correct, a better estimate of this underlying variance is given by $s_e^2$ rather than the sample variance in group $i$. Hence the confidence interval for $\mu_i$, obtained by replacing $s^2$ with $s_e^2$ in (2.11), is

$$\bar{y}_i \pm t_{n-\ell} s_e / \sqrt{n_i}. \tag{9.3}$$

Notice that $t$ has $n - \ell$ d.f. in (9.3) because the error MS, $s_e^2$, has $n - \ell$ d.f. We evaluate $t_{n-\ell}$ at the required percentage level. In (9.3), $s_e/\sqrt{n_i}$ is the estimated standard error of $\bar{y}_i$ from the ANOVA model.

*Example 9.3*    For the hypothetical data in Table 9.1, the error MS is found from Table 9.4 to be 0.035. Each group has the same number of observations and hence each group sample mean has the same standard error of $\sqrt{0.035}/\sqrt{6} = 0.076$. From Table B.4 the 5% critical value of $t_{15}$ is 2.13. To complete the components of (9.3), sample means are taken from Table 9.1. The results are shown in Table 9.5. Vegans are estimated to have the lowest blood cholesterol and omnivores the highest.

### 9.2.5    Comparison of group means

The $F$ test in the ANOVA tells us whether all the population means may be considered equal. Whatever the result of this test, we often wish to compare specific pairs of group means.

**Table 9.5**  Estimated mean cholesterol (mmol/l) with 95% confidence interval for each diet group, data from Table 9.1

| Diet group | Mean (95% confidence interval) |
|---|---|
| Omnivores | 6.32 (6.16, 6.48) |
| Vegetarians | 5.95 (5.79, 6.11) |
| Vegans | 5.67 (5.51, 5.83) |

For instance, we have seen, from Example 9.2, that there is a significant difference between the cholesterol means in the three diet groups but we might still be interested in knowing whether vegan and vegetarian means are significantly different. The $F$ test only tells us whether the whole set of means deviates significantly from the overall mean. It is quite possible to have a significant $F$ test but a non-significant particular pairwise comparison. Conversely, we might have a non-significant $F$ and yet a pair of means that are significantly different. In the latter case we could have one mean above, but not significantly different from, the overall mean (for all the data from the $\ell$ groups) and the second mean below, but again not significantly different from, the overall mean.

To estimate the difference between two specific population means (say, $\mu_i - \mu_k$), we simply compute $\bar{y}_i - \bar{y}_k$. To construct a confidence interval we adapt (2.15) and (2.18), just as in Section 9.2.4, to obtain

$$\bar{y}_i - \bar{y}_k \pm t_{n-\ell}\hat{se}, \qquad (9.4)$$

where the estimated standard error of $\bar{y}_i - \bar{y}_k$ is

$$\hat{se} = s_e\sqrt{1/n_i + 1/n_k}. \qquad (9.5)$$

A $t$ test (Section 2.7.3) follows from computation of $(\bar{y}_i - \bar{y}_k)/\hat{se}$ which is compared to the $t$ distribution with the error d.f. ($n - \ell$ d.f.).

*Example 9.4*  To compare vegetarian and vegan diets for the data of Table 9.1, we find, from Table 9.4 and (9.5),

$$\hat{se} = \sqrt{0.035(1/6 + 1/6)} = 0.108.$$

As seen in Example 9.3, the 5% critical value of $t_{n-\ell} = t_{15}$ is 2.13. Thus, from (9.4), we have the 95% confidence interval for the difference between means given by

$$5.95 - 5.67 \pm 2.13 \times 0.108,$$

that is, $0.28 \pm 0.23$ or $(0.05, 0.51)$. We test this difference by comparing $0.28/0.108 = 2.59$ with $t_{15}$. The $p$ value is 0.02, so there is indeed evidence of a difference in vegetarian and vegan cholesterol means.

An incorrect procedure, sometimes applied when comparing mean values in epidemiology, is to construct the two individual confidence intervals and only reject the null hypothesis if they fail to overlap. Comparing the overlapping vegetarian and vegan confidence intervals in Table 9.5 with the result of Example 9.4 demonstrates the error. This underlines the fact that differences should be compared, as in this section, by taking account of their correct standard error, which, in turn, determines the length of the confidence interval.

A major difficulty with making pairwise comparisons is that this can lead to bias. For instance, if we calculate the sample means and *then* decide to compare the two groups with the largest and smallest means we know (all else being equal) that we are more likely to find a significant result than when other groups are compared. To prevent such bias only pre-planned comparisons should be made, that is contrasts specified *before* data collection. Furthermore, we can expect, just by chance, to find at least one significant result provided enough pairwise comparisons are made. This is easily proven from basic probability theory. A test carried out at the 5% level of significance has a probability of 5/100 of rejecting the null hypothesis (that the two means are equal) when it is true. For the three-group data of Table 9.1 we could carry out three pairwise tests. The chance of at least one of these rejecting a null hypothesis when all three null hypotheses are true is $1 - (95/100)^3 = 0.14$, which is far bigger than the nominal 0.05. In general, with $m$ comparisons this becomes $1 - (95/100)^m$. There is a better than even chance of at least one significant result when $m$ exceeds 13.

Various solutions have been suggested for this problem of **multiple comparisons** (see Steel and Torrie, 1980). The simplest is the **Bonferroni rule**, which states that when $m$ comparisons are made the $p$ value for each individual test should be multiplied by $m$. Thus if Example 9.4 described just one of three comparison tests carried out with the dietary data then the $p$ value would be recomputed as $3 \times 0.02 = 0.06$. Using this method, we would now conclude that the difference between vegetarian and vegan cholesterol levels was not significant at the 5% level.

Two problems with the Bonferroni method are that it often gives values above unity, and that it is conservative (tends to lead to non-significance). In general, it is best to restrict the number of comparisons to a small number, not to exceed the degrees of freedom $(\ell - 1)$, and then report the $p$ values without the correction but possibly with a warning note. If many tests are necessary then a more extreme significance level than usual (say 0.1% rather than 5%) might be taken as the 'cut-point' for decision-making. Using the Bonferroni rule, we would adopt an adjusted significance level of $s/m$, where $s$ is the nominal significance level (say, 5%) and $m$ is the number of comparisons.

## 9.2.6    *Fitted values*

Often it is useful to consider the fitted, or predicted, values determined by a statistical model. To do this we need to consider the mathematical form of the model. In this section we shall derive mathematical expressions for fitted values.

One-way ANOVA assumes that the only systematic component of the model is that due to groups. Note that group membership is a categorical variable (for example, diet has three alphabetic levels in Example 9.1). To be able to provide a mathematical expression for the model that is both easily understandable and generalizable we shall use a set of dummy variables to represent groups.

A **dummy** or **indicator variable** takes only two values, zero or unity. It takes the value unity when the 'parent' categorical variable attains some pre-specified level, and the value zero in all other circumstances. The full set of dummy variables has one variable for each level of the categorical variable. Thus, in the dietary example, the full set of dummy variables is

$$x^{(1)} = \begin{cases} 1 & \text{for omnivores} \\ 0 & \text{otherwise,} \end{cases} \qquad x^{(2)} = \begin{cases} 1 & \text{for vegetarians} \\ 0 & \text{otherwise,} \end{cases}$$

$$x^{(3)} = \begin{cases} 1 & \text{for vegans} \\ 0 & \text{otherwise.} \end{cases}$$

Note the use of superscripts to identify specific dummy variables.

The ANOVA model for the diet example is

$$y = \alpha + \beta^{(1)}x^{(1)} + \beta^{(2)}x^{(2)} + \beta^{(3)}x^{(3)} + \varepsilon, \tag{9.6}$$

where $\alpha$ and each $\beta^{(i)}$ are unknown parameters. Here $\varepsilon$ is the random component which (like $y$) varies from person to person; everything else in (9.6) is the systematic part of the model. For simplicity, unlike (9.1) and (9.2), the $i$ and $j$ subscripts are suppressed in (9.6).

The $\alpha$ and $\beta^{(i)}$ parameters are estimated by the principle of **least squares**. We call their estimates $a$ and $b^{(i)}$, respectively. These are the values in the estimated systematic part of the model expressed by (9.6), that is,

$$\hat{y} = a + b^{(1)}x^{(1)} + b^{(2)}x^{(2)} + b^{(3)}x^{(3)}, \tag{9.7}$$

that minimize the sum of squared differences between the true and fitted values, $\sum(y - \hat{y})^2$. Least squares ensures that the total, and thus the average, distance between the true and predicted value is as small as possible. Squares are required for the same reason that they are required when calculating the variance (Section 2.6.3) – that is, to avoid cancelling out positive and negative differences. See Clarke and Cooke (1992) for mathematical details.

The fitted values – that is, the values of $y$ predicted from the model – are given by (9.7). Because only one $x$ value will be non-zero at any one time, (9.7) can be written in a more extensive, but more understandable, form by considering the three dietary groups separately: for omnivores, $x^{(1)} = 1$, $x^{(2)} = 0$ and $x^{(3)} = 0$, and hence the fitted value is

$$\hat{y}_{\text{omnivore}} = a + b^{(1)};$$

for vegetarians, $x^{(1)} = 0$, $x^{(2)} = 1$ and $x^{(3)} = 0$, giving

$$\hat{y}_{\text{vegetarian}} = a + b^{(2)};$$

for vegans, $x^{(1)} = 0$, $x^{(2)} = 0$ and $x^{(3)} = 1$, giving

$$\hat{y}_{\text{vegan}} = a + b^{(3)}.$$

Notice that the one-way ANOVA model for this example can only produce three different predicted values because it assumes that, apart from random error, cholesterol is solely determined by diet.

One complication arises in the model specification (9.7). We have four unknown parameters ($a$, $b^{(1)}$, $b^{(2)}$ and $b^{(3)}$) but we are only estimating three fitted values. This means that we cannot (mathematically) find values for the parameters unless we introduce a **linear constraint** upon their values. The constraint that we shall adopt concerns the $b$ parameters only and has the general form

$$\sum_{i=1}^{3} w^{(i)} b^{(i)} = w$$

for the dietary example. The $\{w^{(i)}\}$ are a set of weights and $w$ is a scaling factor. A consequence of the necessity for such a constraint is that we need only two dummy variables to determine all the fitted values. This is another way of saying that diet, with three levels, has only 2 d.f. The full expression, (9.7), is said to be **over-parametrized**.

The general form of the $\ell$-group one-way ANOVA model is

$$y = \alpha + \beta^{(1)} x^{(1)} + \beta^{(2)} x^{(2)} + \cdots + \beta^{(\ell)} x^{(\ell)} + \varepsilon. \tag{9.8}$$

The general form of the fitted values from an $\ell$-group one-way ANOVA is

$$\hat{y} = a + b^{(1)} x^{(1)} + b^{(2)} x^{(2)} + \cdots + b^{(\ell)} x^{(\ell)}, \tag{9.9}$$

where

$$x^{(i)} = \begin{cases} 1 & \text{if the group variable attains its } i\text{th level} \\ 0 & \text{otherwise} \end{cases}$$

and

$$\sum_{i=1}^{\ell} w^{(i)} b^{(i)} = w, \tag{9.10}$$

for some $\{w^{(i)}\}$ and $w$.

Various choices can be made for $\{w^{(i)}\}$ and $w$. In statistical textbooks it is usual to take $w^{(i)} = n_i$ for each $i$ (that is, the weight is the sample size within group $i$) and $w = 0$. Then the linear constraint, (9.10), becomes

$$\sum_{i=1}^{\ell} n_i b^{(i)} = 0.$$

The great advantage of this choice is that it makes $\alpha$ become $\mu$ and $\beta^{(i)}$ become $\mu_i - \mu$ in (9.8), and thus $a$ becomes $\bar{y}$ and $b^{(i)}$ becomes $\bar{y}_i - \bar{y}$ in (9.9). These parameters have a direct interpretation, as the grand mean and the deviation of the ith group mean from this grand mean.

### 9.2.7   Using computer packages

Many commercial software packages will fit one-way ANOVA models. Statistical packages allow the models to be fitted in one (or both) of two ways: either by constructing and then fitting the dummy variables, or by a more direct method. The first involves the user setting up $\ell - 1$ dummy variables (for a group variable with $\ell$ levels) and using either a regression procedure or a general linear model procedure (Section 9.6). The second way involves using either a procedure that is specific to the one-way ANOVA (perhaps implementing the equations of Table 9.2 or Table 9.3) or a general linear model procedure with a declaration to tell the computer that the variable which defines the groups is categorical.

We shall not describe the use of dummy variables in computer packages here; details will be given in a similar context in Section 10.4.3. Also we shall not look at computer procedures defined solely to deal with ANOVA models, such as PROC ANOVA in the SAS package. These do not generalize to the more complex situations given in this chapter and should be easy to use and understand using the subsections that precede this one.

We shall concentrate, instead, on software routines to fit general linear models which require the categorical ('group') variable to be defined. Such routines exist, for example, in GENSTAT, GLIM, SAS and SPSS. GENSTAT and GLIM require the categorical variable to be declared as a 'FACTOR',

SPSS also calls it a factor or a 'BY' variable, whilst SAS calls it a 'CLASS' variable.

Unfortunately, different packages adopt different choices for $\{w^{(i)}\}$ and $w$ in (9.10). For instance, GENSTAT and GLIM take $w^{(1)} = 1$ and all other $w^{(i)}$ and $w$ to be zero. Put simply, this constraint is

$$b^{(1)} = 0.$$

We shall be viewing output from SAS which adopts the convention that $w^{(\ell)} = 1$ and all other $w^{(i)}$ and $w$ are zero, that is,

$$b^{(\ell)} = 0.$$

So SAS fixes the parameter for the last level of a categorical variable to be zero, whereas GENSTAT and GLIM fix the first to be zero.

Many users of SPSS will find that a more complex constraint has been used (although SPSS will allow user-defined constraints). This is the so-called 'deviation contrast': $w^{(i)} = 1$ for all $i$ and $w = 0$. With this, (9.10) becomes

$$\sum_{i=1}^{\ell} b^{(i)} = 0.$$

SPSS then prints out results for the first $\ell - 1$ levels, leaving the user to compute the last $b$ parameter (if required) as

$$b^{(\ell)} = -\sum_{i=1}^{\ell-1} b^{(i)}.$$

Whichever method is used we shall arrive at the same fitted values, as Table 9.6 demonstrates (apart from rounding error) for the dietary data. However, it is crucial to discover which method the package selected has used. This is necessary for various tasks, not only the determination of fitted values (several examples appear later). If in doubt, we can run a simple example, such as Example 9.1, through the package. Note that SPSS values for the dietary example's $b^{(i)}$ will be the same as the 'textbook' since $n_i$ is a constant in this example.

Apart from rounding error, the fitted values shown in Table 9.6 are simply the sample means for the three dietary groups, as given in Table 9.1. So the most likely outcome for any future (say) vegan is the mean of all vegans currently observed. The simplicity of this obvious result should not be viewed with cynicism! The methodology of this and the previous subsection is easily generalizable, and demonstrably does give sensible results in the present context.

**Table 9.6**  Parameter estimates and fitted values for three different model formulations, data from Table 9.1

|  | Method | | |
|---|---|---|---|
| Parameter/diet | GENSTAT[a] | SAS[a] | Textbook[b] |
| Parameter estimates | | | |
| $a$ | 6.32 | 5.67 | 5.98 |
| $b^{(1)}$ | 0 | 0.64 | 0.34 |
| $b^{(2)}$ | −0.37 | 0.27 | −0.03 |
| $b^{(3)}$ | −0.64 | 0 | −0.31 |
| Fitted values[c] | | | |
| Omnivores | 6.32 | 6.31 | 6.32 |
| Vegetarians | 5.95 | 5.94 | 5.95 |
| Vegans | 5.67 | 5.67 | 5.67 |

[a] As defined in Section 9.2.7.
[b] As defined at the end of Section 9.2.6.
[c] From (9.7) using the appropriate parameter estimates.

Output 9.1 shows SAS results for Example 9.1 from using the SAS general linear models procedure, PROC GLM. The program to produce this output is given in Appendix A. CHOLEST is the name chosen for the variable that holds cholesterol values. DIET was read in using the codes 1 = omnivore, 2 = vegetarian, 3 = vegan. Notice that (apart from rounding) the ANOVA table has the same numbers as in Table 9.4. SAS provides several decimal places, almost certainly too many for publication purposes. On the other hand, Table 9.4 is almost certainly too brief for accuracy in further calculations. The C.V. is the coefficient of variation (Section 2.6.4), defined as $100s_e/\bar{y}$; MSE is the mean square for error; R-square is discussed in Section 9.3. Note how SAS alerts the user to the fact that the linear constraint it has used is not unique, although the message is somewhat cryptic. In future listings from SAS reproduced here, this message will be suppressed.

Parameter estimates from Output 9.1 have been incorporated into Table 9.6. SAS denotes the parameter $a$ as the 'intercept'; this has a more direct meaning in regression (Section 9.3.1).

Along with each parameter estimate (except $b^{(3)}$, which is fixed to be zero) SAS gives its estimated standard error and a test that the parameter is zero. This is a $t$ test (taking the error d.f. from the ANOVA table) using the test statistic, $T =$ estimate/$\hat{s}$e. Although these tests can be useful, they do require careful interpretation. From (9.7), we can show that

**Output 9.1**   SAS results for Examples 9.1 and 9.2

General Linear Models Procedure

Dependent Variable: CHOLEST

| Source | DF | Sum of Squares | Mean Square | F Value | Pr > F |
|---|---|---|---|---|---|
| Model | 2 | 1.24487778 | 0.62243889 | 17.62 | 0.0001 |
| Error | 15 | 0.52983333 | 0.03532222 | | |
| Corrected Total | 17 | 1.77471111 | | | |

| R-Square | C.V. | Root MSE | CHOLEST Mean |
|---|---|---|---|
| 0.701454 | 3.144012 | 0.1879421 | 5.9777778 |

| Parameter | | Estimate | T for H0: Parameter = 0 | Pr > \|T\| | Std Error of Estimate |
|---|---|---|---|---|---|
| INTERCEPT | | 5.673333333 B | 73.94 | 0.0001 | 0.07672703 |
| DIET | 1 | 0.641666667 B | 5.91 | 0.0001 | 0.10850841 |
| | 2 | 0.271666667 B | 2.50 | 0.0243 | 0.10850841 |
| | 3 | 0.000000000 B | . | . | . |

NOTE: The X'X matrix has been found to be singular and a generalized inverse was used to solve the normal equations. Estimates followed by the letter 'B' are biased, and are not unique estimators of the parameters.

$$a = \hat{y}_{\text{vegan}},$$
$$b^{(1)} = \hat{y}_{\text{omnivore}} - \hat{y}_{\text{vegan}},$$
$$b^{(2)} = \hat{y}_{\text{vegetarian}} - \hat{y}_{\text{vegan}},$$

because of the SAS constraint $b^{(3)} = 0$. Hence $a$ is the predicted cholesterol value for vegans whilst $b^{(1)}$ and $b^{(2)}$ are estimates of the difference in cholesterol between each of the other two groups and vegans. The vegan group is, because of the SAS constraint and due to its being labelled as the last of the three groups, the **base** or **reference group**. Hence the $t$ tests show that: the vegan mean is significantly different from zero ($p < 0.0001$); there is a significant difference between the omnivore and vegan means ($p < 0.0001$); and there is a significant difference between the vegetarian and vegan means ($p = 0.0243$). The last of these three tests agrees with Example 9.4.

If we wish to see all the group means (fitted values) with associated statistics and test all possible differences using SAS we should issue a sub-command for PROC GLM to display the least-squares means (Section 9.4.6).

## 9.3    One quantitative explanatory variable

### 9.3.1    Simple linear regression

Like a one-way ANOVA, a **simple linear regression** (SLR) model relates the outcome variable, $y$, to a single explanatory variable, $x$. The only difference is that $x$ is now a quantitative variable. For instance, whereas a one-way ANOVA model is suitable for relating serum cholesterol to type of diet (Example 9.1), a SLR model might relate serum cholesterol to dietary cholesterol intake (a continuous measure).

The SLR model is

$$y = \alpha + \beta x + \varepsilon, \tag{9.11}$$

where $\alpha$ and $\beta$ are unknown parameters and, as usual, $\varepsilon$ is the random error which is assumed to have a standard normal distribution. The primary aim of an SLR analysis is to produce estimates $a$ and $b$ for $\alpha$ and $\beta$, respectively. That is, the fitted SLR line is

$$\hat{y} = a + bx. \tag{9.12}$$

This fitted model is best understood from a diagram (Figure 9.1). We call this a *linear* regression model because the $x$–$y$ relationship is modelled to follow a straight line; *simple* linear regression is regression with only one $x$ variable.

The parameter $a$ is called the **intercept** because it is the value of $y$ when $x = 0$, when the fitted line intercepts the $y$ (vertical) axis. The parameter $b$ is the slope of the fitted line; the line goes up $b$ units for each unit increase in $x$. If $b$ is negative then the line slopes downwards from left to right, and $y$ will then decrease as $x$ increases.

We can use the method of least squares to produce the estimates $a$ and $b$ from observed data on $n$ pairs of $(x, y)$ observations. Clarke and Cooke (1992) show these estimates to be

$$b = S_{xy}/S_{xx}, \tag{9.13}$$

$$a = \bar{y} - b\bar{x} = \left(\sum y/n\right) - b\left(\sum x/n\right), \tag{9.14}$$

where

$$S_{xx} = \sum_{i=1}^{n} (x - \bar{x})^2 \tag{9.15}$$

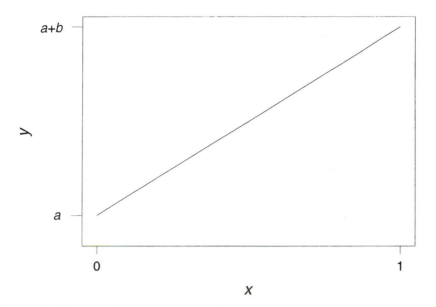

**Figure 9.1**    The simple linear regression model.

and

$$S_{xy} = \sum_{i=1}^{n} (x - \bar{x})(y - \bar{y}). \qquad (9.16)$$

In fact $S_{xx}$ has already been defined as (2.10), in the definition of the sample variance of the $x$ values. Here we shall be interested in the sample variance of the $y$ values, and an additional definition to be made is

$$S_{yy} = \sum_{i=1}^{n} (y - \bar{y})^2. \qquad (9.17)$$

From (2.9) we can see that the sample variance of the $x$ values is $S_{xx}/(n-1)$ and that the sample variance of the $y$ values is $S_{yy}/(n-1)$. We define $S_{xy}/(n-1)$ to be the sample **covariance** between the $x$ and $y$ variables. Whereas the variance measures how a single variable varies from observation to observation (ignoring any other variables), the covariance measures how two variables vary together (Section 9.3.2).

As is clear from (9.12), the SLR model predicts $y$ from $x$. To be precise, we are assuming that when $x$ is fixed at a specific value the value of $y$ is random, but with a systematic component which depends linearly upon $x$. Notice that if we decide subsequently that we should rather predict $x$ from $y$ we *cannot* use the same fitted model. Instead, we would have to fit a new SLR model where the roles of $y$ and $x$ are interchanged. This will, in general, produce a different fitted line.

Just as when $x$ is a categorical variable, it can be shown that (9.11) splits the overall variation in $y$ up into two components: that explained by regression on $x$ and the error (residual, or unexplained, variation). We can summarize this split using the same presentation as in Section 9.2.2, an ANOVA table; see Table 9.7. Apart from the different formulae for all sums of squares and d.f., except those for the total, Table 9.7 is essentially identical to Table 9.2.

To compute Table 9.7 by hand we should calculate $S_{xx}$, $S_{xy}$ and $S_{yy}$ not from (9.15)–(9.17) but rather from the following equivalent expressions which are rather easier to deal with:

$$S_{xx} = \sum x^2 - \left(\sum x\right)^2 / n, \tag{9.18}$$

$$S_{xy} = \sum xy - \left(\sum x\right)\left(\sum y\right) / n, \tag{9.19}$$

$$S_{yy} = \sum y^2 - \left(\sum y\right)^2 / n. \tag{9.20}$$

Also note that the error SS is simply the total SS minus the regression SS.

By analogy with the one-way ANOVA model, the $F$ ratio from Table 9.7 should be compared with one-sided $F$ values on $(1, n-2)$ d.f. This produces a test of $\beta = 0$, the null hypothesis that the slope of the regression line is zero. If the result is significant (say, at the 5% level) then the regression is said to be 'significant'. If $\beta = 0$ then $x$ has no role in predicting $y$ because, in this case, (9.12) generates fitted values,

$$\hat{y} = a$$

which are the same whatever the value of $x$. The fitted model then makes a horizontal straight line.

**Table 9.7**  Analysis of variance table for simple linear regression

| Source of variation | Sum of squares | Degrees of freedom | Mean square | F ratio |
|---|---|---|---|---|
| Regression on $x$ | $S_{xy}^2 / S_{xx}$ | 1 | $s_r^2 = \mathrm{SS}/\text{d.f.}$ | $s_r^2 / s_e^2$ |
| Error | $S_{yy} - (S_{xy}^2 / S_{xx})$ | $n-2$ | $s_e^2 = \mathrm{SS}/d.f.$ | |
| Total | $S_{yy}$ | $n-1$ | | |

The **coefficient of determination**,

$$r^2 = \text{regression SS/total SS}, \tag{9.21}$$

measures how successful the regression has been. We often multiply it by 100, so that it expresses the percentage of the variation in $y$ that has been explained by regression on $x$. For SLR the square root of $r^2$ is the correlation (Section 9.3.2).

Since $a$ and $b$ are sample-based estimates of $\alpha$ and $\beta$, we can specify their precision using confidence intervals. Taking these separately, confidence intervals are

$$a \pm t_{n-2}\hat{\text{se}}(a) \tag{9.22}$$

$$b \pm t_{n-2}\hat{\text{se}}(b), \tag{9.23}$$

respectively, where the estimated standard errors are, respectively,

$$\hat{\text{se}}(a) = \sqrt{s_e^2 \left\{ \frac{1}{n} + \frac{\bar{x}^2}{S_{xx}} \right\}} \tag{9.24}$$

$$\hat{\text{se}}(b) = \sqrt{s_e^2/S_{xx}}, \tag{9.25}$$

and $t_{n-2}$ is the appropriate critical value from the $t$ distribution with the error d.f.

We can also test the null hypothesis that the intercept is zero, $H_0 : \alpha = 0$. This would be useful when we want to see whether the absence of $x$ (that is, $x = 0$) is associated with the absence of $y$ ($y = 0$). However, this is by no means always a sensible test to make. When it is sensible, we compute the test statistic

$$a/\hat{\text{se}}(a), \tag{9.26}$$

to be compared with $t_{n-2}$. Similarly, to test $H_0 : \beta = 0$ we compute

$$b/\hat{\text{se}}(b), \tag{9.27}$$

which is also to be compared with $t_{n-2}$. Notice that (9.27) tests the same thing as the $F$ ratio in Table 9.7. The square of (9.27) is the $F$ ratio and the square of (two-sided) $t_{n-2}$ is (one-sided) $F_{1,n-2}$. In general, $F$ and $t$ tests are only equivalent when the $F$ test has unity for its first d.f. and has its second d.f. in common with the corresponding $t$ test.

A regression model is often used for making predictions, which are easily obtained from (9.12). Suppose we wish to predict $y$ for an individual whose $x$ value is $x_0$. From (9.12), the predicted value is

$$\hat{y}_0 = a + bx_0. \tag{9.28}$$

We can attach confidence limits to our prediction. The confidence interval is

$$\hat{y}_0 \pm t_{n-2}\hat{\text{se}}(\hat{y}_0),  \tag{9.29}$$

where the estimated standard error of the predicted value is

$$\hat{\text{se}}(\hat{y}_0) = \sqrt{s_e^2 \left\{ 1 + \frac{1}{n} + \frac{(x_0 - \bar{x})^2}{S_{xx}} \right\}}.  \tag{9.30}$$

Another possibility is to predict the mean value of $y$ over all individuals whose $x$ value is $x_0$. That is, on average what value can $y$ be expected to take when $x = x_0$? The predicted value is the same as before,

$$\hat{\bar{y}}_0 = \hat{y}_0,$$

where $\hat{y}_0$ is given by (9.28), but the confidence interval is

$$\hat{\bar{y}}_0 \pm t_{n-2}\hat{\text{se}}\left(\hat{\bar{y}}_0\right),  \tag{9.31}$$

where

$$\hat{\text{se}}\left(\hat{\bar{y}}_0\right) = \sqrt{s_e^2 \left\{ \frac{1}{n} + \frac{(x_0 - \bar{x})^2}{S_{xx}} \right\}}.  \tag{9.32}$$

Notice that both (9.30) and (9.32) will get smaller as the sample size, $n$, increases, just as we should expect. They will also be smaller for a chosen $x_0$ that is closer to $\bar{x}$ and will increase as $x_0$ moves away from $\bar{x}$ equally in either direction. This makes intuitive sense: the most accurate prediction is made at the centre of the observed values and the least accurate is at the peripheries. A prediction at a value of $x_0$ beyond the range of observed data is sure to be of dubious quality because we can never be sure that the linear relationship holds in these uncharted regions. This is reflected in the large standard error and thus wide confidence interval for such a prediction.

*Example 9.5*  Table 9.8 shows data on the relationship between sugar consumption and dental caries in the 61 developing countries for which data were available to Woodward and Walker (1994). Sugar consumption was derived from government and industry sources and the average number of decayed, missing or filled teeth (DMFT) at age 12 was obtained from the WHO Oral Disease Data Bank, where the results of national surveys were compiled. Each of these surveys was carried out at some time between 1979 and 1990; sugar consumption has been averaged over the 5 (or sometimes fewer) years previous to the year of the DMFT survey.

**Table 9.8**   Estimates of mean DMFT at age 12 years old and mean sugar consumption (kg/head of population/year) in 61 developing countries

| Country | Sugar | DMFT | Country | Sugar | DMFT |
|---|---|---|---|---|---|
| Algeria | 36.60 | 2.3 | Kuwait | 44.63 | 2.0 |
| Angola | 12.00 | 1.7 | Madagascar | 7.76 | 4.4 |
| Argentina | 34.56 | 3.4 | Malawi | 7.56 | 0.9 |
| Bahamas | 34.40 | 1.6 | Malaysia | 35.10 | 3.9 |
| Bahrain | 34.86 | 1.3 | Maldives | 31.42 | 2.1 |
| Bangladesh | 2.88 | 3.5 | Mali | 5.00 | 2.2 |
| Barbados | 63.02 | 4.4 | Morocco | 32.68 | 1.8 |
| Belize | 49.02 | 4.0 | Myanmar | 1.44 | 1.1 |
| Botswana | 35.60 | 0.5 | Niger | 4.68 | 1.7 |
| Brazil | 46.98 | 6.7 | Nigeria | 10.15 | 2.0 |
| Cameroon | 7.56 | 1.5 | Pakistan | 16.02 | 1.2 |
| China, PR | 4.66 | 0.7 | Philippines | 23.93 | 2.2 |
| Colombia | 37.76 | 4.8 | Saudi Arabia | 38.66 | 1.8 |
| Congo, DR | 2.66 | 1.0 | Senegal | 14.26 | 1.5 |
| Cuba | 62.14 | 3.9 | Sierra Leone | 4.84 | 1.3 |
| Cyprus | 34.10 | 2.5 | Singapore | 49.56 | 2.5 |
| El Salvador | 34.44 | 5.1 | Somalia | 11.82 | 1.3 |
| Ethiopia | 3.92 | 0.4 | Sri Lanka | 18.10 | 1.9 |
| Fiji | 54.24 | 2.8 | Sudan | 24.16 | 2.1 |
| Gambia | 26.56 | 1.6 | Syria | 40.18 | 1.7 |
| Ghana | 4.36 | 0.4 | Tanzania | 4.72 | 0.6 |
| Guatemala | 35.30 | 8.1 | Thailand | 15.34 | 1.5 |
| Guyana | 40.65 | 2.7 | Togo | 10.70 | 0.3 |
| Haiti | 11.17 | 3.2 | Tunisia | 27.30 | 2.1 |
| Hong Kong | 24.18 | 1.5 | Uganda | 0.97 | 1.5 |
| Indonesia | 12.50 | 2.3 | Western Samoa | 19.10 | 2.5 |
| Iraq | 43.00 | 2.7 | Yemen, AR | 30.00 | 3.1 |
| Ivory Coast | 10.74 | 2.9 | Yemen, PDR | 22.32 | 0.7 |
| Jamaica | 45.98 | 6.7 | Zambia | 18.53 | 2.3 |
| Jordan | 44.44 | 1.0 | Zimbabwe | 27.00 | 1.2 |
| Korea, Rep. | 11.56 | 0.9 | | | |

Note: These data are available electronically together with the data in Table 9.18 – see Appendix C.
Source: Woodward and Walker (1994).

The data in Example 9.5 are plotted in Figure 9.2. This type of diagram is called a **scatterplot**. From this scatterplot we see that caries does seem to increase with sugar consumption, although the relationship is not strong due to the high variation in DMFT for small variations in sugar consumption.

As the interesting epidemiological question is whether increased sugar consumption leads to caries, rather than the other way round, we shall regress

DMFT on sugar (as suggested by Figure 9.2). Thus DMFT is the $y$ variable and sugar is the $x$ variable.

From Table 9.8, $n = 61$ and

$$\sum x = 1499.77, \qquad \sum y = 141.50,$$
$$\sum x^2 = 53463.2923, \quad \sum y^2 = 479.51,$$
$$\sum xy = 4258.303.$$

From (9.18) and (9.19),

$$S_{xx} = 53463.2923 - 1499.77^2/61 = 16589.357,$$
$$S_{xy} = 4258.303 - 1499.77 \times 141.50/61 = 779.32833.$$

Thus, from (9.13) and (9.14),

$$b = 779.32833/16589.357 = 0.0469776,$$
$$a = 141.50/61 - 0.0469776 \times 1499.77/61 = 1.16466.$$

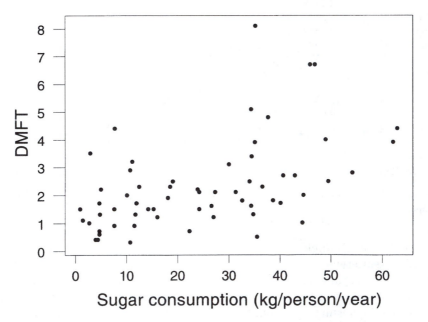

**Figure 9.2**  DMFT against sugar consumption in developing countries, data from Table 9.8.

Hence, after rounding, the fitted regression line is

$$y = 1.165 + 0.0470x.$$

Since $b$ is positive, the line predicts that $y$ will increase with increasing $x$. This can be seen from Figure 9.3 where the fitted line has been superimposed over the raw data.

To construct the ANOVA table we use (9.20) to obtain

$$S_{yy} = 479.51 - 141.50^2/61 = 151.27639.$$

Then Table 9.9 is obtained using the formulae from Table 9.7.

From this we see that $r^2 = 36.609/151.276 = 0.242$, using (9.21). Hence just over 24% of the country-to-country variation in DMFT is due to differences in sugar consumption. The remaining 76% may be attributed to other factors, presumably to include the fluoride content of the water drunk, dental hygiene practice and other aspects of diet. At this point the major weakness of the data for exploring causality is worth noting: the data are merely national averages

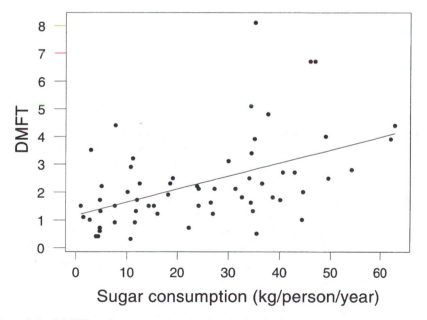

**Figure 9.3** DMFT against sugar consumption in developing countries, showing the fitted simple linear regression line.

**Table 9.9**   Analysis of variance table for DMFT, developing countries

| Source of variation | Sum of squares | Degrees of freedom | Mean square | F ratio | p value |
|---|---|---|---|---|---|
| Regression on sugar | 36.609 | 1 | 36.609 | 18.84 | <0.0001 |
| Error | 114.667 | 59 | 1.9435 | | |
| Total | 151.276 | 60 | | | |

and so we cannot link specific individual outcomes for sugar consumption and caries. An additional problem here is that sugar consumption relates to everyone, whereas DMFT is recorded only for 12-year-olds.

Using (9.25), we find the estimated standard error of the slope of the fitted regression line to be

$$\sqrt{1.9435/16589.357} = 0.0108237.$$

To obtain a 95% confidence interval for the slope from (9.23) we require the two-sided 5% critical value of $t_{59}$. From a statistical computer package, this was found to be 2.001. Hence the interval is

$$0.0469776 \pm 2.001 \times 0.0108237$$

that is, $0.0470 \pm 0.0217$ or $(0.0253, 0.0687)$. If we wish, we can test the null hypothesis that the true slope, $\beta$, is zero using (9.27),

$$0.0469776/0.0108237 = 4.34.$$

Compared to $t_{59} = 2.001$ this is highly significant. From Table B.4, $p < 0.001$, using the nearest available d.f. of 60. In fact the $p$ value, found from a statistical computer package, is even below 0.0001. Hence, there is real evidence to refute the assertion that DMFT does not increase with sugar consumption. The regression 'is significant' at the 0.01% level.

Note that the alternative $F$ test, based on the analysis of variance table (Table 9.9), gives the same result. The square of the $t$ statistic is $4.34^2 = 18.84$, which is the $F$ ratio given in Table 9.9. Comparing 18.84 with $F_{1,59}$ will clearly give a $p$ value below 0.001, by reference to the first column, last row of Table B.5(e).

Using (9.24) we find the estimated standard error of the intercept of the fitted regression line to be

$$\sqrt{1.9435\left\{\frac{1}{61} + \frac{(1499.77/61)^2}{16589.357}\right\}} = 0.3204,$$

leading to a 95% confidence interval for the intercept of

$$1.16466 \pm 2.001 \times 0.3204$$

that is, $1.165 \pm 0.641$ or $(0.524, 1.806)$, using (9.22). To formally test the null hypothesis that the intercept is zero we use (9.26) to obtain the test statistic

$$1.16466/0.3204 = 3.63.$$

Compared to $t_{59}$ this is highly significant ($p = 0.0006$). Hence there is evidence to reject the null hypothesis; when there is zero sugar consumption we can, nevertheless, expect average DMFT to be non-zero in developing countries.

Output 9.2 shows the results obtained when SAS PROC GLM was used to analyse the sugar data. The results agree with the calculations above. PROC GLM labels the regression SS as the 'model SS' and the slope is labelled 'SUGAR', showing that this is the parameter that multiplies this particular $x$ variable.

To illustrate the use of regression for prediction, suppose we know that another developing country has an average annual sugar consumption of 35 kg per head of population. We then wish to predict its DMFT. In (9.28) and (9.30) this requires taking $x_0 = 35$. The predicted DMFT is, from (9.28),

$$1.16466 + 0.0469776 \times 35 = 2.8089,$$

**Output 9.2**    SAS results for Example 9.5

General Linear Models Procedure

Dependent Variable: DMFT

| Source | DF | Sum of Squares | Mean Square | F Value | Pr > F |
|---|---|---|---|---|---|
| Model | 1 | 36.60905137 | 36.60905137 | 18.84 | 0.0001 |
| Error | 59 | 114.66734208 | 1.94351427 | | |
| Corrected Total | 60 | 151.27639344 | | | |

| | R-Square | C.V. | Root MSE | DMFT Mean |
|---|---|---|---|---|
| | 0.242001 | 60.09900 | 1.3940998 | 2.3196721 |

| Parameter | Estimate | T for H0: Parameter = 0 | Pr > \|T\| | Std Error of Estimate |
|---|---|---|---|---|
| INTERCEPT | 1.164680383 | 3.63 | 0.0006 | 0.32043887 |
| SUGAR | 0.046976241 | 4.34 | 0.0001 | 0.01082375 |

which rounds off to 2.81. This agrees with a rough evaluation found from using the fitted line in Figure 9.3. From (9.30) the estimated standard error of this prediction is

$$\sqrt{1.9435\left\{1 + \frac{1}{61} + \frac{(35 - (1499.77/61))^2}{16589.357}\right\}} = 1.4100.$$

The 95% confidence interval for the prediction is, from (9.29),

$$2.8089 \pm 2.001 \times 1.4100$$

that is, $2.81 \pm 2.82$ or $(-0.01, 5.63)$. This illustrates the large error in predicting individual values, especially where they are not close to the mean (which is around 25 in this case).

Suppose, instead, that we wish to predict the average DMFT over *all* countries with an average annual sugar consumption of 35 kg per head. This predicted mean value would still be 2.81, but the estimated standard error of this prediction is found, from (9.32), as

$$\sqrt{1.9435\left\{\frac{1}{61} + \frac{(35 - (1499.77/61))^2}{16589.357}\right\}} = 0.2111.$$

The 95% confidence interval for the predicted average is, from (9.31),

$$2.8089 \pm 2.001 \times 0.2111$$

which is $2.81 \pm 0.42$ or $(2.39, 3.23)$. Since we are now considering errors in predicting an average over several countries, this interval is considerably smaller than that found earlier for predicting the outcome for an individual country. Figure 9.4 shows the boundaries of the 95% confidence intervals for the average predictions at all values of sugar within the range of the observed data in Table 9.8. The predictions themselves are simply the fitted SLR line. The minimum interval is for the prediction when sugar consumption takes its mean value (according to the observed data set). As the sugar value, at which prediction is made, moves away from this mean, the interval increases in size.

### 9.3.2 Correlation

A topic closely related to simple linear regression is that of correlation. **Pearson's product-moment correlation coefficient** is a measure of linear association between two quantitative variables, $y$ and $x$. It is defined as the

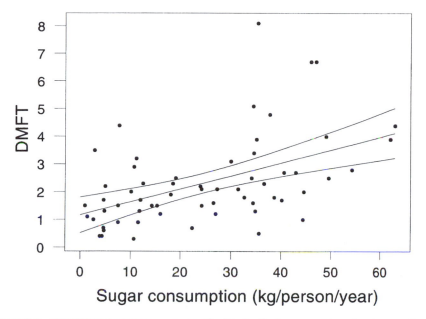

**Figure 9.4**  DMFT against sugar consumption in developing countries, showing predicted mean values and their 95% confidence limits.

covariance divided by the square root of the product of the two variances. Its sample value is defined, using (9.15)–(9.17), as

$$r = \frac{S_{xy}}{\sqrt{S_{xx}S_{yy}}} \tag{9.33}$$

The correlation coefficient takes the value $-1$ for perfectly negatively correlated data, where $y$ goes down as $x$ goes up in a perfect straight line: see Figure 9.5(a). For perfectly positively correlated data, as in Figure 9.5(b), it takes the value unity. The nearer to zero is the correlation coefficient, the less linear association there is between the two variables. Table B.11 gives values of $r$ that provide just sufficient evidence of a non-zero correlation for various sample sizes. Statistical computer packages will produce exact $p$ values.

As the choice of symbol suggests, the correlation coefficient, $r$, is the square root of the coefficient of determination, $r^2$, as defined by (9.21). Hence, for Example 9.5 the correlation coefficient is $\sqrt{0.242} = 0.49$. Here $n = 61$; Table B.11 shows that $p < 0.001$, so there is strong evidence to refute the hypothesis of a lack of linear association between sugar consumption and DMFT in developing countries.

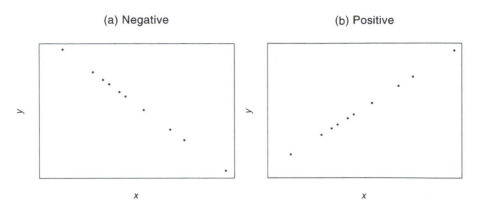

**Figure 9.5** Perfect (a) negative and (b) positive correlation.

Examination of (9.13) and (9.33) shows that

$$r = b\sqrt{\frac{S_{xx}}{S_{yy}}} = b\left\{\frac{\text{standard deviation of } x \text{ values}}{\text{standard deviation of } y \text{ values}}\right\}$$

so that the correlation coefficient and slope of the regression line must vary together. Not surprisingly, tests for significant (i.e. non-zero) correlation and regression are equivalent (Altman, 1991).

Although correlation is a useful summary measure of a relationship, it has drawbacks. First, it tells us nothing about the form this relationship takes, so that, unlike regression, it cannot be used for prediction. Second, a significant correlation merely means that we cannot conclude complete absence of any linear relationship. With the size of data sets that are common in epidemiology, correlations of below ±0.1 may turn out to be significant at extreme levels of significance. This is sometimes erroneously referred to as 'strong correlation'. Third, the significance test assumes that the two variables have a two-dimensional normal distribution. This is not easy to confirm, although it is usually assumed if both the $x$ and $y$ variables are reasonably symmetric (perhaps after a transformation). Fourth, the correlation coefficient can give a misleading summary in certain special circumstances. This includes the cases illustrated by Figure 9.6. Figure 9.6(a) illustrates the case where there is an outlier. There is clearly a negative relationship for the observations without the outlier, and yet application of (9.33) leads to a correlation of $r = 0.97$, quite close to perfect positive correlation. Figure 9.6(b) illustrates the case where the observations cluster

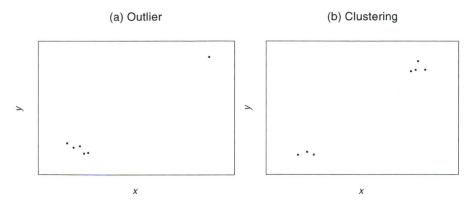

(a) Outlier                                    (b) Clustering

**Figure 9.6** Two situations where use of Pearson's correlation coefficient would be inappropriate.

into two subsets. There is no evidence that $y$ is related to $x$ in either subgroup and yet the correlation is 0.99. Notice that the SLR model would also be inappropriate in these cases; transformations or subgroup analyses may be worth considering when straightforward correlation and SLR are inappropriate. These examples illustrate the need for a scatterplot before deciding upon an appropriate analysis strategy. When the data set is huge some summarization may be required, such as plotting average $y$ values within certain ranges of the $x$ variable.

If we wish to quantify by how much $y$ and $x$ go up (or down) together, without specifying that the relationship follows a straight line, we can use (9.33) with the $x$ and $y$ values replaced by their ranks. The result is called **Spearman's correlation coefficient**. Thus, if the data followed a perfect exponential curve (see Figure 9.7(c)), Spearman's correlation would be exactly unity, whereas Pearson's would be positive but somewhat below unity. For the data of Table 9.8 we find Spearman's correlation coefficient by ranking the 61 $y$ values (Togo $= 1, \ldots$, Guatemala $= 61$) and ranking the 61 $x$ values (Uganda $= 1, \ldots$, Barbados $= 61$). We then apply (9.33) with the $x$ ranks taking the place of $x$, and the $y$ ranks replacing $y$, to give a result of 0.53, slightly bigger than the Pearson correlation.

Spearman's correlation is used, rather than Pearson's, when the $x$ or $y$ data are highly non-normal (including when the data naturally occur in an ordinal form) and transformation cannot help. It is an example of a non-parametric correlation coefficient. Provided that the sample size is even moderately large (say, above 30), Table B.11 may be used to assess the significance of

Spearman's correlation. Conover (1980) gives exact values for use in hypothesis tests when $n \leq 30$.

Further details about correlation, including simple formulae for confidence intervals, are given by Clarke and Cook (1992).


### 9.3.3 Non-linear regression

In Section 9.3.1 we assumed that the relationship between the two quantitative variables being related was linear. Although this is unlikely ever to be exactly true, except in artificial circumstances, it is often a working approximation in epidemiology. Some relationships are, however, certainly not linear and it would then be misleading to describe them by means of linear regression lines. For example, many epidemiological relationships are subject to 'diminishing returns': $y$ increases with $x$ at a continually decreasing rate (see Figure 9.6(d)).

Non-linear regression models may be fitted, although their theory, computation and interpretation can be complex (see Bates and Watts, 1988; Seber and Wild, 1989). In some cases we can find a linear equivalent to the non-linear model through transformation. Only this simple situation will be considered here.

All non-linear modelling procedures begin with inspection of the scatterplot. From this, with some mathematical insight, we hope to deduce the appropriate form of the relationship. For example, if the points on the plot seem to follow the exponential curve (Figure 9.7(c)),

$$\hat{y} = A \exp(Bx), \tag{9.34}$$

for some parameters $A$ and $B$, then this is the non-linear model to fit.

The transformation method works by manipulating the non-linear formula until it takes the linear form. For instance, taking logarithms of both sides in (9.34) gives

$$\log \hat{y} = a + bx, \tag{9.35}$$

which is of the linear form (9.12) if we consider $\log y$ as the outcome variable. Here $a = \log A$ and $b = B$. We use the SLR model to fit the non-linear model by regressing $\log y$ on $x$.

The only drawbacks with this simple procedure are that not all non-linear formulae are linearizable and we must assume that, after transformation, the random error is both normally distributed and additive. For instance, the true values corresponding to (9.35) must satisfy

$$\log y = \alpha + \beta x + \varepsilon,$$

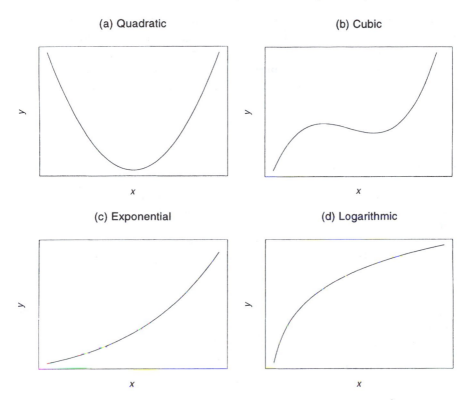

**Figure 9.7**  Some examples of non-linear relationships: (a) $y = A + Bx + Cx^2$; (b) $y = A + Bx + Cx^2 + Dx^3$; (c) $y = A \exp(Bx)$; (d) $y = A + B \log(x)$.

with $\alpha$, $\beta$ and the error term, $\varepsilon$, defined as usual. This assumption of additive normal error is often unreasonable (see Section 9.8 for methods of checking). Sometimes this causes us to switch to an alternative type of regression (Chapters 10 and 11) or to fit, from first principles, a non-linear model with additive normal errors on the original scale. The latter might be attempted using the procedure **PROC NLIN** in the SAS package.

As a guide to choosing an appropriate non-linear equation, Figure 9.7 shows some examples that have been found useful in epidemiological research. Figures 9.7(a) and 9.7(b) are examples of **polynomials**: equations involving integer powers of $x$. The **quadratic**, with terms up to $x^2$, is a second-degree polynomial; the **cubic** is a third-degree polynomial. The first-degree polynomial is the straight line. Polynomials give rise to curves where the number of turning points is equal to the degree of the polynomial minus one. Thus the quadratic has one turning point.

Each example in Figure 9.7 uses values of the parameters ($A$, $B$, etc.) which ensure that $y$ increases as $x$ increases for the biggest values of $x$. Each curve can be flipped over by changing the sign of one or more of the parameters. Each example in Figure 9.7 may be linearized, although the polynomials require a multiple linear regression model (Section 9.7), where the explanatory variables are the powers of $x$.

*Example 9.6*   In Example 9.5 we saw how dental caries depends upon sugar consumption through a linear regression model. In fact, careful scrutiny of Figure 9.2 shows that the linear regression model is not entirely satisfactory for the data given in Table 9.8 (see also Section 9.8), and so a range of non-linear models were considered. One of these was the 'log model', (9.35), which regresses $\log_e$(DMFT) on sugar. To fit this we simply find logs (to base e, although any other base could be used) of all the DMFT values in Table 9.8 and then apply (9.13)–(9.16) taking $y$ as $\log_e$(DMFT) and $x$ as sugar consumption. This results in the fitted regression line

$$\hat{y} = 0.096 + 0.0214x.$$

To obtain the predicted DMFT score at a given value of $x$, say $x = x_0$, we find the antilogs (exponents) of the predicted $y$; thus our prediction is

$$\exp\{0.096 + 0.0214x_0\}.$$

Figure 9.8 shows the predicted DMFT values for each value of sugar consumption within the observed range. As expected, we now have a fitted curve.

Comparing Figure 9.8 with Figure 9.3, the log model does seem to have captured the pattern of the data slightly better. This type of comparison is generally best made through residual plots (Section 9.8).

Table 9.10 gives the ANOVA for the log model. Using (9.21), we find $r^2 = 7.5933/29.1424 = 0.261$. Unfortunately, we cannot compare this directly with the $r^2$ from Table 9.9 (which is smaller) so as to conclude that the log model gives a better fit to the data because the transformation alters the interpretation of $r^2$ on the original scale. Instead, see Example 9.13 for a comparison of the two models. Kvålseth (1985) and Scott and Wild (1991) give a discussion of the $r^2$ problem, whilst Flanders *et al.* (1992) give a general discussion of epidemiological linear regression models with transformations.

It is possible that some other non-linear model might do better for the DMFT data, although it is clear from Figure 9.2 that no mathematical relationship will model the observed DMFT–sugar relationship closely. Considerably better prediction is likely only when other explanatory variables are introduced into the model.

## 9.4   Two categorical explanatory variables

In Section 9.2 we saw how a one-way ANOVA model deals with data that are classified by a single categorical variable or **factor** (as it is often called in this application). The next most complex model of this type would be one with two factors. For example, suppose that we know the sex of each of the subjects

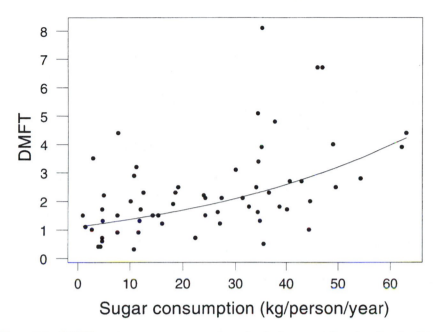

**Figure 9.8**  DMFT against sugar consumption, developing countries, showing the fitted regression curve from the log model.

**Table 9.10**  Analysis of variance table for $\log_e$(DMFT), developing countries

| Source of variation | Sum of squares | Degrees of freedom | Mean square | F ratio | p value |
|---|---|---|---|---|---|
| Regression on sugar | 7.5933 | 1 | 7.5933 | 20.79 | < 0.0001 |
| Error | 21.5491 | 59 | 0.3652 | | |
| Total | 29.1424 | 60 | | | |

identified in Table 9.1. We could then analyse the data to see whether sex or type of diet, or both, influence blood cholesterol. This leads to a **two-way ANOVA**.

### 9.4.1  Model specification

By analogy with (9.6), the two-way ANOVA model for one factor $(x_1)$ with $\ell$ levels and a second $(x_2)$ with $m$ levels may be written as

$$y = \alpha + \beta_1^{(1)}x_1^{(1)} + \beta_1^{(2)}x_1^{(2)} + \cdots + \beta_1^{(\ell)}x_1^{(\ell)}$$
$$+ \beta_2^{(1)}x_2^{(1)} + \beta_2^{(2)}x_2^{(2)} + \cdots + \beta_2^{(m)}x_2^{(m)} + \varepsilon.$$

As always, $y$ and $\varepsilon$ are the outcome variable and random error, respectively. The $\{\beta_1^{(i)}\}$ are a set of $\ell$ parameters representing the effects of each of the levels of $x_1$ and $\{\beta_2^{(i)}\}$ are $m$ parameters representing $x_2$. The $\{x_1^{(i)}\}$ and $\{x_2^{(i)}\}$ are two sets of dummy variables. The intercept term, $\alpha$, is often written as $\beta_0$ to emphasize that it is just another parameter which needs to be estimated. We shall adopt this convention from now on.

As usual, we shall denote the estimated $\beta$s as $b$s. For example, the fitted values from the two-way ANOVA model for the dietary data of Table 9.1 (when sex is known) are given by

$$\hat{y} = b_0 + b_1^{(1)}x_1^{(1)} + b_1^{(2)}x_1^{(2)} + b_1^{(3)}x_1^{(3)} + b_2^{(1)}x_2^{(1)} + b_2^{(2)}x_2^{(2)}, \qquad (9.36)$$

where

$$x_1^{(1)} = \begin{cases} 1 & \text{for omnivores} \\ 0 & \text{otherwise} \end{cases} \qquad x_1^{(2)} = \begin{cases} 1 & \text{for vegetarians} \\ 0 & \text{otherwise} \end{cases}$$

$$x_1^{(3)} = \begin{cases} 1 & \text{for vegans} \\ 0 & \text{otherwise,} \end{cases}$$

$$x_2^{(1)} = \begin{cases} 1 & \text{for men} \\ 0 & \text{for women} \end{cases} \qquad x_2^{(2)} = \begin{cases} 1 & \text{for women} \\ 0 & \text{for men.} \end{cases}$$

To be able to fix the $b$s we need to introduce constraints upon their values, just as in Section 9.2.6. Here we define one constraint for the $b_1$s and another for the $b_2$s. Both will have the general form of (9.10).

## 9.4.2   Model fitting

We shall assume, from now on, that a computer package is available to do the model fitting. The user will need to supply the computer routine with information about $y$, $x_1$ and $x_2$ for each observation. Additionally he or she may have to use the data manipulation facilities within the package to set up two sets of dummy variables (Section 10.4.3), or may have to declare, to the routine that fits models, that $x_1$ and $x_2$ are factors. In the latter case the package will automatically choose its own constraints upon the $b_1$s and $b_2$s, as explained in Section 9.2.7. For example, when PROC GLM in SAS is told that $x_1$ and $x_2$ are CLASS variables it sets the parameters corresponding to the last levels of both $x_1$ and $x_2$ to zero; that is, $b_1^{(\ell)} = 0$ and $b_2^{(m)} = 0$.

The output produced will depend upon the package, and sometimes the particular procedure chosen, where there is a choice. We can certainly expect to see an ANOVA table, but parameter estimates and/or fitted values may only appear after a special sub-command is issued.

### 9.4.3  Balanced data

The data are **balanced** if each level of one factor occurs the same number of times within each level of the second factor. Equivalently, each factor combination must occur the same number of times. Thus in Table 9.1, when we introduce sex as a further factor, the data would be balanced if half of the subjects in each diet group were male. We would then have three replicates of each of the $3 \times 2 = 6$ factor combinations; for instance, there would be three male vegetarians.

The great advantage of balanced data is that we obtain independent estimates of the effect of each factor. This is a great help in the interpretation of results and leads to simple computation procedures (see Clarke and Kempson, 1997). However, epidemiological research rarely produces balanced data by chance; this is normally achieved through design. The only situation where such a design is common is an intervention study. Even then, drop-outs (leading to missing values) can destroy the designed balance.

Most non-statistical commercial software that fits two-way ANOVA models will only deal with balanced data. Due to the simplicity of balance, several specialist statistical packages include a routine that only deals with balanced data. Such routines are straightforward to use, and will not be considered further here. An example (as mentioned already) is PROC ANOVA in SAS.

### 9.4.4  Unbalanced data

As indicated above, unbalanced data are the norm in observational epidemiology (surveys, cohort and case–control studies). In this case, we shall not be able to assess the separate effects of the two factors simultaneously. Instead we can assess their combined effect, through a one-way ANOVA where the 'group SS' will now be called the **model SS**. For a two-way study, without consideration of interaction, the model d.f. will be $(\ell - 1) + (m - 1)$, this being the sum of the d.f. for the $x_1$ and $x_2$ factors.

The combined effect is, however, of limited epidemiological interest: really we would like to split it into its components. We can only do this by considering the factors sequentially, allowing for what went before. The effect of the first factor entered into the model is then obtained unconditionally, but the second is evaluated after allowing for the first. By convention 'bar notation' is used to specify conditional effects, as in 'second|first' (see Table 9.12 for a practical example). Sequential fitting gives rise to a **sequential ANOVA** table where the model SS is split into two components called the **sequential SS** (or, in SAS, the **Type I SS**). The sequential SS will sum to the model SS.

One problem with the sequential approach is that the factors are treated in a different way, which may compromise the interpretation. An alternative is to consider the effect of each factor after allowing for the other. This leads to **cross-adjusted SS** (called **Type III SS** by SAS and **unique SS** by SPSS), which do not total to the model SS (unless the data are balanced). The cross-adjusted approach is used when $t$ tests are provided for the $\beta$ parameters within computer output: for instance, in the two-way ANOVA results of Output 9.9.

Since the cross-adjusted SS, and the second of the sequential SS, measure the effect of one variable adjusted for the other, they give a means for adjustment to deal with confounding (Chapter 4). This topic will be considered further in Section 9.9.

The SAS package prints Type I and III SS by default. The Type II SS may also be useful. These are like the Type III SS except that the cross-adjustment now fails to include any interaction terms.

*Example 9.7*    For the data in Table 9.1, suppose that it turned out that subjects 1, 2, 4, 5 and 6 in the omnivore group, subject 6 in the vegetarian group and subject 1 in the vegan group are men; all others are women. This is illustrated by Table 9.11. The data were read into SAS and the two-way ANOVA model was fitted using PROC GLM. The results appear as Output 9.3 (here SAS results are given without the table of parameter estimates).

The Type I (sequential) and Type III (cross-adjusted) SS list the variables in the order fitted in the model; here DIET was fitted first. The Type I and III SS for the final (second) term fitted (SEX) must always be the same, and thus provide the same test, as indeed they do here: SEX has a significant effect ($p = 0.0087$) even after the effect of diet has been accounted for. The Type I and III SS, and associated tests, for DIET differ: DIET is highly significant ($p < 0.0001$) when considered alone, but not as significant ($p = 0.0021$) when considered in the presence of SEX. Clearly some of the effect of diet on cholesterol is explained by the effect of sex: the non-meat eaters tend to be female, whilst it is men who tend to have higher values of cholesterol (see Table 9.11).

Notice that the Type I SS correctly sum to the model SS, which has three degrees of freedom (two for diet plus one for sex). Table 9.12 is the sequential ANOVA table constructed from Output 9.3. (with rounded values). This shows how the Type I SS split the entire 'model' source of variation into two components, with associated tests based on the usual $F$ ratios using the error MS as the denominator. The error d.f. is most easily understood as the total d.f. less the d.f. of each of the two factors.

**Table 9.11**    Serum total cholesterol (mmol/l) by sex and type of diet

|  | Diet group | | |
|---|---|---|---|
|  | Omnivores | Vegetarians | Vegans |
| Male |  |  |  |
|  | 6.35 | 6.11 | 6.01 |
|  | 6.47 |  |  |
|  | 6.37 |  |  |
|  | 6.11 |  |  |
|  | 6.50 |  |  |
| Mean | 6.360 | 6.110 | 6.010 |
| Female |  |  |  |
|  | 6.09 | 5.92 | 5.42 |
|  |  | 6.03 | 5.44 |
|  |  | 5.81 | 5.82 |
|  |  | 6.07 | 5.73 |
|  |  | 5.73 | 6.62 |
| Mean | 6.090 | 5.912 | 5.606 |
| Overall Mean | 6.315 | 5.945 | 5.673 |

**Output 9.3**    SAS results for Example 9.7

General Linear Models Procedure

Dependent Variable: CHOLEST

| Source | DF | Sum of Squares | Mean Square | F Value | Pr > F |
|---|---|---|---|---|---|
| Model | 3 | 1.4560956 | 0.4853652 | 21.33 | 0.0001 |
| Error | 14 | 0.3186156 | 0.0227583 |  |  |
| Corrected Total | 17 | 1.7747111 |  |  |  |

| | R-Square | C.V. | Root MSE | CHOLEST Mean |
|---|---|---|---|---|
| | 0.820469 | 2.523653 | 0.1509 | 5.9778 |

| Source | DF | Type I SS | Mean Square | F Value | Pr > F |
|---|---|---|---|---|---|
| DIET | 2 | 1.2448778 | 0.6224389 | 27.35 | 0.0001 |
| SEX | 1 | 0.2112178 | 0.2112178 | 9.28 | 0.0087 |

| Source | DF | Type III SS | Mean Square | F Value | Pr > F |
|---|---|---|---|---|---|
| DIET | 2 | 0.4490468 | 0.2245234 | 9.87 | 0.0021 |
| SEX | 1 | 0.2112178 | 0.2112178 | 9.28 | 0.0087 |

**Table 9.12**   Sequential ANOVA table for Example 9.7

| Source of variation | Sum of squares | Degrees of freedom | Mean square | F ratio | p value |
|---|---|---|---|---|---|
| Diet | 1.2447 | 2 | 0.6225 | 27.3 | <0.0001 |
| Sex\|Diet | 0.2112 | 1 | 0.2112 | 9.3 | 0.009 |
| Error | 0.3186 | 14 | 0.0228 | | |
| Total | 1.7747 | 17 | | | |

Of course, the order of fitting terms into the model could be altered so that SEX comes first. This would give rise to a different sequential ANOVA table including a test for the effect of sex uncorrected for diet.

*Example 9.8*   Suppose, instead, that the first three subjects within each diet group in Table 9.1 were male and the rest were female. Output 9.4 gives the results from fitting a two-way ANOVA to this data structure. The data are now balanced and so the Type I and III SS are equal, and both sum to the model SS. The effects of sex and diet can be simultaneously evaluated: diet has a significant effect on cholesterol ($p = 0.0002$) but sex has no discernible effect ($p = 0.5330$).

**Output 9.4**   SAS results for Example 9.8

General Linear Models Procedure

Dependent Variable: CHOLEST

| Source | DF | Sum of Squares | Mean Square | F Value | Pr > F |
|---|---|---|---|---|---|
| Model | 3 | 1.25990000 | 0.41996667 | 11.42 | 0.0005 |
| Error | 14 | 0.51481111 | 0.03677222 | | |
| Corrected Total | 17 | 1.77471111 | | | |

| | R-Square | C.V. | Root MSE | CHOLEST Mean |
|---|---|---|---|---|
| | 0.709918 | 3.207895 | 0.1917608 | 5.9777778 |

| Source | DF | Type I SS | Mean Square | F Value | Pr > F |
|---|---|---|---|---|---|
| DIET | 2 | 1.24487778 | 0.62243889 | 16.93 | 0.0002 |
| SEX | 1 | 0.01502222 | 0.01502222 | 0.41 | 0.5330 |

| Source | DF | Type III SS | Mean Square | F Value | Pr > F |
|---|---|---|---|---|---|
| DIET | 2 | 1.24487778 | 0.62243889 | 16.93 | 0.0002 |
| SEX | 1 | 0.01502222 | 0.01502222 | 0.41 | 0.5330 |

### 9.4.5   Fitted values

As in Section 9.2.7, we can use the parameter estimates produced by the computer package to find the fitted values (model predictions). For instance, Table 9.13 shows the parameter estimates, as produced by SAS PROC GENMOD, for Example 9.7. Notice that the final parameter in each of the two sets is zero because this is the constraint imposed by SAS. Other packages may use different rules, although the method presented here would still be applicable. Results, such as those in Table 9.13, need to be substituted into (9.36). For example, consider the fitted value for male omnivores. Here $x_1^{(1)} = 1$, $x_2^{(1)} = 1$ and all other $x$s are zero. Hence, in (9.36),

$$\hat{y} = 5.62489 + 0.44789 + 0.29067 = 6.3635.$$

For female omnivores the corresponding sum is

$$\hat{y} = 5.62489 + 0.44789 + 0 = 6.0728.$$

These and the remaining predictions are shown in Table 9.14. Notice that these results differ from the sex-specific dietary group sample means shown in Table 9.11.

### 9.4.6   Least-squares means

Fitted values give predictions for the average value in the cross-classes (see Table 9.14), but we often wish to have predictions for one (or both) of the factors alone. We do this by averaging out the effect of the other factor, using

**Table 9.13**   Parameter estimates produced by SAS for Example 9.7

| Intercept $b_0$ | Diet | | | Sex | |
|---|---|---|---|---|---|
| | $b_1^{(1)}$ | $b_1^{(2)}$ | $b_1^{(3)}$ | $b_2^{(1)}$ | $b_2^{(2)}$ |
| 5.62489 | 0.44789 | 0.27167 | 0 | 0.29067 | 0 |

**Table 9.14**   Fitted values for Example 9.7

| Sex | Diet group | | |
|---|---|---|---|
| | Omnivores | Vegetarians | Vegans |
| Male | 6.3635 | 6.1872 | 5.9156 |
| Female | 6.0728 | 5.8966 | 5.6249 |

the fitted values. Since the fitted values are based on least-squares estimation we call these averaged-out values **least-squares means**. They are also known as **adjusted means**.

For example, the least-squares means for diet from Table 9.14 are: for omnivores, $(6.3635 + 6.0728)/2 = 6.218$; for vegetarians, $(6.1872 + 5.8966)/2 = 6.042$; for vegans, $(5.9156 + 5.6249)/2 = 5.770$. These are interpreted as the predicted values of cholesterol for each diet group after taking account of the effect of sex. Hence, if sex were considered a confounder, these could be called confounder-adjusted estimates. Notice that these adjusted estimates differ from the overall means given in Table 9.11, indicating that sex has had some effect.

Although they are of less practical sense here, we could work out least-squares means for sex, adjusted for diet. For instance, the diet-adjusted least-squares mean for men is $(6.3635 + 6.1872 + 5.9156)/3 = 6.155$.

Sometimes it is sensible to test whether a least-squares mean is zero. More often, in epidemiology, we wish to compare least-square means. Computer procedures, such as SAS PROC GLM, can be made to do this. Output 9.5 shows SAS results for diet in Example 9.7 (here the DIET codes are $1 =$ omnivore, $2 =$ vegetarian, $3 =$ vegan, as before). Notice that the means agree with the rounded values derived above. All means are significantly different from zero $(p < 0.0001)$, but this is only to be expected: no one has zero cholesterol. Of more interest are the comparative tests: after allowing for sex effects we see that vegans have significantly lower cholesterol than both omnivores $(p = 0.001)$ and vegetarians $(p = 0.0075)$. As mentioned in Section 9.2.5, caution is advisable with such multiple testing.

**Output 9.5**    Further SAS results for Example 9.7

General Linear Models Procedure

Least Squares Means

| DIET | CHOLEST LSMEAN | Std Err LSMEAN | Pr > |T| H0:LSMEAN = 0 | LSMEAN Number |
|---|---|---|---|---|
| 1 | 6.21811111 | 0.06931465 | 0.0001 | 1 |
| 2 | 6.04188889 | 0.06931465 | 0.0001 | 2 |
| 3 | 5.77022222 | 0.06931465 | 0.0001 | 3 |

Pr > |T| H0: LSMEAN (i) = LSMEAN (j)

| i/j | 1 | 2 | 3 |
|---|---|---|---|
| 1 | . | 0.1246 | 0.0010 |
| 2 | 0.1246 | . | 0.0075 |
| 3 | 0.0010 | 0.0075 | . |

## 9.4.7  Interaction

In Section 4.7 the basic concepts of interaction were introduced. In the current context an interaction would occur if the effect of one factor differed depending upon the value of the second factor. In Example 9.7 there could be a different effect of diet on blood cholesterol for men and women.

The two-way ANOVA, discussed so far, can be extended to include an interaction. Interaction terms are simply the cross-multiplied terms of the constituent or **main effects**. Thus if the two main effects have $\ell$ and $m$ levels respectively, we define the interaction by the $\ell m$ new $x$ variables derived as the cross-products of the dummy variables representing the main effects.

For example, we can extend (9.36) to include a sex by diet interaction by creating variables,

$$x_3^{(11)} = x_1^{(1)}x_2^{(1)} \qquad x_3^{(21)} = x_1^{(2)}x_2^{(1)} \qquad x_3^{(31)} = x_1^{(3)}x_2^{(1)}$$
$$x_3^{(12)} = x_1^{(1)}x_2^{(2)} \qquad x_3^{(22)} = x_1^{(2)}x_2^{(2)} \qquad x_3^{(32)} = x_1^{(3)}x_2^{(2)},$$

each of which is to be multiplied by a corresponding $b_3$ parameter in the fitted model. For instance, using the definition of $x_1^{(1)}$ and $x_2^{(1)}$ given in Section 9.4.1,

$$x_3^{(11)} = \begin{cases} 1 & \text{if } x_1 = 1 \text{ and } x_2 = 1 \\ 0 & \text{otherwise;} \end{cases}$$

so $x_3^{(11)}$ is unity only for male omnivores, otherwise it is zero. The fitted two-way ANOVA model with interaction for this example is

$$\hat{y} = b_0 + b_1^{(1)}x_1^{(1)} + b_1^{(2)}x_1^{(2)} + b_1^{(3)}x_1^{(3)} + b_2^{(1)}x_2^{(1)} + b_2^{(2)}x_2^{(2)}$$
$$+ b_3^{(11)}x_3^{(11)} + b_3^{(21)}x_3^{(21)} + b_3^{(31)}x_3^{(31)} + b_3^{(12)}x_3^{(12)} + b_3^{(22)}x_3^{(22)} + b_3^{(32)}x_3^{(32)}.$$

$$(9.37)$$

The interaction can be fitted on computer using dummy variables exactly as suggested here (Section 10.9) or by including an interaction term in a model declaration made to a procedure that recognizes factors and interactions, such as PROC GLM in SAS. As before, constraints will need to be made to enable estimation, and we must know which method the computer package uses. Since, in general, the first factor has $\ell - 1$ d.f. and the second has $m - 1$, the interaction, defined through their product, has $(\ell - 1)(m - 1)$ d.f. As $\ell m$ terms are used to define the interaction, we therefore need to introduce $\ell m - (\ell - 1)(m - 1) = \ell + m - 1$ independent linear constraints.

Since SAS sets the parameter for the last level of a factor (CLASS variable) to zero, it also sets the corresponding interaction parameters to zero. That is, $b_3^{(ij)}$ is fixed at zero when $i$ is the last level of $x_1$ or $j$ is the last level of $x_2$. Other packages will have similar rules.

Fitted values, and thus least-squares means, from a two-way ANOVA model with interaction simply reproduce the observed sample means (given in Table 9.11).

*Example 9.9*    Output 9.6 shows the Type I SS and parameter estimates from fitting the two-way ANOVA model with interaction to the data of Table 9.11. There is no significant interaction ($p = 0.7024$) in this case. Notice that, for example, the fitted value for male omnivores (DIET = 1, SEX = 1) is found from picking out all the appropriate terms in (9.37); that is, with rounding,

$$5.606 + 0.484 + 0.404 - 0.134 = 6.360.$$

This is the sample mean for male omnivores given in Table 9.11.

## 9.5    Model building

When we have two factors the two-way ANOVA model is not necessarily the appropriate one for the data. An interesting epidemiological question is whether a simpler one-way ANOVA will suffice. If it will, then we can say that one of the two factors is sufficient for predicting the quantitative outcome variable.

**Output 9.6**    SAS results for Example 9.9

General Linear Models Procedure

| Source | DF | Type I SS | Mean Square | F Value | Pr > F |
|---|---|---|---|---|---|
| DIET | 2 | 1.2448778 | 0.6224389 | 24.86 | 0.0001 |
| SEX | 1 | 0.2112178 | 0.2112178 | 8.44 | 0.0132 |
| DIET*SEX | 2 | 0.0182156 | 0.0091078 | 0.36 | 0.7024 |

| Parameter | | Estimate | T for H0: Parameter = 0 | Pr > |T| | Std Error of Estimate |
|---|---|---|---|---|---|
| INTERCEPT | | 5.606000000 B | 79.23 | 0.0001 | 0.07075780 |
| DIET | 1 | 0.484000000 B | 2.79 | 0.0163 | 0.17332051 |
| | 2 | 0.306000000 B | 3.06 | 0.0099 | 0.10006664 |
| | 3 | 0.000000000 B | . | . | . |
| SEX | 1 | 0.404000000 B | 2.33 | 0.0380 | 0.17332051 |
| | 2 | 0.000000000 B | . | . | . |
| DIET*SEX | 1 1 | −0.134000000 B | −0.55 | 0.5946 | 0.24511222 |
| | 1 2 | 0.000000000 B | . | . | . |
| | 2 1 | −0.206000000 B | −0.84 | 0.4171 | 0.24511222 |
| | 2 2 | 0.000000000 B | . | . | . |
| | 3 1 | 0.000000000 B | . | . | . |
| | 3 2 | 0.000000000 B | . | . | . |

There are five possible models that could be adopted when two factors have been observed: the **empty** (or **null**) model (that with no factors); the two one-way ANOVA models; the two-way ANOVA; and the two-way with interaction. In epidemiological research we may often find it useful to fit all possible models because this provides insight into the relationships between the outcome variable and the factors, and gives precise information for model selection. The empty model, which assumes that no factors have any effect (that is, $\hat{y} = \bar{y}$), is so simple that it may well be unnecessary to fit it. Having fitted all the models, we sometimes wish to decide upon one model that is, in some sense, 'best'. We can use $F$ tests from ANOVA tables to help make our decision.

Thus, for the balanced data of Example 9.8, we would reject the two-factor model, and conclude that the simpler one-way model with diet alone will suffice (that is, sex can be ignored in determining cholesterol). However, notice that we have not tested for an interaction in Example 9.8; it would be dangerous to delete a variable before considering its role within interactions.

Whenever we fit an ANOVA model that includes all possible interactions between all the factors included in the model, the fitted values must equal the sample means, because there is no source of variation left unaccounted for, between groups. This has already been seen in the one-way ANOVA of Section 9.2.7 (where there can be no interactions) and the two-way ANOVA with interaction of Section 9.4.7.

*Example 9.10*    Table 9.15 gives data from a random sample of 150 subjects from the Scottish Heart Health Study (SHHS). In this exercise we wish to see how body mass index (BMI) depends upon both cigarette smoking history and a person's sex. Table 9.16 gives some summary statistics calculated from Table 9.15.

Taking BMI as the $y$ variable, sex as $x_1$ and smoking as $x_2$, we have four possible (non-empty) models:
1.  $y$ versus $x_1$ (BMI depends upon sex alone);
2.  $y$ versus $x_2$ (BMI depends upon smoking alone);
3.  $y$ versus $x_1$ and $x_2$ (BMI depends upon both sex and smoking);
4.  $y$ versus $x_1, x_2$ and their interaction (BMI depends upon smoking status in a different way for men and women).

Models 1 and 2 are both one-way ANOVA models, model 3 is a two-way (unbalanced) ANOVA and model 4 is a two-way ANOVA with interaction.

We could fit models 1 and 2 using formulae given in Section 9.2, where $\ell$ (the number of groups) is 2 and 3, respectively. Instead of this, we shall view SAS output. The data from Table 9.15 were read into SAS; Outputs 9.7 and 9.8 show excerpts from the SAS results from fitting models 1 and 2, respectively. As both are one-term models (they have a single $x$ variable), Types I and III sums of squares and mean squares are irrelevant; they simply repeat the model SS and MS, and so are omitted here. Parameter estimates are easily interpreted by reference to the marginal (row and column) totals of Table 9.16 (see Section 9.2.7 for explanation).

**Table 9.15**  Body mass index (kg/m$^2$), sex and cigarette smoking status for a random sample of 150 subjects in the SHHS. Codes for sex are 1 = male, 2 = female. Codes for smoking are 1 = current, 2 = ex, 3 = never

| Body mass index | Sex | Smoking status | Body mass index | Sex | Smoking status | Body mass index | Sex | Smoking status |
|---|---|---|---|---|---|---|---|---|
| 30.25 | 1 | 3 | 24.34 | 1 | 2 | 29.01 | 1 | 3 |
| 24.16 | 1 | 3 | 26.85 | 1 | 2 | 24.74 | 1 | 1 |
| 23.29 | 1 | 1 | 26.75 | 1 | 1 | 28.73 | 1 | 1 |
| 24.11 | 1 | 1 | 26.58 | 1 | 2 | 25.95 | 1 | 3 |
| 21.20 | 1 | 1 | 28.65 | 1 | 2 | 27.10 | 1 | 1 |
| 26.67 | 1 | 2 | 24.46 | 1 | 3 | 28.03 | 1 | 2 |
| 25.93 | 1 | 2 | 24.57 | 1 | 2 | 24.45 | 1 | 1 |
| 26.59 | 1 | 3 | 19.72 | 1 | 1 | 20.55 | 1 | 1 |
| 21.72 | 1 | 2 | 30.85 | 1 | 3 | 23.80 | 1 | 2 |
| 25.10 | 1 | 1 | 25.26 | 1 | 3 | 32.18 | 1 | 3 |
| 27.78 | 1 | 1 | 27.18 | 1 | 2 | 25.39 | 2 | 3 |
| 25.07 | 2 | 2 | 25.16 | 2 | 2 | 28.38 | 1 | 3 |
| 21.45 | 2 | 1 | 32.87 | 2 | 3 | 25.22 | 2 | 3 |
| 23.53 | 2 | 1 | 23.50 | 2 | 3 | 26.03 | 2 | 2 |
| 22.94 | 2 | 1 | 34.85 | 2 | 2 | 25.56 | 2 | 2 |
| 22.03 | 2 | 3 | 23.88 | 2 | 2 | 26.90 | 2 | 2 |
| 27.12 | 2 | 2 | 26.72 | 2 | 3 | 26.90 | 2 | 3 |
| 24.39 | 2 | 2 | 26.85 | 1 | 1 | 25.96 | 2 | 3 |
| 24.24 | 2 | 2 | 26.02 | 2 | 1 | 24.75 | 2 | 1 |
| 28.35 | 2 | 2 | 20.80 | 1 | 3 | 21.45 | 2 | 1 |
| 27.03 | 2 | 3 | 28.34 | 1 | 1 | 22.55 | 1 | 3 |
| 30.12 | 2 | 3 | 24.00 | 2 | 1 | 25.96 | 1 | 3 |
| 27.97 | 1 | 3 | 28.84 | 2 | 3 | 23.80 | 2 | 3 |
| 24.77 | 2 | 1 | 26.35 | 1 | 1 | 21.91 | 2 | 2 |
| 23.89 | 1 | 3 | 22.77 | 2 | 3 | 20.55 | 2 | 3 |
| 19.29 | 2 | 1 | 18.72 | 2 | 3 | 21.61 | 2 | 2 |
| 24.24 | 2 | 3 | 26.13 | 2 | 1 | 24.52 | 2 | 2 |
| 22.46 | 2 | 2 | 20.32 | 2 | 1 | 22.38 | 2 | 2 |
| 26.44 | 2 | 3 | 25.56 | 2 | 3 | 24.46 | 2 | 2 |
| 23.44 | 2 | 1 | 23.05 | 2 | 1 | 23.83 | 2 | 1 |
| 28.09 | 1 | 3 | 25.01 | 1 | 1 | 29.00 | 1 | 2 |
| 28.67 | 1 | 2 | 15.55 | 1 | 1 | 25.31 | 1 | 2 |
| 26.99 | 1 | 2 | 24.34 | 1 | 1 | 23.30 | 1 | 1 |
| 31.31 | 1 | 2 | 22.57 | 1 | 2 | 24.91 | 1 | 1 |
| 25.83 | 1 | 1 | 29.03 | 1 | 2 | 29.48 | 1 | 2 |
| 29.37 | 1 | 1 | 23.99 | 1 | 1 | 29.04 | 1 | 1 |
| 28.96 | 1 | 2 | 27.16 | 1 | 1 | 24.82 | 1 | 1 |
| 21.91 | 1 | 2 | 25.88 | 1 | 2 | 24.05 | 1 | 3 |
| 32.42 | 1 | 1 | 28.74 | 1 | 2 | 33.08 | 1 | 3 |

**Table 9.15**   *cont.*

| Body mass index | Sex | Smoking status | Body mass index | Sex | Smoking status | Body mass index | Sex | Smoking status |
|---|---|---|---|---|---|---|---|---|
| 25.22 | 1 | 3 | 24.76 | 1 | 2 | 31.96 | 1 | 1 |
| 35.74 | 1 | 2 | 31.21 | 1 | 1 | 26.51 | 1 | 3 |
| 29.71 | 1 | 3 | 24.90 | 1 | 2 | 19.96 | 1 | 1 |
| 29.94 | 2 | 3 | 25.39 | 2 | 1 | 30.12 | 2 | 3 |
| 33.95 | 2 | 3 | 25.15 | 2 | 1 | 32.02 | 2 | 3 |
| 21.17 | 2 | 1 | 33.75 | 2 | 3 | 22.77 | 2 | 3 |
| 20.57 | 2 | 1 | 21.91 | 2 | 1 | 22.52 | 2 | 1 |
| 20.81 | 2 | 1 | 27.14 | 2 | 2 | 28.16 | 2 | 1 |
| 29.27 | 2 | 3 | 21.36 | 2 | 3 | 28.80 | 2 | 3 |
| 32.05 | 2 | 3 | 24.01 | 2 | 1 | 27.46 | 1 | 1 |
| 26.61 | 2 | 3 | 22.94 | 2 | 1 | 24.91 | 2 | 3 |

Note: These data are available electronically – see Appendix C.

The $F$ test in Output 9.7 shows that sex is important as a predictor of BMI (it is only just non-significant at the customary 5% significance level; $p = 0.0512$). Output 9.8 shows that smoking is very significant ($p = 0.0019$). Hence both sex and smoking are 'needed' in the absence of the other, although smoking is the most important predictor of the two.

Output 9.9 gives the results of fitting model 3. The model SS has three degrees of freedom, made up of one from SEX (since it has two levels) and two from SMOKING (since it has three levels). The model terms are significant ($p = 0.0004$) when taken together, but this fact does not lead to a simple epidemiological interpretation. We need to break up the SS (and d.f.) in order to provide useful results.

The first break-up gives the Type I (sequential) SS. The $x$ terms SEX and SMOKING were introduced in this order and so the Type I SS shows the effect of SEX alone and then the effect of SMOKING after accounting for SEX. Both are significant at the 5% level. So SEX is a useful predictor by itself and SMOKING is useful even when we have accounted for SEX. The sequential ANOVA table, constructed from the SAS results, is given as Table 9.17.

**Table 9.16**   Mean BMI (kg/m$^2$) by cigarette smoking status and sex (sample size given in brackets), data from Table 9.15

| Smoking status | Sex | | |
|---|---|---|---|
| | 1 (Male) | 2 (Female) | Total |
| 1 (Current) | 25.53 (31) | 23.23 (24) | 24.53 (55) |
| 2 (Ex) | 26.83 (26) | 25.34 (18) | 26.22 (44) |
| 3 (Never) | 26.90 (21) | 26.74 (30) | 26.81 (51) |
| Total | 26.33 (78) | 25.22 (72) | 25.80 (150) |

**Output 9.7**   SAS results from fitting model 1 of Example 9.10

General Linear Models Procedure

Dependent Variable: BMI

| Source | DF | Sum of Squares | Mean Square | F Value | Pr > F |
|---|---|---|---|---|---|
| Model | 1 | 46.279129 | 46.279129 | 3.86 | 0.0512 |
| Error | 148 | 1772.354349 | 11.975367 | | |
| Corrected Total | 149 | 1818.633477 | | | |

| | R-Square | C.V. | Root MSE | BMI Mean |
|---|---|---|---|---|
| | 0.025447 | 13.41393 | 3.4605 | 25.798 |

| Parameter | Estimate | T for H0: Parameter = 0 | Pr > \|T\| | Std Error of Estimate |
|---|---|---|---|---|
| INTERCEPT | 25.22000000 B | 61.84 | 0.0001 | 0.40782906 |
| SEX   1 | 1.11179487 B | 1.97 | 0.0512 | 0.56555715 |
|         2 | 0.00000000 B | . | . | . |

**Output 9.8**   SAS results from fitting model 2 of Example 9.10

General Linear Models Procedure

Dependent Variable: BMI

| Source | DF | Sum of Squares | Mean Square | F Value | Pr > F |
|---|---|---|---|---|---|
| Model | 2 | 148.47252 | 74.23626 | 6.53 | 0.0019 |
| Error | 147 | 1670.16095 | 11.36164 | | |
| Corrected Total | 149 | 1818.63348 | | | |

| | R-Square | C.V. | Root MSE | BMI Mean |
|---|---|---|---|---|
| | 0.081640 | 13.06569 | 3.3707 | 25.798 |

| Parameter | Estimate | T for H0: Parameter = 0 | Pr > \|T\| | Std Error of Estimate |
|---|---|---|---|---|
| INTERCEPT | 26.80647059 B | 56.79 | 0.0001 | 0.47199284 |
| SMOKING   1 | −2.27937968 B | −3.48 | 0.0007 | 0.65524995 |
|           2 | −0.58828877 B | −0.85 | 0.3977 | 0.69353897 |
|           3 | 0.00000000 B | . | . | . |

The Type III (cross-adjusted) SS show the effect of SEX accounting for SMOKING and SMOKING accounting for SEX. The latter, of course, repeats the corresponding Type I result. The new result here is that SEX is important even when we know SMOKING (indeed it is even more important since $p = 0.0158$ now, rather than 0.0420).

Notice that the model SS in Output 9.9 is greater than the sum of those in Outputs 9.7 and 9.8 (214.04 > 46.28 + 148.47), showing that sex and smoking do not act independently.

**Output 9.9**    SAS results from fitting model 3 of Example 9.10

General Linear Models Procedure

Dependent Variable: BMI

| Source | DF | Sum of Squares | Mean Square | F Value | Pr > F |
|---|---|---|---|---|---|
| Model | 3 | 214.03997 | 71.34666 | 6.49 | 0.0004 |
| Error | 146 | 1604.59351 | 10.99037 | | |
| Corrected Total | 149 | 1818.63348 | | | |

| | R-Square | C.V. | Root MSE | | BMI Mean |
|---|---|---|---|---|---|
| | 0.117693 | 12.85043 | 3.3152 | | 25.798 |

| Source | DF | Type I SS | Mean Square | F Value | Pr > F |
|---|---|---|---|---|---|
| SEX | 1 | 46.27913 | 46.27913 | 4.21 | 0.0420 |
| SMOKING | 2 | 167.76084 | 83.88042 | 7.63 | 0.0007 |

| Source | DF | Type III SS | Mean Square | F Value | Pr > F |
|---|---|---|---|---|---|
| SEX | 1 | 65.56745 | 65.56745 | 5.97 | 0.0158 |
| SMOKING | 2 | 167.76084 | 83.88042 | 7.63 | 0.0007 |

| Parameter | | Estimate | T for H0: Parameter=0 | Pr > \|T\| | Std Error of Estimate |
|---|---|---|---|---|---|
| INTERCEPT | | 26.25471312 B | 50.86 | 0.0001 | 0.51626231 |
| SEX | 1 | 1.33998243 B | 2.44 | 0.0158 | 0.54860663 |
| | 2 | 0.00000000 B | . | . | . |
| SMOKING | 1 | −2.48288503 B | −3.82 | 0.0002 | 0.64981850 |
| | 2 | −0.82833910 B | −1.20 | 0.2313 | 0.68915699 |
| | 3 | 0.00000000 B | . | . | . |

**Table 9.17**    Sequential ANOVA table for BMI $(kg/m^2)$, data from Table 9.15, results taken from Output 9.9

| Source of variation | Sum of squares | Degrees of freedom | Mean square | F ratio | p value |
|---|---|---|---|---|---|
| Sex | 46.28 | 1 | 46.28 | 4.21 | 0.04 |
| Smoking\|Sex | 167.76 | 2 | 83.88 | 7.63 | 0.0007 |
| Error | 1604.59 | 146 | 10.99 | | |
| Total | 1818.63 | 149 | | | |

Indeed, they seem to act antagonistically (Section 4.7), explaining the increasing significance of sex after accounting for smoking. The model SS in Output 9.7 is, as it should be, the Type I SS for SEX in Output 9.9 and the two Type I SS in Output 9.9 correctly add to the model SS in the same display.

**Output 9.10**    SAS results from fitting model 4 of Example 9.10

General Linear Models Procedure

Dependent Variable: BMI

| Source | DF | Sum of Squares | Mean Square | F Value | Pr > F |
|---|---|---|---|---|---|
| Model | 5 | 243.82337 | 48.76467 | 4.46 | 0.0008 |
| Error | 144 | 1574.81011 | 10.93618 | | |
| Corrected Total | 149 | 1818.63348 | | | |

| R-Square | C.V. | Root MSE | BMI Mean |
|---|---|---|---|
| 0.134070 | 12.81872 | 3.3070 | 25.798 |

| Source | DF | Type I SS | Mean Square | F Value | Pr > F |
|---|---|---|---|---|---|
| SEX | 1 | 46.27913 | 46.27913 | 4.23 | 0.0415 |
| SMOKING | 2 | 167.76084 | 83.88042 | 7.67 | 0.0007 |
| SMOKING*SEX | 2 | 29.78340 | 14.89170 | 1.36 | 0.2595 |

| Source | DF | Type III SS | Mean Square | F Value | Pr > F |
|---|---|---|---|---|---|
| SEX | 1 | 62.70666 | 62.70666 | 5.73 | 0.0179 |
| SMOKING | 2 | 162.40502 | 81.20251 | 7.43 | 0.0009 |
| SMOKING*SEX | 2 | 29.78340 | 14.89170 | 1.36 | 0.2595 |

| Parameter | | Estimate | T for H0: Parameter = 0 | Pr > \|T\| | Std Error of Estimate |
|---|---|---|---|---|---|
| INTERCEPT | | 26.74033333 B | 44.29 | 0.0001 | 0.60377096 |
| SEX | 1 | 0.16061905 B | 0.17 | 0.8647 | 0.94090909 |
| | 2 | 0.00000000 B | . | . | . |
| SMOKING | 1 | −3.50700000 B | −3.87 | 0.0002 | 0.90565645 |
| | 2 | −1.40533333 B | −1.43 | 0.1562 | 0.98595385 |
| | 3 | 0.00000000 B | . | . | . |
| SMOKING*SEX | 1 1 | 2.13475730 B | 1.64 | 0.1031 | 1.30144695 |
| | 1 2 | 0.00000000 B | . | . | . |
| | 2 1 | 1.33399634 B | 0.96 | 0.3365 | 1.38329241 |
| | 2 2 | 0.00000000 B | . | . | . |
| | 3 1 | 0.00000000 B | . | . | . |
| | 3 2 | 0.00000000 B | . | . | . |

Output 9.10 is for model 4. The crucial test in this listing is that for the SMOKING by SEX interaction (written with an asterisk in SAS notation) after accounting for the two constituent main effects. As this was introduced last into the model, the result can be read either from the Type I or Type III SS. Otherwise the Type III SS have no useful interpretation here. The interaction is clearly not significant ($p = 0.2595$), and so we conclude that smoking status does not act differently on BMI for men and women. Although we must thus reject model 4, for completeness the parameter estimates have been shown. Notice the effect of the SAS rule, that the parameter for the last level of any group is set to zero, on these

estimates. We can find fitted values for any combination of SEX and SMOKING by picking out and adding the appropriate terms. For example, for female never-smokers (SMOKING = 3, SEX = 2) the predicted BMI (in rounded figures) is

$$26.74 + 0 + 0 + 0 = 26.74\,\text{kg/m}^2.$$

This requires the least complex arithmetic. One of the most complex examples is for male ex-smokers (SMOKING = 2, SEX = 1) giving

$$26.74 + 0.16 - 1.41 + 1.33 = 26.82\,\text{kg/m}^2.$$

Apart from rounding error, all six fitted values generated this way must agree with the cross-classified group sample means shown in Table 9.16, as they do.

Although we have built up the model from simplest to most complex, a sounder strategy would be to start with model 4 and only work 'backwards' if the interaction is not significant. This can save unnecessary work.

Given our results, we conclude that person-to-person variation in BMI depends upon both the person's sex and smoking status, each of which is still important after the other has been accounted for (that is, model 3 is 'best'). Supposing that it is the effect of smoking (and giving up smoking) that is of key interest, it would be useful to see least-squares means for smoking after correcting for the sex effect. These are sensible summaries of the effect of smoking, given that there is no evidence of a sex interaction in this case. To obtain these, model 3 was refitted, this time requesting SAS to show least-squares means for smoking. Results are shown in Output 9.11. In fact, these are broadly similar to the uncorrected, raw, means in Table 9.16, although the difference between current and never smokers is increased. Smoking appears to provide a benefit in reducing BMI, much of which goes after quitting. See Bolton-Smith and Woodward (1997) for an analysis of the complete SHHS data set.

**Output 9.11**  SAS results from refitting model 3 of Example 9.10 with terms in reverse order

General Linear Models Procedure

| Source | DF | Type I SS | Mean Square | F Value | Pr > F |
|---|---|---|---|---|---|
| SMOKING | 2 | 148.47252 | 74.23626 | 6.75 | 0.0016 |
| SEX | 1 | 65.56745 | 65.56745 | 5.97 | 0.0158 |

Least Squares Means

| SMOKING | BMI LSMEAN | Std Err LSMEAN | Pr > \|T\| H0:LSMEAN=0 | LSMEAN Number |
|---|---|---|---|---|
| 1 | 24.4418193 | 0.4483789 | 0.0001 | 1 |
| 2 | 26.0963652 | 0.5022633 | 0.0001 | 2 |
| 3 | 26.9247043 | 0.4667339 | 0.0001 | 3 |

Pr > |T| H0: LSMEAN (i) = LSMEAN(j)

| i/j | 1 | 2 | 3 |
|---|---|---|---|
| 1 | . | 0.0148 | 0.0002 |
| 2 | 0.0148 | . | 0.2313 |
| 3 | 0.0002 | 0.2313 | . |

So as to provide further insight, Output 9.11 has been generated by introducing the terms into the model in the opposite order to that used for Output 9.9. Both fit the same model, model 3, and hence almost all the SAS results are identical and so are not presented here. The exception is the sequential SS display, and so this is shown. As they must, the two Type I SS sum to the model SS in Output 9.9; the SMOKING Type I SS is the same as the model SS in Output 9.8; the SEX given SMOKING Type I SS is the same as the equivalent Type III SS in Output 9.9.

## 9.6    General linear models

In Section 9.2 we introduced a model using a single categorical variable, which was generalized to deal with two categorical variables in Section 9.4. We could now go on to generalize the model for a single quantitative variable given in Section 9.3.1. However, the similarity of the models and the ANOVA tables in Sections 9.2 and 9.3 show this to be unnecessary. Both models take the form

$$y = \alpha + \beta x + \varepsilon,$$

except that a categorical $x$ variable needs to be represented by a set of dummy variables and associated $\beta$ parameters. That is, $\beta x$ needs to be expanded out.

A bivariate linear regression model takes the form

$$y = \beta_0 + \beta_1 x_1 + \beta_2 x_2 + \varepsilon, \tag{9.38}$$

which is exactly as for the two-way ANOVA model, except that the latter expands $\beta_1 x_1$ and $\beta_2 x_2$ into their component sets (Section 9.4.1). The bivariate regression ANOVA table, sequential and cross-adjusted SS have exactly the same interpretation as in Section 9.4, and model building proceeds as in Section 9.5. Interaction is represented as the product of the $x_1$ and $x_2$ variables. Fitted values are generated in a similar way (see Example 9.14), but now go up gradually, rather than in steps.

From now on we shall deliberately blur the distinction between categorical and quantitative variables in the right-hand side of the model equation. We shall consider models where the variables can be of either type. Provided the model is linear in structure and the error is additive and normally distributed, as in (9.38), then we call such models **general linear models**. Notice that these should not be confused with generalized linear models which, for one thing, allow the error to be non-normal (see Chapter 10). A general linear model is a special case of a generalized linear model.

Much of the terminology from general linear models arises from regression analysis. For example, the parameters (multipliers of the $x$ variables) in (9.36) and (9.38) are called **partial regression coefficients**, meaning that they represent the effect of the corresponding $x$ variable, when all other $x$ variables are kept fixed. In a sense all ANOVA models *are* regression models, once the dummy variables are defined. Thus (9.36) is a linear regression model with five $x$ variables and (9.37) is a linear regression model with 11 $x$ variables. The only difference is that the $x$ variables must be bound in sets within an ANOVA model: it makes no sense to fit a subset of the dummy variables for one particular categorical variable.

All specialist statistical software packages of any pedigree will fit general linear models. In some cases, such as MINITAB, SAS and SPSS, there are also separate procedures to deal exclusively with ANOVA models and others to deal exclusively with regression models. Some packages, such as GENSTAT, GLIM, MINITAB, SAS and SPSS, expect the terms within the general linear model to be defined according to type: quantitative or categorical. Others, such as MLN and STATA, expect dummy variables to be used for categorical variables.

When the explanatory variable of major interest is quantitative, but in the analysis we assess the confounding or interaction effects of a subsidiary categorical explanatory variable, the procedure is called a **comparison of regressions** (Example 9.11). When the explanatory variable of major interest is categorical and the subsidiary is quantitative we call this an **analysis of covariance**. However, these terms are largely redundant and reflect the separate historical development of ANOVA and regression models.

*Example 9.11*   The publication used in Example 9.5 gave separate results for developing and industrialized countries. Table 9.18 shows the data for the 29 industrialized countries considered in the paper. Taking this together with Table 9.8, we have 90 observations on national sugar consumption and dental caries.

Since we found a better regression fit when the logarithm of DMFT was regressed on sugar for developing countries (Example 9.6) we shall take the $y$ variable to be $\log_e$(DMFT) in this example. There are two $x$ variables: let $x_1$ be sugar consumption and $x_2$ type of country. Four regression models will be considered:

1. $y$ versus $x_1$ (DMFT depends upon sugar alone);
2. $y$ versus $x_2$ (DMFT depends upon type of country alone);
3. $y$ versus $x_1$ and $x_2$ (DMFT depends upon sugar and type of country);
4. $y$ versus $x_1, x_2$ and their interaction (DMFT depends upon sugar in a different way in developing and industrialized nations).

Model 1 is a simple linear regression model fitted to the 90 (developing and industrialized) observations. Model 2 is a one-way analysis of variance model for a factor with two levels. Model 3 is a general linear model with two variables, one of which is quantitative, the other categorical. Model 4 is another general linear model, but with an interaction term added.

The four models were fitted in SAS PROC GLM, having declared TYPE (of country) as a CLASS variable. LOGDMFT was defined as $\log_e$(DMFT) and fitted as the $y$ variable. Results are given as Outputs 9.12–9.15. Although we shall ultimately choose only one of the models to describe our data, each model will be described in turn, both so as to provide interpretation of SAS output and to illustrate differences between the models.

**Table 9.18**   Estimates of mean DMFT at age 12 years and mean sugar consumption (kg/ head of population/year) in 29 industrialized countries

| Country | Sugar | DMFT | Country | Sugar | DMFT |
|---|---|---|---|---|---|
| Albania | 22.16 | 3.4 | Japan | 23.32 | 4.9 |
| Australia | 49.96 | 2.0 | Malta | 47.62 | 1.6 |
| Austria | 47.32 | 4.4 | Netherlands | 53.54 | 2.5 |
| Belgium | 40.86 | 3.1 | New Zealand | 50.16 | 2.4 |
| Canada | 42.12 | 4.3 | Norway | 41.28 | 2.7 |
| Czechoslovakia | 49.92 | 3.6 | Poland | 49.28 | 4.4 |
| Denmark | 48.28 | 1.6 | Portugal | 33.48 | 3.2 |
| Finland | 41.96 | 2.0 | Sweden | 45.60 | 2.2 |
| France | 37.40 | 3.0 | Switzerland | 44.98 | 2.4 |
| Germany, West | 39.42 | 5.2 | Turkey | 28.32 | 2.7 |
| Greece | 33.30 | 4.4 | UK | 43.95 | 3.1 |
| Hungary | 48.98 | 5.0 | USA | 32.14 | 1.8 |
| Iceland | 51.62 | 6.6 | USSR | 48.92 | 3.0 |
| Ireland | 48.56 | 2.9 | Yugoslavia | 37.86 | 6.1 |
| Italy | 30.74 | 3.0 | | | |

Source: Woodward and Walker (1994).

Output 9.12 gives the fitted linear regression model (after rounding) as

$$\hat{y} = 0.1511 + 0.0212x_1,$$

which is illustrated by Figure 9.9(a). Since this is a one-term model the Type I and III (sequential and cross-adjusted) SS and MS are both equal to the model SS and MS, and so

**Output 9.12**   SAS results from fitting model 1 of Example 9.11

General Linear Models Procedure

Dependent Variable: LOGDMFT

| Source | DF | Sum of Squares | Mean Square | F Value | Pr > F |
|---|---|---|---|---|---|
| Model | 1 | 10.97728939 | 10.97728939 | 34.99 | 0.0001 |
| Error | 88 | 27.60682128 | 0.31371388 | | |
| Corrected Total | 89 | 38.58411068 | | | |

| R-Square | C.V. | Root MSE | LOGDMFT Mean |
|---|---|---|---|
| 0.284503 | 70.99216 | 0.5601017 | 0.7889627 |

| Parameter | Estimate | T for H0: Parameter = 0 | Pr > \|T\| | Std Error of Estimate |
|---|---|---|---|---|
| INTERCEPT | 0.1511479867 | 1.23 | 0.2221 | 0.12292940 |
| SUGAR | 0.0211598620 | 5.92 | 0.0001 | 0.00357711 |

are not shown. The slope is significantly different from zero ($p < 0.0001$). However, the intercept is not significantly different from zero at the 5% level ($p = 0.2221$).

Output 9.13 gives the results of fitting the one-way ANOVA model. We can only interpret the parameter estimates given in Output 9.13 if we know how the categorical variable $x_2$ (TYPE) was read into SAS. In fact TYPE took the value 1 for industrialized and 2 for developing countries in the data set read into SAS. Hence the fitted model (after rounding) defined by the estimates at the bottom of Output 9.13 is

$$\hat{y} = 0.6215 + 0.5196x_2^{(1)} + 0x_2^{(2)}$$

where

$$x_2^{(1)} = \begin{cases} 1 & \text{for industrialized countries} \\ 0 & \text{for developing countries,} \end{cases} \qquad x_2^{(2)} = \begin{cases} 1 & \text{for developing countries} \\ 0 & \text{for industrialized countries.} \end{cases}$$

The predicted $y$ for industrialized countries is thus

$$\hat{y} = 0.6215 + 0.5196 + 0 = 1.1411,$$

and for developing countries is

$$\hat{y} = 0.6215 + 0 + 0 = 0.6215.$$

Thus $\log_e(\text{DMFT})$, and consequently DMFT itself, is higher in industrialized countries. This difference is significant ($p = 0.0003$) according to the two equivalent tests shown in Output 9.13. These two tests are an $F$ test on (1, 88) d.f. and a $t$ test on 88 d.f. As explained in Section 9.3.1, these two tests are equivalent because the first d.f. for $F$ is 1 and the second is equal to the d.f. for the $t$ test. The intercept, which is now the predicted $\log_e(\text{DMFT})$ value for developing countries, is significantly different from zero ($p < 0.0001$). Figure 9.9(b) illustrates the fitted model.

**Output 9.13**   SAS results from fitting model 2 of Example 9.11

General Linear Models Procedure

Dependent Variable: LOGDMFT

| Source | DF | Sum of Squares | Mean Square | F Value | Pr > F |
|---|---|---|---|---|---|
| Model | 1 | 5.30737923 | 5.30737923 | 14.04 | 0.0003 |
| Error | 88 | 33.27673144 | 0.37814468 | | |
| Corrected Total | 89 | 38.58411068 | | | |
| | R-Square | C.V. | Root MSE | LOGDMFT Mean | |
| | 0.137553 | 77.94218 | 0.6149347 | 0.7889627 | |

| Parameter | Estimate | T for H0: Parameter = 0 | Pr > \|T\| | Std Error of Estimate |
|---|---|---|---|---|
| INTERCEPT | 0.6215250932 B | 7.89 | 0.0001 | 0.07873432 |
| TYPE 1 | 0.5196338074 B | 3.75 | 0.0003 | 0.13870315 |
| 2 | 0.0000000000 B | . | . | . |

Output 9.14 shows results for model 3. The fitted two-variable model (after rounding from Output 9.14) is

$$\hat{y} = 0.1703 + 0.0184x_1 + 0.2032x_2^{(1)} + 0x_2^{(2)},$$

where $x_2^{(1)}$ and $x_2^{(2)}$ are as before. Hence, for industrialized countries (where $x_2^{(1)} = 1$ and $x_2^{(2)} = 0$), we have

$$\hat{y} = 0.1703 + 0.0184x_1 + 0.2032 + 0 = 0.3735 + 0.0184x_1.$$

For developing countries (where $x_2^{(1)} = 0$ and $x_2^{(2)} = 1$),

$$\hat{y} = 0.1703 + 0.0184x_1 + 0 + 0 = 0.1703 + 0.0184x_1.$$

Figure 9.9(c) illustrates this fitted model (a 'parallel lines' model).

In Output 9.14 the model SS of 11.60 (rounded) splits sequentially into 10.98 (for SUGAR) and 0.62 (for TYPE). SUGAR, the first term entered into the model, is highly significant ($p < 0.0001$) by itself, but TYPE is not significant ($p = 0.1616$) after accounting for SUGAR. The Type III SS show that SUGAR is still highly significant after accounting for TYPE. Hence we do not seem to require TYPE, once we know SUGAR, to predict LOGDMFT. This is despite the fact that TYPE is a significant predictor when taken in isolation (as seen in Output 9.13).

**Output 9.14**   SAS results from fitting model 3 of Example 9.11

General Linear Models Procedure

Dependent Variable: LOGDMFT

| Source | DF | Sum of Squares | Mean Square | F Value | Pr > F |
|---|---|---|---|---|---|
| Model | 2 | 11.59555941 | 5.79777971 | 18.69 | 0.0001 |
| Error | 87 | 26.98855126 | 0.31021323 | | |
| Corrected Total | 89 | 38.58411068 | | | |

| | R-Square | C.V. | Root MSE | LOGDMFT Mean |
|---|---|---|---|---|
| | 0.300527 | 70.59496 | 0.5569679 | 0.7889627 |

| Source | DF | Type I SS | Mean Square | F Value | Pr > F |
|---|---|---|---|---|---|
| SUGAR | 1 | 10.97728939 | 10.97728939 | 35.39 | 0.0001 |
| TYPE | 1 | 0.61827002 | 0.61827002 | 1.99 | 0.1616 |

| Source | DF | Type III SS | Mean Square | F Value | Pr > F |
|---|---|---|---|---|---|
| SUGAR | 1 | 6.28818018 | 6.28818018 | 20.27 | 0.0001 |
| TYPE | 1 | 0.61827002 | 0.61827002 | 1.99 | 0.1616 |

| Parameter | Estimate | T for H0: Parameter = 0 | Pr > \|T\| | Std Error of Estimate |
|---|---|---|---|---|
| INTERCEPT | 0.1703433216 B | 1.38 | 0.1696 | 0.12299546 |
| SUGAR | 0.0183506278 | 4.50 | 0.0001 | 0.00407585 |
| TYPE  1 | 0.2032214738 B | 1.41 | 0.1616 | 0.14394967 |
|       2 | 0.0000000000 B | . | . | . |

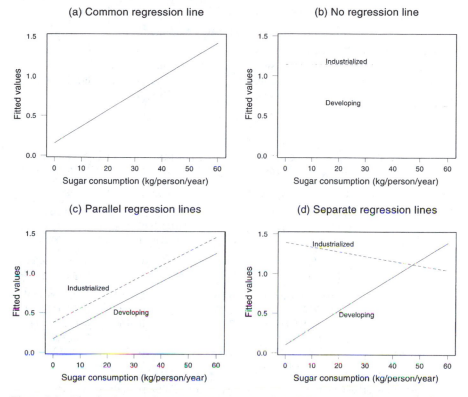

**Figure 9.9**  Fitted values against sugar consumption (a)–(d) for models 1–4 respectively, as specified in the text.

Output 9.15 shows results for model 4. The fitted model when the interaction between the $x$ terms is included is obtained from Output 9.15 (after rounding) as

$$\hat{y} = 0.0955 + 0.0214x_1 + 1.2916x_2^{(1)} + 0x_2^{(2)} - 0.0273x_1x_2^{(1)} + 0x_1x_2^{(2)},$$

with $x_2^{(1)}$ and $x_2^{(2)}$ as before. Hence, for industrialized countries (where $x_2^{(1)} = 1$ and $x_2^{(2)} = 0$) we have

$$\hat{y} = 0.0955 + 0.0214x_1 + 1.2916 - 0.0273x_1 = 1.3871 - 0.0059x_1.$$

For developing countries (where $x_2^{(1)} = 0$ and $x_2^{(2)} = 1$),

$$\hat{y} = 0.0955 + 0.0214x_1.$$

The fitted model (a 'separate lines' model) is illustrated by Figure 9.9(d).

The Type III SS are not useful here (and so are not shown), since we would not wish to consider either main effect after accounting for their interaction. The Type I SS show, crucially, that the interaction *is* significant at the 5% level ($p = 0.03$) after accounting for the two main effects. That is, the interaction truly adds to the predictive power of the model. Hence, model 4 is the one to adopt: $\log_e(\text{DMFT})$, and hence DMFT itself, depends upon sugar in a different

**Output 9.15**   SAS results from fitting model 4 of Example 9.11

General Linear Models Procedure

Dependent Variable: LOGDMFT

| Source | DF | Sum of Squares | Mean Square | F Value | Pr > F |
|---|---|---|---|---|---|
| Model | 3 | 12.97276317 | 4.32425439 | 14.52 | 0.0001 |
| Error | 86 | 25.61134750 | 0.29780637 | | |
| Corrected Total | 89 | 38.58411068 | | | |

| R-Square | C.V. | Root MSE | LOGDMFT Mean |
|---|---|---|---|
| 0.336220 | 69.16885 | 0.5457164 | 0.7889627 |

| Source | DF | Type I SS | Mean Square | F Value | Pr > F |
|---|---|---|---|---|---|
| SUGAR | 1 | 10.97728939 | 10.97728939 | 36.86 | 0.0001 |
| TYPE | 1 | 0.61827002 | 0.61827002 | 2.08 | 0.1533 |
| SUGAR*TYPE | 1 | 1.37720376 | 1.37720376 | 4.62 | 0.0343 |

| Parameter | Estimate | T for H0: Parameter = 0 | Pr > \|T\| | Std Error of Estimate |
|---|---|---|---|---|
| INTERCEPT | 0.095506602 B | 0.76 | 0.4485 | 0.12543488 |
| SUGAR | 0.021394414 B | 5.05 | 0.0001 | 0.00423693 |
| TYPE 1 | 1.291599971 B | 2.46 | 0.0160 | 0.52539846 |
| 2 | 0.000000000 B | . | . | . |
| SUGAR*TYPE 1 | −0.027274207 B | −2.15 | 0.0343 | 0.01268294 |
| 2 | 0.000000000 B | . | . | . |

way in the two types of countries. Since the slope for industrialized countries is virtually zero, it seems that DMFT has a relationship with sugar only in developing countries. This is an example of a unilateral interaction (Section 4.7). The epidemiological explanation for this may be the greater use of fluoride toothpastes, and other dental hygiene products, in more developed nations. From the $R^2$ value in Output 9.15, the best model accounts for almost 34% of the country-to-country variation in caries (on the log scale).

Due to the significant interaction, prediction depends upon type of country even though its main effect is not significant, after accounting for the effect of sugar, in both Output 9.14 and Output 9.15. It would *not* be correct to drop this non-significant main effect from the model, because the interaction term should always be accompanied by its corresponding main effects.

To emphasize the effect of using $\log_e(\text{DMFT})$ as the dependent variable, Figure 9.10 shows the predicted values from the best model, model 4, on the original scale. The observed values are also given for comparison. Fitted values are only shown for the observed ranges of sugar consumptions.

## 9.7   Several explanatory variables

So far we have been restricted to one or two explanatory variables in our models. The principles thus established, for model interpretation and evalu-

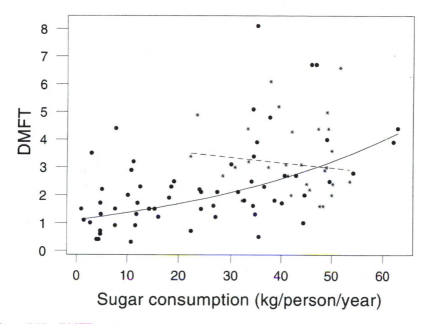

**Figure 9.10**  DMFT against sugar consumption, showing the fitted curves from model 4 in the text. Asterisks denote industrialized countries, dots denote developing countries.

ation, carry over to the multiple-variable situation, which is common in epidemiology. For instance, we can evaluate the importance of a specific explanatory variable, adjusting for the effect of several others which are confounding variables, by fitting it last into the multiple-variable model. The final sequential SS gives the desired test, whilst the adjusted estimates are derived from the parameter estimates for the variable of interest. We shall return to this issue in Section 9.9.

A more complex situation is where we have several candidate risk factors and we wish to know which of them is required to predict the outcome variable. For instance, we could have five risk factors (say, $x_1$ to $x_5$) but we wish to know whether some subset of the five will suffice for predicting $y$. Those variables not in the selected subset may be omitted because they have no real relationship with $y$, or because they are highly correlated with one or more of the selected variables.

Most statistical computer packages include automatic routines to select an appropriate subset of explanatory variables. These operate on the principle of parsimony; precise details are given by Draper and Smith (1981). One *modus operandi* would be to begin by fitting all the separate single-variable models that relate $y$ to an $x$ variable, and select that $x$ variable which gives the most highly significant result (from its one-way ANOVA table). Provided this most significant result is more extreme than some predetermined level (say 5%) then we enter the variable into our selected subset and continue. At the second stage we could test each other variable for an effect conditional on the variable already selected (using $F$ tests from the sequential ANOVAs), and select that which is most significant, provided that there is one significant at 5%. At the next stage we evaluate each remaining variable conditional on these first two selected, etc. We stop when we fail to find a significant addition. This is a simple kind of **forward selection** procedure. **Backward selection** works in the reverse order, starting with all explanatory variables and deleting (if possible) the least important at each stage. **Stepwise selection** is a mixture of these two approaches; as such it may also be used as a generic name for these automatic selection methods.

Automatic selection procedures have the advantage of simplicity of operation. However, they are not guaranteed to find the 'best' model in any statistical sense. More importantly, they may prevent the researcher from understanding his or her data completely. For example, it will not be clear how interrelationships between the variables affect the epidemiological interpretation. Often researchers treat the selected subset as the only variables that have any effect on the outcome variable, failing to recognize that an excluded variable may still be important when some of the selected variables are unadjusted for. The justification for adjustments should be epidemiological rather than statistical. Other problems are discussed by Greenland (1989).

Unfortunately the alternative, to fit all possible models, can be a daunting task. For instance, even if we ignore interactions, with five explanatory variables there are 26 models to fit (5 with one $x$ variable, 10 with two, 10 with three, 5 with four and 1 with all five). When we consider that we could have anything up to five-way interactions as well, the number of models appears to be prohibitively large. However, we can often reduce the scale of the problem by using our experience (to delete uninteresting or unlikely combinations), common sense (perhaps to delete multi-way interactions because they are extremely difficult to interpret) or by thinking carefully about what we wish to achieve (for instance, we may always want certain variables, such as age and sex, in the model because they are fundamental confounders). Furthermore, modern computing facilities make it particularly easy to fit several models to the same set of data with little effort.

Supposing that we can fit all the models that interest us, how should we compare them (perhaps to find the best overall model)? A common mistake is to do this through the coefficient of determination (the ratio of the model to the total SS, often multiplied by 100). When many variables are involved this is usually called the $R^2$ **statistic**, to distinguish it from the corresponding $r^2$ statistic which involves only one explanatory variable: see (9.21). Unfortunately $R^2$ will *always* grow as extra explanatory variables are added to the model. This is a mathematical certainty, whatever the importance of the added variable. For quantitative explanatory variables, $R^2$ can only be used to compare models with the same number of terms.

Various statistics have been proposed to replace $R^2$ when comparing models with different degrees of freedom (see Montgomery and Peck, 1992). Many computer packages produce an **adjusted** $R^2$ to serve this purpose; effectively it corrects $R^2$ for the d.f. A simple and effective method of comparison is to find the model with the smallest error MS. Since this is the unexplained variation standardized by its d.f., it will serve as an overall measure of lack of explanatory power. Often models with slightly higher error MS but fewer $x$ terms are compared with the minimum error MS model through sequential ANOVA table $F$ tests, so as to enable non-significant terms to be deleted. Hence, a more parsimonious model may result.

As described in Section 9.6, when the multiple-variable model includes categorical variables we should consider the set of dummy variables for any one categorical variable to be bound together. We either keep or delete the entire set from a model; the sets should not be broken up. If all the variables are quantitative we have a **multiple regression model**. This title is sometimes used for any many-variate general linear model. Epidemiological investigators often use 'multivariate analysis' as a synonym for multiple regression (of any kind). This should be avoided, because the term has a different meaning in statistics.

*Example 9.12*  Bolton-Smith *et al.* (1991) use data from the SHHS to ascertain dietary and non-dietary predictors of high-density lipoprotein (HDL) cholesterol. Here some of their analyses are reproduced using further survey data unavailable at the time of their report, but using fewer variables and restricting the analysis to men. The data to be used are records of serum HDL cholesterol, age, alcohol, dietary cholesterol and fibre consumption for 4897 men. These data are available electronically: see Appendix C.

As a first step to exploring the relationship between the variables (which are all quantitative), consider Table 9.19. We see that the outcome variable, HDL cholesterol, is only highly correlated with alcohol. Although there are significant correlations with cholesterol and (negatively) with fibre, the actual correlations are low. There are reasonably high negative correlations between alcohol and both age and fibre and positive correlations between cholesterol and both alcohol and fibre.

We might consider that age is really a confounding variable: we would then like to assess the effect of dietary risk factors after having allowed for age. We might then wish to look at **partial correlation coefficients**: correlations between the other variables adjusted for age. These may be found as the correlations between the residuals (Section 9.8) from the separate SLRs of each of the other four variables on age. Statistical computer packages will produce

426    Modelling quantitative outcome variables

**Table 9.19**  Pearson correlation matrix for serum HDL cholesterol, age, alcohol, cholesterol and fibre consumption, SHHS men

|  | HDL | Age | Alcohol | Cholesterol | Fibre |
|---|---|---|---|---|---|
| HDL | 1 | −0.006 | 0.328 | 0.058 | −0.041 |
| Age |  | 1 | −0.124 | −0.033 | −0.017 |
| Alcohol |  |  | 1 | 0.146 | −0.133 |
| Cholesterol |  |  |  | 1 | 0.102 |
| Fibre |  |  |  |  | 1 |

Note: Values given in *italics* are not significantly different from zero ($p > 0.05$).

the partial correlations by more direct methods. Continuing, we may then fit all possible regressions with the proviso that age is present in all models.

Rather than do this, we shall treat age just as for the other three explanatory variables. Table 9.20 gives the results of all the regression fits. Using the $R^2$ criterion within subsets of models that have the same number of variables, the best one-variable model regresses HDL cholesterol on alcohol (as we already know from Table 9.19), the best two-variable model has the $x$ variables alcohol and age, and the best three-variable model has alcohol, age and cholesterol.

**Table 9.20**  Results of fitting all possible (non-empty) regression models, using age (in years) and consumption of alcohol (units/week), cholesterol (mg/day) and fibre (g/day), to predict HDL cholesterol (mmol/l), SHHS men

| Number of x variables | $R^2$ (%) | Error mean square | Intercept | Age | Alcohol | Cholesterol | Fibre |
|---|---|---|---|---|---|---|---|
| 1 | 0.0037 | 0.13478 | 1.4086 | −0.0021 |  |  |  |
| 1 | **10.7632** | 0.12027 | 1.2607 |  | 0.0062 |  |  |
| 1 | 0.3309 | 0.13434 | 1.3106 |  |  | 0.00014 |  |
| 1 | 0.1714 | 0.13455 | 1.4086 |  |  |  | −0.00206 |
| 2 | **10.8859** | **0.12013** | 1.1477 | 0.0022 | 0.0063 |  |  |
| 2 | 0.3327 | 0.13436 | 1.3239 | −0.0027 |  | 0.00014 |  |
| 2 | 0.1759 | 0.13457 | 1.4301 | −0.0004 |  |  | −0.00206 |
| 2 | 10.7729 | 0.12029 | 1.2518 |  | 0.0062 | 0.00002 |  |
| 2 | 10.7637 | 0.12030 | 1.2583 |  | 0.0062 |  | 0.00011 |
| 2 | 0.5569 | 0.13406 | 1.3566 |  |  | 0.00015 | −0.00238 |
| 3 | **10.8966** | 0.12014 | 1.1379 | 0.0023 | 0.0063 | 0.00002 |  |
| 3 | 10.8870 | 0.12016 | 1.1435 | 0.0023 | 0.0063 |  | 0.00017 |
| 3 | 0.5592 | 0.13408 | 1.3721 | −0.0003 |  | 0.00015 | −0.00238 |
| 3 | 10.7730 | 0.12031 | 1.2508 |  | 0.0062 | 0.00002 | 0.00005 |
| 4 | **10.8970** | 0.12017 | 1.1355 | 0.0023 | 0.0063 | 0.00002 | 0.00011 |

Note: Values given in **bold** are the best (see text for criteria). Values given in *italics* are not significant ($p > 0.05$).

As they must, these models also have the lowest error MS within their set. Overall, the best model seems to be that with alcohol and age, because it has the lowest error MS of all.

We should consider whether the age plus alcohol model might be replaced by something simpler (that is, with fewer variables). In this case a simpler model could only be one with a single $x$ variable, and the sensible choice, from such models, is that with alcohol alone, since this is the SLR model with highest $R^2$ (by far). To make the comparison, we fit the bivariate regression model with age and alcohol, making sure alcohol is fitted first so that we can ascertain whether age has a significant *extra* effect. The sequential ANOVA table is given as Table 9.21. From this we see that age is necessary after allowing for alcohol (although alcohol is clearly much more important). Thus the age plus alcohol model is considered to be the best for predicting HDL cholesterol in men. From Table 9.20 we see that age and alcohol together explain about 11% of the person-to-person variation in HDL cholesterol.

Notice that, just because age plus alcohol gives the best model, our analyses show that this does *not* mean that cholesterol and fibre have no effect on HDL cholesterol. Indeed, they have a stronger statistical effect than age when taken alone, according to Table 9.19. From Table 9.20 we can see that their statistical effect is removed by alcohol. What epidemiological conclusions we can reach depends upon our understanding of the causal pathways (Section 4.3). If we can assume that heavier drinking just happens to go with a diet that is higher in cholesterol and lower in fibre, then we might conclude that the (small) effects of cholesterol and fibre are explained by confounding with alcohol.

Having fitted all the models, we can see precisely how the variables interrelate. Of particular interest here is the variable age. From Table 9.20 we see that it is only ever significant (and then has a positive effect) when considered with alcohol; indeed, it has a small negative effect unless alcohol is allowed for. From Table 9.19, we would not even consider it further if we based our analysis on simple correlations, and yet it has appeared in the 'best' model.

Another point of interest is the effect of alcohol; this is all but unchanged regardless of which other variables are allowed for in the analysis. Hence there are no variables that act as confounders for alcohol. Not only is alcohol the strongest predictor of HDL cholesterol, but also its effect is not influenced by any of the other explanatory variables considered.

## 9.8  Model checking

As indicated in Section 9.1, the model adopted should have isolated the systematic and the random components of the outcome variable. After fitting

**Table 9.21**  Sequential ANOVA table for Example 9.12

| Source of variation | Sum of squares | Degrees of freedom | Mean square | F ratio | p value |
|---|---|---|---|---|---|
| Alcohol | 71.01 | 1 | 71.01 | 591.10 | < 0.0001 |
| Age\|Alcohol | 0.81 | 1 | 0.81 | 6.74 | 0.0095 |
| Error | 587.94 | 4894 | 0.12 | | |
| Total | 659.76 | 4896 | | | |

the model we can see how successful we have been by examining the differences between the observed and fitted values, $y - \hat{y}$. These errors generated by the model are called the **residuals**. If the model has been successful the residuals will be both small and truly random. Furthermore, because we have assumed (when developing significance tests etc.) that the random error has a normal distribution with zero mean and constant variance, the residuals should be a random sample from this distribution.

A very useful way of examining the residuals is to plot them against the fitted values: the resultant diagram is called a **residual plot**. If the residual plot shows an obvious pattern, such as the points appearing to make a 'U' shape, then the residuals have a systematic component. This violates the assumption of the model, and suggests that a different model should be fitted (probably a quadratic regression in the example of the 'U' shape cited). If the residual plot shows one or more very large, or very small, values then we should be concerned about the effect of the corresponding $x$–$y$ values as **outliers**. These are points that are a long way from the fitted line (should it have been drawn on the original scatterplot). They may have seriously affected the fit of the regression line, and will certainly have inflated the error MS. It is always worth checking outliers in case they have been wrongly recorded, or in case they come from a source that is so special that it might sensibly be considered separately.

Since size may be hard to judge objectively, the residuals are often divided by their standard error before their examination begins. The standard error is estimated by the square root of the error MS from the ANOVA table for the model. Hence the **standardized residuals** are

$$(y - \hat{y})/s_e \tag{9.39}$$

for each observation. The standardized residuals should follow the standard normal distribution if the model is 'good'. Hence, we expect only 5% of their values to exceed $\pm 1.96$, from Table B.2. Any standardized residual that is less than $-1.96$ or greater than $1.96$ may be considered an outlier. We can check the normality assumption by constructing a normal plot (Section 2.7.1) of either the residuals or standardized residuals.

*Example 9.13* For the sugar and caries data from developing countries, as analysed in Example 9.5, we have the observed, $y$, values in Table 9.8. The fitted values (estimated systematic component) come from the regression line

$$\hat{y} = 1.165 + 0.0470x.$$

To calculate the residuals (estimated random component), one for each country, we find $\hat{y}$ and subtract the result from the corresponding $y$. For instance, the fitted value for Algeria ($x = 36.60$) is

$$\hat{y} = 1.165 + 0.0470 \times 36.60 = 2.89.$$

The residual is thus

$$y - \hat{y} = 2.3 - 2.89 = -0.59.$$

On Figure 9.3 we could measure this residual by sending up a vertical line at a sugar consumption of 36.60. The vertical distance between the dot (observed value) and the line (fitted value) is 0.59. This residual is negative because the dot lies below the fitted regression line.

From Table 9.9 the error MS is $s_e^2 = 1.9435$. From (9.39), the standardized residual for Algeria is

$$-0.59/\sqrt{1.9435} = -0.42.$$

Figure 9.11 shows the residual plot, using standardized residuals, including a useful reference line at zero. The point for Algeria has coordinates (2.89, −0.42). There is no obvious pattern in the plot except slight evidence of increasing residual variability with increasing $\hat{y}$. There is one very large standardized residual (that for Guatemala). We have no reason to suppose that this is based on erroneous data, nor any other good reason to treat this country separately. Three other countries also provide outliers. Since all four are positive outliers (beyond +1.96), the residual plot is unbalanced, with roughly two-thirds of standardized residuals taking negative values.

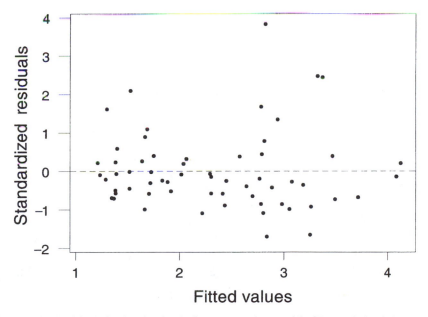

**Figure 9.11**   Residual plot for the simple linear regression model of Example 9.5 (DMFT on original scale).

Figure 9.12 is the normal plot for this problem. Here there is obvious curvature, akin to an elongated 'S' shape. We conclude that the standardized residuals do not arise from the required standard normal distribution.

Figures 9.13 and 9.14 show equivalents, to the last two plots, for log-transformed DMFT regressed on sugar, as in Example 9.6. In Figure 9.13 we see a random pattern in the residuals with no one gross outlier nor any indication of growth of residual variation, unlike before. Almost exactly half of the residuals (30/61) are negative. However, there are still a number of outliers. The pattern of Figure 9.14 is fairly close to a straight line, although there is a problem in the tails.

We can conclude that the log model is slightly better than the model on the original scale. The log regression model seems to satisfy the model requirements reasonably well. As noted in Example 9.6, a better model may be available; we can only find out by trial-and-error fitting and residual examination. However, inspection of the scatterplot (Figure 9.2), shows that no very precise regression model can be fitted to these data because the points are dispersed in a generally non-systematic fashion.

Residual plots will look somewhat different when ANOVA models have been fitted. Since fitted values go up in steps (at the levels of the group variable(s)) there will be several residuals at each fitted value. Hence the residual plot will be a series of columns of points. Problems with the model would be diagnosed if the columns had very different averages or ranges.

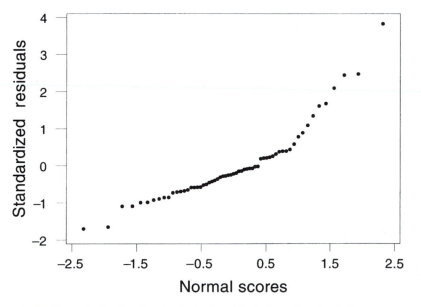

**Figure 9.12**  Normal plot for the standarized residuals from the simple linear regression model of Example 9.5 (DMFT on orginal scale).

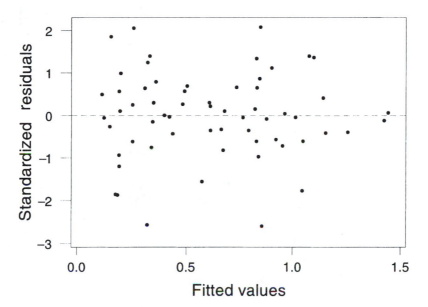

**Figure 9.13**  Residual plot for the transformed simple linear regression model of Example 9.6 (DMFT on log scale).

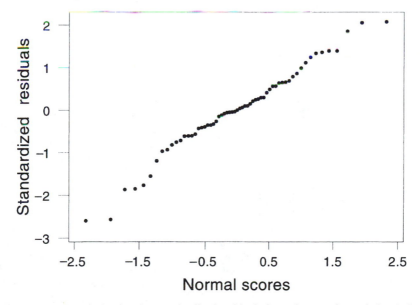

**Figure 9.14**  Normal plot for the standardized residuals from the transformed simple linear regression model of Example 9.6 (DMFT on log scale).

Another issue when considering the fit of quantitative explanatory variables is that of **influence**. An influential value is one which has a serious impact on the regression parameter estimates – that is, where the line sits (for simple linear regression). If we draw an analogy with a see-saw, where a child exerts greater turning moment the further he or she sits from the centre, we see that it is extreme values of $x$ (far from their mean) that exert greatest influence on the regression fit – for example, the $x$ values of over 60 kg of sugar per head per annum in Figure 9.2 (from Cuba and Barbados). An objective measure of influence is **Cook's distance**, computed by many statistical software packages. See Cook and Weisberg (1982) for details.

For further details of the theory of model checking see Belsley et al. (1980), Draper and Smith (1981) and Cook and Weisberg (1982). More applied accounts are given by Chatterjee and Price (1991) and Montgomery and Peck (1992).

### 9.9   Confounding

In most of the preceding we have assumed that all the explanatory variables are of equal status. If, instead, one of them is the variable of interest and the rest are confounders, it is unlikely to be sensible to think about the 'best' model as in Sections 9.5 and 9.7. Instead, we may well wish to fit the variable of interest alone, then with certain important confounders and finally with all confounders and compare the results, just as was done in a different context in Table 4.8.

*Example 9.14*   We shall now consider an example that is part of an investigation reported by McDonagh et al. (1997). This followed an intriguing suggestion by Patel et al. (1995) that *Helicobacter pylori* infection may be related to the level of plasma fibrinogen. McDonagh et al. (1997) used data from the third Glasgow MONICA study to see, first, if this relationship held in their data and, second, whether it could be explained by confounding. Here we shall only consider the MONICA data for men, of whom 510 had their fibrinogen and *H. pylori* status recorded. These data are available electronically: see Appendix C.

Initially, fibrinogen was compared amongst those men who had and did not have *H. pylori*. Results are given in Table 9.22. In this table the $Q$s are the quartiles (defined in Section 2.6.1). Since there is clear right skew in these data, all further analyses were carried out on log-transformed fibrinogen.

The 95% confidence interval for the difference between the two $\log_e$(fibrinogen) means (positive–negative) is (0.01, 0.10). The test to compare log means has a $p$ value of 0.012. Hence *H. pylori* status does, indeed, appear to be related to fibrinogen: men with positive *H. pylori* have higher values.

**Table 9.22**    Fibrinogen (g/l) by *H. pylori* status, MONICA men (s.e. = standard error)

| *H. pylori* status | *n* | *Mean (s.e.)* | $Q_1$ | $Q_2$ | $Q_3$ |
|---|---|---|---|---|---|
| Positive | 361 | 2.93 (0.038) | 2.43 | 2.84 | 3.35 |
| Negative | 149 | 2.76 (0.059) | 2.33 | 2.55 | 3.07 |

Age is a potential confounding factor in the relationship between *H. pylori* and fibrinogen, because both variables are known to increase with age. For the MONICA data this is confirmed because the Pearson correlation between age and $\log_e$(fibrinogen) is 0.34, whilst summary statistics for age by *H. pylori* status, given in Table 9.23, show that those with the infection are, on average, a few years older.

To explore the effect of age further, $\log_e$(fibrinogen) was compared to *H. pylori* within each separate 10-year age group. Since the MONICA study sampled people aged 25–74 years, there are five age groups. Results for $\log_e$(fibrinogen) are given in Table 9.24. The results of the *t* tests for each age group suggest that there is no age-specific effect of *H. pylori* status on fibrinogen. Hence, we may expect to find no effect of *H. pylori* on fibrinogen levels, after adjustment for age.

To adjust the relationship between $\log_e$(fibrinogen) and *H. pylori* for age, the model

$$y = \beta_0 + \beta_1 x_1 + \beta_2^{(1)} x_2^{(1)} + \beta_2^{(2)} x_2^{(2)} + \varepsilon$$

was fitted, where $x_1$ is age, $x_2$ represents *H. pylori* status, $y$ is $\log_e$(fibrinogen) and $\varepsilon$ is the random error. The dummy variables for *H. pylori* are

$$x_2^{(1)} = \begin{cases} 1 & \text{for negatives} \\ 0 & \text{for positives,} \end{cases} \qquad x_2^{(2)} = \begin{cases} 1 & \text{for positives} \\ 0 & \text{for negatives.} \end{cases}$$

**Table 9.23**    Age (in years) by *H. pylori* status, MONICA men (s.e. = standard error)

| *H. pylori* status | *n* | *Mean (s.e.)* | $Q_1$ | $Q_2$ | $Q_3$ |
|---|---|---|---|---|---|
| Positive | 361 | 53.4 (0.71) | 42 | 55 | 65 |
| Negative | 149 | 47.0 (1.10) | 37 | 46 | 57 |

**Table 9.24**    $\log_e$(fibrinogen) mean (and standard error in parentheses) by age group and *H. pylori* status, MONICA men

| Age group (*years*) | *n* | *H. pylori* status | | *p value* |
|---|---|---|---|---|
| | | Positive | Negative | |
| 25–34 | 65 | 0.86 (0.041) | 0.87 (0.033) | 0.86 |
| 35–44 | 100 | 0.99 (0.032) | 0.97 (0.030) | 0.60 |
| 45–54 | 107 | 1.00 (0.024) | 1.00 (0.039) | 0.99 |
| 55–64 | 122 | 1.10 (0.022) | 1.10 (0.052) | 0.89 |
| 65–74 | 116 | 1.13 (0.025) | 1.03 (0.059) | 0.09 |

To ensure that a test for *H. pylori* after adjusting for age was produced, age was entered first into the model. PROC GLM in SAS produced the following fitted model:

$$\hat{y} = 0.7319 + 0.0059x_1 - 0.0206x_2^{(1)} + 0x_2^{(2)}$$

with ANOVA table as given by Table 9.25. The key line here is that for *H. pylori* given age. Since the $F$ test has a $p$ value of 0.36, we can conclude that there is no difference between the average $\log_e$(fibrinogen) levels by *H. pylori* status, after allowing for age. Hence the relationship seen earlier can be explained by both variables changing with increasing age.

Age-adjusted $\log_e$(fibrinogen) means by *H. pylori* status come from calculating the fitted values, $\hat{y}$, for each level of *H. pylori*, $x_2$; for *H. pylori* negatives we have

$$\hat{y} = 0.7319 + 0.0059x_1 - 0.0206 = 0.7113 + 0.0059x_1,$$

and for *H. pylori* positives

$$\hat{y} = 0.7319 + 0.0059x_1.$$

To obtain age-adjusted (least squares) means by *H. pylori* status we evaluate $\hat{y}$ at the mean age in the sample; that is, we find fitted values keeping age fixed at its mean. Since the mean age of the 510 MONICA men was 51.56, the age-adjusted $\log_e$(fibrinogen) means are, for *H. pylori* negatives,

$$0.7113 + 0.0059 \times 51.56 = 1.01$$

and for *H. pylori* positives,

$$0.7319 + 0.0059 \times 51.56 = 1.03$$

which are very similar. This emphasizes the lack of association between fibrinogen and *H. pylori* after allowing for the effect of age. Notice the different way that least-squares means are calculated when adjusting for a quantitative variable, such as age, compared to a categorical variable, such as sex (Section 9.4.6).

We can, of course, obtain these least-squares means directly from PROC GLM in SAS. As we have seen previously, this also gives the standard errors of the least-squares means. We can use these to find a 95% confidence interval for the age-adjusted mean $\log_e$(fibrinogen) as

$$\text{least-squares mean} \pm 1.96 \times \text{standard error} \tag{9.40}$$

for each *H. pylori* group. We can find the corresponding interval for fibrinogen itself (on the original scale) by back-transformation; in this case we raise the lower and upper limits in (9.40) to the exponential power.

**Table 9.25**  Sequential ANOVA table for $\log_e$(fibrinogen) in Example 9.14

| Source of variation | Sum of squares | Degrees of freedom | Mean square | F ratio | p value |
|---|---|---|---|---|---|
| Age | 3.459 | 1 | 3.459 | 66.86 | <0.0001 |
| *H. pylori*\|Age | 0.043 | 1 | 0.043 | 0.83 | 0.36 |
| Error | 26.229 | 507 | 0.052 | | |
| Total | 29.730 | 509 | | | |

One final point to make is that we have taken fibrinogen to be the outcome variable, which is saying that *H. pylori* (and age) determines fibrinogen. It *may* be that the epidemiological hypothesis is that fibrinogen (and age) determines the risk of *H. pylori*. Although the basic principles of dealing with the confounder (age) will remain the same, it would not be sensible to fit a general linear model with *H. pylori* as the outcome variable, because this variable is binary and certainly not normally distributed. The correct approach is described in Chapter 10.

### 9.9.1   Adjustment using residuals

Given a suitable computer package, the easiest way to adjust for a single confounder is to fit it first in a bivariate model. There is an alternative procedure which uses only single-variable models, which is worth reporting if only as an aid to interpretation.

To explain this method, suppose that we wish to find the effect of $x$ on the outcome variable, $y$, adjusting for the confounder, $c$. We proceed by fitting the model that relates $y$ to $c$; call this model's residuals $e_y$. Then we fit the model that relates $x$ to $c$; call these residuals $e_x$. Confounder-adjusted results then come from fitting the model that relates $e_y$ to $e_x$. So, whereas the unadjusted analysis stems from the model that fits $x$ to the outcome variable $y$, the adjusted analysis stems from the model that fits the $x$ residuals to the $y$ residuals. Both residuals measure the remaining effect *after* taking account of the confounding variable, and so we have a logical method for removing the effect of confounding from the $x$–$y$ relationship.

The residuals method leads to the same result as the bivariate (or, in general, many-variable) modelling approach using sequential sums of squares and fitted values, in the context of general linear models. A demonstration of this is provided by Kahn and Sempos (1989). Unfortunately, there is no such simple equivalence in other statistical modelling situations, such as that met in Chapter 10. Then the multiple variable modelling approach is generally used.

## 9.10   Non-normal alternatives

With the exception of Spearman's correlation coefficient, all the foregoing procedures in this chapter assume that data, or at least the residuals from the model fitted to the data, arise from a normal distribution. Alternative methods exist for cases where normality may not be reasonably assumed, or induced by transformation. As with Spearman's correlation, several of these utilize the ranks of the data. One example is the **Kruskal–Wallis test**, which is a direct generalization of the two-sample Wilcoxon test (Section 2.8.2) to cover several samples. Just as the Wilcoxon test is a non-parametric (distribution-free) alternative to the $t$ test, so the Kruskal–Wallis test is a non-parametric alternative to the one-way ANOVA.

Several non-parametric alternatives to the methods of this chapter are described by Conover (1980); Härdle (1990) is concerned solely with non-parametric regression. As described in Section 2.8.2, these methods will be less powerful than the methods given earlier in this chapter when normality is (at least roughly) true. Other approaches to dealing with lack of normality and other problems with model assumptions are described by Tiku et al. (1986) and Birkes and Dodge (1993).

Due to space limitations, we shall consider only the Kruskal–Wallis test here. This requires data to be classified into $\ell$ groups, as in the one-way ANOVA. The null hypothesis can be taken as 'the medians are equal in all the groups', and the alternative is 'at least one median is different' . When $\ell = 2$ the Kruskal–Wallis test reduces to the Wilcoxon test of Section 2.8.2. As with the Wilcoxon test, we begin by ranking the entire set of data. Let $R_{ij}$ be the rank of the $j$th subject in group $i$, $n_i$ be the size of group $i$, $n = \sum n_i$ be the total sample size and $T_i = \sum_{j=1}^{n_i} R_{ij}$ be the sum of ranks for group $i$. If there are no tied ranks, the Kruskal–Wallis test statistic is

$$\frac{12}{n(n+1)} \sum_{i=1}^{\ell} \frac{T_i^2}{n_i} - 3(n+1). \tag{9.41}$$

When there are ties, we take the average rank for each tied rank in a set (as in Section 2.8.2) and compute

$$d = \frac{1}{n-1} \left\{ \sum_{i=1}^{\ell} \sum_{j=1}^{n_i} R_{ij}^2 - \frac{(n+1)^2 n}{4} \right\}. \tag{9.42}$$

The test statistic is then

$$\frac{1}{d} \left\{ \sum_{i=1}^{\ell} \frac{T_i^2}{n_i} - \frac{(n+1)^2 n}{4} \right\}. \tag{9.43}$$

If there are few ties then (9.41) is a reasonable, and much simpler, approximation to (9.43). Whether (9.41) or (9.43) is used, the Kruskal–Wallis test statistic is compared to chi-square with $\ell - 1$ d.f. This is an approximate procedure. For small sample sizes an exact procedure is required; exact tables are given by Iman et al. (1975).

*Example 9.15* Consider the dietary data of Table 9.1. This time we shall test whether average serum total cholesterol differs between dietary groups without assuming any specific probability distribution. The entire data were ranked in ascending order; Table 9.26 shows the results, arranged as in Table 9.1.

Here $n = 18$ and $n_i = 6$, for $i = 1, 2, 3$; thus

$$\sum \frac{T_i^2}{n_i} = \frac{91.5^2}{6} + \frac{53^2}{6} + \frac{26.5^2}{6} = 1980.5833.$$

Ignoring the presence of ties, the simple formula, (9.41), gives the test statistic

$$\frac{12}{18 \times 19} 1980.5833 - 3 \times 19 = 12.49.$$

Alternatively, we can use the more complex procedure which does take account of the ties. First find

$$\sum \sum R_{ij}^2 = 15^2 + 17^2 + \cdots + 3^2 = 2108,$$

$$(n+1)^2 n/4 = 19^2 \times 18/4 = 1624.5.$$

Then, using (9.42),

$$d = \frac{1}{17}(2108 - 1624.5) = 28.4412.$$

The test statistic, (9.43), is thus

$$\frac{1}{28.4412}(1980.5833 - 1624.5) = 12.52.$$

In this case, with 4/18 tied ranks, the two approaches give virtually the same result. In both cases, comparing the test statistic with $\chi_2^2$ leads to a $p$ value of 0.02. Hence there is a real difference in cholesterol medians between dietary groups. Compare this to the $p$ value of less than 0.001, reported in Section 9.2.3, for the corresponding one-way ANOVA.

**Table 9.26**    Ranks for the dietary data of Table 9.1

| Subject no. (*within group*) | Diet group | | |
| | *Omnivores* | *Vegetarians* | *Vegans* |
| --- | --- | --- | --- |
| 1 | 15 | 8 | 9 |
| 2 | 17 | 10 | 1 |
| 3 | 12 | 6 | 2 |
| 4 | 16 | 11 | 7 |
| 5 | 13.5 | 4.5 | 4.5 |
| 6 | 18 | 13.5 | 3 |
| Total | 91.5 | 53 | 26.5 |

## Exercises

(Some of these require the use of a computer package with appropriate procedures.)

9.1    Use one-way ANOVA to test whether the mean cholesterol is the same for those with and without coronary heart disease in the Scottish Heart Health Study data of Table 2.10. Compare your result with that of Example 2.10.

9.2    For the third MONICA Survey data from north Glasgow in Table C.2, construct the one-way ANOVA table for protein S by alcohol group.
   (i)     Use this to test whether mean protein S differs between the five alcohol groups.
   (ii)    Find a 99% confidence interval for the mean protein S for non-drinkers.
   (iii)   Find a 99% confidence interval for the difference between mean protein S in heavy and non-drinkers.
   (iv)    Repeat the test in (i), but this time using a Kruskal–Wallis test. Compare the two test results.

9.3    In a case–control study of coronary heart disease (CHD) and consumption of hydrogenated marine oils, Thomas (1992) obtained fat specimens at necropsy from 136 men who died from CHD and another 95 men who died from other, unrelated, causes. Data were collected from nine areas of England and Wales. He published a sequential ANOVA table for the percentage hydrogenated menhaden in adipose tissue, part of which is given below.

| Source of variation | Sum of squares |
|---|---|
| Areas | 2.3203 |
| Case–control status\|Areas | 0.4089 |
| Interaction\|Main effects | 0.1675 |
| Error | |
| Total | 10.3117 |

   (i)     Complete the ANOVA table, including the test results.
   (ii)    Interpret your results.
   (iii)   Is there any prior analysis that you would have wished to perform before constructing the ANOVA table?

9.4    Data have been collected from 12 people in a study of how smoking affects the desire for healthy eating. Each person's smoking status was recorded: two were never smokers, four were ex-smokers, three were classified as light smokers and three as heavy smokers. Consumption of antioxidant vitamins was also recorded, measured on a combined and standardized scale. The one-way ANOVA model relating antioxidant score to smoking status was fitted using three computer packages and by hand calculation using the method given in a statistics textbook (you do not need to know how any of these methods works to be able to answer the questions). The fitted model (in each case) was:

$$\hat{y} = a + b^{(1)}x^{(1)} + b^{(2)}x^{(2)} + b^{(3)}x^{(3)} + b^{(4)}x^{(4)},$$

where all terms are as in (9.9) and the superscripts 1–4 denote never, ex-, light and heavy smokers, respectively. The four sets of parameter estimate results are given as follows.

| Parameter estimates | GENSTAT | SAS | SPSS | Textbook |
|---|---|---|---|---|
| $a$ | 1.8 | 0.3 | 1.025 | 1.0 |
| $b^{(1)}$ | 0 | 1.5 | 0.775 | 0.8 |
| $b^{(2)}$ | −0.3 | 1.2 | 0.475 | 0.5 |
| $b^{(3)}$ | −1.3 | 0.2 | −0.525 | −0.5 |
| $b^{(4)}$ | −1.5 | 0 | −0.725 | −0.7 |

(i)   Confirm that all four methods give the same fitted values (estimated means) for the antioxidant score in each smoking group. Write down these fitted values.

(ii)   What must the observed mean antioxidant scores have been in each smoking group?

(iii)   Use your results in (ii) to compute the total observed antioxidant score for each smoking group. Add these together and divide by 12 to find the overall mean score. Check that this agrees with the appropriate value in the 'Textbook' column in the table.

(iv)   Suppose that a new computer package became available, which chooses the constraint upon the $b$ parameters that $b^{(2)} = 0$. Write down the set of parameter estimates which this package would produce for the problem described here.

9.5   Refer to the epilepsy data given in Table C.11.

(i)   Fit a two-way ANOVA model without interaction to the BO test results. Give the sequential ANOVA table with diagnosis introduced first. Interpret your results.

(ii)   Find the standardized residuals from the model fitted in (i). Plot these against the fitted values. Also produce a normal plot of the standardized residuals. Identify any unusual values.

(iii)   Find the fitted values from the model of (i). Use these to calculate the least-squares BO test means by duration of treatment, adjusted for diagnosis.

(iv)   Fit the two-way ANOVA model with interaction. Is there any evidence of interaction?

(v)   Define a new variable, 'combination', which specifies the combination of diagnosis and duration for each child (for example, children 1, 4 and 11 make up the group with the combination of PS and one year's duration). Fit the one-way ANOVA model that relates BO test to combination. Show that the combination sum of squares is equal to the sum of the three sequential sums of squares for the model of (iv).

9.6   Kiechl et al. (1996) give observed and adjusted mean values for $\gamma$-glutamyltransferase (U/l) by alcohol status (average daily consumption in grams) for 820 subjects in a cross-sectional survey carried out in Bruneck, Italy. Results are shown below.

| Alcohol group (g) | Observed | Adjusted[a] |
|---|---|---|
| Abstainers | 14.9 | 17.9 |
| 1–50 | 17.4 | 18.6 |
| 51–99 | 31.8 | 30.0 |
| ≥100 | 40.2 | 38.4 |

[a] For sex, age, smoking, body mass index, physical activity and social status.

Discuss the consequences of these results with regard to the use of γ-glutamyltransferase as a biochemical marker of alcohol consumption.

9.7    For the Glasgow MONICA data in Table C.2.
   (i)     Plot Protein S against Protein C.
   (ii)    Find the Pearson correlation between Protein C and Protein S.
   (iii)   Repeat (i), but after transforming Protein C by using the inverse reciprocal transformation defined in Section 2.8.1. How much difference has this made? Test for a significant non-zero correlation. Why is it more likely that the test is valid when this transformed variable is used?
   (iv)    Find the Spearman correlation between Protein C and Protein S. How would this result alter if Protein C was first transformed?
   (v)     Fit the simple linear regression of Protein S (the $y$ variable) on Protein C. Test for a significant regression using an $F$ test and specify the coefficient of determination.
   (vi)    Calculate the standardized residuals and fitted values for each observation from (v). Hence construct a residual plot. Does this suggest any problems with the model?
   (vii)   Find the normal scores of the standardized residuals. Use these to construct a normal plot. What does this tell you, and why is this result important in the current context?
   (viii)  Test the null hypothesis that the true intercept (for the regression model) is zero.
   (ix)    Find a 95% confidence interval for the true intercept.
   (x)     Test the null hypothesis that the true slope is zero using a $t$ test. Compare your results with the $F$ test in (v).
   (xi)    Find a 95% confidence interval for the true slope.
   (xii)   Predict Protein S when Protein C is 100 iu/dl. Give a 95% confidence interval for this prediction.
   (xiii)  Predict the mean value of Protein S for all men with a Protein C value of 100 iu/dl. Give a 95% confidence interval for your prediction.

9.8    For the SHHS data of Table 2.10, regress systolic on diastolic blood pressure. Identify any regression outlier using standardized residuals. Refit the model with the outlier removed.

9.9    Cotinine is an objective biochemical marker of tobacco smoke inhalation. For the SHHS data of Table 2.10, plot cotinine against self-reported daily cigarette consumption. Discuss the problems of using standard simple linear regression analysis to predict the average amount of cotinine per cigarette smoked with these data.

9.10   Consider the ozone exposure data of Table C.12. It would be of interest to establish whether age, height or weight are important predictors of ozone exposure effects. This will assist in the efficient design of future studies of ozone exposure. Fit the three possible simple linear regression models to the data of Table C.12 in order to address this issue. What do you conclude?

9.11   Refer to the anorexia data of Table C.13.
   (i)     Estimate the mean BPI for cases and for controls.
   (ii)    Compare the two distributions (cases and controls) using boxplots.
   (iii)   Do your results in (i) and (ii) support the prior hypothesis of the researchers, that cases have a lower BPI? Consider the danger involved in carrying out a one-sided test, as this prior hypothesis might suggest. Test the null hypothesis that cases and controls have the same BPI, using a two-sided test.

(iv)    One possible confounding variable in this example is the true width, since the relative error in perception (that is, the BPI) might differ with increasing body size. Plot BPI against true width, marking cases and controls with different symbols or colours. Does BPI seem to change with true width? If so, how? Does it appear that a different regression line will be required for cases and controls?

(v)    From a general linear model, test the effect of case–control status adjusted for true width.

(vi)    Write down the equation of the fitted bivariate model from (v). Find the mean true width. Hence compute the least-squares means (adjusted for true width) for cases and controls.

(vii)    Fit the simple linear regressions of (a) BPI on true width, (b) case–control status on true width. Find the (raw) residuals from (a) and (b) and fit the simple linear regression of the (a) residuals on the (b) residuals. Compare the slope parameter from this model with that for case–control status in (vi). You should find a close relationship: why?

(viii)    Compare the results in (v) and (vii) with those in (ii) and (iii). What effect has adjustment for true width had? Are there any other potential confounding variables that might be worth considering, were data available?

9.12    Returning to the MONICA data of Table C.2 (following on from Exercise 9.2), fit all remaining general linear models (without interaction) to predict Protein S from any of age, alcohol group and Protein C. Summarize your overall findings. Do any of these three variables have an important effect in the presence of the other two?

9.13    Using the SHHS data in Table 2.10, fit all possible multiple regression models (without interactions) that predict the $y$ variable serum total cholesterol from diastolic blood pressure, systolic blood pressure, alcohol, carbon monoxide and cotinine. Scrutinize your results to understand how the $x$ variables act in conjunction. For these data, which is the 'best' multiple regression model for cholesterol? What percentage of variation does it explain ?

9.14    For the UK population data of Table C.14, fit the simple linear regression of population on year. Calculate the $r^2$ statistic. Is this model a good fit to the data? Note that it will be easier to fit 'year' as $1, 2, 3, \ldots$, allowing for the missing year at 1941.

# 10

# Modelling binary outcome data

## 10.1  Introduction

In epidemiology we are most often concerned with deciding how a risk factor is related to disease (or death). If we decide to develop statistical models to represent the relationship between risk factor and disease, it is natural to take the risk factor as the $x$ variable and the disease outcome as the $y$ variable in the regression model. Implicitly, it is the $x$ variable that is a potential cause of the $y$ variable, and not vice versa.

Consider now the nature of this $y$ variable. In the most straightforward situation, it measures whether or not the individual concerned has contracted the disease; hence, it is a binary variable. Raw data, collected from $n$ individuals, will be of the form of Table 10.1, where the risk factor values may be quantitative or qualitative. If we consolidate the data, by counting how often disease occurs at each distinct value of $x$, we obtain the alternative view of the data given in Table 10.2, where the risk factor values are now all unique (assumed to be $\ell$ in all). This is rather easier to deal with.

Of the $n_i$ people with the $i$th risk factor value $x_i$, $e_i$ have the disease, giving a proportion with disease of $r_i = e_i/n_i$. The notation is chosen with epidemiological practice in mind, and is consistent with earlier chapters of this book. The proportion of people who experience an event $(e_i/n_i)$ will give the risk $(r_i)$ of disease, for people with the $i$th value of the risk factor. With a continuous risk factor the risk factor variable may be grouped, so as to produce large numbers for the $n_i$. The problem of modelling disease outcome may now be seen to be one of modelling the relationship between $r$ and $x$.

*Example 10.1*  Table 10.3 shows data from the *Helicobacter pylori* study of McDonagh *et al.* (1997) described in Example 9.14. Figure 10.1 shows a scatterplot of the proportion with prevalent disease against social class. In the main, the chance of *H. pylori* seems to increase as we go across the social classifications (that is, with increasing deprivation). We might seek to quantify this relationship through regression modelling.

**Table 10.1**   Raw data on risk factor values and disease outcome

| Risk factor value | Disease? |
|---|---|
| $x_1$ | Yes |
| $x_2$ | No |
| . | . |
| . | . |
| . | . |
| $x_n$ | No |

**Table 10.2**   Grouped data on risk factor values and disease outcome

| Risk factor value | Number with disease | Total number | Proportion with disease |
|---|---|---|---|
| $x_1$ | $e_1$ | $n_1$ | $r_1$ |
| $x_2$ | $e_2$ | $n_2$ | $r_2$ |
| . | . | . | . |
| . | . | . | . |
| . | . | . | . |
| $x_\ell$ | $e_\ell$ | $n_\ell$ | $r_\ell$ |

**Table 10.3**   Prevalent *Helicobacter pylori* and occupational social class amongst men in north Glasgow in the third MONICA survey

| | Number | | |
|---|---|---|---|
| Occupational social class (rank) | With H. pylori | Total | Proportion with H. pylori |
| I     Non-manual, professional (1) | 10 | 38 | 0.26 |
| II    Non-manual, intermediate (2) | 40 | 86 | 0.46 |
| IIIn Non-manual, skilled (3) | 36 | 57 | 0.63 |
| IIIm Manual, skilled (4) | 226 | 300 | 0.75 |
| IV    Manual, partially skilled (5) | 83 | 108 | 0.77 |
| V     Manual, unskilled (6) | 60 | 73 | 0.82 |

*Example 10.2*   The Scottish Heart Health Study (SHHS) recruited 5754 men aged 40–59. Table 10.4 shows the number and percentage of deaths within an average of 7.7 years of follow-up, by age of man at baseline (time of recruitment). Although we have seen, in Section 5.2, that some subjects were observed for longer durations than others in the SHHS, we shall ignore these differences throughout this chapter: that is, we assume that this is a fixed cohort. The data are illustrated by Figure 10.2. There is clearly a tendency for risk of death to increase with age, as would be expected, but some individual age groups have more (or fewer) deaths than would be expected according to the general pattern. Presumably this is due to random variation. Regression modelling should be useful both to summarize the relationship shown in Table 10.4 and to smooth out the random variation.

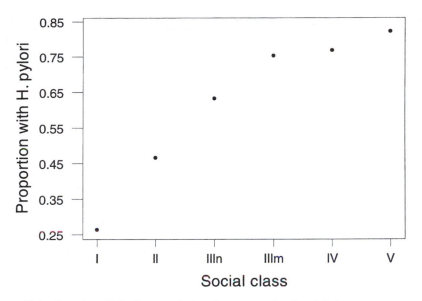

**Figure 10.1**   Prevalent *Helicobacter pylori* against occupational social class amongst men in north Glasgow in the third MONICA survey.

## 10.2   Problems with standard regression models

The relationship between $r$ and $x$ could be modelled using simple linear regression (or, since $x$ could be qualitative, more generally by the general linear model), as described in Chapter 9. Computationally this is quite possible, but there are three problems which cause this approach to be inappropriate.

### 10.2.1   The r–x relationship may well not be linear

Proportions (including risks) must lie between 0 and 1 inclusive. When the observed proportions scan most of this allowable range, as in Table 10.3, the pattern in the scatterplot is generally non-linear, as in Figure 10.1. This is because there tends to be 'squashing up' as proportions approach the asymptotes (barriers) at either 0 or 1. The problem is not so acute in Figure 10.2 because the percentages (restricted to between 0 and 100) only cover a small part of the allowable range. Nevertheless, some levelling out at the left-hand side may be seen.

**Table 10.4** Deaths by age at baseline in the SHHS

| | Number | | |
| | Dying | Total | Percentage |
| Age (years) | | | dying |
|---|---|---|---|
| 40 | 1 | 251 | 0.4 |
| 41 | 12 | 317 | 3.8 |
| 42 | 13 | 309 | 4.2 |
| 43 | 6 | 285 | 2.1 |
| 44 | 10 | 236 | 4.2 |
| 45 | 8 | 254 | 3.1 |
| 46 | 10 | 277 | 3.6 |
| 47 | 12 | 278 | 4.3 |
| 48 | 10 | 285 | 3.5 |
| 49 | 14 | 276 | 5.1 |
| 50 | 15 | 274 | 5.5 |
| 51 | 14 | 296 | 4.7 |
| 52 | 19 | 305 | 6.2 |
| 53 | 36 | 341 | 10.6 |
| 54 | 26 | 305 | 8.5 |
| 55 | 21 | 276 | 7.6 |
| 56 | 28 | 325 | 8.6 |
| 57 | 41 | 302 | 13.6 |
| 58 | 38 | 260 | 14.6 |
| 59 | 49 | 302 | 16.2 |

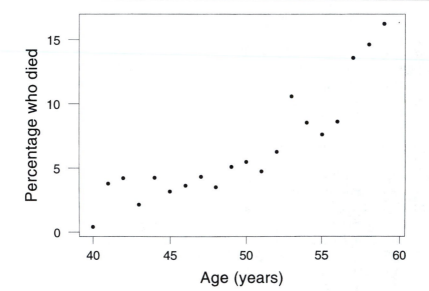

**Figure 10.2** Percentage of deaths against age at baseline in the SHHS.

*10.2.2    Predicted values of the risk may be outside the valid range*

The fitted linear regression model for $r$ regressed on $x$ is given by (9.12) as

$$\hat{r} = a + bx.$$

This can lead to predictions of risks that are negative or are greater than unity, and so impossible.

*Example 10.3*    Fitting a linear regression line to the data in Table 10.4 and Figure 10.2, using (9.13) and (9.14), gives the equation,

$$\hat{r} = -25.394 + 0.645 \times \text{age}.$$

Here both the constant and slope are highly significant ($p < 0.001$) and the model explains 97% of the variation in risk. Hence the regression model appears to be very successful. However, suppose the model was used to predict the risk of death for someone aged 39. This prediction would be

$$\hat{r} = -25.394 + 0.645 \times 39 = -0.239,$$

a negative risk! To be fair, extrapolation from regression lines is never a good idea. However, here we are only extrapolating by one year and we would hope that the regression model would behave well this close to the observed range of ages. Furthermore, similar problems are found with confidence limits for predicted risks *within* the range of the observed data for this example. With other data sets, the predicted risks can take impossible values even within the range of observations.

*10.2.3    The error distribution is not normal*

In simple linear regression we fit the model

$$r = \alpha + \beta x + \varepsilon,$$

where $\varepsilon$ arises from a standard normal distribution. This is (9.11) but where the $y$ variable is the proportion with the disease (the risk). Proportions are not likely to have a normal distribution; they are likely to arise from a **binomial** distribution. We would expect to detect this lack of normality if we carried out model checking (Section 9.8), for instance in the situation of Example 10.3.

If we ignore this problem we can still fit the simple linear regression model, but any inferences drawn from it would be inaccurate. For example, the confidence interval for the slope of the regression line is calculated using $t$ statistics which make an assumption of normality. Furthermore, simple linear regression assumes that each observation is equally precise, and thus should be given equal weight. The proportion $r_i = e_i/n_i$ will have estimated variance

$r_i(1 - r_i)/n_i$ (the binomial variance), which is certainly not constant for all $i$ even if the sample sizes within each level, $n_i$, are fixed.

One way round the distributional problem may be to transform the data; if the $n_i$ are all reasonably similar the arcsine square root transformation (Section 2.8.1) should be useful, since this makes the variance reasonably constant. However, this method is, at best, approximate.

## 10.3    Logistic regression

Figure 10.3 shows the shape of the logistic function,

$$y = \{1 + \exp(-b_0 - b_1 x)\}^{-1},  \tag{10.1}$$

relating some variable, $y$, to another variable, $x$, through the constants $b_0$ and $b_1$. The elongated S shape of the logistic function is a good match to the types of relationship we wish to measure: solving the problem of Section 10.2.1. There is an asymptote at $y = 0$ and at $y = 1$: solving the problem of Section 10.2.2. Hence the fitted regression equation,

$$\hat{r} = \{1 + \exp(-b_0 - b_1 x)\}^{-1},  \tag{10.2}$$

where, as usual, $\hat{r}$ is the fitted (or predicted) value, $b_0$ is the sample estimate of the true 'intercept', $\beta_0$, and $b_1$ is the sample estimate of the true 'slope', $\beta_1$,

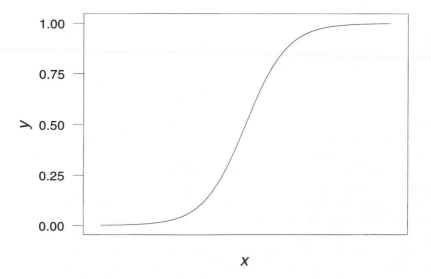

**Figure 10.3**    The logistic function, defined by (10.1).

should provide a useful model in the current context, provided we can treat the random variation appropriately. As far as the practitioner is concerned, this simply means telling the computer that the data have binomial rather than normal error, when using standard commercial software (thus solving the problem of Section 10.2.3). Such software will produce maximum likelihood estimates (see Clayton and Hills, 1993) of the $\beta$ coefficients using iterative calculations.

We can manipulate (10.2) into:

$$\log_e\left(\frac{\hat{r}}{1-\hat{r}}\right) = b_0 + b_1 x \tag{10.3}$$

which is the most often quoted form of the logistic regression equation. The left-hand side of (10.3) is called the **logit**. By reference to Section 3.2, we see that the logit is the log of the odds of disease. Hence the logistic regression model postulates a relationship between the log odds of disease and the risk factor. This makes this model of key importance in epidemiology. The right-hand side of (10.3) is exactly as for a simple linear regression model, and is called the **linear predictor**. Note that (10.3) should strictly be called the 'simple linear logistic regression' equation because there is only one $x$ variable, and it is assumed to have a linear effect on the logit.

The odds of disease, for any specified value of $x$, come from raising the result of (10.3), with $b_0$ and $b_1$ supplied by a computer package, to the power e. Suppose that we wished to estimate the odds ratio, $\psi$, for $x = x_1$ compared to $x = x_0$. Thus, in the context of Example 10.2, we might wish to find the odds of death for a man aged 59 compared to a man aged 40. Here $x_1 = 59$ and $x_0 = 40$. Obviously, we could do this by calculating the two separate odds, from (10.3), and dividing. A quicker method is to use the fact that the log of a ratio is the difference between the logs of the two components of that ratio, and hence

$$\log(\hat{\psi}) = \log(\hat{\text{odds}}_1/\hat{\text{odds}}_0) = \log(\hat{\text{odds}})_1 - \log(\hat{\text{odds}})_0$$
$$= \hat{\text{logit}}_1 - \hat{\text{logit}}_0$$
$$= b_0 + b_1 x_1 - (b_0 + b_1 x_0)$$
$$= b_1(x_1 - x_0),$$

so that

$$\hat{\psi} = \exp\{b_1(x_1 - x_0)\}. \tag{10.4}$$

That is, the odds ratio ($x_1$ compared to $x_0$) is the exponent of the slope parameter ($b_1$) times the difference between $x_1$ and $x_0$. Its standard error is

$$se\left(\log \hat{\psi}\right) = (x_1 - x_0)\, se(b_1). \qquad (10.5)$$

Hence, the 95% confidence interval for $\psi$ has limits

$$\exp\{b_1(x_1 - x_0) - 1.96(x_1 - x_0)\hat{se}(b_1)\}$$
$$\exp\{b_1(x_1 - x_0) + 1.96(x_1 - x_0)\hat{se}(b_1)\}. \qquad (10.6)$$

Standard errors, and thus confidence intervals, are more difficult to obtain for odds, risk and relative risk. We shall delay consideration of these until Section 10.4.1.

## 10.4    Interpretation of logistic regression coefficients

In this section we shall consider how to use the estimates of the logistic regression coefficients to make useful inferences in epidemiological research. We shall consider four different types of $x$ variable: binary, quantitative, categorical and ordinal.

### 10.4.1    Binary risk factors

*Example 10.4*    Consider the data from the Pooling Project given in Table 3.2. These data were entered into SAS and analysed using PROC GENMOD, one of the SAS procedures that may be used to fit logistic regression models. As in several other examples, the computer program is given in Appendix A. Part of the output is given in Table 10.5. This tells us that the model

$$\hat{\text{logit}} = -2.3283 + 0.3704x \qquad (10.7)$$

has been fitted. To interpret this we need to know that the codes used for smoking status, the $x$ variable, were

$$x = \begin{cases} 1 & \text{for smokers} \\ 0 & \text{for non-smokers.} \end{cases}$$

From (10.4), the odds ratio for a coronary event, comparing smokers to non-smokers, is

$$\exp\{0.3704(1 - 0)\} = \exp(0.3704) = 1.448.$$

**Table 10.5**    Excerpt derived from SAS output for Example 10.4

| Parameter | Estimate | Standard error |
|---|---|---|
| INTERCEPT | −2.3283 | 0.1482 |
| SMOKING | 0.3704 | 0.1698 |

Thus the odds ratio for exposure compared to non-exposure is particularly easy to derive when exposure is coded as 1 and non-exposure as 0 in the logistic regression model. All we have to do is to raise the slope parameter estimate, $b_1$, to the power e.

Also, from Table 10.5, the estimated standard error of this log odds ratio is 0.1698. From (10.6), an approximate 95% confidence limit for the odds ratio may be calculated as

$$\exp\{0.3704 \pm 1.96 \times 0.1698\},$$

that is, (1.038, 2.020).

We can also use (10.7) to find the odds in Example 10.4, if so desired. The odds of a coronary event come directly from (10.7), since the logit is the log odds. For smokers $(x = 1)$, the log odds are

$$-2.3283 + 0.3704 \times 1 = -1.9579,$$

giving odds of 0.1412. For non-smokers $(x = 0)$, the odds are

$$\exp(-2.3283 + 0) = 0.0975.$$

We can estimate the risk, $r$, of a coronary event for smokers from (10.2) and (10.7). That is,

$$\hat{r} = \{1 + \exp(2.3283 - 0.3704 \times 1)\}^{-1} = 0.1237.$$

In fact it is slightly easier to note that

$$\hat{r} = \left\{1 + \exp(-\widehat{\text{logit}})\right\}^{-1}. \tag{10.8}$$

So, for non-smokers,

$$\hat{r} = \{1 + \exp(2.3283)\}^{-1} = 0.0889.$$

The estimated relative risk for smokers compared to non-smokers is then most easily found as the ratio: $0.1237/0.0889 = 1.39$. Note that all the answers given here agree with those found by simple methods in Examples 3.1 and 3.2.

Standard errors, and thus confidence limits, for odds are generally not so straightforward to obtain. This is because they may involve more than one parameter, and, since the parameters are not independent, **covariances** between parameters need to be accounted for. For example, the variance of the logit when $x = 1$ (smokers in Example 10.4) is

$$V(b_0) + V(b_1) + 2C(b_0, b_1),$$

where the Vs denote variances and C covariance. SAS PROC GENMOD and other computer software can be asked to produce the **variance-covariance matrix** (sometimes simply called the **covariance matrix**) of parameter estimates. This is a square matrix with both rows and columns labelled by the parameters. Diagonal elements are the covariances of each parameter with itself; that is, the

**Table 10.6**  Variance-covariance matrix for Example 10.4

|        | $b_0$     | $b_1$     |
|--------|-----------|-----------|
| $b_0$  | 0.02195   | −0.02195  |
| $b_1$  |           | 0.02882   |

variances. Off-diagonals are the covariances: since these are equal above and below the diagonal, only one of them needs to be reported. In Example 10.4, the variance-covariance matrix is given by Table 10.6. From this,

$$\hat{V}(\widehat{logit}_{smokers}) = 0.02195 + 0.02882 + 2 \times -0.02195 = 0.00687$$

and so

$$\hat{se}(\widehat{logit}_{smokers}) = \sqrt{0.00687} = 0.0829,$$

and the 95% confidence interval for the odds of a coronary event amongst smokers is

$$\exp\{-1.9579 \pm 1.96 \times 0.0829\}$$

which is (0.120, 0.166).

Standard errors of risks and relative risks are difficult to obtain because they are non-linear functions of the model parameters, $b_0$ and $b_1$. In general, the variance of a non-linear function is *not* the same function of the variances. For example, even if we know $V(risk_{smokers})$ and $V(risk_{non\text{-}smokers})$, we cannot easily find the variance of $\lambda$, the relative risk for smokers compared to non-smokers, since

$$V(\lambda) \neq V(risk_{smokers})/V(risk_{non\text{-}smokers}).$$

As a consequence, only *approximate* standard errors of risk and relative risk may be derived. Even these are messy to derive and consequently are omitted here. Hence, it is best to use odds ratios (and odds, if required) as the outcome measures whenever logistic regression is used, whatever the form of the explanatory variable.

### 10.4.2    Quantitative risk factors

*Example 10.5*  Consider the data in Table 10.4. The parameter estimates from using SAS PROC GENMOD with these data are presented in Table 10.7. Hence, the fitted model is:

$$\widehat{logit} = -8.4056 + 0.1126x, \tag{10.9}$$

**Table 10.7**  Results produced by SAS for Example 10.5

| Parameter | Estimate | Standard error |
|---|---|---|
| INTERCEPT | −8.4056 | 0.5507 |
| AGE | 0.1126 | 0.0104 |

where the logit is the log odds of death and $x$ is the age of the man. The interpretation of $b_1$ = 0.1126 is very easy in this case; it is simply the slope of the regression line, directly analogous to the situation in simple linear regression. Reference to (10.4) shows that for each increase in age of 1 year the logit is estimated to increase by 0.1126. Figure 10.4 illustrates observed and fitted logit values and percentages. The logistic regression has smoothed out the irregularities (particularly at age 40) in the observed data. This may be easier to see from the logits, where the fitted values necessarily follow a straight line. However, interpretation is more immediate for the percentages. Observed logits are calculated from the definition of odds, (3.8); fitted percentages (risks multiplied by 100) come from (10.2).

To best understand the practical implications of the fitted model we should transform the fitted logits. For example, we have already posed the question, 'What is the odds ratio for men aged 59 relative to age 40?'. From (10.4) and (10.9), this is

$$\hat{\psi} = \exp\{0.1126(59 - 40)\} = 8.49.$$

Men aged 59 are approximately eight and half times as likely to die in the next 7.7 years as those aged 40. To calculate the 95% confidence interval for $\psi$ we use (10.6), substituting the estimated value of $se(b_1) = 0.0104$,

$$\exp\{0.1126(59-40) \pm 1.96(59-40)0.0104\},$$

or (5.77, 12.51). Thus we are 95% confident that the interval from 5.77 to 12.51 contains the true odds ratio.

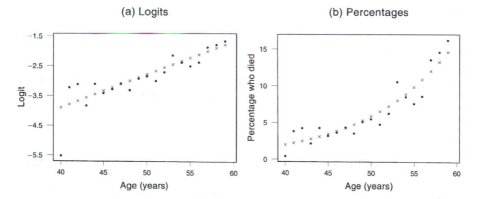

**Figure 10.4**  Observed and fitted (a) logits, and (b) percentages, from a logistic regression model for the data in Table 10.4. Observed values are indicated by dots, fitted values by crosses.

### 10.4.3    Categorical risk factors

When the $x$ variable is categorical with $\ell$ levels, the fitted logistic regression model becomes

$$\hat{\text{logit}} = b_0 + b_1^{(1)}x^{(1)} + b_1^{(2)}x^{(2)} + \cdots + b_1^{(\ell)}x^{(\ell)}, \tag{10.10}$$

where each $x^{(i)}$ variable is defined as

$$x^{(i)} = \begin{cases} 1 & \text{if } x \text{ takes its } i\text{th level} \\ 0 & \text{otherwise.} \end{cases}$$

That is, the $\{x^{(i)}\}$ are dummy variables (Section 9.2.6), which together represent the variable $x$. In fact, because $x$ will have $\ell - 1$ degrees of freedom these $x^{(i)}$ variables cannot be independent, since there are $\ell$ of them. Hence, they must be fitted subject to one, arbitrary, linear constraint, just as in Section 9.2.6. We will see the effect of the choice of constraint in Example 10.6. From (10.10), the estimated logit for level $i$ is

$$\hat{\text{logit}}^{(i)} = b_0 + b_1^{(i)},$$

subject to the linear constraint chosen.

Then the odds ratio for level $i$ compared to level $j$, which we shall call $\psi^{(ij)}$, may be found in much the same way as (10.4) was derived from (10.3). That is,

$$\hat{\text{logit}}^{(i)} - \hat{\text{logit}}^{(j)} = b_1^{(i)} - b_1^{(j)},$$

whence

$$\hat{\psi}^{(ij)} = \exp\left(b_1^{(i)} - b_1^{(j)}\right). \tag{10.11}$$

Furthermore,

$$\text{se}\left(\hat{\text{logit}}^{(i)} - \hat{\text{logit}}^{(j)}\right) = \sqrt{V\left(b_1^{(i)}\right) + V\left(b_1^{(j)}\right) - 2C\left(b_1^{(i)}, b_1^{(j)}\right)}. \tag{10.12}$$

Unfortunately, this requires knowledge of $C(b_1^{(i)}, b_1^{(j)})$. In the special case when $b_1^{(j)} = 0$, (10.11) and (10.12) reduce to the much simpler forms:

$$\hat{\psi}^{(ij)} = \exp\left(b_1^{(i)}\right), \tag{10.13}$$

$$\text{se}\left(\hat{\text{logit}}^{(i)} - \hat{\text{logit}}^{(j)}\right) = \text{se}\left(b_1^{(i)}\right). \tag{10.14}$$

Whether (10.12) or (10.14) is used, the 95% confidence interval for $\psi^{(ij)}$ is

$$\exp\left\{\left(b_1^{(i)} - b_1^{(j)}\right) \pm 1.96 \,\hat{\text{se}}\left(\hat{\text{logit}}^{(i)} - \hat{\text{logit}}^{(j)}\right)\right\}. \tag{10.15}$$

*Example 10.6* The data in Table 10.3 are for an explanatory variable (social class) with six categorical levels. In such cases there are several ways in which odds ratios, to summarize the relationship between risk factor and disease status, may be defined. For example, any one of the six social class levels could be defined as the base level and all other classes would be compared to this reference. This gives rise to five prevalence odds ratios. Any other choice of base would give five different odds ratios, although appropriate multiplication of these would reproduce the original set (Section 3.6).

When categorical variables are fitted in computer packages the natural choice of base level will vary with the package chosen (Section 9.2.7). The data in Table 10.3 were fitted in SAS PROC GENMOD by entering the social class rank from Table 10.3 as the variable RANK, declared as a categorical variable ('CLASS' variable in SAS notation). The parameter estimates produced are presented in Table 10.8. That is, the fitted model is, by reference to (10.10),

$$\hat{\text{logit}} = 1.5294 - 2.5590x^{(1)} - 1.6692x^{(2)} - 0.9904x^{(3)}$$
$$- 0.4129x^{(4)} - 0.3294x^{(5)} + 0x^{(6)},$$

where

$$x^{(i)} = \begin{cases} 1 & \text{if the social class rank is } i \\ 0 & \text{otherwise} \end{cases}$$

are the relevant dummy variables and the computer package has supplied values for the $\{b_1^{(i)}\}$.

From this we can see, as previously explained in Section 9.2.7, that SAS fixes the parameter for the *last* level of any categorical variable to be zero. This implies that the linear constraint imposed by SAS on (10.10) is $b_1^{(\ell)} = 0$. Consequently SAS expects odds ratios to be calculated relative to the *highest* level; that is, the social class with rank = 6 is the base. Hence, for example, the odds ratio contrasting social class II (rank 2) to social class V (rank 6) is, from (10.13),

$$\hat{\psi}^{(26)} = \exp(-1.6692) = 0.188,$$

with 95% confidence interval, from (10.14) and (10.15),

$$\exp\{-1.6692 \pm 1.96 \times 0.3746\}$$

or (0.090, 0.393). Other odds ratios relative to social class V are similarly easy to derive.

**Table 10.8** Results produced by SAS for Example 10.6

| Parameter | Estimate | Standard error |
|---|---|---|
| INTERCEPT | 1.5294 | 0.3059 |
| RANK 1 | −2.5590 | 0.4789 |
| RANK 2 | −1.6692 | 0.3746 |
| RANK 3 | −0.9904 | 0.4111 |
| RANK 4 | −0.4129 | 0.3340 |
| RANK 5 | −0.3294 | 0.3816 |
| RANK 6 | 0.0000 | 0.0000 |

Suppose that we prefer our odds ratios to use the first social class as the base. This might be because we expect this class to have the lowest prevalence odds, or simply because we are more comfortable making comparisons against the 'lowest' group (in terms of numbering or otherwise). For example, consider comparing social class II (rank 2) to social class I (rank 1). From (10.11),

$$\hat{\psi}^{(21)} = \exp\left(b_1^{(2)} - b_1^{(1)}\right) = \exp(-1.6692 - (-2.5590))$$

$$= e^{0.8898} = 2.43.$$

An alternative way of deriving this from the table of parameter estimates is to notice that

$$\hat{\psi}^{(21)} = \hat{\psi}^{(26)}\hat{\psi}^{(61)} = \hat{\psi}^{(26)}/\hat{\psi}^{(16)}$$

$$= \exp(-1.6692)/\exp(-2.5590)$$

$$= \exp(-1.6692 - (-2.5590))$$

as before.

To obtain the 95% confidence interval for $\hat{\psi}^{(21)}$ we must first obtain the variance-covariance matrix. The matrix produced by SAS PROC GENMOD is presented as Table 10.9. Note that $b_1^{(6)}$ is fixed by SAS, so has no variance. Then, by (10.12),

$$\hat{se}\left(\hat{logit}^{(2)} - \hat{logit}^{(1)}\right) = \sqrt{0.14033 + 0.22930 - 2 \times 0.09359} = 0.4271.$$

Thus the 95% confidence interval for $\hat{\psi}^{(21)}$ is, from (10.15),

$$\exp\{-1.6692 - (-2.5590) \pm 1.96 \times 0.4271\},$$

that is, $\exp\{0.8898 \pm 0.8371\}$ or (1.05, 5.62).

As may be seen from Example 10.6, there is a great advantage to having a 'slope' parameter of zero for the chosen base level. As a consequence, it is sensible to force the computer package to do this, and so avoid the more extensive calculations made at the end of Example 10.6. To be able to force the most convenient mode of fitting, we must know the linear constraint that is used by whatever computer package we choose to use. For instance, we have seen that SAS PROC GENMOD fixes the last level to have a 'slope' parameter of zero, $b_1^{(\ell)} = 0$. As we saw in Section 9.2.7, some packages (including GENSTAT and GLIM), by contrast, will fix the *first* level to have a 'slope'

**Table 10.9**    Variance-covariance matrix produced by SAS for Example 10.6

|            | $b_0$    | $b_1^{(1)}$ | $b_1^{(2)}$ | $b_1^{(3)}$ | $b_1^{(4)}$ | $b_1^{(5)}$ |
|------------|----------|-------------|-------------|-------------|-------------|-------------|
| $b_0$        | 0.09359  | -0.09359    | -0.09359    | -0.09359    | -0.09359    | -0.09359    |
| $b_1^{(1)}$  |          | 0.22930     | 0.09359     | 0.09359     | 0.09359     | 0.09359     |
| $b_1^{(2)}$  |          |             | 0.14033     | 0.09359     | 0.09359     | 0.09359     |
| $b_1^{(3)}$  |          |             |             | 0.16899     | 0.09359     | 0.09359     |
| $b_1^{(4)}$  |          |             |             |             | 0.11153     | 0.09359     |
| $b_1^{(5)}$  |          |             |             |             |             | 0.14564     |

parameter of zero, $b_1^{(1)} = 0$. Hence the estimate and estimated standard error of $\psi^{(21)}$ for Example 10.6 would come directly from these packages, only requiring 'RANK' to be declared as a categorical variable. Some packages, such as SPSS, allow the user a degree of choice in setting the base level.

There are two ways to force the chosen package to use a base that is not the one that the package automatically chooses when the levels are entered in their natural numerical order. The easiest way is to present the package with levels of the $x$ variable that are appropriately reordered.

*Example 10.7*   Consider the problem at the end of Example 10.6 again, and suppose that SAS PROC GENMOD is to be used. If we wish to use social class I as the base for all the odds ratios we use the coding in Table 10.10 for the new variable 'SOCLASS' derived from the old variable 'RANK'. The lowest RANK is now the highest SOCLASS; everything else is left unaltered. The parameter estimates from SAS for the logistic regression using SOCLASS are shown in Table 10.11. Now, from (10.13), (10.14) and (10.15) we see immediately that

$$\hat{\psi}^{(21)} = \exp(0.8899) = 2.43,$$

with a 95% confidence interval of

$$\exp\{0.8899 \pm 1.96 \times 0.4271\}$$

or (1.05, 5.62) as before. Indeed, all $\hat{\psi}^{(i1)}$ are easy to deal with; the complete set of odds ratios and their 95% confidence intervals are shown in Figure 10.5. Keeping the odds for social

**Table 10.10**   Social class coding (SOCLASS) which is suitable for treating the lowest rank (RANK) as the base group when considered as a CLASS variable in SAS

| Social class | RANK | SOCLASS |
|---|---|---|
| I | 1 | 7 |
| II | 2 | 2 |
| IIIn | 3 | 3 |
| IIIm | 4 | 4 |
| IV | 5 | 5 |
| V | 6 | 6 |

**Table 10.11**   Results produced by SAS for Example 10.7

| Parameter | Estimate | Standard error |
|---|---|---|
| INTERCEPT | −1.0296 | 0.3684 |
| SOCLASS 2 | 0.8899 | 0.4271 |
| SOCLASS 3 | 1.5686 | 0.4595 |
| SOCLASS 4 | 2.1461 | 0.3920 |
| SOCLASS 5 | 2.2296 | 0.4333 |
| SOCLASS 6 | 2.5590 | 0.4789 |
| SOCLASS 7 | 0.0000 | 0.0000 |

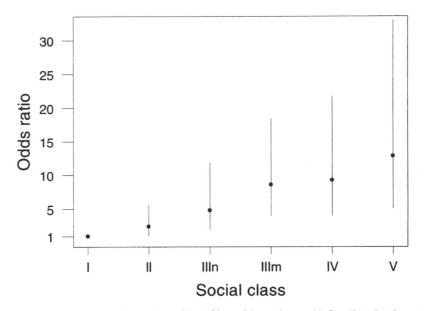

**Figure 10.5**    Prevalence odds ratios (with 95% confidence intervals) for *H. pylori* by social class group.

class I fixed as 1, we can see how the prevalence odds ratio of *H. pylori* increases with 'increasing' social class (increasing deprivation).

The other way to change the default choice of base is to employ dummy variables. SAS PROC GENMOD, GENSTAT, GLIM and SPSS (and others) allow the explanatory variable to be declared as categorical. Several other computer packages, or individual procedures, do not have this facility. When using such software, categorical variables must be defined as a set of dummy variables. Even when a categorical declaration *is* available we can choose not to make this declaration, because the linear constraint used is inconvenient, and define convenient dummy variables instead. Given a categorical variable with $\ell$ levels, we shall need to define and fit $\ell - 1$ dummy variables. This is because the group variable has only $\ell - 1$ d.f. (Section 9.2.6).

*Example 10.8*    Consider again the problem of calculating odds ratios relative to the base of social class I for Example 10.6. This time SAS PROC GENMOD was used without the CLASS declaration to denote RANK (Example 10.6) or SOCLASS (Example 10.7) as categorical. Instead five dummy variables, X2–X6, were defined out of the original RANK variable, X$i$ having value 1 if RANK $= i$ and 0 otherwise. The consequent data set, arising from Table 10.3, for input to SAS is given as Table 10.12, where $E$ is the number with disease

**Table 10.12**  Data for Example 10.8 including the dummy variables for social class (X2–X6)

| RANK | X2 | X3 | X4 | X5 | X6 | E | N |
|------|-----|-----|-----|-----|-----|-----|-----|
| 1 | 0 | 0 | 0 | 0 | 0 | 10 | 38 |
| 2 | 1 | 0 | 0 | 0 | 0 | 40 | 86 |
| 3 | 0 | 1 | 0 | 0 | 0 | 36 | 57 |
| 4 | 0 | 0 | 1 | 0 | 0 | 226 | 300 |
| 5 | 0 | 0 | 0 | 1 | 0 | 83 | 108 |
| 6 | 0 | 0 | 0 | 0 | 1 | 60 | 73 |

**Table 10.13**  Results produced by SAS for Example 10.8

| Parameter | Estimate | Standard error |
|-----------|----------|----------------|
| INTERCEPT | −1.0296 | 0.3684 |
| X2 | 0.8899 | 0.4271 |
| X3 | 1.5686 | 0.4595 |
| X4 | 2.1461 | 0.3920 |
| X5 | 2.2296 | 0.4333 |
| X6 | 2.5590 | 0.4789 |

and $N$ is the total number at each level. Note that, for example, X4 is zero unless RANK = 4. The five explanatory variables X2–X6 were fitted using PROC GENMOD. Table 10.13 gives the results, which are exactly as in Table 10.11, as they should be.

Notice that the lowest level (RANK = 1) is the base level in Example 10.8. This is because all the X variables are zero when RANK = 1. This makes all the X variables, when fitted together, into a set of contrasts with RANK = 1.

### 10.4.4  Ordinal risk factors

Our logistic regression models for Table 10.3 have, so far, ignored the ordering of the categories (levels). It might be sensible to consider a logistic regression model for the ranks themselves, rather than the categories they represent. This requires treating 'rank' as a quantitative measure; we may then proceed exactly as in Section 10.4.2.

*Example 10.9*  The *H. pylori* data in Table 10.3 were, once more, analysed with SAS PROC GENMOD, but now treating RANK as continuous (that is to say, no CLASS declaration was made and dummy variables were not defined). The estimated intercept was −1.0893 and slope was 0.5037. Hence the model fitted is

$$\hat{\text{logit}} = -1.0893 + 0.5037x,$$

where $x$ is the rank. Notice that this implies a linear trend in the log odds by increasing rank score (Figure 10.6(a)), hence this is a linear trend model of a certain kind.

If we consider the odds ratio for a unit increase in the rank score, (10.4) gives

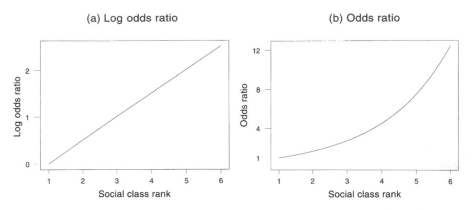

**Figure 10.6**   Fitted values for (a) the log odds ratio, and (b) the odds ratio, when social class I (rank = 1) is fixed to have an odds of unity.

$$\hat{\psi} = e^{0.5037} = 1.65.$$

Hence we estimate that the odds go up by a factor of 1.65 for each step along the social scale. That is, we have fitted a model for a constant multiplicative increase in odds by social class. This is emphasized by Figure 10.6(b). The odds ratio for a step of $s$ units is $1.65^s$. Recall that, due to the way occupational social class groups are defined, a higher-numbered group represents increased deprivation.

If the ordinal (linear trend) model is adequate we would expect the estimates of the odds from this model to be close to those from the categorical model (where they are not assumed to have a fixed relationship with each other) fitted in Example 10.7. For example, the odds in social class III are 1.71 for the categorical model (from Table 10.13) and 1.52 for the ordinal model, which are fairly close. Since the odds ratio is scaled, so that its value in the base group (social class I) is unity, separately for each model, we cannot expect close agreement when comparing sizes of odds ratios in Figures 10.5 and 10.6(b) even when the linear trend model is appropriate. Thus the odds ratio for social class III compared to I is 4.80 for the categorical model but only 2.74 for the ordinal model; this difference does not prove lack of appropriateness of the linear trend assumption. We consider the lack of fit of the ordinal model in Example 10.24.

## 10.5   Generic data

Up to now we have assumed that the data are supplied to the computer package in a grouped form (as in Table 10.2). However, as mentioned at the outset in Section 10.1, raw data are usually ungrouped, simply recording the risk factor level and disease status for each individual separately. This is the **generic** (or **case-by-case** or **binary**) **data** format, as represented by Table 10.1.

In practice, generic data are easier to deal with than grouped data; it is simply easier to describe the methodology using the grouped format. With generic data we code our disease status variable as 1 if disease is present and 0 if disease is absent. We can fit logistic regression models just as before, except that, in the notation of Section 10.1, $n_i = 1$ for each $i$ (each individual),

$$e_i = \begin{cases} 1 & \text{if individual } i \text{ has the disease} \\ 0 & \text{otherwise} \end{cases}$$

and hence $r_i = e_i/n_i = e_i$.

*Example 10.10*   Table 10.4 presents a summarized version of the SHHS data on age and death. The original database for the study is, conceptually, a rectangular matrix of individuals against variables. When we select out the age and death status variables only, we obtain a matrix with 5754 rows and two columns (AGE and DEATH, coded as 0 for no, 1 for yes). These data are available electronically: see Appendix C. We need to define a third column which is made up of 5754 entries of the number 1. These three columns then take the place of the first three columns in Table 10.4, although 'age' will now have many duplicate values and will not be sorted in order. These three columns of generic data can be input to a computer package and a logistic regression model fitted.

SAS PROC GENMOD was used in this way. Output 10.1 gives part of the full output. The estimates and their standard errors will be seen to agree with those found using the grouped data of Table 10.4, as presented in Table 10.7. The degrees of freedom column in Output 10.1 is redundant here, and in all future examples, except that it will show a result of zero when the corresponding parameter is fixed to be zero. The chi-square test given in Output 10.1 will be explained in Section 10.7.4.

As Example 10.10 demonstrates, we obtain the same estimates from generic and grouped data. There will be differences when we consider ideas of lack of fit of logistic regression models in Section 10.7.1.

## 10.6   Multiple logistic regression models

Just as with standard regression models, logistic models may be specified with several explanatory variables, rather than only one. Given $k$ explanatory

**Output 10.1**   SAS results for Example 10.10

The GENMOD Procedure

Analysis of Parameter Estimates

| Parameter | DF | Estimate | Std. Err | ChiSquare | Pr > Chi |
|-----------|----|----------|----------|-----------|----------|
| INTERCEPT | 1 | −8.4056 | 0.5507 | 232.9962 | 0.0001 |
| AGE | 1 | 0.1126 | 0.0104 | 116.9216 | 0.0001 |

variables, the multiple logistic regression model is, by analogy with (10.3),

$$\log_e\left(\frac{\hat{r}}{1-\hat{r}}\right) = b_0 + b_1 x_1 + b_2 x_2 + \cdots + b_k x_k,$$

where $\hat{r}$ is the estimated risk of disease. The right-hand side of the model equation is now a multiple linear predictor.

If, say, $x_i$ is a categorical variable with $\ell$ levels then we replace $b_i x_i$ with

$$b_i^{(1)} x_i^{(1)} + b_i^{(2)} x_i^{(2)} + \cdots + b_i^{(\ell)} x_i^{(\ell)},$$

where

$$x_i^{(j)} = \begin{cases} 1 & \text{if } x_i \text{ takes its } j\text{th level} \\ 0 & \text{otherwise,} \end{cases}$$

subject to an arbitrary linear constraint (such as $b_i^{(\ell)} = 0$). All this, apart from the differences identified in Section 10.3, is exactly as for general linear models. Logistic regression is an example of a **generalized linear model** (see McCullagh and Nelder, 1989), a class of models which includes the general linear model (standard regression and analysis of variance).

Multiple logistic models are dealt with in much the same way as single-variable models, but (as with multiple-variable general linear models) allow for a wider range of inferences. Basic analyses are now explained by example.

*Example 10.11*    Table 10.14 presents data on coronary heart disease (CHD), blood pressure and cholesterol from the cohort phase of the SHHS. As in Example 10.2, we are considering this as a fixed cohort study with a follow-up period of 7.7 years. This time, data are only shown for the 4095 men with no evidence of CHD at baseline, for whom systolic blood pressure and serum total cholesterol were measured. The blood pressure and cholesterol groups chosen in Table 10.14 are the fifths for the entire set of male data, that is before those with CHD at baseline were deleted.

These data were read into SAS, denoting the systolic blood pressure (SBP) variable as SBP5TH and the total cholesterol variable as CHOL5TH. They were then analysed in PROC GENMOD, fixing the lowest level of SBP5TH and CHOL5TH respectively to have a log

**Table 10.14**   Ratio of CHD events to total number by systolic blood pressure (SBP) and cholesterol fifths for men in the SHHS who were free of CHD at baseline

| SBP (mmHg) | Serum total cholesterol (mmol/l) | | | | |
|---|---|---|---|---|---|
| | ≤ 5.41 | 5.42–6.01 | 6.02–6.56 | 6.57–7.31 | > 7.31 |
| ≤ 118 | 1/190 | 0/183 | 4/178 | 8/157 | 4/132 |
| 119–127 | 2/203 | 2/175 | 6/167 | 10/166 | 11/137 |
| 128–136 | 5/173 | 9/176 | 9/181 | 8/167 | 11/164 |
| 137–148 | 5/139 | 3/156 | 10/154 | 13/174 | 16/174 |
| > 148 | 5/123 | 8/123 | 12/144 | 13/179 | 23/180 |

odds of zero (odds of unity). The parameter estimates produced by SAS (after relabelling, as explained in Section 10.4.3) are given in Table 10.15.

From Table 10.15 the fitted model is

$$\widehat{\text{logit}} = -4.5995 + 0x_1^{(1)} + 0.6092x_1^{(2)} + 0.8697x_1^{(3)} + 1.0297x_1^{(4)} + 1.3425x_1^{(5)}$$
$$+ 0x_2^{(1)} + 0.2089x_2^{(2)} + 0.8229x_2^{(3)} + 1.0066x_2^{(4)} + 1.2957x_2^{(5)}, \tag{10.16}$$

where $x_1^{(i)}$ represents the $i$th level of SBP and $x_2^{(i)}$ represents the $i$th level of cholesterol, for $i$ running from 1 to 5 in rank order in each case. Since the highest estimate is for the highest fifth in each case, we can immediately see that it is most dangerous to be in the top fifth of both SBP and cholesterol.

We can estimate the log odds of CHD for a man in the highest level of SBP ($>148\,\text{mmHg}$) and highest level of cholesterol ($>7.31\,\text{mmol/l}$) to be, from (10.16),

$$\widehat{\text{logit}} = \exp\{-4.5995 + 1.3425 + 1.2957\} = -1.9613.$$

The odds are thus $e^{-1.9613} = 0.1407$.

We can estimate the risk for a man in these two extreme levels using (10.8),

$$\hat{r} = \{1 + \exp(1.9613)\}^{-1} = 0.1233.$$

So the chance of a coronary event in a follow-up period of 7.7 years is 0.1233 for middle-aged Scotsmen with the highest levels (by fifths) of both SBP and cholesterol.

We can estimate the log odds ratio for a man in the combination of highest levels (5, 5) relative to the combination of lowest levels (1, 1) (SBP $\leq 118\,\text{mmHg}$; cholesterol $\leq 5.41\,\text{mmol/l}$) from (10.16) as

$$\log\hat{\psi} = \widehat{\text{logit}}^{(5,5)} - \widehat{\text{logit}}^{(1,1)}$$
$$= (-4.5995 + 1.3425 + 1.2957) - (-4.5995)$$
$$= 1.3425 + 1.2957 = 2.6382,$$

whence the odds ratio is $e^{2.6382} = 14.0$. Notice that the constant term ($-4.5995$) simply cancels out, as it must do whenever any odds ratio is calculated.

The relative risk for the same contrast is

**Table 10.15**  Estimates for Example 10.11, as produced by SAS

| Parameter | | Estimate |
|---|---|---|
| INTERCEPT | | $-4.5995$ |
| SBP5TH | 1 | 0.0000 |
| SBP5TH | 2 | 0.6092 |
| SBP5TH | 3 | 0.8697 |
| SBP5TH | 4 | 1.0297 |
| SBP5TH | 5 | 1.3425 |
| CHOL5TH | 1 | 0.0000 |
| CHOL5TH | 2 | 0.2089 |
| CHOL5TH | 3 | 0.8229 |
| CHOL5TH | 4 | 1.0066 |
| CHOL5TH | 5 | 1.2957 |

$$\hat{r}^{(5,5)}/\hat{r}^{(1/1)},$$

which turns out to be $0.1233/0.009957 = 12.4$. Notice that this is similar to the odds ratio, as would be expected since CHD is reasonably unusual, even in the high-risk group.

It is interesting to see how the two risk factors behave when varied alone, to compare with the combined effect seen already. From Table 10.15, the odds ratio comparing level 5 of SBP to level 1, keeping cholesterol fixed, is $e^{1.3425} = 3.8$. It is quite correct to ignore all the estimates for cholesterol in deriving this. To see this, consider the odds ratio for the 5th compared to the 1st fifth for SBP keeping cholesterol fixed at its 3rd fifth. This is the same as finding the odds ratio for the combination of (SBP, cholesterol) as (5, 3) relative to (1, 3). From (10.16),

$$\text{lo}\hat{\text{g}}\text{it}^{(5,3)} = -4.5995 + 1.3425 + 0.8229$$

$$\text{lo}\hat{\text{g}}\text{it}^{(1,3)} = -4.5995 + 0 + 0.8229.$$

Hence the log odds are $\text{lo}\hat{\text{g}}\text{it}^{(5,3)} - \text{lo}\hat{\text{g}}\text{it}^{(1,3)} = 1.3425$ and $\hat{\psi} = e^{1.3425}$, as stated. The constant term and the slope parameter for level 3 of cholesterol have cancelled out.

Similarly, for comparing between extreme levels of cholesterol, keeping SBP fixed, the odds ratio is $e^{1.2957} = 3.7$. Notice that $3.8 \times 3.7 = 14.1$, which is very similar to the combined odds ratio of 14.0 found earlier, suggesting that there is little interaction between these two risk factors (see Sections 4.8.2 and 10.9).

Confidence intervals for comparisons where only one variable's levels are varied follow exactly as in Section 10.4.3. When the levels of two (or more) variables are varied we shall need the variance-covariance matrix. For instance, the standard error of the log odds ratio comparing (5, 5) to (1, 1) in Example 10.11 is

$$\text{se}\left\{\text{lo}\hat{\text{g}}\text{it}^{(5,5)} - \text{lo}\hat{\text{g}}\text{it}^{(1,1)}\right\} = \text{se}\left\{b_0 + b_1^{(5)} + b_2^{(5)} - \left(b_0 + b_1^{(1)} + b_2^{(1)}\right)\right\}$$

$$= \text{se}\left\{b_1^{(5)} + b_2^{(5)}\right\}$$

$$= \sqrt{\text{V}\left(b_1^{(5)}\right) + \text{V}\left(b_2^{(5)}\right) + 2\text{C}\left(b_1^{(5)}, b_2^{(5)}\right)}.$$

Using this, the 95% confidence interval is, as usual,

$$\text{estimate} \pm 1.96\hat{\text{se}}.$$

*Example 10.12*   A rather more substantial example is provided by fitting six risk factors for the SHHS data on men with no prior history of CHD. This time SBP and cholesterol were both fitted as quantitative variables, since Table 10.15 suggests that both of their effects are linear (see also Section 10.7.3). The other variables fitted were age, body mass index (BMI: weight/square of height), smoking status and self-reported activity in leisure. Age and BMI are quantitative; smoking is coded as $1 =$ never smoked, $2 =$ ex-smoker, $3 =$ current smoker; activity in leisure is also categorical, coded as $1 =$ active, $2 =$ average, $3 =$ inactive. As in Example 10.11, any man for whom at least one variable has a missing value is not included. The data used are available electronically: see Appendix C.

With so many variables it is very time-consuming to create the multi-way table (which needs to be six-dimensional here) corresponding to Table 10.14. Furthermore, the quantitative variables would give rise to huge tables, since we are not grouping them here. Hence, the data were input to SAS in generic form: 4049 lines each containing data for the seven variables, AGE, TOTCHOL, BMI, SYSTOL, SMOKING, ACTIVITY and CHD, where

$$CHD = \begin{cases} 1 & \text{if the individual had a CHD event} \\ 0 & \text{if not,} \end{cases}$$

and the variables have obvious names. PROC GENMOD was used to fit the logistic regression model with base levels 1 (active) for activity in leisure and 1 (never smoked) for smoking status. As explained in Section 10.5, a further column consisting of 4049 copies of the number 1 was created to hold the $n_i$. The parameter estimates produced are given in Table 10.16.

The fitted model is thus

$$\text{log\^{}it} = -10.1076 + 0.0171x_1 + 0.3071x_2 + 0.0417x_3 + 0.0204x_4$$
$$+ 0x_5^{(1)} + 0.3225x_5^{(2)} + 0.7296x_5^{(3)} + 0x_6^{(1)} - 0.1904x_6^{(2)} - 0.1011x_6^{(3)}, \quad (10.17)$$

where the $x$ variables and units of measurement are as defined in Table 10.16.

As in the single-variable situation, the parameter for a quantitative variable represents the increase in log odds for a unit increase in the variable, but now keeping all other variables fixed. Hence the increase in log odds for an increase of 1 mmol/l in cholesterol, keeping the other five variables fixed, is 0.3071; the log odds for an increase of 2 mmol/l in cholesterol, keeping all else fixed, is $2 \times 0.3071 = 0.6142$; the odds ratio for a cholesterol of $x + s$ relative to $x$, keeping all else fixed, is $\exp(0.3071s)$ regardless of the value of $x$.

Similar interpretations follow for categorical variables. Thus 0.3225 is the log odds ratio for ex-smokers compared to never smokers, keeping all the other five variables fixed at some arbitrary values. Notice that the negative signs for estimates of ACTIVITY give unexpected

**Table 10.16**  Parameter estimates for Example 10.12, as produced by SAS

| | Variable name/symbol | Units of measurement/code | Parameter estimate |
|---|---|---|---|
| – | INTERCEPT | – | −10.1076 |
| $x_1$ | AGE | years | 0.0171 |
| $x_2$ | TOTCHOL | mmol/l | 0.3071 |
| $x_3$ | BMI | kg/m$^2$ | 0.0417 |
| $x_4$ | SYSTOL | mmHg | 0.0204 |
| $x_5^{(1)}$ | SMOKING 1 | never smoker | 0.0000 |
| $x_5^{(2)}$ | SMOKING 2 | ex-smoker | 0.3225 |
| $x_5^{(3)}$ | SMOKING 3 | current smoker | 0.7296 |
| $x_6^{(1)}$ | ACTIVITY 1 | active | 0.0000 |
| $x_6^{(2)}$ | ACTIVITY 2 | average | −0.1904 |
| $x_6^{(3)}$ | ACTIVITY 3 | inactive | −0.1011 |

inferences in our example: those who are average and inactive have a lower odds of CHD than those who are active in their leisure time. This may be a result of bias caused by self-assessment of activity level.

As in Example 10.11, we can use the multiple logistic regression model to make inferences about combinations of variable outcomes. For example, the log odds for a 50-year-old active male ex-smoker who is currently free of CHD and has a serum total cholesterol value of 6.0 mmol/l, BMI of $25\,\text{kg/m}^2$ and SBP of $125\,\text{mmHg}$ is

$$\text{logit} = -10.1076 + 0.0171 \times 50 + 0.3071 \times 6.0$$
$$+ 0.0417 \times 25 + 0.0204 \times 125 + 0.3225 + 0 = -3.4950,$$

from which the odds are $e^{-3.495} = 0.030$ and, using (10.8), the risk is $\{1 + e^{3.495}\}^{-1} = 0.029$. Hence we expect around 3% of such men to experience a coronary event during a period of 7.7 years.

Consider a similar man with all as before, except that he is a current smoker and has an SBP of 150. The log odds for such a man compared to the previous type is easily found by finding the difference in logits, ignoring any terms that must cancel out:

$$0.0204(150 - 125) + 0.7296 - 0.3225 = 0.9171.$$

Thus $\hat{\psi} = e^{0.9171} = 2.50$. The second type of man has two and a half times the odds of a CHD event compared to the first type.

## 10.7    Tests of hypotheses

So far we have only considered the issue of estimating the effect of a risk factor upon disease outcome in our discussion of logistic regression. As in other branches of statistical analysis, we will often be interested in whether the effect observed is attributable to chance. Three particular types of hypothesis will be described here: tests of lack of fit of the overall model (which are unsuitable for generic data); tests of effect of any one risk factor contained within the model; and tests of the linear effect of ordered categorical risk factors.

All of these tests use a quantity called the **deviance**, which is calculated whenever a generalized linear model is fitted by a statistical computer package. The deviance, in turn, is calculated from the **likelihood**, which is a measure of how likely a particular model is, given the observed data. Complete details, and many examples, are given in Clayton and Hills (1993). The deviance is, essentially, a measure of the difference between the postulated model and the model which, by definition, is a perfect fit to the data (called the **full** or **saturated** model). To be precise, it is given by

$$D = -2\{\log \hat{L} - \log \hat{L}_\text{F}\}$$

where $L$ is the likelihood for the postulated model and $L_\text{F}$ is the likelihood for the full model. The larger the value of the deviance, the greater the difference between the likelihood of the current model and that of the model which has perfect fit. When the data have a normal distribution (the general linear model), the deviance may be shown to be the residual sum of squares.

As far as the practical epidemiologist is concerned, the deviance may be regarded simply as a test statistic, akin to Student's $t$ statistic, the chi-square statistic and many others. The interested reader is referred to McCullagh and Nelder (1989) for a full explanation, and to Collett (1991) for an explanation in the context of logistic regression.

### 10.7.1 Lack of fit

If the data are grouped – that is, not in generic form – the deviance of the model can be used to test for lack of fit of the model to the data. However, if the data are in generic form, this is not possible for theoretical reasons (see Collett, 1991). It can be shown that the test for lack of fit requires comparison of the deviance with chi-square on the same d.f. as that of the deviance.

In order to understand how the model deviance may be used, Table 10.17 shows the model deviance and d.f. for all the examples used so far. The d.f. for a model deviance is calculated just as for the residual term in the general linear model, that is,

d.f. = number of data items − number of independent parameters in the

fitted model,

where the number of independent parameters is 1 for the intercept (constant) term, 1 for a quantitative variable and $\ell - 1$ for a categorical variable with $\ell$ levels, and the 'data items' each correspond to a distinct definition of $n$ (denominator for the calculation of risk). For example, there are 20 data items in Example 10.2. Table 10.18 shows how the d.f. for the deviance is calculated for each of the seven examples listed in Table 10.17. With the generic data format (Examples 10.10 and 10.12), the number of data items is simply the sample size.

As already stated, we can make no use of the model deviance to determine lack of fit when the data are analysed in generic form: hence no $p$ value is given in Table 10.17 for Examples 10.10 and 10.12. However, notice that the deviance and d.f. are quite different for Examples 10.5 and 10.10, which (as we have already seen) produce the same fitted models. The model deviance is similarly of no use when it turns out to be zero. In fact this signifies that the full model must have been fitted. This is always the case when a single categorical variable is recorded and fitted to grouped data, as in Examples 10.4 and 10.6. As Table 10.18 shows, we have 'used up' all the degrees of freedom in the

**Table 10.17**  Model deviance and brief descriptions for all prior examples: *p* values are found from a computer package, comparing the deviance to chi-square with d.f. as for the deviance

| Example number | Brief description | Type of Variable | Data | Model Deviance | d.f. | p value |
|---|---|---|---|---|---|---|
| 10.1/6/7/8 | MONICA *H. pylori* | Categorical | Grouped | 0 | 0 | – |
| 10.9 | MONICA *H. pylori* | Quantitative | Grouped | 6.55 | 4 | 0.17 |
| 10.2/3/5 | SHHS Deaths | Quantitative | Grouped | 23.46 | 18 | 0.17 |
| 10.10 | SHHS Deaths | Quantitative | Generic | 2683.67 | 5752 | – |
| 10.4 | Pooling CHD | Categorical | Grouped | 0 | 0 | – |
| 10.11 | SHHS CHD | Categorical | Grouped | 18.86 | 16 | 0.28 |
| 10.12 | SHHS CHD | Mixed | Generic | 1481.34 | 4040 | – |

**Table 10.18**   Derivation of d.f. for model deviances

| Example number | Number of data items | Variables (number of indep. parameters) | Difference = d.f. |
|---|---|---|---|
| 10.1/6/7/8 | 6 | constant (1) social class (5) | $6 - 1 - 5 = 0$ |
| 10.9 | 6 | constant (1) social class (1) | $6 - 1 - 1 = 4$ |
| 10.2/3/5 | 20 | constant (1) age (1) | $20 - 1 - 1 = 18$ |
| 10.10 | 5754 | constant (1) age (1) | $5754 - 1 - 1 = 5752$ |
| 10.4 | 2 | constant (1) smoking (1) | $2 - 1 - 1 = 0$ |
| 10.11 | 25 | constant (1) SBP (4) cholesterol (4) | $25 - 1 - 4 - 4 = 16$ |
| 10.12 | 4049 | constant (1) age (1) cholesterol (1) BMI (1) SBP (1) smoking (2) activity (2) | $4049 - 1 - 1 - 1 - 1 - 1 - 2 - 2 = 4040$ |

models fitted in these examples: no other sources of variability remain. By definition, such models have perfect fit and lack of fit is not an issue.

For Examples 10.5, 10.9 and 10.11 we can evaluate lack of fit. In Examples 10.5 and 10.9 a quantitative variable is used to summarize the effect of the $x$ variable; this does *not* give rise to a full model because there is remaining variation about the fitted line (Figure 10.4). Neither of these models has a significant deviance ($p > 0.10$), and hence we may conclude that the fitted models show no problems of lack of fit.

In Example 10.11 the remaining variation, not modelled, is the interaction between SBP and cholesterol. This interaction will have $(5 - 1)(5 - 1) = 16$ d.f. because both SBP and cholesterol have five levels. However, again $p > 0.10$, and so we can safely conclude that the model with only the two main effects is a satisfactory fit to the data. In fact, the probable lack of interaction in this problem was remarked upon in Example 10.11.

If lack of fit is found we might suspect that further explanatory variables are needed to predict disease, or that we have, in some way, inadequately modelled the effect of the current variables. Absence of evidence for lack of fit does not necessarily mean that the fit cannot be improved by adding new variables to the model, or that problems, such as outliers, do not occur in the data (Section 10.10). Indeed, tests of lack of fit are really of limited use; generally it is much more meaningful to test for specific effects.

### 10.7.2   Effect of a risk factor

Now we consider a test of the effect of a risk factor, rather than the adequacy of the overall model which contains this risk factor and other terms (including the constant). As a preliminary, the concept of model **nesting** will be defined: model A is said to be nested within model B if model B contains all the variables of model A plus at least one other. In this context the constant is thought of as a variable. Examples of nesting are given in Table 10.19.

When model A is nested within model B we can test the hypothesis that the extra terms in B have no effect by calculating the difference between the deviances of models A and B, denoted $\Delta D$, and comparing this with chi-square on d.f. given by the difference in d.f., denoted $\Delta$d.f., between the two models. This procedure (relying upon an approximate theoretical derivation) works for generic, as well as grouped, data.

*Example 10.13*   We return to the data on *H. pylori* and social class in Table 10.3, as analysed in Examples 10.6–10.8. We will be interested in knowing whether a man's social class has any effect on his chance of having *H. pylori*. So far we have fitted the model that assumes that it does:

$$\text{logit} = b_0 + b^{(1)}x^{(1)} + b^{(2)}x^{(2)} + b^{(3)}x^{(3)} + b^{(4)}x^{(4)} + b^{(5)}x^{(5)} + b^{(6)}x^{(6)}. \tag{10.18}$$

Let us consider the null hypothesis, $H_0 : b^{(j)} = 0$ for all $j$, against the alternative, $H_1$ : some $b^{(j)} \neq 0$. The null hypothesis states that no social class has any effect on the log odds of *H. pylori* different from the overall average effect (encapsulated by the constant term). Under $H_0$,

$$\text{logit} = b_0, \tag{10.19}$$

which is equivalent to saying that each social class has the same effect. Model (10.19) is clearly nested within model (10.18): the difference between them is the set of variables for the risk factor 'social class'. In Example 10.6 we found that (10.18) is

**Table 10.19**   Some examples of nesting (model A is nested within model B)

| Example number | Model A | Model B |
| --- | --- | --- |
| 10.6 | constant | constant + social class |
| 10.11 | constant + SBP | constant + SBP + cholesterol |
| 10.12 | constant + age + cholesterol + BMI + smoking | constant + age + cholesterol + BMI + SBP + smoking + activity in leisure |

$$\text{loĝit} = 1.5294 - 2.5590x^{(1)} - 1.6692x^{(2)} - 0.9904x^{(3)} - 0.4129x^{(4)} - 0.3294x^{(5)},$$

and the deviance for this model is 0 on 0 d.f. (see Tables 10.17 and 10.18, or simply note that this is the full model). Fitting (10.19) gives

$$\text{loĝit} = 0.7876,$$

with deviance 64.44 on 5 d.f. Notice that the $b_0$ in model (10.19) is different from that in model (10.18); just because the models are nested certainly does not suggest that the estimates of any common effects are, in any way, close. Here

$$\Delta D = 64.44 \text{ on } \Delta\text{d.f.} = 5 \text{ d.f.}$$

Comparing to $\chi_5^2$ the $p$ value for this is below 0.0001. Hence the test is extremely significant; we reject $H_0$ and conclude that there is, indeed, some effect of social class.

*Example 10.14*   Consider Example 10.11 once more. There are four models (not involving interactions) that may be fitted:

1. $\text{loĝit} = b_0$
2. $\text{loĝit} = b_0 + b_1^{(1)}x_1^{(1)} + b_1^{(2)}x_1^{(2)} + b_1^{(3)}x_1^{(3)} + b_1^{(4)}x_1^{(4)} + b_1^{(5)}x_1^{(5)}$
3. $\text{loĝit} = b_0 + b_2^{(1)}x_2^{(1)} + b_2^{(2)}x_2^{(2)} + b_2^{(3)}x_2^{(3)} + b_2^{(4)}x_2^{(4)} + b_2^{(5)}x_2^{(5)}$
4. $\text{loĝit} = b_0 + b_1^{(1)}x_1^{(1)} + b_1^{(2)}x_1^{(2)} + b_1^{(3)}x_1^{(3)} + b_1^{(4)}x_1^{(4)} + b_1^{(5)}x_1^{(5)}$
    $+ b_2^{(1)}x_2^{(1)} + b_2^{(2)}x_2^{(2)} + b_2^{(3)}x_2^{(3)} + b_2^{(4)}x_2^{(4)} + b_2^{(5)}x_2^{(5)},$

where $x_1 = $ SBP and $x_2 = $ cholesterol, both fitted as a categorical variable with five levels. As just seen, $b_j^{(i)}$ will vary from model to model for each value of $i$ and $j$ because it represents the effect of $x_j^{(i)}$ adjusted for all other $x$ variables included in the specific model. Results of fitting these models may be presented in an **analysis of deviance table** (Table 10.20).

We can assess the significance of SBP by comparing models 1 and 2; cholesterol by comparing models 1 and 3; SBP and cholesterol together by comparing models 1 and 4; SBP *over and above* cholesterol by comparing models 3 and 4; cholesterol *over and above* SBP by comparing models 2 and 4. As in Section 9.5, this gives us scope for answering several types of question that are common in epidemiology.

Results are given in Table 10.21. In this table, the vertical line means 'given', as is standard notation (introduced in Section 9.4.4). The $p$ values come from comparing $\Delta D$ and $\chi^2$ with $\Delta$d.f. Notice that the $\Delta$d.f. are as would be expected in each case: four when one of the five-level effects is assessed and eight when both are assessed. In general, the assessment of one variable at a time will be more illuminating than multiple assessments (such as that on 8 d.f. given here). Hence future analysis of deviance tables will only show $\Delta D$s for single effects.

**Table 10.20**   Analysis of deviance table for Example 10.14

| Model | Deviance | d.f. |
|---|---|---|
| 1 constant | 84.83 | 24 |
| 2 constant + SBP | 56.73 | 20 |
| 3 constant + cholesterol | 49.48 | 20 |
| 4 constant + SBP + cholesterol | 18.86 | 16 |

**Table 10.21**   Further analysis of deviance table for Example 10.14

| Effect | $\Delta D$ | $\Delta d.f.$ | p value |
|---|---|---|---|
| SBP | 84.83 − 56.73 = 28.10 | 24 − 20 = 4 | < 0.0001 |
| cholesterol | 84.83 − 49.48 = 35.35 | 24 − 20 = 4 | < 0.0001 |
| SBP + cholesterol | 84.83 − 18.86 = 65.97 | 24 − 16 = 8 | < 0.0001 |
| SBP\|cholesterol | 49.48 − 18.86 = 30.62 | 20 − 16 = 4 | < 0.0001 |
| cholesterol\|SBP | 56.73 − 18.86 = 37.87 | 20 − 16 = 4 | < 0.0001 |

All of the tests are highly significant, implying that both variables have an effect on CHD, whether or not the effect of the other is already accounted for. Notice that, whenever we analyse two (or more) variables together, we should also consider their interaction (Section 10.9).

*Example 10.15*   Turning now to Example 10.12, there are six risk factors, and hence 64 possible models that could be fitted (without interactions). We could use an automatic variable selection algorithm to choose a 'best' model, but (as in Section 9.7) more insight will be gained by building the final model rather more carefully.

Consider, first, the raw effects of each of the six variables. To assess these we fit the constant alone, and then the constant plus each variable in turn. Subtracting each other deviance obtained from the first in turn, and comparing to $\chi^2$ with $\Delta d.f.$ degrees of freedom gives the required tests (Table 10.22).

From this we can conclude that activity in leisure is not an important risk factor: its effect is nowhere near significant, since $p \gg 0.05$. In fact this is comforting, because (as already noted) the estimates found in Example 10.12 are not what would be expected: those who are average in activity were found to have the least, and those who are active the most, risk of CHD. Now we know that the differences are explainable by chance variation. It could well be that self-reported level of activity is simply not a very accurate measure of true activity.

All the remaining variables are significant ($p < 0.05$). Of these, age seems to be the least important, perhaps because of the restricted age range and because prevalent cases of CHD were excluded. Total cholesterol and SBP are the most important.

Next, we consider fitting the model with the five variables that have raw (univariate) significance, and deleting one variable at a time to see whether that variable is needed in the presence of the remainder (Table 10.23). We see that age is not significant ($p = 0.22$) in the presence of the other four variables. If we take strict 5% significance, BMI may also be dropped, but as it is almost significant ($p = 0.057$) in the presence of the remaining four, and is very significant by itself, we shall keep it in our predictive model. Total cholesterol, SBP and smoking status are all highly significant in the presence of each other, age and BMI.

Continuing by fitting the four variables that seem important, and then dropping terms one by one, gives Table 10.24 (here the first row repeats results from the previous analysis of deviance table). The results are almost exactly as before, as far as p values are concerned. If we use the 6.2% significance level, all four remaining variables are significant in the presence of the other three. So none can be dropped.

As a final step, we should try bringing 'activity' back into the model: adding that to the four previously chosen gives a non-significant $\Delta D$ ($p = 0.58$). Hence, we conclude that the

**Table 10.22**  First analysis of deviance table for Example 10.15

| Model | Fit details | | Test details | | | Effect |
| --- | --- | --- | --- | --- | --- | --- |
| | $D$ | d.f. | $\Delta D^a$ | $\Delta d.f.^a$ | p value | |
| constant | 1569.37 | 4048 | – | – | – | |
| constant + AGE | 1563.46 | 4047 | 5.91 | 1 | 0.015 | AGE |
| constant + TOTCHOL | 1534.56 | 4047 | 34.81 | 1 | <0.0001 | TOTCHOL |
| constant + BMI | 1560.43 | 4047 | 8.94 | 1 | 0.003 | BMI |
| constant + SBP | 1528.01 | 4047 | 41.36 | 1 | <0.0001 | SBP |
| constant + SMOKING | 1556.22 | 4046 | 13.15 | 2 | 0.0014 | SMOKING |
| constant + ACTIVITY | 1569.06 | 4046 | 0.31 | 2 | 0.86 | ACTIVITY |

[a]Relative to the first model.

**Table 10.23**   Second analysis of deviance table for Example 10.15

| Model (each including the constant) | Fit details | | Test details | | | Effect |
|---|---|---|---|---|---|---|
| | $D$ | d.f. | $\Delta D^{a}$ | $\Delta d.f.^{a}$ | p value | |
| AGE + TOTCHOL + BMI + SBP + SMOKING | 1482.47 | 4042 | — | — | — | |
| TOTCHOL + BMI + SBP + SMOKING | 1484.00 | 4043 | 1.53 | 1 | 0.22 | AGE\|others |
| AGE + BMI + SBP + SMOKING | 1507.72 | 4043 | 25.25 | 1 | < 0.0001 | TOTCHOL\|others |
| AGE + TOTCHOL + SBP + SMOKING | 1486.09 | 4043 | 3.62 | 1 | 0.057 | BMI\|others |
| AGE + TOTCHOL + BMI + SMOKING | 1509.03 | 4043 | 26.56 | 1 | < 0.0001 | SBP\|others |
| AGE + TOTCHOL + BMI + SBP | 1496.34 | 4044 | 13.87 | 2 | 0.001 | SMOKING\|others |

[a]Relative to the first model.

**Table 10.24** Third analysis of deviance table for Example 10.15

| Model (each including the constant) | Fit details | | Test details | | | Effect |
|---|---|---|---|---|---|---|
| | $D$ | $d.f.$ | $\Delta D^{a}$ | $\Delta d.f.^{a}$ | $p$ value | |
| TOTCHOL + BMI + SBP + SMOKING | 1484.00 | 4043 | – | – | – | |
| BMI + SBP + SMOKING | 1509.00 | 4044 | 25.00 | 1 | < 0.0001 | TOTCHOL\|others |
| TOTCHOL + SBP + SMOKING | 1487.48 | 4044 | 3.48 | 1 | 0.062 | BMI\|others |
| TOTCHOL + BMI + SMOKING | 1515.37 | 4044 | 31.37 | 1 | < 0.0001 | SBP\|others |
| TOTCHOL + BMI + SBP | 1497.40 | 4045 | 13.40 | 2 | 0.001 | SMOKING\|others |

[a]Relative to the first model.

model that best represents the log odds of CHD is that found from fitting total cholesterol, BMI, systolic blood pressure and smoking. The fitted model turns out to be

$$\hat{\text{logit}} = -9.4572 + 0.3035 \times \text{TOTCHOL} + 0.0401 \times \text{BMI}$$
$$+ 0.0214 \times \text{SBP} + 0.3291 \times \text{ex} + 0.7094 \times \text{current}$$

where 'ex' = 1 only for ex-smokers and 'current' = 1 only for current smokers.

### 10.7.3    Tests for linearity and non-linearity

In Section 10.4.4 we saw how to fit a linear trend in the log odds for an ordered categorical explanatory variable. We can test for lack of fit (for grouped data) or for the significance of the linear trend, just as for other logistic regression models. Indeed, we can go further. Since the linear trend model specifies a summary (1 d.f.) relationship (straight line) between the $\ell$ levels of the ordered categorical variable (on $\ell - 1$ d.f.), the linear trend model is nested within the overall model. The $\Delta D$ between the two models can be used to test for non-linearity, when compared to chi-square with $\ell - 2$ d.f.

*Example 10.16*   For the *H. pylori* data of Table 10.3, social class was fitted as a categorical variable in Example 10.6 and as an ordinal variable in Example 10.9 (the model that assumes a linear trend on the log scale). The analysis of deviance table for the combined analysis (which repeats some results from Example 10.13) is given as Table 10.25. Here there are two $\Delta D$s calculated using the linear trend model. These are the test statistic for linear trend: deviance of the linear model subtracted from the deviance of the constant model, and the test statistic for non-linearity: deviance of linear trend model less the deviance of the categorical model. In fact, because the categorical model happens to be the full model in this example, the latter is also the test for lack of fit of the linear trend model, which is intuitively reasonable. Clearly there is a significant effect of social class (upon prevalence of *H. pylori*), and the effect seems to be well summarized by a linear trend, since there is no evidence of non-linearity ($p = 0.17$).

However, we have to be careful when we use such a general test for non-linearity. Consider a single explanatory variable, $x$. The 'non-linearity' is a combination of several effects, and can be broken down into distinct polynomial components (Section 9.3.3). These components, each with 1 d.f., are the effects of different powers of $x$ – that is, $x^2, x^3$, etc. It may be that one (or more) of these is significant, but when its effect is combined into the total, this is swamped by the non-significant (usually higher-order) terms.

In Example 10.16 there does seem to be some curvature in the response: although *H. pylori* undoubtedly goes up with social class, the prevalence has a 'local peak' in the middle classes (Figure 10.1). This may be explained by a second-degree polynomial (quadratic) term, $x^2$. A quadratic curve has one turning point, either a U shape or its reverse (Figure 9.7(a)). If the quadratic term is significant, but the linear is not, then the outcome variable goes up and then down, or vice versa. Such responses are relatively unusual in epidemi-

**Table 10.25** Analysis of deviance table for Example 10.16

| Model | Fit details | | Test details | | | Effect |
|---|---|---|---|---|---|---|
| | $D$ | d.f. | $\Delta D$ | $\Delta$d.f. | p value | |
| 1 constant | 64.44 | 5 | – | – | – | |
| 2 constant + social class | 0 | 0 | 64.44 | 5 | < 0.0001 | social class |
| 3 constant + linear trend | 6.46 | 4 | 57.98[a] | 1 | < 0.0001 | linear trend |
| | | | 6.46[b] | 4 | 0.17 | non-linearity |

[a]Relative to model 1. [b]Relative to model 2.

ology, but see Section 3.6.3. In Figure 10.1 it appears that the U shape is superimposed on a straight line, so that the upward trend has a 'wobble'. Some other types of non-linearity might be modelled by using a transformation, exactly as for normal regression models (Section 9.3.3).

*Example 10.17*   To test for all polynomial effects in Example 10.16, the quintic polynomial (highest order possible, since social class has five degrees of freedom) was fitted, along with all polynomials of lower orders. Let $x$ denote the social class rank, as defined in Example 10.9, and $c =$ constant. Results are given in Table 10.26. Note that the sum of the $\Delta D$s for all the non-linear effects $(x^2, x^3, x^4,$ and $x^5)$ in Table 10.26 is $5.76 + 0.05 + 0.43 + 0.22 = 6.46$, the $\Delta D$ for non-linearity found in Table 10.25. All we have done here is to partition this $\Delta D$, and its $\Delta$d.f., into four components, each representing a different type of effect.

The significant effects here are $x$ and $x^2$. Hence the quadratic model

$$\text{lo}\hat{\text{g}}\text{it} = b_0 + b_1 x + b_2 x^2$$

is suggested. The global test for non-linearity in Example 10.16 has been misleading. After fitting the model to determine the $b$ coefficients, Figure 10.7 was produced. Observed and expected values are reasonably close, as we would hope (see also Example 10.24).

Epidemiologists often split quantitative variables into categories before analysis, typically using quintiles (as in Example 10.11) or some other

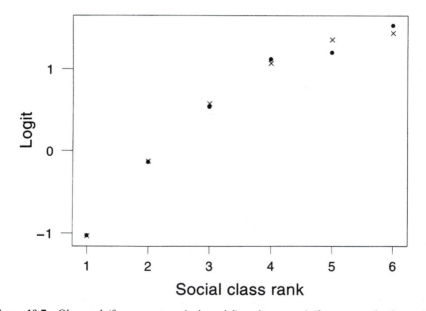

**Figure 10.7**   Observed (from a categorical model) and expected (from a quadratic model) logits for *H. pylori* by social class group. Observed values are indicated by dots, expected values by crosses.

**Table 10.26** Analysis of deviance table for Example 10.17

| Model | Fit details | | Test details | | | Effect |
|---|---|---|---|---|---|---|
| | $D$ | d.f. | $\Delta D^a$ | $\Delta d.f.^a$ | p value | |
| $c$ | 64.44 | 5 | – | – | | |
| $c + x$ | 6.46 | 4 | 57.98 | 1 | < 0.0001 | linear |
| $c + x + x^2$ | 0.70 | 3 | 5.76 | 1 | 0.02 | quadratic |
| $c + x + x^2 + x^3$ | 0.65 | 2 | 0.05 | 1 | 0.82 | cubic |
| $c + x + x^2 + x^3 + x^4$ | 0.22 | 1 | 0.43 | 1 | 0.51 | quartic |
| $c + x + x^2 + x^3 + x^4 + x^5$ | 0 | 0 | 0.22 | 1 | 0.64 | quintic |

[a] relative to the polynomial model of one less degree.

percentiles. This is because the consequent set of odds ratios is easy to understand and gives a greater insight into the risk profile than if the variables were left in their raw form. Tests for linear trend then explore, as in Example 10.16, whether there is a linear effect on the log scale, from (say) fifth to fifth. If the variable is very skewed this does not imply that there is a linear trend across the true range of the data, because the quintiles are then not even approximately equally spaced over this range. If the idea is to explore possible linearity in the variable itself, probably to ascertain whether it would be appropriate to fit it in its raw, quantitative form, then the values used for the ordinal variable should be some appropriate summary of the categorical groups, such as the medians of each fifth (as suggested in Section 3.6.2) in the context of Example 10.11. Notice that it would not be correct to compare the deviances for the models with the variable in grouped and ungrouped (quantitative) form because these are not nested models.

### 10.7.4    Tests based upon estimates and their standard errors

In Sections 10.4–10.6 we saw several examples in which an estimate was quoted with its estimated standard error. Provided that the estimator is approximately normally distributed, we can use this information (as in other statistical procedures) to provide a simple test of the null hypothesis that the true value of the parameter estimated is zero, adjusting for all other effects in the model. Under this null hypothesis,

$$\left(\frac{\text{estimate}}{\hat{se}}\right)^2$$

comes from a chi-square distribution with 1 d.f. (at least approximately). This is equivalent to calculating the confidence interval and simply checking whether zero is inside it. This procedure generally gives a result that is slightly different from the recommended method using deviances. In practice, the difference is unlikely to be important unless more fundamental problems are present, such as a very small sample size.

*Example 10.18*    In Example 10.6 we found the 95% confidence interval for the logit that compares social class II to social class I to be $0.8898 \pm 0.8371 = (0.053, 1.727)$. As zero is outside this interval we can conclude that there is a significant difference ($p < 0.05$) in the prevalence of *H. pylori* between these two social class groups. We can do slightly better by looking at the square of the ratio between the estimate and its estimated standard error, $(0.8898/0.4271)^2 = 4.34$, giving a $p$ value of 0.02 when compared to $\chi_1^2$.

Notice that we could also use the confidence interval for the odds ratio, rather than the logit, but in this case a significant result is a consequence of *unity* lying outside the confidence interval.

**Output 10.2**   SAS results for Example 10.19

The GENMOD Procedure

Analysis of Parameter Estimates

| Parameter | | DF | Estimate | Std Err | ChiSquare | Pr > Chi |
|---|---|---|---|---|---|---|
| INTERCEPT | | 1 | −10.1076 | 0.9972 | 102.7451 | 0.0000 |
| AGE | | 1 | 0.0171 | 0.0136 | 1.5741 | 0.2096 |
| TOTCHOL | | 1 | 0.3071 | 0.0597 | 26.4681 | 0.0000 |
| BMI | | 1 | 0.0417 | 0.0214 | 3.7998 | 0.0513 |
| SYSTOL | | 1 | 0.0204 | 0.0038 | 28.4114 | 0.0000 |
| SMOKING | 2 | 1 | 0.3225 | 0.2506 | 1.6570 | 0.1980 |
| SMOKING | 3 | 1 | 0.7296 | 0.2192 | 11.0815 | 0.0009 |
| SMOKING | 4 | 0 | 0.0000 | 0.0000 | . | . |
| ACTIVITY | 2 | 1 | −0.1904 | 0.1801 | 1.1184 | 0.2903 |
| ACTIVITY | 3 | 1 | −0.1011 | 0.2335 | 0.1874 | 0.6651 |
| ACTIVITY | 4 | 0 | 0.0000 | 0.0000 | . | . |

*Example 10.19*   The 'Analysis of Parameter Estimates' produced by SAS PROC GENMOD for Example 10.12 is given as Output 10.2. Here SMOKING 4 and ACTIVITY 4 are the relabelled *lowest* levels (never smoker and active, respectively), as explained in Example 10.7. Here SAS has done the necessary division and squaring to obtain the chi-square test statistics (using more decimal places than shown for the individual components). For the quantitative variables (age, total cholesterol, BMI and SBP), and indeed any variable (with the exception of the constant) that has 1 d.f., the tests shown are directly comparable to the $\Delta D$ in dropping that term from the model fitted.

For instance, in Table 10.17 we saw that the deviance for the model of Example 10.12 is 1481.34 on 4040 d.f. When BMI was dropped from the model – that is, the remaining four variables were fitted – the deviance grew to 1485.04 on 4041 d.f. Thus $\Delta D = 3.70$, slightly smaller than the value 3.7998 obtained in the approximate chi-square test in Output 10.2. Similarly, the $p$ value from the $\Delta D$ test is slightly bigger at 0.0544, compared to 0.0513, although differences in the third decimal place are not at all important.

For variables with more than 1 d.f. (smoking and activity in this example) the chi-square test statistics give a set of 1 d.f. tests that partition the entire d.f., rather like the polynomial partition in Example 10.17. Here, because of the SAS rules and the labelling of levels adopted, other levels of the categorical variables are contrasted with the lowest level. We can see that the only significant ($p < 0.05$) difference in CHD risk is between SMOKING 3 (current smokers) and SMOKING 4 (never smokers).

## 10.7.5   Problems with missing values

In all the examples used here the issue of missing values has not arisen because anyone with any missing value has been deleted in all examples. In most large-scale epidemiological investigations there are some missing values, and we must be careful how we deal with them. It is assumed that a method for imputing missing values is not to be used and, instead, the standard method of deleting observations with missing values is to be used (see the comments in Section 2.2.1).

Often we build up multiple regression models by getting so far and then wondering if a newly introduced variable will alter the inference. If this new variable has missing values, which lead us to delete additional observations, then we *cannot* compare the deviance of the extended model with any model that has gone before. This is because the models with differing sets of observations (subjects) are not nested. Instead we shall have to refit previous models, possibly including that with the constant alone, using only those individuals with complete data. These will provide suitable reference models for calculation of $\Delta D$.

## 10.8   Confounding

As with general linear models, adjustment for confounding variables is achieved through logistic modelling by fitting the confounder with and without the risk factor (Section 9.9). Comparison of deviances, for the model with the confounder against the model with the confounder plus the risk factor, gives an indication of whether the risk factor is still important after allowing for the confounder. Comparison of odds ratios from these two models indicates the effect of the confounder. There is no formal significance test to see whether or not a potential confounder is truly a confounder: this is not entirely a statistical issue. However, we could reasonably conclude no confounding in the study at hand if the odds ratios, unadjusted and adjusted, were very similar.

*Example 10.20*   Consider the problem of Examples 10.11 and 10.14 again. Suppose we wished to consider SBP as a potential confounding factor for the cholesterol–CHD relationship. We obtain a test of the null hypothesis that cholesterol has no effect on CHD after adjustment for SBP by comparing models 2 and 4 in Example 10.14. As we have already seen, this involves a test on the difference in deviances, which turns out to be extremely significant ($p < 0.0001$). Thus SBP does not remove the effect of cholesterol (as already seen in Example 10.14), and we can judge that cholesterol has an effect that is over and above that of SBP.

This is not sufficient for us to conclude that SBP does not confound the cholesterol–CHD relationship: it could still be that the direction or magnitude of the relationship is altered by the presence or absence of SBP. To consider this we could look at the odds ratios for fifths of cholesterol with and without adjustment for SBP. Parameter estimates from fitting statistical models produced by computer packages (unless specifically stated otherwise) always adjust each term for all other terms fitted, and in Example 10.11 the only terms fitted (besides the constant) are cholesterol and SBP fifths. Note that this is model 4 in Example 10.14. Thus the cholesterol estimates given in Table 10.15 are adjusted for SBP, and vice versa. To get unadjusted estimates we fit model 3 of Example 10.14 again. Results are given in Table 10.27.

**Table 10.27** CHD odds ratios for cholesterol, unadjusted and adjusted for systolic blood pressure for men in the Scottish Heart Health Study who were CHD-free at baseline

| Serum total cholesterol fifth | Odds ratio | |
|---|---|---|
| | Unadjusted | Adjusted |
| 1 | 1 | 1 |
| 2 | 1.25 | 1.23 |
| 3 | 2.36 | 2.28 |
| 4 | 2.96 | 2.74 |
| 5 | 4.05 | 3.65 |

For ease of interpretation, odds ratios are shown (slope parameter estimates raised to the power e).

The two sets of odds ratios are very similar (in both cases the base odds ratio is, of course, fixed at unity). There is little evidence of any important confounding effect. Nevertheless, the adjusted odds ratios are smaller: accounting for another major coronary risk factor has reduced the effect for cholesterol. We would expect this, since there is a tendency for poor lifestyle factors to cluster together.

## 10.9 Interaction

As with general linear models, we deal with interaction by introducing one or more terms into the logistic regression model which are the cross-multiplications of the constituent variables. Here we shall consider interactions involving two variables. Higher-order interactions would be defined, and dealt with, in a similar way. In turn, we shall consider interactions between two categorical variables, a quantitative and a categorical variable and (briefly) two quantitative variables. As described in Section 4.9, whenever an interaction turns out to be significant the main effects of the constituent terms (for example, simple one-factor odds ratios) are likely to be misleading, and thus should not be used.

### 10.9.1 Between two categorical variables

Given a categorical variable $A$ with $\ell$ levels we can define its effect by $\ell - 1$ dummy variables (Example 10.8). Given a second categorical variable, $B$, with $m$ levels and therefore $m - 1$ dummy variables, the interaction is represented by the set of $(\ell - 1)(m - 1)$ variables formed by cross-multiplication of the two individual sets of dummy variables. The interaction has $(\ell - 1)(m - 1)$ d.f. We test by calculating $\Delta D$ for the model that includes the two main effects ($A$ and $B$) compared with the model that includes these and the interaction (written $A*B$).

*Example 10.21*   Table 10.28 shows some more data from the SHHS, this time for both sexes. Bortner score (Bortner, 1969) is a measure of personality (Type A behaviour). Although a high Bortner score has been thought to be a bad thing, Table 10.28 shows that the opposite is true in the SHHS. CHD incidence seems to come down with increasing Bortner score, but much more rapidly for women. Hence we might suspect that there is an interaction between Bortner score and sex. We will test this using dummy variables, and taking Bortner score in grouped form, grouping being by quarters (as in the table).

Dummy variables, X1–X3 for Bortner quarter and X4 for sex, are defined in Table 10.29. The interaction variables, X5–X7, defined by cross-multiplying the relevant components of Table 10.29, are given in Table 10.30. Table 10.31 shows the consequent full data set; the number with CHD positive is the number of events (denoted *e* in Section 10.1) out of *n* trials (sample size for the Bortner quarter/sex group).

**Table 10.28**   CHD status, after follow-up of 7.7 years, by Bortner score quarter at baseline for those in the SHHS with Bortner score measured who were CHD-free at baseline

| Quarter of Bortner score | Male | | Female | | |
|---|---|---|---|---|---|
| | No CHD | CHD | No CHD | CHD | Total |
| 1 (≤ 144) | 1022 | 57 (5.3%) | 915 | 30 (3.2%) | 2024 |
| 2 (145–169) | 918 | 56 (5.8%) | 1081 | 20 (1.8%) | 2075 |
| 3 (170–194) | 927 | 39 (4.0%) | 1066 | 10 (0.9%) | 2042 |
| 4 (> 194) | 1022 | 46 (4.3%) | 938 | 10 (1.0%) | 2016 |
| Total | 3889 | 198 (4.8%) | 4000 | 70 (1.7%) | 8157 |

**Table 10.29**   Dummy variables for Bortner score and for sex

| Bortner quarter | X1 | X2 | X3 | Sex | X4 |
|---|---|---|---|---|---|
| 1 | 0 | 0 | 0 | Female | 0 |
| 2 | 1 | 0 | 0 | Male | 1 |
| 3 | 0 | 1 | 0 | | |
| 4 | 0 | 0 | 1 | | |

**Table 10.30**   Interaction variables for Bortner score by sex (derived from Table 10.29)

| Bortner quarter | X5 | | X6 | | X7 | |
|---|---|---|---|---|---|---|
| | Sex | | Sex | | Sex | |
| | Female | Male | Female | Male | Female | Male |
| 1 | 0 | 0 | 0 | 0 | 0 | 0 |
| 2 | 0 | 1 | 0 | 0 | 0 | 0 |
| 3 | 0 | 0 | 0 | 1 | 0 | 0 |
| 4 | 0 | 0 | 0 | 0 | 0 | 1 |

**Table 10.31** Specification of data (M = male, F = female)

| Bortner quarter | Sex | Dummy variables representing | | | | | | | CHD | |
| | | Bortner quarter | | | Sex | Interaction | | | | |
| | | X1 | X2 | X3 | X4 | X5 | X6 | X7 | Positive | n |
|---|---|---|---|---|---|---|---|---|---|---|
| 1 | M | 0 | 0 | 0 | 1 | 0 | 0 | 0 | 57 | 1079 |
| 1 | F | 0 | 0 | 0 | 0 | 0 | 0 | 0 | 30 | 945 |
| 2 | M | 1 | 0 | 0 | 1 | 1 | 0 | 0 | 56 | 974 |
| 2 | F | 1 | 0 | 0 | 0 | 0 | 0 | 0 | 20 | 1101 |
| 3 | M | 0 | 1 | 0 | 1 | 0 | 1 | 0 | 39 | 966 |
| 3 | F | 0 | 1 | 0 | 0 | 0 | 0 | 0 | 10 | 1076 |
| 4 | M | 0 | 0 | 1 | 1 | 0 | 0 | 1 | 46 | 1068 |
| 4 | F | 0 | 0 | 1 | 0 | 0 | 0 | 0 | 10 | 948 |

Table 10.32 is the analysis of deviance table for these data. All effects are significant ($p < 0.05$), including the interaction. Hence model 5 should be adopted:

$$\widehat{\text{logit}} = b_0 + b_1 X1 + b_2 X2 + b_3 X3 + b_4 X4 + b_5 X5 + b_6 X6 + b_7 X7$$

and the odds ratios will thus be examined separately for the two sexes. The $\{b_i\}$ produced by SAS PROC GENMOD are presented in Table 10.33.

Consider the fitted logit for Bortner quarter 1, male sex. By Table 10.31, $X4 = 1$ and all other X variables are zero. Hence the logit is

$$-3.4177 + 0.5313 \times 1.$$

Continuing in this fashion, we can produce all the logits. A sensible set of odds ratios to summarize the findings would be comparisons of the other three Bortner quarters against the first, separately for each sex. As usual, log odds ratios are the differences between the logit for the numerator and denominator of the odds ratio. For example, the log odds ratio for Bortner 4 versus 1, male sex, is

$$\{-3.4177 + (-1.1234 \times 1) + 0.5313 \times 1 + 0.9090 \times 1\} - \{-3.4177 + 0.5313 \times 1\}$$
$$= -1.1234 + 0.9090 = -0.2144.$$

Notice that the constant and sex terms cancel out. Continuing in this way, we find the complete set of log odds ratios, and hence odds ratios. Table 10.34 shows the latter, together with associated confidence intervals.

Confidence intervals for female odds ratios (relative to Bortner quarter 1) are easy to construct because each is calculated from only one $b$ parameter. For instance, the log odds ratio for Bortner 4 versus 1, female sex, is $-1.1234$ with estimated standard error $0.3681$, giving a 95% confidence interval for the odds ratio of

$$\exp\{-1.1234 \pm 1.96 \times 0.3681\}.$$

Calculation of confidence intervals for the male odds ratios is more complex because each involves two $b$ parameters. For instance, we have already seen this when finding the estimated odds ratio for Bortner 4 versus 1, where all but two terms cancelled out. In this situation we need to have the variance-covariance matrix, as in Example 10.6. Alternatively, we could refit model 5 using a new definition of X4 that makes $X4 = 1$ for females and 0 for males (X5–X7 will also change as a consequence). Then it is the male standard errors, rather than the female, that can be calculated directly from the standard errors of the $b$. This method will be described in detail in Example 10.22.

Our conclusion from Table 10.34 is that Bortner score has little effect on the incidence of CHD for men, but increasing score implies decreasing risk (with the highest two quarters virtually the same) for women.

If the computer package used allows interactions to be specified as part of the model directly *and* allows categorical variables to be declared, then much work can be saved since the dummy variables do not need to be constructed. SAS PROC GENMOD was used in this way, defining BORT to be the Bortner quarter, except that the first quarter has BORT = 5 so as to make it the reference group (Example 10.7). Sex was read in as SEX = 1 for men and 2 for women, the CLASS declaration was used for both BORT and SEX, and BORT*SEX was included in the model statement. Output 10.3 shows the parameter estimates produced when model 5 of Table 10.32 was fitted. The non-zero parameter estimates and their standard errors are exactly as in Table 10.33, as they should be.

**Table 10.32**  Analysis of deviance table for Example 10.21

| | Fit details | | Test details | | | |
| Model | D | d.f. | $\Delta D$ | $\Delta d.f.$ | p value | Effect |
|---|---|---|---|---|---|---|
| 1 constant | 86.63 | 7 | – | – | – | |
| 2 constant + X1 to X3 | 72.49 | 4 | 14.14[a] | 3 | 0.003 | Bortner |
| 3 constant + X4 | 21.40 | 6 | 65.23[a] | 1 | < 0.0001 | sex |
| 4 constant + X1 to X4 | 8.15 | 3 | 64.34[b] | 1 | < 0.0001 | sex\|Bortner |
| | | | 13.25[c] | 3 | 0.004 | Bortner\|sex |
| 5 constant + X1 to X7 | 0 | 0 | 8.15[d] | 3 | 0.043 | interaction\|Bortner, sex |

[a]Relative to model 1.
[b]Relative to model 2.
[c]Relative to model 3.
[d]Relative to model 4.

**Table 10.33**  Parameter estimates for model 5 in Table 10.32, as produced by SAS

| Parameter | Estimate | Standard error |
|---|---|---|
| INTERCEPT | −3.4177 | 0.1855 |
| X1 | −0.5722 | 0.2921 |
| X2 | −1.2514 | 0.3679 |
| X3 | −1.1234 | 0.3681 |
| X4 | 0.5313 | 0.2301 |
| X5 | 0.6618 | 0.3505 |
| X6 | 0.9694 | 0.4250 |
| X7 | 0.9090 | 0.4204 |

**Table 10.34**  Odds ratios (95% confidence intervals) by sex and Bortner quarter for SHHS subjects who were free of CHD at baseline

| Bortner quarter | Sex | |
|---|---|---|
| | Male | Female |
| 1 | 1 | 1 |
| 2 | 1.09 (0.75, 1.60) | 0.56 (0.32, 1.00) |
| 3 | 0.75 (0.50, 1.12) | 0.29 (0.14, 0.59) |
| 4 | 0.81 (0.55, 1.20) | 0.33 (0.16, 0.67) |

**Output 10.3**  SAS results for Example 10.21, model 5

The GENMOD Procedure

Analysis of Parameter Estimates

| Parameter | | | DF | Estimate | Std Err | ChiSquare | Pr > Chi |
|---|---|---|---|---|---|---|---|
| INTERCEPT | | | 1 | −3.4177 | 0.1855 | 339.3010 | 0.0000 |
| BORT | 2 | | 1 | −0.5722 | 0.2921 | 3.8358 | 0.0502 |
| BORT | 3 | | 1 | −1.2514 | 0.3679 | 11.5680 | 0.0007 |
| BORT | 4 | | 1 | −1.1234 | 0.3681 | 9.3150 | 0.0023 |
| BORT | 5 | | 0 | 0.0000 | 0.0000 | . | . |
| SEX | 1 | | 1 | 0.5313 | 0.2301 | 5.3304 | 0.0210 |
| SEX | 2 | | 0 | 0.0000 | 0.0000 | . | . |
| BORT*SEX | 2 | 1 | 1 | 0.6618 | 0.3505 | 3.5661 | 0.0590 |
| BORT*SEX | 2 | 2 | 0 | 0.0000 | 0.0000 | . | . |
| BORT*SEX | 3 | 1 | 1 | 0.9694 | 0.4250 | 5.2036 | 0.0225 |
| BORT*SEX | 3 | 2 | 0 | 0.0000 | 0.0000 | . | . |
| BORT*SEX | 4 | 1 | 1 | 0.9090 | 0.4204 | 4.6756 | 0.0306 |
| BORT*SEX | 4 | 2 | 0 | 0.0000 | 0.0000 | . | . |
| BORT*SEX | 5 | 1 | 0 | 0.0000 | 0.0000 | . | . |
| BORT*SEX | 5 | 2 | 0 | 0.0000 | 0.0000 | . | . |

## 10.9.2  Between a quantitative and a categorical variable

When one variable is quantitative and the other is categorical (with $\ell$ levels) the interaction is represented by the set of variables defined by the product of the quantitative variable and each of the dummy variables for the categorical variable. We shall need to define $\ell - 1$ interaction dummy variables because the interaction has $\ell - 1$ d.f.

*Example 10.22*  The problem of Example 10.21 could have been addressed by retaining Bortner score in its original quantitative form. Using the generic form of the data, the set of models from before was refitted with quantitative Bortner score using SAS PROC GENMOD. Sex was declared as a CLASS (categorical) variable with values 1 for men and 2 for women. Results are shown in Table 10.35. The data are available electronically: see Appendix C.

As in the previous example, all effects are significant (note that the unadjusted effect of sex is just as in Table 10.32, apart from rounding error). Hence the interaction needs to be accounted for; model 5 is the 'best'. SAS results for model 5 are given as Output 10.4. The fitted model is

$$\hat{\text{logit}} = b_0 + b_1^{(1)}\text{SEX}^{(1)} + b_1^{(2)}\text{SEX}^{(2)} + b_2 x + b_3^{(1)}\text{SEX}^{(1)}x + b_3^{(2)}\text{SEX}^{(2)}x, \qquad (10.20)$$

where $x =$ Bortner score and

$$\text{SEX}^{(1)} = \begin{cases} 1 & \text{for men} \\ 0 & \text{for women,} \end{cases} \qquad \text{SEX}^{(2)} = \begin{cases} 1 & \text{for women} \\ 0 & \text{for men.} \end{cases}$$

In the special parametrization used by SAS, the last levels of everything arising from a CLASS statement, including terms that contribute to interactions, are set to zero. Hence SEX 2 and BORTNER*SEX 2 are set to zero in Output 10.4. The general logit for men is, from (10.20),

$$\hat{\text{logit}}_M = b_0 + b_1^{(1)} + b_2 x + b_3^{(1)}x$$
$$= \left(b_0 + b_1^{(1)}\right) + \left(b_2 + b_3^{(1)}\right)x;$$

whilst the general logit for women is

$$\hat{\text{logit}}_F = \left(b_0 + b_1^{(2)}\right) + \left(b_2 + b_3^{(2)}\right)x.$$

**Output 10.4**  SAS results for Example 10.22, model 5

The GENMOD Procedure

Analysis of Parameter Estimates

| Parameter | | DF | Estimate | Std Err | ChiSquare | Pr > Chi |
|---|---|---|---|---|---|---|
| INTERCEPT | | 1 | −1.9644 | 0.4982 | 15.5453 | 0.0001 |
| SEX | 1 | 1 | −0.6266 | 0.5821 | 1.1584 | 0.2818 |
| SEX | 2 | 0 | 0.0000 | 0.0000 | . | . |
| BORTNER | | 1 | −0.0129 | 0.0032 | 16.5674 | 0.0001 |
| BORTNER*SEX | 1 | 1 | 0.0106 | 0.0036 | 8.5432 | 0.0035 |
| BORTNER*SEX | 2 | 0 | 0.0000 | 0.0000 | . | . |

**Table 10.35**   Analysis of deviance table for Example 10.22

| Model | Fit details | | Test details | | | Effect |
|---|---|---|---|---|---|---|
| | $D$ | d.f. | $\Delta D$ | $\Delta d.f.$ | p value | |
| 1 constant | 2357.88 | 8156 | – | – | – | – |
| 2 constant + Bortner | 2347.61 | 8155 | 10.27[a] | 1 | 0.001 | Bortner |
| 3 constant + sex | 2292.66 | 8155 | 65.22[a] | 1 | <0.0001 | sex |
| 4 constant + sex + Bortner | 2283.07 | 8154 | 64.54[b] | 1 | <0.0001 | sex\|Bortner |
| | | | 9.59[c] | 1 | 0.002 | Bortner\|sex |
| 5 constant + sex + Bortner + Bortner*sex | 2274.58 | 8153 | 8.49[d] | 1 | 0.004 | interaction\| Bortner, sex |

[a]Relative to model 1.
[b]Relative to model 2.
[c]Relative to model 3.
[d]Relative to model 4.

In this example these become:

$$\text{logit}_M = (-1.9644 - 0.6266) + (-0.0129 + 0.0106)x$$
$$= -2.5910 - 0.0023x,$$
$$\text{logit}_F = (-1.9644 + 0) + (-0.0129 + 0)x$$
$$= -1.9644 - 0.0129x.$$

We have two straight lines of different intercept and slope. The odds ratios for a unit increase in $x$ are then

$$\hat{\psi}_M = \exp(-0.0023) = 0.998$$

for men and

$$\hat{\psi}_F = \exp(-0.0129) = 0.987$$

for women, because the constant term will cancel out when the appropriate logits are subtracted.

Just as in Example 10.21, the confidence interval is easy to obtain for any odds ratio which uses only one of the $b$ parameters in its estimation. Here female odds ratios only use $b_2$ (all other terms are fixed at zero or cancel out). Thus, from Output 10.4, the 95% confidence interval for a unit increase in Bortner score for women is

$$\exp\{-0.0129 \pm (1.96)(0.0032)\}$$

or (0.981, 0.993).

Since any odds ratio for men uses both $b_2$ and $b_3^{(1)}$, we either need the variance-covariance matrix or to refit the model but this time forcing the male sex to be the last, in numerical order, entered to SAS. We will use the latter method. Similar 'tricks' will work with other packages.

If we define a new variable,

$$\text{SEX2} = 3 - \text{SEX}$$

then

$$\text{SEX2} = 3 - 1 = 2 \quad \text{when SEX} = 1 \text{ (men)}$$
$$\text{SEX2} = 3 - 2 = 1 \quad \text{when SEX} = 2 \text{ (women)},$$

so that SEX2 takes its highest level for men. SAS will, consequently, fix the parameter estimates for men to be zero.

Results from SAS are given as Output 10.5. Notice how the parameters involving sex in Outputs 10.4 and 10.5 have a different sign, but the same magnitude. Other parameters are completely different, although the fitted model will turn out to be exactly the same as before. Straightaway we see that

$$\hat{\psi}_M = \exp(-0.0023) = 0.998$$

(just as before), with 95% confidence interval,

$$\exp\{-0.0023 \pm 1.96 \times 0.0018\}$$

or (0.994, 1.001). Both the male and female odds ratios indicate a drop of odds with increasing Bortner score, but the rate of decrease is greater for women. The trend is only

**Output 10.5**   SAS results for Example 10.22, model 5, using a different variable to represent sex compared to that used in Output 10.4

The GENMOD Procedure

Analysis of Parameter Estimates

| Parameter | | DF | Estimate | Std Err | ChiSquare | Pr > Chi |
|-----------|---|----|----------|---------|-----------|----------|
| INTERCEPT | | 1 | −2.5910 | 0.3011 | 74.0573 | 0.0000 |
| SEX2 | 1 | 1 | 0.6266 | 0.5821 | 1.1584 | 0.2818 |
| SEX2 | 2 | 0 | 0.0000 | 0.0000 | . | . |
| BORTNER | | 1 | −0.0023 | 0.0018 | 1.7152 | 0.1903 |
| BORTNER*SEX2 | 1 | 1 | −0.0106 | 0.0036 | 8.5432 | 0.0035 |
| BORTNER*SEX2 | 2 | 0 | 0.0000 | 0.0000 | . | . |

significant $(p < 0.05)$ for women (from checking whether the 95% confidence interval contains unity). This agrees with the findings in Example 10.21.

### 10.9.3   Between two quantitative variables

Interactions between two quantitative variables are easy to fit: the $A * B$ interaction is literally the product of $A$ and $B$, on a case-by-case basis. Using a computer package, if variable $A$ is in one column and $B$ in another, we simply ask the package to multiply the two columns to form the interaction variable's column.

However, such interactions may be difficult to interpret: a significant result means that there is a linear effect of $A \times B$ after allowing for linear effects of both $A$ and $B$. Generally it is more helpful to categorize either or (more likely) both the variables and proceed as in Section 10.9.1 or 10.9.2.

## 10.10   Model checking

### 10.10.1   Residuals

In Section 10.7.1 we saw how to test for lack of fit with grouped data. Such a test, even when possible, is insufficient to determine whether the model is appropriate. Just as in general linear models (Section 9.8), we need also to examine model residuals. In this section we shall consider residual analysis for grouped data. When the data are generic the residuals will, by definition, be of a special binary form, requiring more complex analyses (see Collett, 1991).

There are several different types of residual that have been suggested for use with logistic regression models. The simplest is the **raw residual**. Using the definition of $e_i$ in Section 10.1, the $i$th raw residual, $resid_i$, is

$$\text{resid}_i = \text{observed } (e_i) - \text{expected } (e_i) = e_i - \hat{e}_i, \tag{10.21}$$

as in general linear models. In logistic regression

$$\hat{e}_i = n_i \hat{r}_i, \tag{10.22}$$

where $\hat{r}_i$ is the predicted risk from the model.

Unfortunately the raw residual is difficult to interpret because its size depends on the variability of both $e_i$ and $\hat{e}_i$. Various ways of standardizing the raw residual have been suggested: see Collett (1991) for an extensive description. One of these leads to the **deviance residual**, which is derived from components of the deviance. The $i$th deviance residual is

$$\text{devres}_i = \{\text{sign}[\text{resid}_i]\} \left\{ \sqrt{2e_i \log_e \left( \frac{e_i}{\hat{e}_i} \right) + 2(n_i - e_i) \log_e \left( \frac{n_i - e_i}{n_i - \hat{e}_i} \right)} \right\}, \tag{10.23}$$

where the first term on the right-hand side denotes that we take the sign of the deviance residual to be the sign of the $i$th residual. Then

$$\text{model deviance} = \sum (\text{devres}_i)^2.$$

Much more useful is the **standardized deviance residual**, defined by

$$\text{stdevres}_i = d_i / \sqrt{(1 - h_i)} \tag{10.24}$$

where

$$h_i = n_i \hat{r}_i (1 - \hat{r}_i) V(\widehat{\text{logit}}_i). \tag{10.25}$$

Here we introduce $h_i$, called the **leverage**. The standardized deviance residuals have variance unity, and so are easy to interpret for size. Further, provided the $n_i$ are not small, these residuals will, approximately, have a standard normal distribution when the model is correct. Thus we should be wary of stdevres values larger than 1.96 or less than $-1.96$, the upper and lower $2\frac{1}{2}\%$ percentage points from the standard normal distribution. Some computer packages will produce residuals automatically; with others they will have to be derived from any of (10.21)–(10.25).

Whichever residuals are chosen, we expect to find values close to zero and without any systematic pattern, for the model to be acceptable. As in general linear models, we can check for systematic patterns by plotting the residuals. In logistic modelling, residuals are often plotted against the observation number (giving an **index plot**), the linear predictor and/or each explanatory variable. The latter two will be equivalent if there is only one explanatory variable. The plots will identify any observations with large residuals (outliers). The great advantage of standardized deviance residuals (as with standardized residuals in general linear models) is that we have limits to guide our subjective concept of size.

*Example 10.23*  We shall carry out model checking of Example 10.5. First we evaluate, as a specific example, residuals for the first observation (men aged 40).

Here $i = 1$ and, by observation, $e_1 = 1$ and $n_1 = 251$. By (10.2) and using the estimates from Table 10.7, the predicted risk of death,

$$\hat{r}_1 = \{1 + \exp(8.4056 - 0.1126 \times 40)\}^{-1} = 0.019809.$$

By (10.22) and Table 10.4, the predicted number of deaths, $\hat{e}_1 = 251 \times 0.019809 = 4.972$. Then, by (10.21) and Table 10.4, the raw residual, $\text{resid}_1 = 1 - 4.972 = -3.972$. Then, by (10.23), the deviance residual,

$$\text{devres}_1 = -\sqrt{2 \times 1 \times \log_e\left(\frac{1}{4.972}\right) + 2(251 - 1)\log_e\left(\frac{251 - 1}{251 - 4.972}\right)} = -2.191.$$

To obtain the leverage, $h_1$, we need the variance of $\hat{\text{logit}}_1$. We can get this from the variance-covariance matrix of model parameters as

$$V(b_0 + b_1 x) = V(b_0) + x^2 V(b_1) + 2x\, C(b_0, b_1),$$

where $x = 40$. For brevity we simply quote the answer here to be 0.020207. Then, by (10.25), $h_1 = 251 \times 0.019809(1 - 0.019809)0.020207 = 0.098480$. Finally, by (10.24), the first standardized deviance residual,

**Table 10.36**  Residuals and death statistics for the model fitted in Example 10.5

| Age | Number of deaths | | Residuals | | |
| --- | --- | --- | --- | --- | --- |
| | Observed | Expected | Raw | Deviance | Standardized deviance |
| 40 | 1  | 4.96  | −3.96 | −2.19 | −2.30 |
| 41 | 12 | 7.00  | 5.00  | 1.74  | 1.85  |
| 42 | 13 | 7.62  | 5.38  | 1.80  | 1.91  |
| 43 | 6  | 7.84  | −1.84 | −0.69 | −0.73 |
| 44 | 10 | 7.24  | 2.76  | 0.99  | 1.03  |
| 45 | 8  | 8.69  | −0.69 | −0.24 | −0.25 |
| 46 | 10 | 10.56 | −0.56 | −0.18 | −0.18 |
| 47 | 12 | 11.81 | 0.19  | 0.06  | 0.06  |
| 48 | 10 | 13.48 | −3.48 | −1.02 | −1.05 |
| 49 | 14 | 14.53 | −0.53 | −0.14 | −0.15 |
| 50 | 15 | 16.04 | −1.04 | −0.27 | −0.28 |
| 51 | 14 | 19.26 | −5.26 | −1.30 | −1.34 |
| 52 | 19 | 22.04 | −3.04 | −0.69 | −0.71 |
| 53 | 36 | 27.34 | 8.66  | 1.65  | 1.72  |
| 54 | 26 | 27.10 | −1.10 | −0.22 | −0.23 |
| 55 | 21 | 27.16 | −6.16 | −1.29 | −1.35 |
| 56 | 28 | 35.38 | −7.38 | −1.36 | −1.46 |
| 57 | 41 | 36.32 | 4.68  | 0.81  | 0.89  |
| 58 | 38 | 34.50 | 3.50  | 0.63  | 0.70  |
| 59 | 49 | 44.15 | 4.85  | 0.78  | 0.91  |

$$\text{stdevres}_1 = -2.191/\left(\sqrt{1 - 0.098480}\right) = -2.31.$$

Table 10.36 shows the full set of residuals, of the three types mentioned, plus observed and expected deaths. This analysis has been done using a computer retaining a considerable number of decimal places. Consequently the results for age 40 are slightly more accurate than those just derived.

The three residuals always have the same sign, but the rank ordering for raw residuals is quite different from that of the other two. Consideration of Figure 10.4(a) would lead us to expect the first residual to be the largest. Whilst it is for the other two, it is nowhere near the largest (in absolute terms) amongst the raw residuals. This illustrates the problem with raw residuals. The first standardized deviance residual is less than $-1.96$, indicating a real problem with the model. The result for age 40 is an outlier.

As a consequence, men of age 40 were deleted and the model refitted. To predict deaths from men aged 41–59 the fitted model turned out to be

$$\hat{\text{logit}} = -8.0827 + 0.1067x$$

where $x$ is age. Compare this with (10.9).

Figure 10.8 shows the standardized deviance residuals plotted against age for this revised model. There are no unusually extreme residuals, nor any obvious patterns. The logistic regression model seems to produce adequate predictions of chances of death for those aged 41–59 years.

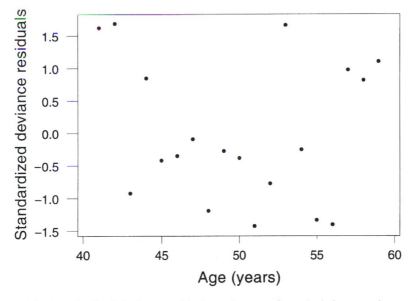

**Figure 10.8** Standardized deviance residuals against age for a logistic regression model fitted to the data of Table 10.4, after first omitting age 40 years.

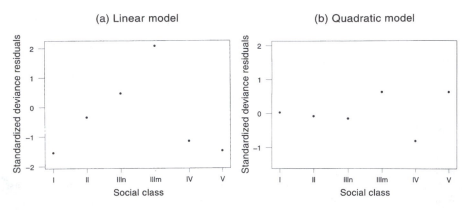

**Figure 10.9** Standardized deviance residuals against social class for logistic regression models with (a) only a linear term, (b) linear and quadratic terms, using the data of Table 10.3.

*Example 10.24* In Example 10.17 we saw the inadequacy of the linear model for predicting *H. pylori* prevalence by social class. Figure 10.9(a) shows the plot of standardized deviance residuals against social class for this model. The upside-down U pattern is obvious, suggesting that the systematic effect of social class has not yet been captured fully. Figure 10.9(b) shows the same plot for the quadratic model; this model is acceptable since there is no pattern (and no unacceptably large residuals).

### 10.10.2  Influential observations

As in general linear models, outliers are not the only kind of problematic observations. Additional diagnostic tests are required to identify those observations which have a substantial impact on the fit of the logistic model. Refer to Collett (1991) for details and examples.

### 10.10.3  Heterogeneity

A logistic regression model will be inadequate if the model does not take proper account of the variability in the observed data. Problems can arise, for instance, when there are correlations between the responses of individuals within the study. For example, people sampled from the same locality may influence each other's response, especially if the outcome measure is some subjective measure of disease status. Alternatively, the sample may consist of several sub-samples, each of which would give different responses to the same value of the explanatory variable(s). For example, the Pooling Project

(Example 10.4) is an amalgamation of different studies. It is possible that, say, serum total cholesterol may have been measured differently between studies so that, even though the cholesterol–CHD relationship is really consistent, the relationship between *recorded* cholesterol and CHD varies by individual study.

Problems such as these come under the general heading of **heterogeneity**. When grouped data seem to fit the data well, according to residual plots, and yet there is still lack of fit (Section 10.7.1) it may be that heterogeneity needs to be accounted for. In this case the deviance will be much greater than its degrees of freedom: this is called **overdispersion**. Sometimes heterogeneity is apparent from the deviance being much less than the d.f. This is called **underdispersion** – that is, the variation in the data is less than would be expected under the logistic regression (binomial) assumption. In practice this is unusual. In the logistic regression context heterogeneity is sometimes referred to as **extra-binomial variation**.

Whatever the cause, or direction, of heterogeneity, the statistical tools to allow for it are the same. The simplest of these defines a dispersion parameter which multiplies the standard binomial variance (see Williams, 1982). Many commercial computer routines, including PROC GENMOD in SAS, will allow such a parameter to be included in the specification of the logistic model. If there is known clustering within the data, for example in the Pooling Project (an example of **meta-analysis**: combining individual studies) or where sampling has been carried out in a hierarchical fashion (for example, selected individuals within selected hospitals within selected towns), a **multi-level model** (see Goldstein, 1995) will be appropriate. Such models allow for variation at several levels of aggregation, and can accept variables that are only defined at cluster, as opposed to individual, level – for instance, the size of a hospital or the average level of air pollution in a town, in the example above. Multi-level models may be defined for other statistical models besides logistic regression, including standard regression, Poisson regression and survival analysis.

## 10.11   Case–control studies

Logistic regression may be used to analyse case–control studies, but, just as when only descriptive statistics are used, the range of analyses possible is restricted. Matched studies, whatever the design framework, require special analyses. Since matching is most frequently done within case–control studies, we shall consider logistic models for matching within this context.

### 10.11.1   Unmatched studies

Suppose that we define case–control status to be the outcome variable, with a 'case' outcome taken to be the positive event, and exposure status to be the explanatory variable. Then we can analyse the case–control study by logistic regression in much the same way as for data arising by cross-sectional survey, cohort study or intervention. The only proviso is that we *cannot* construct estimates of the risk, relative risk or odds of disease. In the context of logistic regression, this is proved mathematically by Collett (1991). Hence (10.8) does not hold and, whilst (10.3) still defines the logit, the logit is no longer the log odds (more precisely, it is no longer a valid estimate of the population log odds).

What we *can* do is estimate the odds ratio, exactly as for any other type of study design: for instance, (10.4) is still usable. Similarly, those procedures for testing with deviances and model checking described earlier still hold good. So, as long as we make all inferences in terms of odds ratios, which is the natural thing to do using a logistic model in any case, unmatched case–control studies give no new problem. Notice that all these comments are consistent with the material of Section 6.2.1.

*Example 10.25*   The data of Table 6.2 (showing case–control status for melanoma and sun protection status) are presented in Table 10.37, this being of the typical format of this chapter. In the notation of Table 10.2, 'cases' $= e$ and 'total' $= n$. SAS PROC GENMOD returned the following estimate (and estimated standard error) for protection:

$$-0.3315 \ (\hat{se} = 0.1563).$$

This gives the estimated odds ratio as $\exp(-0.3315) = 0.72$, with 95% confidence interval

$$\exp\{-0.3315 \pm 1.96 \times 0.1563\}$$

or (0.53, 0.98), which agrees with the result found without the logistic regression model in Example 6.3.

The $\Delta$deviance for comparing the model with sun protection status to the empty model (with a constant term only) is 4.53 with 1 d.f. ($p = 0.03$). This result is very similar to the chi-square test statistic of 4.19 ($p = 0.04$) reported in Example 6.3.

When there are several exposure variables, possibly in addition to confounding and interaction variables, we simply take each to be an

**Table 10.37**   Sun protection during childhood against case–control status for cutaneous melanoma

| Sun protection? | Cases | Controls | Total |
|---|---|---|---|
| Yes | 99 | 132 | 231 |
| No | 303 | 290 | 593 |

explanatory variable in a multiple logistic regression model (as usual). If any of the explanatory variables is continuous we would normally wish to analyse the data in generic form. The outcome variable would then take the value 1 for cases and 0 for controls.

### 10.11.2  Matched studies

Matched studies give rise to **conditional logistic regression models**. These are obtained from maximum likelihood analysis, conditioning on the observed set of explanatory variables in any one matched set being allocated to that set, although not necessarily to the same individuals within the set (see Breslow and Day, 1980). In general, this leads to relatively complex analyses (see Breslow *et al.*, 1978) and special computer routines are needed. In the special case of 1 : 1 matching the conditional likelihood can be reduced to the standard likelihood, and thus standard logistic regression procedures can be used (see Collett, 1991). In SAS matched analyses may be carried out using **PROC PHREG**, a procedure designed primarily for use with Cox regression (Section 11.6), provided that the DISCRETE option is selected. Whatever package is used, it will be necessary to declare the matching information, usually by defining a unique number for each matched set.

*Example 10.26*   The paired data of Table 6.11 were read into SAS in generic form: for each individual the set (pair) number (1–109), case–control status (1 = case, 0 = control) and family history status (1 = yes, 0 = no) were read. The conditional logistic regression analysis performed by **PROC PHREG** gave the following estimate (and estimated standard error) for family history:

$$0.733969 \ (\hat{se} = 0.35119).$$

This gives the estimated odds ratio as $\exp(0.733969) = 2.08$, with 95% confidence interval

$$\exp\{0.733969 \pm 1.96 \times 0.35119\}$$

or (1.05, 4.15). The odds ratio is exactly as given in Example 6.8, although the confidence interval is slightly narrower than the exact interval found previously. The test results also turn out to be very similar to those found in Example 6.8. Note that there is no need to include any of the concordant pairs in the data input and analysis.

*Example 10.27*   In Example 6.11 we analysed data from a many : many matched synthetic case–control study of myocardial infarction (MI). As well as the risk factor, D-dimer (recorded as low/high), a number of potential confounding variables were available for each study participant. One of these was systolic blood pressure (SBP). In Section 6.6.4 we saw how to determine the effect of D-dimer on MI (case–control status). Now we shall also see how to assess the adjusted effect of D-dimer, accounting for the effect of SBP. Table 10.38 shows the data required as input to the computer; as in Table 6.19, the sets have been sorted by increasing size.

**Table 10.38**   Results from a matched case–control study on MI: case–control status is 0 for a control and 1 for a case; D-dimer status is 0 for low and 1 for high ('exposed'); SBP = systolic blood pressure

| Set no. | Case/ control | D-dimer status | SBP (mmHg) | Set no. | Case/ control | D-dimer status | SBP (mmHg) |
|---|---|---|---|---|---|---|---|
| 1 | 0 | 0 | 142 | 15 | 0 | 1 | 147 |
| 1 | 0 | 1 | 105 | 15 | 0 | 1 | 163 |
| 1 | 1 | 0 | 142 | 15 | 0 | 1 | 206 |
| 2 | 0 | 0 | 131 | 15 | 0 | 0 | 152 |
| 2 | 0 | 0 | 117 | 15 | 0 | 1 | 143 |
| 2 | 0 | 0 | 120 | 15 | 0 | 0 | 120 |
| 2 | 1 | 0 | 130 | 15 | 0 | 1 | 180 |
| 3 | 0 | 0 | 126 | 15 | 1 | 1 | 200 |
| 3 | 0 | 1 | 109 | 15 | 1 | 0 | 147 |
| 3 | 0 | 0 | 103 | 16 | 0 | 0 | 163 |
| 3 | 1 | 1 | 179 | 16 | 0 | 0 | 147 |
| 4 | 0 | 1 | 138 | 16 | 0 | 0 | 143 |
| 4 | 0 | 1 | 124 | 16 | 0 | 0 | 123 |
| 4 | 0 | 1 | 136 | 16 | 0 | 1 | 153 |
| 4 | 1 | 1 | 147 | 16 | 1 | 0 | 148 |
| 5 | 0 | 1 | 127 | 16 | 1 | 1 | 127 |
| 5 | 0 | 1 | 143 | 16 | 0 | 1 | 155 |
| 5 | 0 | 1 | 136 | 16 | 0 | 0 | 149 |
| 5 | 0 | 0 | 160 | 17 | 1 | 1 | 156 |
| 5 | 1 | 0 | 127 | 17 | 0 | 0 | 159 |
| 6 | 0 | 1 | 155 | 17 | 0 | 1 | 190 |
| 6 | 0 | 1 | 125 | 17 | 0 | 1 | 131 |
| 6 | 0 | 0 | 184 | 17 | 0 | 1 | 152 |
| 6 | 0 | 0 | 165 | 17 | 0 | 1 | 164 |
| 6 | 1 | 1 | 177 | 17 | 0 | 1 | 160 |
| 7 | 0 | 1 | 123 | 17 | 0 | 1 | 135 |
| 7 | 0 | 1 | 139 | 17 | 0 | 1 | 169 |
| 7 | 1 | 0 | 133 | 17 | 1 | 0 | 137 |
| 7 | 0 | 0 | 153 | 18 | 0 | 1 | 174 |
| 7 | 0 | 0 | 131 | 18 | 1 | 1 | 141 |
| 8 | 0 | 0 | 154 | 18 | 0 | 0 | 137 |
| 8 | 0 | 0 | 138 | 18 | 0 | 0 | 144 |
| 8 | 0 | 1 | 164 | 18 | 0 | 0 | 152 |
| 8 | 1 | 0 | 150 | 18 | 0 | 0 | 150 |
| 8 | 0 | 0 | 161 | 18 | 0 | 0 | 185 |
| 9 | 0 | 0 | 113 | 18 | 0 | 1 | 134 |
| 9 | 0 | 1 | 125 | 18 | 1 | 1 | 134 |
| 9 | 1 | 1 | 112 | 18 | 0 | 1 | 134 |
| 9 | 0 | 1 | 150 | 19 | 0 | 0 | 122 |
| 9 | 0 | 1 | 139 | 19 | 0 | 0 | 141 |

**Table 10.38**   *cont.*

| Set no. | Case/ control | D-dimer status | SBP (mmHg) | Set no. | Case/ control | D-dimer status | SBP (mmHg) |
|---|---|---|---|---|---|---|---|
| 10 | 0 | 0 | 125 | 19 | 0 | 0 | 130 |
| 10 | 0 | 1 | 130 | 19 | 0 | 0 | 142 |
| 10 | 0 | 0 | 151 | 19 | 0 | 1 | 131 |
| 10 | 0 | 0 | 129 | 19 | 0 | 0 | 140 |
| 10 | 1 | 1 | 152 | 19 | 1 | 0 | 146 |
| 11 | 0 | 0 | 129 | 19 | 0 | 0 | 122 |
| 11 | 0 | 0 | 92 | 19 | 0 | 1 | 136 |
| 11 | 1 | 0 | 131 | 19 | 0 | 0 | 129 |
| 11 | 0 | 1 | 137 | 19 | 0 | 1 | 153 |
| 11 | 0 | 0 | 105 | 19 | 0 | 1 | 140 |
| 12 | 0 | 0 | 109 | 19 | 1 | 1 | 181 |
| 12 | 0 | 0 | 108 | 19 | 1 | 0 | 207 |
| 12 | 0 | 0 | 139 | 20 | 0 | 1 | 148 |
| 12 | 0 | 1 | 110 | 20 | 0 | 0 | 125 |
| 12 | 1 | 1 | 129 | 20 | 0 | 0 | 147 |
| 13 | 0 | 1 | 113 | 20 | 0 | 1 | 142 |
| 13 | 0 | 0 | 161 | 20 | 0 | 0 | 134 |
| 13 | 0 | 0 | 121 | 20 | 0 | 1 | 128 |
| 13 | 0 | 0 | 104 | 20 | 1 | 1 | 132 |
| 13 | 1 | 0 | 131 | 20 | 0 | 0 | 143 |
| 14 | 0 | 1 | 151 | 20 | 0 | 1 | 144 |
| 14 | 0 | 0 | 117 | 20 | 1 | 0 | 189 |
| 14 | 0 | 0 | 120 | 20 | 0 | 1 | 134 |
| 14 | 0 | 0 | 135 | 20 | 0 | 1 | 149 |
| 14 | 0 | 1 | 181 | 20 | 0 | 1 | 111 |
| 14 | 0 | 1 | 171 | 20 | 0 | 1 | 113 |
| 14 | 0 | 0 | 148 | 20 | 1 | 1 | 115 |
| 14 | 1 | 1 | 145 | | | | |

Note: These data are available electronically – see Appendix C.

Three conditional logistic regression models were fitted using PROC PHREG: D-dimer alone, SBP alone and both together. The minus twice log likelihoods (Section 10.7) for these models were reported as 96.966, 92.899 and 92.713, respectively; furthermore, the empty model (reported automatically by PROC PHREG) has the value 97.239.

D-dimer, with two levels, has 1 d.f. Hence we may test for D-dimer unadjusted and adjusted by comparing $97.239 - 96.966 = 0.273$ and $92.899 - 92.713 = 0.186$, respectively, with $\chi_1^2$. Clearly neither is significant at any reasonable level. Hence we may conclude that D-dimer appears to have no effect on MI, whether or not we adjust for SBP. The estimated odds ratio (with 95% confidence interval) is 1.26 (0.53, 2.96) unadjusted and 1.22 (0.50, 2.94) adjusted, showing that adjustment has no real effect. Notice that the continuous variable SBP is a significant risk factor for MI in its own right since its effect is evaluated from comparing $97.239 - 92.899 = 4.34$ with $\chi_1^2$ ($p = 0.04$).

The unadjusted results from maximum likelihood methodology recorded here are similar to the Mantel–Haenszel results given in Example 6.11. The test statistic is slightly bigger than the continuity-corrected test statistic in Example 6.11, although without the continuity correction the two results are only 0.001 apart. The estimate and lower confidence limit for $\psi$ are identical; the upper limit is 2.96, compared to 3.02 in Example 6.11.

## 10.12    Outcomes with several ordered levels

Up to now we have assumed that disease outcome is measured as either 'yes' or 'no'. In some instances it may be possible to define the severity of disease – for example, 'no disease', 'little', 'moderate', 'severe' and 'death'. Then the outcome is ordinal; the $y$ variable is an ordered categorical variable. Although this is outside the intended scope of this chapter, it is so closely related to the preceding material that it is appropriate to consider this situation here.

Armstrong and Sloan (1989) give an example of an ordered categorical outcome variable arising from a study of miners exposed to tremolite fibres where the outcome is the profusion of small opacities on a chest X-ray recorded on a 12-point ordered scale. Hastie *et al.* (1989) give a similar example where a combined osteoporosis score is constructed for each subject from individual grades of osteoporosis of the sacrium, ilium, pelvis and ischium. In such cases standard regression modelling is inappropriate because the $y$ variable is not normally distributed. Non-parametric procedures, such as the two-sample Wilcoxon test (Section 2.8.2) are applicable, but cannot make allowance for several explanatory variables, as would a statistical model. It would be possible to collapse the outcomes into a binary variable – for example, 'below 6' and 'above 6' for the problem of Armstrong and Sloan (1989) – and then use logistic regression modelling. However, this would throw away information on the precise severity of disease.

What is required is a modelling procedure that falls somewhere between standard and logistic regression. Several such models for ordered categorical outcomes have been suggested (see Agresti, 1996). One of these is the **proportional odds model** (see McCullagh, 1980), which is easy to fit using commercial software, such as SAS.

### 10.12.1    The proportional odds assumption

Consider a simple problem where each individual is recorded as either 'exposed' or 'unexposed' to a solitary risk factor. This is just as in Section 10.4.1, but now disease severity is recorded, say, on an $\ell$-point ordinal scale. Table 10.39 shows the form of the data: this is a direct extension of Table 3.1.

**Table 10.39**    Disease severity ($D_\ell$ most, $D_1$ least) against risk factor status

| Risk factor status | Disease severity | | | | | Total |
|---|---|---|---|---|---|---|
| | $D_\ell$ | $D_{\ell-1}$ | $\dots$ | $D_2$ | $D_1$ | |
| Exposed | $e_\ell$ | $e_{\ell-1}$ | | $e_2$ | $e_1$ | |
| Not exposed | $u_\ell$ | $u_{\ell-1}$ | | $u_2$ | $u_1$ | |
| Total | | | | | | $n$ |

Consider combining the severity classes $(D)$ into two groups. For example we could take $D_\ell$ by itself as one group and the rest ($D_{\ell-1}$ to $D_1$) as the other. Then Table 10.39 would reduce to Table 3.1 such that

$$a = e_\ell, \quad b = e_1 + e_2 + \cdots + e_{\ell-1},$$
$$c = u_\ell, \quad d = u_1 + u_2 + \cdots + u_{\ell-1}.$$

We could then apply (3.9) to find the odds ratio for most severe disease status (perhaps death) against any less severe disease status (perhaps survival) as

$$\psi_\ell = \frac{e_\ell(u_1 + u_2 + \cdots + u_{\ell-1})}{(e_1 + e_2 + \cdots + e_{\ell-1})u_\ell}. \tag{10.26}$$

We can group columns of Table 10.39 in $\ell - 1$ other ways so as to produce $2 \times 2$ tables (each akin to Table 3.1) with 'more severe' in the left-hand and 'less severe' in the right-hand column. We simply keep moving the point of separation one step to the right each time, within the $D$ columns of Table 10.39. Each time an odds ratio may be calculated just as for (10.26): the odds ratio for the $j$ most severe classes of disease versus the $\ell - j$ least severe is, from (3.9),

$$\psi_{\ell-j+1} = \frac{(e_{\ell-j+1} + e_{\ell-j+2} + \cdots + e_\ell)(u_1 + u_2 + \cdots + u_{\ell-j})}{(e_1 + e_2 + \cdots + e_{\ell-j})(u_{\ell-j+1} + u_{\ell-j+2} + \cdots + u_\ell)}. \tag{10.27}$$

The proportional odds assumption is that (10.27) is the same whatever the value of $j$ ($j$ varies from 1 to $\ell - 1$). That is, the relative odds of more severe disease are the same, whatever the definition of 'more severe'.

*Example 10.28*    Woodward *et al.* (1995) describe an application of the proportional odds method to CHD prevalence for the baseline SHHS. Prevalent CHD was defined on a four-point graded scale: MI, angina grade II, angina grade I, no CHD (in decreasing order of severity). In several previous analyses the three grades of CHD had been combined and logistic regression analysis used. The new analysis made use of the more detailed information about the extent of disease.

As an example, we illustrate here a proportional odds analysis of parental history (before age 60) of CHD as a risk factor for CHD in men. This was one of several factors looked at by

Woodward *et al.* (1995). Table 10.40 shows baseline CHD severity against parental history status for every man in the SHHS from whom the relevant information was obtained. Note that this includes data from three Scottish districts that were unavailable to Woodward *et al.* (1995).

To check the proportional odds assumption we (conceptually) divide the disease columns of Table 10.40 into (i) MI versus the rest; (ii) MI plus angina II versus angina I plus no CHD; (iii) any CHD versus no CHD. This produces the following tables:

$$
\begin{array}{llllll}
\text{(i)} & 104 & 892 & \text{(ii)} & 121 & 875 & \text{(iii)} & 166 & 830 \\
& 192 & 3528 & & 222 & 3498 & & 344 & 3376
\end{array}
$$

Then we can calculate the three odds ratios either from (3.9) or (10.27) as: (i) 2.14; (ii) 2.18; (iii) 1.96. These are reasonably similar, and we can conclude that the proportional odds assumption seems to be acceptable. We might report some kind of average of these three as *the* odds ratio for CHD severity (Example 10.29). Certainly those men whose parents had CHD are more likely to have a relatively severe form of CHD themselves.

### 10.12.2    The proportional odds model

The proportional odds regression model is a direct generalization of the logistic regression model, using the proportional odds assumption. Suppose that there are, as before, $\ell$ disease severity categories. Logistic regression could then be used to model $\ell - 1$ logits (just as (10.27) defines $\ell - 1$ odds ratios). These are combined in the proportional odds model: the $i$th logit is estimated as

$$
\widehat{\text{logit}}_i = b_{0i} + b_1 x, \quad i = 1, 2, \ldots, \ell - 1. \tag{10.28}
$$

Notice that the constant term, $b_{0i}$, varies with $i$ (the choice of cut-point amongst the disease categories), but the slope parameter, $b_1$, is independent of $i$. The latter is the mathematical encapsulation of the proportional odds assumption.

If there are several risk factors or confounders, possibly plus interaction terms, the proportional odds model is a multiple regression version of (10.28):

$$
\widehat{\text{logit}}_i = b_{0i} + b_1 x_1 + b_2 x_2 + \cdots + b_k x_k, \quad i = 1, 2, \ldots, \ell - 1, \tag{10.29}
$$

for some $k > 1$.

**Table 10.40**  Prevalent CHD against parental history of CHD for men in the SHHS

| Parental history of CHD? | CHD disease category | | | | |
|---|---|---|---|---|---|
| | MI | Angina II | Angina I | No CHD | Total |
| Yes | 104 | 17 | 45 | 830 | 996 |
| No | 192 | 30 | 122 | 3376 | 3720 |
| Total | 296 | 47 | 167 | 4206 | 4716 |

Computer packages will give estimates of the $b$ coefficients and model deviances, which are used exactly as in Section 10.7. The SAS package procedure PROC LOGISTIC will fit proportional odds models provided the NOSIMPLE option is declared. This also prints out the result of a formal test (described by Peterson, 1990) of the proportional odds assumption. Since this test appears to be very sensitive to small departures from the assumption, only very extreme significance levels (such as $p < 0.01$) should be used as evidence to reject the proportional odds assumption with large samples.

*Example 10.29*   SAS PROC LOGISTIC was used to analyse the data of Example 10.28. The data were entered to SAS with CHD severity coded in rank order (MI coded as 1,..., no CHD as 4). The binary explanatory variable, parental CHD (PARNTS = 1 if yes, 0 if no), was not declared as a categorical variable. Results appear in Output 10.6.

First, we can see that the test of the proportional odds assumption is not significant ($p = 0.2964$), so we have an objective justification for our analysis. The maximum likelihood estimates include INTERCP terms, which are the three separate $b_{0i}$ in (10.28). Of more interest is the PARNTS line, which tells us that the estimate of $b_1$ in (10.28) is 0.6843, which gives an odds ratio of $e^{0.6843} = 1.982$. This is the estimated odds ratio for more severe CHD, comparing those with to those without parental history of CHD. This is an average (although not a simple arithmetic mean) of the three individual odds ratios calculated in Example 10.28.

We can use the INTERCP terms to estimate odds or risks if these are meaningful. For example, the logit for all CHD versus no CHD, for those with parental history of CHD is, by (10.28),

$$-2.2858 + 0.6843 \times 1 = -1.6015,$$

where INTERCP3 is chosen because all CHD : no CHD is the third split (Example 10.28). Then, by (10.8), the estimated prevalence risk is

$$\hat{r} = \{1 + \exp(1.6015)\}^{-1} = 0.17.$$

Since we have fitted the full model we can check this from Table 10.40 (or its third split). Observed data give the prevalence of CHD for those with parental history of CHD as

**Output 10.6**   SAS results for Example 10.29

The LOGISTIC Procedure

Score Test for the Proportional Odds Assumption

Chi-Square = 2.4323 with 2 DF ($p = 0.2964$)

Analysis of Maximum Likelihood Estimates

| Variable | DF | Parameter Estimate | Standard Error | Wald Chi-Square | Pr > Chi-Square | Odds Ratio |
|---|---|---|---|---|---|---|
| INTERCP1 | 1 | −2.8844 | 0.0683 | 1783.7098 | 0.0001 | 0.056 |
| INTERCP2 | 1 | −2.7251 | 0.0647 | 1771.6573 | 0.0001 | 0.066 |
| INTERCP3 | 1 | −2.2858 | 0.0566 | 1629.7623 | 0.0001 | 0.102 |
| PARNTS | 1 | 0.6843 | 0.1017 | 45.3058 | 0.0001 | 1.982 |

$$(104 + 17 + 45)/996 = 166/996 = 0.17,$$

as anticipated.

## Exercises

(Most of these exercises require a computer package with a logistic regression procedure.)

10.1 For the data of Exercise 3.1, find the odds of cardiovascular death for binge beer drinkers and for non-bingers, and the odds ratio comparing the former to the latter, using a logistic regression model. Also find 95% confidence limits for the odds ratio and test the null hypothesis that the odds ratio is unity. Compare your results with those in Exercise 3.1.

10.2 A 12-year study of coronary heart disease (CHD) collected data from men aged 35–54 years. Five variables are available for analysis: CHD outcome (yes/no); age group (35–39/40–44/45–49/50–54 years); diastolic blood pressure (mmHg); serum total cholesterol (mmol/l); cigarette smoking status (never/current/ex). When a logistic regression model was fitted to these data, with CHD as the outcome variable, the parameter estimates shown below were found:

| Effect | Estimate |
|---|---|
| Constant (intercept) | −5.777 |
| Age 35–39 | 0 |
| Age 40–44 | 1.102 |
| Age 45–49 | 1.275 |
| Age 50–54 | 2.070 |
| Diastolic blood pressure | −0.0006598 |
| Serum total cholesterol | 0.2414 |
| Never smoked | 0 |
| Current smoker | 1.190 |
| Ex-smoker | 0.7942 |
| Age 40–44*current smoker | −0.4746 |
| Age 40–44*ex-smoker | −0.7009 |
| Age 45–49*current smoker | −0.2109 |
| Age 45–49*ex-smoker | 0.4739 |
| Age 50–54*current smoker | −0.6831 |
| Age 50–54*ex-smoker | 0.06005 |

Note: * denotes an interaction.

(i) Which levels of the two categorical explanatory variables have been fixed as the base, or reference, levels?

(ii) From the fitted model, estimate the odds ratio of CHD for a man aged 47 who currently smokes cigarettes compared to a man of the same age who has never smoked cigarettes.

(iii) From the fitted model, estimate the probability that a man aged 47 who currently smokes cigarettes, has a diastolic blood pressure of 90 mmHg and a serum total cholesterol level of 6.20 mmol/l will develop CHD within 12 years.

10.3 In a survey of the prevalence of asthma in schoolchildren, Strachan (1988) calculated a bronchial liability index as the forced expiratory volume in 1 second after exercise divided by that before exercise. Results for the liability index, classified by whether or not there was mould in the child's room, were presented as ratios of number with wheeze in the past year divided by total number of children, as shown below.

| Liability index | No mould | Mould |
|---|---|---|
| <0.8 | 17/35 | 3/5 |
| 0.8–0.89 | 7/63 | 4/9 |
| 0.9–0.99 | 34/383 | 10/30 |
| ≥1.0 | 20/303 | 5/34 |

Use logistic regression modelling in working through the following.
(i) Ignoring liability index altogether, find an odds ratio for mould compared with no mould, together with a 95% confidence interval.
(ii) Confirm that mould and liability index do not interact in their effect upon asthma.
(iii) Find the odds ratio for mould compared with no mould, together with a 95% confidence interval, adjusting for liability index. Compare your answer with that in (i). Interpret the result.
(iv) Find odds ratios for the liability index groups, taking the '< 0.8' group as base, adjusting for mould status. Give 95% confidence limits in each case.
(v) Test whether there appears to be a linear effect across the four liability groups, adjusting for mould status. Estimate and interpret the linear effect. Give a 95% confidence interval for the estimate.

10.4 Refer to the data in Table C.3. In the following, use logistic regression models.
(i) Find prevalence risks, odds, relative risk and odds ratio (high versus low) by factor IX status by sex group. Give 95% confidence intervals for the odds ratios. Test for an association between factor IX and cardiovascular disease (CVD) for each sex separately using model deviances. Compare your answers with those to Exercise 3.4.
(ii) Find an age-adjusted, a sex-adjusted and an age/sex-adjusted odds ratio for high versus low factor IX status. Compare your results with those for Exercise 4.7.
(iii) Test for a sex by factor IX and an age group by factor IX interaction. Compare your answers with those to Exercise 4.7.
(iv) Check whether there is a three-way interaction between sex, age group and factor IX status in predicting CVD.

10.5 Swan (1986) gives the following data from a study of infant respiratory disease. The numbers show the proportion of children developing bronchitis or pneumonia in their first year of life by sex and type of feeding.

| Sex | Bottle only | Breast + supplement | Breast only |
|---|---|---|---|
| Boys | 77/458 (0.17) | 19/147 (0.13) | 47/494 (0.10) |
| Girls | 48/384 (0.13) | 16/127 (0.13) | 31/464 (0.07) |

The major question of interest is whether the risk of illness is affected by the type of feeding. Also, is the risk the same for both sexes and, if there are differences between the feeding groups, are these differences the same for boys and girls?

(i) Fit all possible linear logistic regression models to the data. Use your results to answer all the questions posed above through significance testing. Summarize your findings using odds ratios with 95% confidence intervals.

(ii) Fit the model with explanatory variables sex and type of feeding (but no interaction). Calculate the residuals, deviance residuals and standardized deviance residuals and comment on the results.

10.6 Saetta *et al.* (1991) carried out a prospective, single-blind experiment to determine whether gastric content is forced into the small bowel when gastric-emptying procedures are employed with people who have poisoned themselves. Sixty subjects were recruited; each was asked to swallow twenty barium-impregnated polythene pellets. Of the 60, 20 received a gastric lavage, 20 received induced emesis and 20 (controls) received no gastric decontamination. The number of residual pellets counted, by X-ray, in the intestine after ingestion for each subject was, for the induced emesis group,

$$0, 15, 2, 0, 0, 15, 1, 16, 0, 1, 1, 0, 6, 0, 0, 1, 0, 16, 7, 11;$$

for the gastric lavage group,

$$9, 3, 4, 15, 3, 5, 0, 0, 2, 11, 0, 0, 0, 0, 7, 5, 9, 0, 0, 0;$$

and for the control group,

$$0, 9, 0, 0, 4, 5, 0, 0, 13, 0, 0, 12, 0, 0, 1, 0, 4, 4, 6, 7.$$

(i) Is there a significant difference between treatment groups?

(ii) Is the control group significantly different from the other two?

10.7 A cohort study has been carried out to investigate the supposed health benefits of consuming antioxidant vitamins. A large number of men were studied: at baseline their daily antioxidant vitamin consumption (denoted AOX below) was categorized as 1 = low, 2 = medium or 3 = high. Also, at baseline, their daily alcohol consumption (ALC: 1 = none, 2 = occasional drinker, 3 = moderate drinker, 4 = heavy drinker) and smoking status (SMO: 1 = non-smoker, 2 = current smoker) were recorded. Over a 10-year follow-up period each death amongst the cohort was recorded. Logistic regression analysis was used to analyse the data.

(i) When the following sets of explanatory variables were fitted, using a certain computer package (SAS, or some equivalent), the deviances shown below were found:

| Terms fitted | Deviance |
|---|---|
| Constant only | 309.62 |
| AOX | 211.38 |
| SMO | 227.43 |
| ALC | 270.01 |
| AOX + SMO | 173.28 |
| AOX + ALC | 195.53 |
| AOX + SMO + ALC | 171.84 |
| AOX + SMO + AOX*SMO | 144.09 |

Note: * denotes an interaction.
All models include a constant term (intercept).

Write a report to describe the findings, including a table to show the results of appropriate significance tests. Are there any other models which you would suggest should be fitted? If so, state what these models are, and what you would hope to discover by fitting them.

(ii) When the last model in the above table was fitted, the package also produced the estimates and variance-covariance matrix shown below. Here the package has been forced to take AOX = 1 and SMO = 1 as the reference groups for antioxidants and smoking, respectively. The number in parentheses denotes the level of the variable. The parameters corresponding to the first level must be zero.

**Estimates**

| Parameter | Estimate | Standard error |
|---|---|---|
| Constant | −2.38 | 0.16 |
| AOX(2) | −0.37 | 0.22 |
| AOX(3) | −0.91 | 0.34 |
| SMO(2) | 1.19 | 0.18 |
| AOX(2)*SMO(2) | −0.31 | 0.37 |
| AOX(3)*SMO(2) | −0.94 | 0.38 |

**Variance-covariance matrix**

| | Constant | AOX(2) | AOX(3) | SMO(2) | AOX(2)* SMO(2) | AOX(3)* SMO(2) |
|---|---|---|---|---|---|---|
| Constant | 0.026 | | | | | |
| AOX(2) | −0.041 | 0.048 | | | | |
| AOX(3) | −0.052 | 0.017 | 0.116 | | | |
| SMO(2) | −0.080 | 0.038 | 0.041 | 0.032 | | |
| AOX(2)*SMO(2) | −0.011 | 0.057 | 0.059 | 0.064 | 0.137 | |
| AOX(3)*SMO(2) | −0.003 | 0.043 | 0.071 | 0.019 | −0.008 | 0.144 |

Estimate the odds ratios, together with corresponding 95% confidence limits, for antioxidant vitamin consumption, using low consumption as the base, for smokers and non-smokers separately.

10.8 A researcher has carried out a case–control study of risk factors for leukaemia amongst children. He has been told, by a colleague, that he should be using logistic regression to analyse his data. He remembers, from his days at medical school, how to calculate chi-square significance tests and relative risks from contingency tables, and he has done this for all the variables (potential risk factors) in his data set (both continuous and categorical). He comes to you for help, and asks two questions:

(i) 'What is the advantage of using logistic regression rather than simple chi-square tests and relative risks?'

(ii) 'How can I interpret the results of a logistic regression analysis obtained from the SAS package?'

How would you answer these two questions?

10.9 Heinrich *et al.* (1994) describe a study of the effects of fibrinogen on CHD in which healthy men aged 40–65 were followed up for 6 years. In the paper the ratio of CHD events to total numbers is given for subgroups defined by equal thirds of fibrinogen and LDL cholesterol, one of several other variables measured in the study that may affect the fibrinogen–CHD relationship. These ratios are presented below (taking account of a revision subsequent to initial publication).

| Fibrinogen third | LDL cholesterol third | | |
|---|---|---|---|
| | *Lowest* | *Middle* | *Highest* |
| Lowest | 5/263 | 3/215 | 9/186 |
| Middle | 5/230 | 6/219 | 14/213 |
| Highest | 3/178 | 8/217 | 27/262 |

Analyse the data and write a short report of your findings so as to address the study aim.

10.10 Repeat the analysis of Exercise 6.1, the unmatched case–control study of oral contraceptive use and breast cancer, using logistic regression modelling. Compare results.

10.11 Repeat the analysis of Example 6.4, the unmatched case–control study of ethnicity and *E. coli*, using logistic regression modelling. Compare results.

10.12 Repeat the analysis of Example 6.9, the 1 : 5 matched case–control study of BCG vaccination and tuberculosis, using logistic regression modelling. Compare results.

10.13 Refer to the venous thromboembolism matched case–control study of Table C.6.
   (i) Use logistic regression to repeat the analysis of Exercise 6.12. Compare results.
   (ii) Table C.6 also includes data on body mass index (BMI), a potential confounding factor in the relationship between HRT and venous thromboembolism. Test for a significant effect of HRT on venous thromboembolism, adjusting for BMI. Estimate the odds ratio for HRT users versus non-users, adjusting for BMI. Does BMI appear to have a strong confounding effect?

10.14 A colleague plans to undertake a study to investigate the risk factors for Creutzfeldt–Jakob disease, which is a very rare disease. He comes to you to seek advice before he begins data collection. What follows is a series of questions which he asks you. In each case you should answer the question, and provide a brief justification of your answer.
   (i) 'I plan to do a case–control study. Is this a suitable choice of design? If not, what should I do instead?'
   (ii) 'I am considering calculating a series of relative risks for each risk factor I measure. Is this sensible? If not, what should I do instead?'
   (iii) 'I am pretty sure that an individual's age affects his chance of having Creutzfeldt–Jakob disease, and age is related to several of the risk factors that I am interested in. Hence I was thinking of doing separate analyses for each age group. The only problem is that the numbers are likely to get rather small. What can I do to avoid this problem?'

(iv)  'I suspect that a couple of my risk factors act differently for men and women. Is it OK to give a simple average value over the sexes in these cases, or should I do some sort of weighting?'

(v)  'Once I have done all the analyses you have suggested to me, how should I present my results?'

# 11

# Modelling follow-up data

## 11.1 Introduction

In this chapter we consider statistical models for data collected from follow-up (cohort or intervention) studies which involve censoring or where, even in the absence of censoring, the time to an event is regarded as the outcome variable of interest. The methods follow from the basic ideas introduced in Chapter 5; models for survival data occupy Sections 11.2–11.8, whilst models for person-years data are found in Section 11.9.

### 11.1.1 Models for survival data

Two types of regression model for survival data are in general use in epidemiology: **parametric** and **semi-parametric**. Parametric models require a theoretical probability model to be specified for the data. Two useful probability models are introduced in Section 11.4; these are used to create parametric regression models in Section 11.7. The Cox semi-parametric regression model is defined in Sections 11.5 and 11.6. This makes no probability distribution assumption. The reader who wishes only to use the Cox model can omit Sections 11.4, 11.7 and parts of Section 11.8.

## 11.2 Basic functions of survival time

### 11.2.1 The survival function

In Section 5.3 we defined the estimated survival function, which may be calculated from observed survival data, as the estimated cumulative probability of survival. If we let $T$ be the random variable denoting the survival time then the survival function, $S$, evaluated at some specific time, $t$, is

$$S(t) = P(T > t); \tag{11.1}$$

That is, $S(t)$ gives the probability that survival time (follow-up duration without an event) exceeds $t$ time units.

### 11.2.2  The hazard function

The **hazard** is the instantaneous probability of failure (the opposite to survival) within the next small interval of time, having already survived to the start of the interval. As an illustration, consider the entire human life-span and take the event of interest to be death from any cause. The chance of death within the next small interval of time will be relatively high for a new-born baby, but will progressively decrease for children who have already survived past the early days of high risk. For older children and young to middle-aged adults the chance of death in the next small interval of time should be fairly constant, although there may be slight variations due, for example, to death from misadventure amongst older teenagers. For older adults the chance of death will be expected to increase with age, due to increasing frailty. Hence we might expect to see, at least approximately, the hazard function shown in Figure 11.1, in which survival time is age (time since birth). This is a graph of the **hazard function**, or a **hazard plot**.

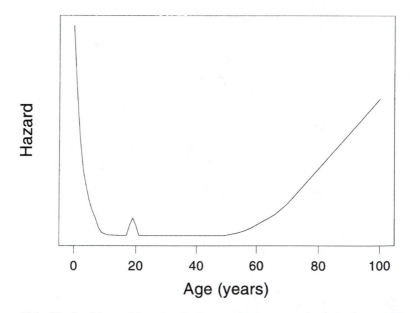

**Figure 11.1**  Idealized hazard function for human death across the entire human life-span (assumed to peak at age 100).

The precise mathematical definition of the hazard evaluated at time $t, h(t)$, is given by Collett (1994). In words, it is the probability of failure during an interval of time, conditional upon survival to the start of the interval (time $t$), divided by the size of the interval, in the limit as the size of the interval tends to zero.

## 11.3    Estimating the hazard function

We shall now consider how to estimate the hazard function from observed data. This will complement the methods for estimation of the survival function given in Chapter 5. As its definition suggests, the hazard is a special type of rate (Section 3.8), and the three methods of calculation described here all use this fact in their derivation.

### 11.3.1    Kaplan–Meier estimation

In Section 5.4 we saw how to estimate the survival function by the Kaplan–Meier (KM) method. The same approach can be used to estimate the hazard function under the assumption that the hazard is constant between successive failure times in the observed data set. These failure times are the distinct times at which events (for example, deaths) occur; where two or more events occur at the same time they all define the same failure time.

As in Chapter 5, let $e_t$ be the number of events at time $t$, where $t$ is one of the failure times, and let $n_t$ be the number at risk (that is, survivors) at time $t$. Now suppose that the next failure time (in rank order) is $u_t$ time units away. We will then estimate the hazard during the time interval from $t$ to $t + u_t$ to be the risk per unit time during the interval,

$$h_t = \frac{e_t}{n_t u_t}. \tag{11.2}$$

This defines a step function which can change (up or down) at successive failure times. Strictly speaking, $t$ is the time *just before* the $e_t$ events occur (just as in Section 5.4). If there were no repeated failure times $e_t$ would always be 1.

*Example 11.1*   Karkavelas *et al.* (1995) give the following survival times (in rank order) for 27 subjects with glioblastoma multiforme:

$$10, 12, 13, 15, 16, 20, 20, 24, 24, 26, 26, 27, 39, 42,$$
$$45, 45, 48, 52, 58, 60, 61, 62, 73, 75, 77, 104, 120.$$

Survival time is recorded as the number of weeks between initiation of cisplatin treatment and death. No subjects were recorded as being censored. Table 11.1 shows the failure times together with the estimated survival and hazard functions and the elements used in their calculation through (5.3) and (11.2). The two functions are plotted in Figures 11.2 and 11.3.

**Table 11.1** Data and survival and hazard function estimation for subjects with glioblastoma multiforme

| Time<br>$t$ | Survivors<br>$n_t$ | Deaths<br>$e_t$ | Interval<br>$u_t$ | Survival<br>$s_t$ | Hazard<br>$h_t$ |
|---|---|---|---|---|---|
| 0 | 27 | 0 | 10 | 1 | 0 |
| 10 | 27 | 1 | 2 | 0.9630 | 0.0185 |
| 12 | 26 | 1 | 1 | 0.9259 | 0.0385 |
| 13 | 25 | 1 | 2 | 0.8889 | 0.0200 |
| 15 | 24 | 1 | 1 | 0.8519 | 0.0417 |
| 16 | 23 | 1 | 4 | 0.8148 | 0.0109 |
| 20 | 22 | 2 | 4 | 0.7407 | 0.0227 |
| 24 | 20 | 2 | 2 | 0.6667 | 0.0500 |
| 26 | 18 | 2 | 1 | 0.5926 | 0.1111 |
| 27 | 16 | 1 | 12 | 0.5556 | 0.0052 |
| 39 | 15 | 1 | 3 | 0.5185 | 0.0222 |
| 42 | 14 | 1 | 3 | 0.4815 | 0.0238 |
| 45 | 13 | 2 | 3 | 0.4074 | 0.0513 |
| 48 | 11 | 1 | 4 | 0.3704 | 0.0227 |
| 52 | 10 | 1 | 6 | 0.3333 | 0.0167 |
| 58 | 9 | 1 | 2 | 0.2963 | 0.0556 |
| 60 | 8 | 1 | 1 | 0.2593 | 0.1250 |
| 61 | 7 | 1 | 1 | 0.2222 | 0.1429 |
| 62 | 6 | 1 | 11 | 0.1852 | 0.0152 |
| 73 | 5 | 1 | 2 | 0.1481 | 0.1000 |
| 75 | 4 | 1 | 2 | 0.1111 | 0.1250 |
| 77 | 3 | 1 | 27 | 0.0741 | 0.0123 |
| 104 | 2 | 1 | 16 | 0.0370 | 0.0313 |
| 120 | 1 | 1 | | | |

The survival plot (Figure 11.2) shows a rapid drop in estimated survival probability up to week 27, with 46% loss between weeks 10 and 27. Thereafter there is little attrition for 18 weeks until the former pattern is re-established, but with somewhat less consistency. There is a long 'tail' in the survival plot because of the relatively long survival of the last couple of subjects. The hazard plot (Figure 11.3) necessarily mirrors these changes. The hazards appear to be very different over time: the hazard (for death) is greatest in the periods around 25, 60 and 75 weeks and broadly seems to increase with increasing survival time.

### 11.3.2 Person-time estimation

One disadvantage with the KM approach is that the hazard function tends to be spiked, as in Figure 11.3. An alternative approach is first to divide the time continuum into a number of intervals (as in a life table) and then take the person-years event rate, (5.18), as the estimate of the hazard within any

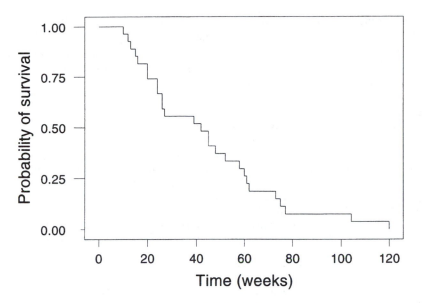

**Figure 11.2** Estimated survival function for subjects with glioblastoma multiforme.

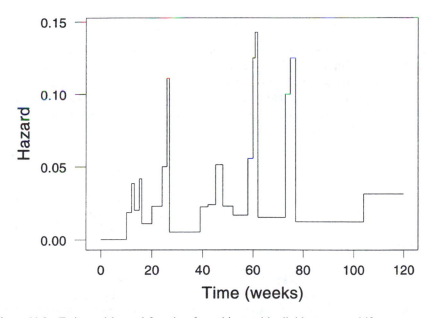

**Figure 11.3** Estimated hazard function for subjects with glioblastoma multiforme.

particular interval. Because time may be recorded in some unit other than years we shall take (5.18) to be the person-time event rate in this context. Provided that the intervals are larger, on average, than the durations between failure times, this method will tend to produce a smoother hazard plot, which is easier to interpret.

*Example 11.2*    Suppose that the survival times in Example 11.1 were grouped into 10-week intervals: 0–9, 10–19, 20–29 weeks, ... The estimated hazard during (for instance) the second of these intervals is, by (5.18), the number of deaths, $e$, divided by the number of person-weeks, $y$. From Table 11.1, $e = 5$. Person-time is easier to calculate separately for those who survive the interval and those who die within the interval (and, when they exist, those who are censored within the interval). The components are then summed. From Table 11.1 we see that deaths occur in weeks 10, 12, 13, 15 and 16. Thus the number of person-weeks for deaths within the second interval is $0 + 2 + 3 + 5 + 6 = 16$. The number of person-weeks for survivors is calculated as the number of survivors (to week 20) times the length of the interval: $22 \times 10 = 220$. Hence the estimated hazard (per week) in the second interval is

$$h_t = \frac{5}{16 + 220} = 0.0212.$$

This is roughly in line with the individual hazards given for times between 10 and 19 weeks in Table 11.1, as it must be. When the complete set of such hazards is plotted they show a similar overall pattern to that seen in Figure 11.3, although with fewer 'bumps'.

### 11.3.3    Actuarial estimation

When survival analysis is performed using the life table approach with the actuarial approximation, (5.8), we can find an estimate of the hazard that is analogous to (11.2). Suppose now that $u_t$ is the length of the interval in the life table that begins at time $t$. Taking $e_t$ as in (11.2) and $n_t^*$ as in (5.8), we find the average number of person-time units at risk in the interval beginning at $t$ to be $(n_t^* - \frac{1}{2}e_t)u_t$. This leads to an estimated hazard of

$$h_t = \frac{e_t}{(n_t^* - \frac{1}{2}e_t)u_t}. \tag{11.3}$$

*Example 11.3*    The hazard in the first year of follow-up for men with known housing accommodation status in the Scottish Heart Health Study (SHHS) may be estimated from Table 5.3. Here $t = 0$ and $n_0^* = 4398.5$, $e_0 = 17$ and $u_0 = 365$ (in days). Hence, by (11.3), the estimated hazard in the first year is

$$h_0 = \frac{17}{(4398.5 - 17/2)365} = 0.00001061.$$

Notice that we could have taken $u_0 = 1$, which would give a hazard per year; daily rates are more in keeping with the hazard as an instantaneous failure rate. We then assume that this estimate applies to each of the first 365 days after baseline.

Given that we have the individual event and censoring times (from Example 5.6) a more accurate picture of daily hazard (allowing it to vary) may be obtained for the problem of Example 11.3 from applying (11.2). Calculations then mirror those used in Table 11.1, except that $n_t$ now decreases due to censoring as well as events. Alternatively, we could apply (5.18) on a person-day basis. We shall not consider actuarial methods in the remainder of this chapter, since these are inferior when we have complete survival information.

## 11.4   Probability models

One approach to modelling survival data is to construct a realistic probability model which seems to fit the data reasonably well. Inferences, such as predictions of average survival time (for example, average time to death), may then be made from the probability model. As in other applications, the advantages are that the probability model has a mathematical form, which may be manipulated as required, and has a 'smoother' form than the observed data. In this context, predictions of intermediate survival probabilities (at times between the observed values) would be made from a smooth curve rather than a step function (such as Figure 5.8). This seems a sensible approach to interpolation.

### 11.4.1   The probability density and cumulative distribution functions

Suppose, now, that we seek to define a probability distribution for survival time – that is, a complete prediction of the survival probabilities at all possible times. Any probability distribution may be specified by its **probability density function** (p.d.f.), denoted $f$, or its **cumulative distribution function** (c.d.f.), $F$. In survival analysis $f(t)$, the p.d.f. evaluated at time $t$, is the probability that an event occurs within a very small interval of time following time $t$. This differs from the hazard function in that the latter is evaluated only for those people who have already survived to time $t$; that is to say, the hazard is a conditional probability. A graphical plot of $f(t)$ against $t$ gives an **event density** curve. Mathematically, $F$ is the integral of $f$ – that is, the area (to the left of a fixed point) under the event density curve. For example, the p.d.f. of the normal distribution is illustrated by Figure 2.11. Table B.1 gives the values from the c.d.f. of the standard normal distribution. Data-based analogues of these two theoretical concepts are, respectively, the histogram and the area under the histogram to the left of any fixed point divided by the total area enclosed by the histogram.

Consider a probability distribution that represents survival data. By definition, the c.d.f. evaluated at time $t$ is

$$F(t) = P(T \leq t) \qquad (11.4)$$

so that the area under the p.d.f. to the left of $t$ is the probability of a survival time of $t$ or less. Now (11.1) and (11.4) show that $S(t)$ and $F(t)$ are complementary probabilities; that is,

$$S(t) = 1 - F(t). \qquad (11.5)$$

Since the total area under a p.d.f. curve is always unity, (11.5) requires $S(t)$ to be the area to the right of the point $t$ under the p.d.f. curve. Figure 11.4 shows the relationships between $S$, $f$ and $F$ for an arbitrary probability model for survival time. Different models will produce different curves, and hence different enclosed areas to the left or right. A number of useful relationships between $h(t)$ and $S(t)$, $f(t)$ and $F(t)$ may be derived, such as

$$h(t) = f(t)/S(t). \qquad (11.6)$$

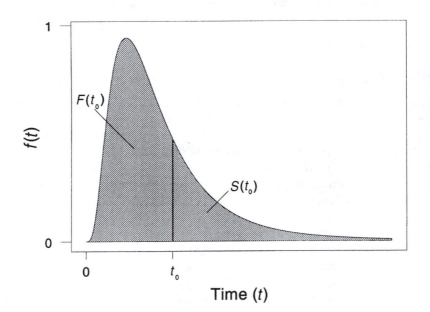

**Figure 11.4** Relationship between the survival function, $S(t)$, the probability density function, $f(t)$, and the cumulative distribution function, $F(t)$, for survival times, $t$. $S(t)$ and $F(t)$ are evaluated at a specific time $t = t_0$.

*11.4.2   Choosing a model*

Due to its pre-eminence in statistics, the obvious probability model to consider first is the normal distribution. This would be a particularly easy model to deal with because of the values of $F(t)$ given, at least after standardization, by Table B.1. However, the normal distribution is unsuitable because survival times tend to have a skewed distribution. For example, Figure 11.5 shows the histogram of the survival times from Example 11.1. The bell-shaped, symmetrical, normal curve of Figure 2.11 would not be a good fit to these data.

We seek a probability distribution whose shape mirrors that of typical survival data, a situation directly analogous to that met in Section 10.2 for data in the form of proportions. In the current context we have several ways in which a candidate probability distribution could be investigated for goodness of fit. As we have just seen, one method is to look at the shape of the curve defined by the p.d.f. of the probability distribution and compare that with the outline of a histogram of the data. Another is to calculate the survival function, $S$, defined by the probability distribution and compare this with the observed survival function. A third is to compare the shape of the theoretical and observed hazard functions. Due to the mathematical relationships between the different functions of survival time, such as (11.6), we should be able to take

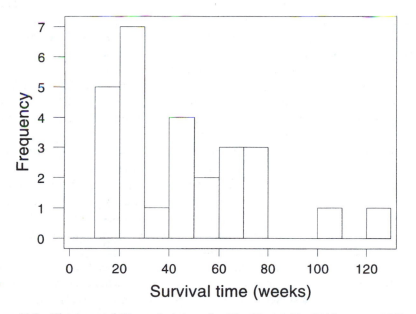

**Figure 11.5**   Histogram of the survival times for 27 subjects with glioblastoma multiforme.

any of these three approaches and still be able to specify the fitted survival and hazard functions, the p.d.f. and c.d.f. (as required).

### 11.4.3    The exponential distribution

The simplest realistic probability model for survival times assumes that they follow an **exponential** distribution. The exponential has p.d.f.

$$f(t) = \lambda e^{-\lambda t}, \tag{11.7}$$

for $t \geq 0$, where $\lambda$ is a constant which could be estimated from observed data. Throughout this chapter $\lambda$ is used to represent an unknown parameter (as is common in the current context); this should not be confused with its use as the relative risk elsewhere in the book. By calculus we may use (11.7) to show that

$$F(t) = 1 - e^{-\lambda t}$$

and hence, by (11.5),

$$S(t) = e^{-\lambda t}. \tag{11.8}$$

Also, by substituting (11.7) and (11.8) into (11.6), we obtain

$$h(t) = \lambda. \tag{11.9}$$

Figure 11.6 shows the shape of the three functions defined by (11.7)–(11.9) for an arbitrary choice of $\lambda$. The exponential p.d.f., $f(t)$, captures the right skewness which is typical of survival data. In fact this $f(t)$ has extreme right skew. The exponential survival function, $S(t)$, has the essential elements of the observed survival plots that we have seen in Chapter 5: it takes the value 1 at $t = 0$, it is non-increasing as $t$ increases and it is never negative. However, the latter two properties would hold whatever the probability model chosen. The exponential hazard function, $h(t)$, defines a straight line with zero slope. Both $f(t)$ and $h(t)$ take the value $\lambda$ when $t = 0$.

Notice that $h(t)$ does not depend upon time, $t$. This means that whenever we adopt the exponential distribution we are assuming that the hazard is constant at all follow-up times. According to Figure 11.1, this might be a reasonable assumption if we wish to model time to death amongst young to middle-aged adults. In many practical applications of survival analysis in epidemiology this is an unreasonable restriction and consequently the exponential distribution is rarely used, despite its attractive simplicity.

Since the mean of the exponential distribution is $1/\lambda$ (see Clarke and Cooke, 1992) the mean survival time is assumed to be $1/\lambda$ whenever we adopt the exponential model for survival time. This gives a simple way of estimating $\lambda$ from sample data when there is no censoring: we estimate $\lambda$ by

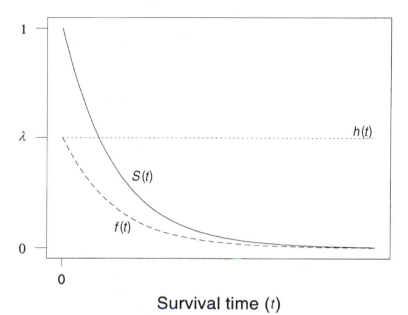

**Figure 11.6**  Probability density function, $f(t)$, survival function, $S(t)$, and hazard function, $h(t)$, for the exponential distribution.

$$\hat{\lambda} = 1/\bar{t}, \qquad (11.10)$$

where $\bar{t}$ is the mean of the observed survival times. When there is censoring we estimate $\lambda$ by

$$\hat{\lambda} = e/\sum t_i$$

where $e$ is the total number of events and $\sum t_i$ is the sum of all the follow-up times, survival times for those who experience an event and censoring times for those who are censored. As with (11.10), gives this a maximum likelihood estimate for $\lambda$.

If we wish to summarize the exponentially distributed survival data, we should use the median rather than the mean, due to the skewness. The median survival time from the exponential model is easily found. Let $t_m$ be the median survival time. Then

$$S(t_m) = 0.5,$$

because half of the subjects will have survival times above the median. Then, by (11.8),

$$0.5 = e^{-\lambda t_m},$$

leading to the result

$$t_m = \frac{1}{\lambda} \log_e 2 = \frac{0.69315}{\lambda}. \tag{11.11}$$

Other percentiles may be derived in a similar way.

*Example 11.4*  To fit an exponential distribution to the data given in Example 11.1 (where there is no censoring) we first find the sample mean of the survival times,

$$\bar{t} = (10 + 12 + 13 + \cdots + 120)/27 = 44.22.$$

Then, by (11.10),

$$\hat{\lambda} = 1/44.22 = 0.0226.$$

The model p.d.f. is thus, from (11.7),

$$f(t) = 0.0226 \, e^{-0.0226t};$$

the survival function is, from (11.8),

$$S(t) = e^{-0.0226t};$$

and the (constant) hazard function is, from (11.9),

$$h(t) = 0.0226.$$

From (11.11) the median survival time from the exponential model is

$$t_m = 0.69315/0.0226 = 30.7 \text{ weeks.}$$

We could evaluate the goodness of fit of the exponential model in Example 11.4 by comparing the plot of $S(t)$ with Figure 11.2. We delay such a comparison to Example 11.5. A further graphical test is described in Section 11.8.1. The theoretical hazard and probability density functions cannot be compared to their observed analogues (Figures 11.3 and 11.5) in terms of size because the scales used are different. However, they can be compared for shape. The exponential assumption of constant hazard does not seem to agree with Figure 11.3, where there appears to be some tendency for the hazard to grow with time. Furthermore, the histogram of Figure 11.5 suggests a peak that is offset from the left edge, unlike the exponential p.d.f. shown in Figure 11.6. Notice also that the median survival time from the exponential model is well below the sample median of 42 weeks which may be calculated from the raw data given in Example 11.1. There is, then, evidence that the exponential model is inappropriate for the glioblastoma multiforme data.

### 11.4.4    The Weibull distribution

A common probability model for survival data employs the **Weibull** distribution. This distribution has p.d.f.

$$f(t) = \lambda\gamma(t^{\gamma-1})\exp\{-\lambda(t^{\gamma})\}, \tag{11.12}$$

for $t \geq 0$, where $\lambda$ and $\gamma$ are constants which may be estimated from sample data. $\lambda$ is called the **scale parameter** and $\gamma$ is the **shape parameter**. Figure 11.7 illustrates the different shapes that the Weibull p.d.f. can take as $\gamma$ changes. It is the great flexibility of the Weibull that makes it such a useful probability model. Notice that some values of $\gamma$ reproduce the right skew typical of survival data.

The survival function corresponding to (11.12) is

$$S(t) = \exp\{-\lambda(t^{\gamma})\}. \tag{11.13}$$

Figure 11.8 gives the Weibull survival functions for two values of $\gamma$ which were chosen so as to illustrate the two major types of curvature that are possible with the model.

The hazard function corresponding to (11.12) and (11.13) is

$$h(t) = \lambda\gamma(t^{\gamma-1}), \tag{11.14}$$

which encompasses a wide range of shapes as $\gamma$ changes (see Figure 11.9), including decreasing ($\gamma < 1$), increasing ($\gamma > 1$) and static ($\gamma = 1$) hazards.

When $\gamma = 1$, (11.12)–(11.14) reduce to (11.7)–(11.9), respectively. This shows that the exponential is simply a special case of the Weibull: that in which the

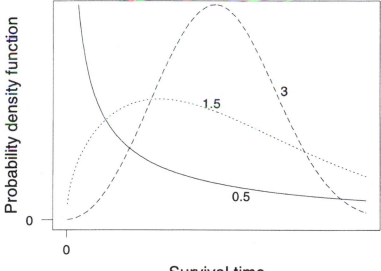

**Figure 11.7**  The probability density function for the Weibull distribution with $\gamma = 0.5, 1.5$ and 3.

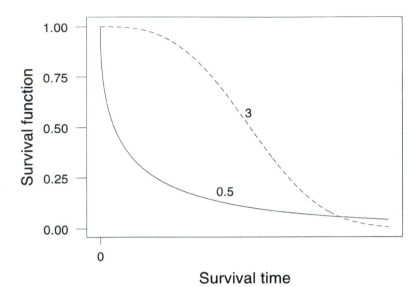

**Figure 11.8**    The survival function for the Weibull distribution with $\gamma = 0.5$ and 3.

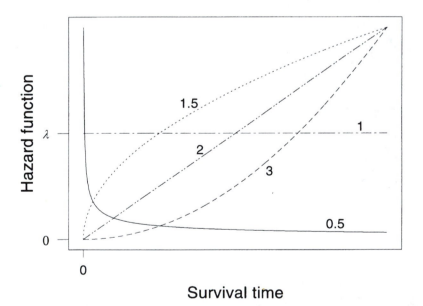

**Figure 11.9**    The hazard function for the Weibull distribution with $\gamma = 0.5$, 1, 1.5, 2 and 3.

shape parameter is unity. This can also be seen from comparing the straight line for $\gamma = 1$, which crosses the vertical axis at $\lambda$, in Figure 11.9 with the exponential hazard function shown in Figure 11.6.

The median survival time, according to the Weibull model, is found, from (11.13), to be

$$t_{\mathrm{m}} = \left\{ \frac{0.69315}{\lambda} \right\}^{1/\gamma}. \tag{11.15}$$

The estimation of $\lambda$ and $\gamma$ for the Weibull model is, unfortunately, not as straightforward as the estimation procedure for the exponential (described in Section 11.4.3). An iterative approach is necessary to find the maximum likelihood estimates. Normally this is done by computer, although Parmar and Machin (1995) give a numerical example. Some commercial statistical packages adopt a generalized approach to fitting various probability distributions which uses a **log-linear representation** (see Collett, 1994). Essentially this means that a different, but equivalent, formulation of the Weibull is used rather than (11.12)–(11.14). This new formulation is, for the hazard function,

$$h(t) = \frac{1}{\xi} \left( t^{\frac{1}{\xi}-1} \right) \exp(-\alpha/\xi). \tag{11.16}$$

Comparing (11.16) to (11.14), we see that

$$\begin{aligned} \lambda &= \exp(-\alpha/\xi), \\ \gamma &= 1/\xi, \end{aligned} \tag{11.17}$$

so that it is reasonably simple to convert from one formulation to the other. PROC LIFEREG in the SAS package uses the representation in (11.16) and refers to $\alpha$ as the 'intercept' and $\xi$ as (confusingly) the 'scale' parameter.

*Example 11.5*   A Weibull model was fitted to the data in Example 11.1 using SAS PROC LIFEREG. As in several other examples, the computer program used is given in Appendix A. The output included estimates of the intercept (3.90749388) and the scale (0.59727071). Taking these as $\alpha$ and $\xi$ in (11.17) gives

$$\lambda = \exp(-3.90749388/0.59727071) = 0.00144,$$
$$\gamma = 1/0.59727071 = 1.674.$$

Thus the fitted Weibull model for the glioblastoma multiforme data has, by (11.12)–(11.15),

$$\begin{aligned} f(t) &= 0.00241 t^{0.674} \exp\left(-0.00144 t^{1.674}\right), \\ S(t) &= \exp\left(-0.00144 t^{1.674}\right), \\ h(t) &= 0.00241 t^{0.674}, \\ t_{\mathrm{m}} &= 40.0 \text{ weeks.} \end{aligned}$$

Figure 11.10 shows the observed (as in Figure 11.2) and fitted (Weibull) survival functions. These seem to be in close agreement. Further support for the Weibull model in this example comes from comparing Figure 11.7, which suggests a right-skewed p.d.f. curve when $\gamma$ is around 1.5 (as here), with Figure 11.5. The fitted hazard function increases with increasing $t$, which broadly agrees with Figure 11.3. Finally, the Weibull median survival time is quite close to the observed value, calculated from Example 11.1, of 42 weeks.

Another graphical test of the suitability of the Weibull is given in Section 11.8.1, where we shall also compare the exponential and Weibull fits. It appears (by informal comparison with Example 11.4) that the Weibull is a better fit to the glioblastoma multiforme data than is the exponential.

### 11.4.5   Other probability models

The Weibull and its special case, the exponential, are the most common probability distributions used to model survival data. However, despite its flexibility, the Weibull cannot reproduce all possible shapes. For example, it cannot produce a hazard that rises to a peak and then falls. Other probability distributions may capture such shapes; the **log-logistic** distribution is a possible model for the example just raised. See Collett (1994) for details of the log-logistic model and other possible probability models for survival data.

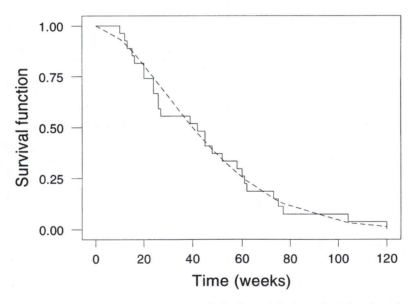

**Figure 11.10**   Observed (solid line) and Weibull (dashed line) survival functions for the glioblastoma multiforme data.

## 11.5   Proportional hazards regression models

### 11.5.1   Comparing two groups

When two groups are to be compared (say, those exposed and those unexposed to some risk factor), an assumption often made in survival analysis is that the ratio of the group-specific hazards (say, exposed divided by unexposed) is the same at all possible survival times. This is called the **proportional hazards** (PH) assumption. We have already encountered this in the context of the log-rank test in Section 5.5.3; here we use the PH assumption in the definition of regression models. An example of PH would occur in the study of survival across the entire human life-span (as in Figure 11.1) if two racial groups were studied and the hazard for death at any particular time for those in one racial group was always the same multiple of the hazard at the equivalent age in the other group.

Let the hazards in the two groups at time $t$ be $h_0(t)$ and $h_1(t)$. Then PH implies that

$$\frac{h_1(t)}{h_0(t)} = \phi \tag{11.18}$$

at all survival times, $t$. Here $\phi$ is a constant that is invariant over time. This constant is called the **hazard ratio** or **relative hazard**. The hazard that appears in the denominator, $h_0(t)$, is called the **baseline hazard**. A plot of the logarithm of the hazard against time, showing the two groups separately, would produce parallel curves separated by a distance of $\log \phi$.

Since hazards are always positive, a more convenient expression for the hazard ratio is

$$\phi = e^{\beta},$$

where $\beta$ is some parameter that has no restrictions (that is, it could be negative or positive), and so is easier to deal with. Equivalently,

$$\log_e \phi = \beta. \tag{11.19}$$

### 11.5.2   Comparing several groups

When several (say, $\ell$) groups are to be compared (for example, the $\ell$ distinct levels of a risk factor) we choose one of the groups to be the base group and compare all other groups against this one. The PH assumption then becomes

$$\frac{h_i(t)}{h_0(t)} = \phi^{(i)}, \tag{11.20}$$

where $i = 1, 2, \ldots, \ell - 1$. That is, the hazard ratio comparing group $i$ to group 0 is a constant, independent of time, but that constant may vary with the choice of the comparison group (that used in the numerator of the ratio). Figure 11.11 illustrates the PH assumption for four groups. The curve shown is an arbitrary choice, but the log hazards must stay parallel (that is, the vertical separation between the curves must stay constant).

As in the two-group situation, we prefer to let

$$\phi^{(i)} = \exp\left(\beta^{(i)}\right)$$

for some unrestricted parameter $\beta^{(i)}$. Hence

$$\log_e \phi^{(i)} = \beta^{(i)}, \tag{11.21}$$

for $i = 1, 2, \ldots, \ell - 1$. Rather than having $\ell - 1$ equations, the set of equations making up (11.21) may be rewritten as

$$\log_e \phi = \beta^{(1)} x^{(1)} + \beta^{(2)} x^{(2)} + \cdots + \beta^{(\ell-1)} x^{(\ell-1)}, \tag{11.22}$$

where

$$x^{(i)} = \begin{cases} 1 & \text{if the comparison group} = i \\ 0 & \text{otherwise.} \end{cases} \tag{11.23}$$

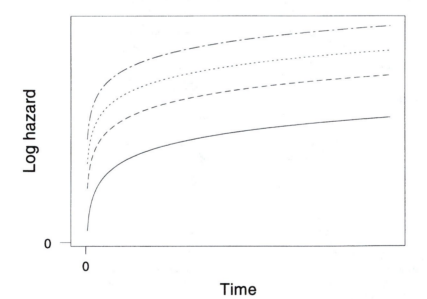

**Figure 11.11**   The proportional hazards assumption for a categorical risk factor with four levels.

This defines a linear regression model for the logarithm of the hazard ratio, where the dummy variables $\{x^{(i)}\}$ are the explanatory variables and the $\{\beta^{(i)}\}$ are the 'slope' parameters. Notice that this linear model has no intercept term, unlike the general linear model for normally distributed data (see, for example, (9.8)). No intercept is necessary here provided that we are only concerned with estimating $\phi$, because it is subsumed within the baseline hazard. That is, (11.20) and (11.22) give

$$\log_e\{h_i(t)\} = \log_e\{h_0(t)\} + \beta^{(1)}x^{(1)} + \beta^{(2)}x^{(2)} + \cdots + \beta^{(\ell-1)}x^{(\ell-1)},$$

so that a constant added to (11.22) could be eliminated by a redefinition of $h_0(t)$.

When sample data are available we may use them to find an estimate, $b^{(i)}$, of $\beta^{(i)}$ for all $i$. The logarithm of the hazard ratio is then estimated to be, by comparison with (11.22),

$$\log_e \hat{\phi} = b^{(1)}x^{(1)} + b^{(2)}x^{(2)} + \cdots + b^{(\ell-1)}x^{(\ell-1)}. \tag{11.24}$$

To fit the model we would first have to set up the dummy variables defined by (11.23). That is, for anyone in group $i$ (for $i > 0$) each $x$ variable takes the value zero except for $x^{(i)}$, which takes the value unity. Some computer packages will do this automatically after being given key commands, just as we saw for logistic regression in Section 10.4.3. For those in the base group $x^{(i)} = 0$ for all $i$, since then (11.20) and (11.22) give, for the comparison of the base group with itself,

$$\log_e \phi = \log_e \phi^{(0)} = \log_e\left\{\frac{h_0(t)}{h_0(t)}\right\} = \log_e\{1\} = 0 + 0 + \cdots + 0 = 0,$$

which is consistent, since $\log 1 = 0$.

Different PH models make different assumptions about $h_0(t)$, the baseline hazard. This leads to different estimates of the $\{\beta^{(i)}\}$. One approach is to assume a particular probability distribution model for $h_0(t)$: in Section 11.7 we shall assume the Weibull model. An alternative approach is to leave $h_0(t)$ totally unspecified: this leads to the Cox model of Section 11.6. Whichever approach is used, there is much in common as far as data analysis is concerned. The remainder of this section will be concerned with useful common methodology; specific examples are dealt with in Sections 11.6 and 11.7. The PH assumption is tested in Section 11.8.

Using (11.23) and (11.24), the hazard ratio for group $i$ compared to group 0 is estimated by

$$\hat{\phi} = \hat{\phi}^{(i)} = \exp\left\{b^{(i)} \times 1\right\} = \exp\left\{b^{(i)}\right\}. \tag{11.25}$$

An approximate 95% confidence interval for $\beta^{(i)}$ is given by

$$b^{(i)} \pm 1.96 \hat{se}\left(b^{(i)}\right),$$

and hence an approximate 95% confidence interval for $\phi^{(i)}$ is given by

$$\exp\left\{b^{(i)} \pm 1.96 \hat{se}\left(b^{(i)}\right)\right\}. \tag{11.26}$$

Notice that (11.18) and (11.19) are special cases of (11.20) and (11.21) where $i$ can only take one value. If we let $b^{(1)} = b$ and $x^{(1)} = x$ then, when $\ell = 2$, (11.24) becomes

$$\log_e \hat{\phi} = bx, \tag{11.27}$$

where the dummy variable $x$ takes the value unity for group 1 and zero for group 0. Consequently the PH regression model for a two-group comparison, (11.27), is a special case of (11.24). Hence (11.25) and (11.26) can equally well be applied to the two-group problem.

### 11.5.3  Modelling with a quantitative variable

When the single explanatory variable is quantitative the PH model is (11.27), where $x$ represents the continuous variable. The baseline hazard is the hazard when $x = 0$, since then (11.27) gives

$$\log_e \hat{\phi} = \log_e\left\{\frac{\hat{h}_0(t)}{\hat{h}_0(t)}\right\} = \log_e\{1\} = b \times 0 = 0,$$

where $\hat{h}$ is the estimated hazard.

The slope parameter $b$ estimates the amount by which $\log \phi$ goes up as $x$ increases from 0 to 1. That is, $b$ estimates the amount by which the log hazard at $x = 1$ exceeds the log hazard at $x = 0$. The PH assumption requires that this amount is the same at all survival times.

Since the hazard at $x = 0$ may be difficult to interpret, we may wish to redefine the baseline hazard by setting $z = x - \bar{x}$ and taking $z$ as the explanatory variable. The baseline hazard will then be for $x = \bar{x}$ and $\phi$ will measure hazards relative to the hazard at the average value of $x$.

Note that, by applying (11.27) at two specific values of $x$, $s$ units apart, and raising the difference to the exponential power, the estimated hazard ratio for an increase in $x$ of $s$ units is

$$\exp(bs). \tag{11.28}$$

An approximate 95% confidence interval for this hazard ratio is given by

$$\exp\{bs \pm 1.96s(\hat{se}(b))\}. \tag{11.29}$$

### 11.5.4   Modelling with several variables

When there is more than one explanatory variable we can define a multiple PH regression model. With $k$ variables this is

$$\log_e \hat{\phi} = b_1 x_1 + b_2 x_2 + \cdots + b_k x_k. \tag{11.30}$$

Some of these $x$ variables may be categorical, in which case a set of dummy variables may be defined, as in (11.23), and used to represent them (a different set is needed for each different categorical variable). This is exactly as we have seen already for general linear models (Chapter 9) and logistic regression (Chapter 10). The baseline hazard in (11.30) is the hazard for someone whose quantitative variables all take the value zero and who is in the base group for each of the categorical variables.

*Example 11.6*   Suppose $k = 3$, $x_1$ represents the categorical variable 'alcohol status' (non-drinkers/light drinkers/heavy drinkers), $x_2$ represents age and $x_3$ represents body mass index (BMI, defined as weight divided by the square of height). By reference to (11.23), two dummy variables are needed to represent $x_1$. For instance,

$$x_1^{(1)} = \begin{cases} 1 & \text{for moderate drinkers} \\ 0 & \text{otherwise,} \end{cases} \qquad x_1^{(2)} = \begin{cases} 1 & \text{for heavy drinkers} \\ 0 & \text{otherwise.} \end{cases}$$

The PH regression model, (11.30), is

$$\log_e \hat{\phi} = b_1^{(1)} x_1^{(1)} + b_1^{(2)} x_1^{(2)} + b_2 x_2 + b_3 x_3,$$

and the baseline hazard is for those non-drinkers who have age zero and body mass index zero. Since zero values are meaningless we may choose to transform $x_2$ and $x_3$, as suggested in Section 11.5.3.

Once we have the values for $\{b\}$ (and their estimated standard errors), from a computer package, we can calculate an estimated hazard ratio (and 95% confidence interval) corresponding to any $x$ variable just as in Section 11.5.2 or 11.5.3, depending upon the form of $x$. The only difference here is that this would be the hazard ratio when all other $x$ variables are fixed at zero or the base level. By repeated use of (11.30) this may be shown to be the hazard ratio when all other $x$ variables are fixed at any values or levels. That is, we obtain **adjusted** hazard ratios.

Interactions are modelled by including appropriate terms in (11.30), just as in Sections 9.4.7 and 10.9. For instance, the interaction between alcohol status and age in Example 11.6 is modelled by two new $x$ variables: $x_4^{(1)} = x_1^{(1)} x_2$ and $x_4^{(2)} = x_1^{(2)} x_2$. The interaction between BMI and age requires only one new term, $x_5 = x_2 x_3$. The estimated hazard ratios for combinations of outcomes of risk factors relative to base combinations follow by picking out from the linear model for $\log_e \hat{\phi}$ those terms that are both non-zero and do not appear in both the numerator and denominator hazard (and thus cancel out). See Section 10.9 for more details.

We can compare nested models (defined in Section 10.7.2) through the **likelihood ratio test**. For each model to be considered, this requires calculation of the statistic $-2 \log L$, where $L$ is the likelihood function evaluated at the values of the maximum likelihood estimates of all parameters in the model. If $L_v$ is the likelihood for a model with $v$ terms and $L_{v+u}$ is the likelihood for a model with the same $v$ terms plus a further $u$ terms then, under the null hypothesis that the $\beta$ coefficients for all these extra $u$ terms are zero,

$$\Delta = -2 \log L_v - (-2 \log L_{v+u}) \qquad (11.31)$$

follows a chi-square distribution with $u$ d.f. Hence we can test whether these $u$ terms are needed in the model, adjusting for the effect of the other $v$ terms, by comparing (11.31) against $\chi_u^2$.

In Example 11.6 we might wish to test for the effect of BMI ($x_3$) adjusting for alcohol status and age ($x_1$ and $x_2$). This involves comparing the model with all four terms against that with three terms (the two dummy variables for $x_1$ plus the quantitative variable $x_2$). Here $v = 3$, $u + v = 4$ and hence we compare $\Delta$ with $\chi_1^2$.

Notice that this procedure mimics that of Section 10.7.2 where (11.31) defines $\Delta D$. Collett (1994) explains why $-2 \log L$ should not be called a deviance in the current context. Nevertheless, the distinction is unnecessary in practical applications. Alternatives to the likelihood ratio test in survival analysis are reviewed by Parmar and Machin (1995).

## 11.6    The Cox proportional hazards model

The PH model introduced by Cox (1972) is the most widely used regression model in survival analysis. Its great advantage is that it requires no particular form for the survival times; in particular, the baseline hazard is unspecified. The theory behind the Cox approach is explained by Collett (1994) and set within a general epidemiological modelling context by Clayton and Hills (1993). Here we are purely concerned with its use in practice. As the Cox approach requires iterative calculations to fit the model, practical applications require the use of a computer. Several commercial statistical software packages have Cox regression procedures, including BMDP, EGRET, SPSS, STATA and SYSTAT. As in earlier chapters, we shall only view results from SAS. Within SAS, Cox regression is carried out by the procedure PROC PHREG.

*Example 11.7*   The patients with glioblastoma multiforme who were the subject of Example 11.1 were classified according to cellularity in Karkavelas *et al.* (1995). The survival times (in weeks) for those with low cellularity (below 300 nuclei) were

$$12, 15, 16, 20, 24, 26, 27, 39, 42, 45, 45, 58, 60, 61, 62, 73, 77, 104, 120;$$

for those with high cellularity (300 nuclei or more) survival times were

$$10, 13, 20, 24, 26, 48, 52, 75.$$

A variable defining group membership (CELLULAR = 1 for low and 2 for high) and another for survival time were read into SAS PROC PHREG. Output 11.1 shows the SAS results. Notice that the binary explanatory variable CELLULAR has been read in as if it were a quantitative variable (we can always do this with a binary variable). The 'slope' parameter, $b$, will thus estimate the effect of a unit increase in CELLULAR: 2 versus 1, or high versus low.

Here $b = 0.557912$ and $\hat{se}(b) = 0.43710$. From (11.28), when $s = 1$, the estimated hazard ratio is

$$\exp(0.557912) = 1.75;$$

and from (11.29) the 95% confidence interval for the hazard ratio is

$$\exp\{0.557912 \pm 1.96 \times 0.43710\},$$

that is, $\exp\{0.557912 \pm 0.856716\}$ or (0.74, 4.11). Hence we estimate that the hazard, at any time, is 1.75 times as great for those with high, compared to low, cellularity. However, the wide confidence interval contains unity, so we cannot claim that there is sufficient evidence to conclude extra risk from high cellularity with this small data set.

The remaining output from SAS provides two tests of the null hypothesis that the hazard ratio is unity. The 'model chi-square' is the difference in $-2 \log L$ (where $L$ is the likelihood) on adding the variable (or 'covariate') CELLULAR to the null model (that with no explanatory variables). The $p$ value for the likelihood ratio test is shown to be 0.2174. An alternative procedure is to divide the estimate of $\beta$ by its standard error and square the result; SAS calls this the **Wald chi-square**. The Wald test statistic is compared to chi-square with

**Output 11.1**   SAS results for Example 11.7

The PHREG Procedure

Testing Global Null Hypothesis: BETA = 0

| Criterion | Without Covariates | With Covariates | Model Chi-Square |
|---|---|---|---|
| −2 LOG L | 129.585 | 128.064 | 1.521 with 1 DF (p = 0.2174) |

Analysis of Maximum Likelihood Estimates

| Variable | DF | Parameter Estimate | Standard Error | Wald Chi-Square | Pr > Chi-Square |
|---|---|---|---|---|---|
| CELLULAR | 1 | 0.557912 | 0.43710 | 1.62918 | 0.2018 |

1 d.f. As explained in Section 10.7.4, this procedure is related to checking whether unity is inside the confidence interval. SAS shows the $p$ value to be 0.2018, very similar to the likelihood ratio test result. We conclude that there is no evidence of an effect of cellularity.

The glioblastoma multiforme data set has the advantages of being small and not involving censoring, but epidemiological studies rarely have either of these qualities. The remaining examples of the Cox model will use the extensive SHHS data set, in which the majority of subjects are censored. In Chapter 10 we ignored the fact that baseline times varied between subjects and treated the SHHS as a simple fixed cohort. Here we use the information on true survival times – elapsed time from recruitment to an event or censoring – just as we did in Chapter 5.

We shall now carry out Cox regression analyses of the problems already described by Examples 10.11 and 10.14 (in Example 11.8), 10.12 and 10.15 (in Example 11.10), 10.21 (in Example 11.11) and 10.22 (in Example 11.12). In each case the data used are available electronically: see Appendix C. What we shall find, throughout, is that the estimates and confidence intervals for the hazard ratio are very similar to those found earlier for the odds ratio. Similarly, the likelihood ratio test results are mostly very similar to the results from analysis of deviance tables found in the corresponding examples of Chapter 10. The agreements are due to the nature of the SHHS (see the discussion in Section 5.2), and cannot be expected in general.

*Example 11.8*   Consider the analysis of serum total cholesterol and systolic blood pressure (SBP) as risk factors for coronary heart disease (CHD) for men who were free of CHD at baseline in the SHHS. Both cholesterol and SBP have been divided into their fifths (as in Table 10.14). Here we have a multiple regression problem with two explanatory variables, both of which are categorical with five groups. The baseline hazard will be chosen as that for someone in the lowest fifth of both cholesterol and SBP. Dummy variables (as in Section 10.4.3) CHOL2, CHOL3, CHOL4 and CHOL5 were defined for cholesterol, and similarly SBP2, SBP3, SBP4 and SBP5 for SBP. For instance,

$$CHOL3 = \begin{cases} 1 & \text{for someone in the 3rd cholesterol fifth} \\ 0 & \text{otherwise} \end{cases}$$

and

$$SBP4 = \begin{cases} 1 & \text{for someone in the 4th SBP fifth} \\ 0 & \text{otherwise.} \end{cases}$$

There are three possible Cox models for the logarithm of the hazard ratio, as specified by (11.30): first, the model with cholesterol alone; then the model with SBP alone; and finally the model with both. Note that we are not considering interactions here.

As we saw in Example 11.7, SAS PROC PHREG returns the value of $\Delta$ in (11.31) for comparing the current model against the null model. By differencing the $\Delta$s for two models that we wish to compare we can produce a new $\Delta$ that is appropriate for the required comparison. For instance, Table 11.2 shows the '$\Delta$ versus null' values returned by SAS PROC PHREG. These are differenced to produce the contrasts required: SBP alone; cholesterol alone (both requiring no further differencing), and the adjusted effects

**Table 11.2**  Likelihood ratio test results for Example 11.8

| | | *Test details* | | | |
| --- | --- | --- | --- | --- | --- |
| *Model* | $\Delta$ *versus null (d.f.)* | $\Delta$ | *d.f.* | *p value* | *Effect* |
| 1 SBP | 39.017 (4) | 39.017 | 4 | < 0.0001 | SBP |
| 2 Cholesterol | 45.026 (4) | 45.026 | 4 | < 0.0001 | cholesterol |
| 3 SBP + Cholesterol | 76.508 (8) | 37.491[a] | 4 | < 0.0001 | cholesterol\|SBP |
| | | 31.482[b] | 4 | < 0.0001 | SBP\|cholesterol |

[a]Relative to model 1. [b]Relative to model 2.

(cholesterol adjusted for SBP and vice versa). Similar differencing is required for the d.f. All effects in Table 11.2 are highly significant. Thus, we conclude that both cholesterol and SBP have an important effect on the hazard for CHD; neither removes the effect of the other. That is, we require the following model:

$$\log_e \hat{\phi} = b_1^{(2)}\text{CHOL2} + b_1^{(3)}\text{CHOL3} + b_1^{(4)}\text{CHOL4} + b_1^{(5)}\text{CHOL5}$$
$$+ b_2^{(2)}\text{SBP2} + b_2^{(3)}\text{SBP3} + b_2^{(4)}\text{SBP4} + b_2^{(5)}\text{SBP5}.$$

This is model 3 in Table 11.2. The parameter estimates supplied by SAS are shown in Output 11.2. Notice that the four levels of each risk factor, other than the base level, are numbered 2–5 here rather than 1–4, as used in (11.22) and elsewhere. These numbers are arbitrary; the base group is defined by the dummy variables (all dummy variables take the value zero when the base level is attained).

The estimated hazard ratio (for example) for someone in the 2nd fifth of SBP compared to the 1st, keeping cholesterol fixed, is

$$\exp(0.602368) = 1.83,$$

with associated 95% confidence interval

$$\exp\{0.602368 \pm 1.96 \times 0.30181\}$$

**Output 11.2**   SAS results for Example 11.8, model 3

The PHREG Procedure

Analysis of Maximum Likelihood Estimates

| Variable | DF | Parameter Estimate | Standard Error | Wald Chi-Square | Pr > Chi-Square |
| --- | --- | --- | --- | --- | --- |
| SBP2 | 1 | 0.602368 | 0.30181 | 3.98331 | 0.0460 |
| SBP3 | 1 | 0.850155 | 0.28756 | 8.74081 | 0.0031 |
| SBP4 | 1 | 1.007984 | 0.28338 | 12.65228 | 0.0004 |
| SBP5 | 1 | 1.328101 | 0.27494 | 23.33415 | 0.0001 |
| CHOL2 | 1 | 0.202506 | 0.31789 | 0.40582 | 0.5241 |
| CHOL3 | 1 | 0.804170 | 0.28292 | 8.07923 | 0.0045 |
| CHOL4 | 1 | 0.975949 | 0.27403 | 12.68447 | 0.0004 |
| CHOL5 | 1 | 1.256328 | 0.26722 | 22.10338 | 0.0001 |

**Table 11.3**  Estimated hazard ratios (95% confidence intervals) for total serum cholesterol (base = 1st fifth) and systolic blood pressure (base = 1st fifth) for SHHS men who were free of CHD at baseline

| Fifth | Total serum cholesterol | Systolic blood pressure |
|---|---|---|
| 1 | 1 | 1 |
| 2 | 1.22 (0.66, 2.28) | 1.83 (1.01, 3.30) |
| 3 | 2.24 (1.28, 3.89) | 2.34 (1.33, 4.11) |
| 4 | 2.65 (1.55, 4.54) | 2.74 (1.57, 4.77) |
| 5 | 3.51 (2.08, 5.93) | 3.77 (2.20, 6.47) |

or (1.01, 3.30), using (11.25) and (11.26). Table 11.3 gives the complete set of estimated hazard ratios and 95% confidence intervals.

The estimates of the 'slope' parameters in Output 11.2 and Table 10.15 are fairly close. The chi-square test statistics in Table 11.2 ($\Delta$) and Table 10.21 ($\Delta D$) are not quite as close, but this is due to the use of grouped data in Example 10.14. In Examples 11.10–11.12, which consider problems where generic data were used in Chapter 10, the agreements are much better (although no further comments on such comparisons will be included).

Table 11.3 suggests that there is a dose-response effect for both cholesterol and SBP. The evidence for causality would be strengthened by considering a linear trend effect for each variable. To demonstrate this idea we shall, for simplicity, only consider the linear trend for SBP here.

*Example 11.9*  By analogy with Section 10.7.3, we can represent the linear trend in the log hazard ratio of SBP by introducing a quantitative variable to represent the SBP fifths. For simplicity we take this variable (SBP5TH in Output 11.3) to be 1 in the 1st fifth of SBP, 2 in the 2nd fifth, etc.

Output 11.3 gives an extract from the results when SBP5TH was fitted as the only explanatory variable in a Cox model using SAS. From this we see that the likelihood ratio test, comparing the linear trend to the null model, is significant ($p < 0.0001$). Hence there is evidence of a linear trend in the log hazard ratio by increasing fifth of SBP. The $\Delta$ value that compares the categorical SBP (model 1 in Table 11.2) with the linear is $39.017 - 37.790 = 1.227$. Comparing this to chi-square on $4 - 1 = 3$ d.f. we get a test for a non-linear response of SBP on CHD. Here this is not significant and, furthermore, $\Delta$ is so small that no specific polynomial effect can be important (unlike Example 10.16). Thus we conclude that the effect of SBP upon CHD acts through a linear trend on the log scale; from Output 11.3 and (11.28) the hazard for CHD is estimated to be multiplied by $\exp(0.320276) = 1.38$ when one SBP fifth is compared with the next lowest. By (11.29), a 95% confidence interval for this multiplicative constant is

$$\exp\{0.320276 \pm 1.96 \times 0.05345\}$$

or (1.24, 1.53). As anticipated from the likelihood ratio test, this interval excludes unity.

*Example 11.10*  A more substantial example from the SHHS, again only taking men with no CHD at baseline and with no missing values ($n = 4049$), comes from fitting the model

**Output 11.3**  SAS results for Example 11.9

The PHREG Procedure

Testing Global Null Hypothesis: BETA = 0

| Criterion | Without Covariates | With Covariates | Model Chi-Square |
|---|---|---|---|
| −2 LOG L | 3247.392 | 3209.603 | 37.790 with 1 DF (p = 0.0001) |

Analysis of Maximum Likelihood Estimates

| Variable | DF | Parameter Estimate | Standard Error | Wald Chi-Square | Pr > Chi-Square |
|---|---|---|---|---|---|
| SBP5TH | 1 | 0.320276 | 0.05345 | 35.91049 | 0.0001 |

**Output 11.4**  SAS results for Example 11.10

The PHREG Procedure

Analysis of Maximum Likelihood Estimates

| Variable | DF | Parameter Estimate | Standard Error | Wald Chi-Square | Pr > Chi-Square |
|---|---|---|---|---|---|
| AGE | 1 | 0.018023 | 0.01318 | 1.87110 | 0.1713 |
| TOTCHOL | 1 | 0.286062 | 0.05499 | 27.05831 | 0.0001 |
| BMI | 1 | 0.038101 | 0.02052 | 3.44862 | 0.0633 |
| SYSTOL | 1 | 0.020049 | 0.00364 | 30.34720 | 0.0001 |
| SMOKE2 | 1 | 0.312110 | 0.24409 | 1.63500 | 0.2010 |
| SMOKE3 | 1 | 0.699888 | 0.21344 | 10.75228 | 0.0010 |
| ACT2 | 1 | −0.188577 | 0.17315 | 1.18607 | 0.2761 |
| ACT3 | 1 | −0.109753 | 0.22417 | 0.23971 | 0.6244 |

Analysis of Maximum Likelihood Estimates

Conditional Risk Ratio and
95% Confidence Limits

| Variable | Risk Ratio | Lower | Upper |
|---|---|---|---|
| AGE | 1.018 | 0.992 | 1.045 |
| TOTCHOL | 1.331 | 1.195 | 1.483 |
| BMI | 1.039 | 0.998 | 1.081 |
| SYSTOL | 1.020 | 1.013 | 1.028 |
| SMOKE2 | 1.366 | 0.847 | 2.205 |
| SMOKE3 | 2.014 | 1.325 | 3.059 |
| ACT2 | 0.828 | 0.590 | 1.163 |
| ACT3 | 0.896 | 0.577 | 1.390 |

$$\log_e \phi = b_1 x_1 + b_2 x_2 + b_3 x_3 + b_4 x_4 + b_5^{(2)} x_5^{(2)} + b_5^{(3)} x_5^{(3)} + b_6^{(2)} x_6^{(2)} + b_6^{(3)} x_6^{(3)}, \qquad (11.32)$$

where $x_1$ = age (in years), $x_2$ = serum total cholesterol (mmol/l), $x_3$ = BMI (kg/m$^2$), $x_4$ = SBP (mmHg), $x_5^{(2)}$ and $x_5^{(3)}$ are two dummy variables representing smoking status (never/ ex/current) and $x_6^{(2)}$ and $x_6^{(3)}$ are two dummy variables representing activity in leisure (active/average/inactive):

$$x_5^{(2)} = \begin{cases} 1 & \text{for ex-smokers} \\ 0 & \text{otherwise,} \end{cases} \qquad x_5^{(3)} = \begin{cases} 1 & \text{for current smokers} \\ 0 & \text{otherwise;} \end{cases}$$

$$x_6^{(2)} = \begin{cases} 1 & \text{for average activity} \\ 0 & \text{otherwise,} \end{cases} \qquad x_6^{(3)} = \begin{cases} 1 & \text{for the inactive} \\ 0 & \text{otherwise.} \end{cases}$$

The baseline hazard is the hazard for subjects with $x_1 = x_2 = x_3 = x_4 = 0$ who have never smoked and are active in their leisure time. Output 11.4 gives the results from fitting (11.32) using SAS PROC PHREG. This time SAS has been asked to exponentiate the $\beta$ estimate and its confidence interval (as we have done for ourselves in Examples 11.7–11.9). This is the final part of the output, where SAS loosely refers to the hazard ratio as the 'risk ratio'. As declared to SAS: $x_1$ = AGE, $x_2$ = TOTCHOL, $x_3$ = BMI, $x_4$ = SYSTOL, $x_5^{(2)}$ = SMOKE2, $x_5^{(3)}$ = SMOKE3, $x_6^{(2)}$ = ACT2 and $x_6^{(3)}$ = ACT3 in (11.32).

As an example of the interpretation of parameters for quantitative variables, consider the variable 'total cholesterol'. Output 11.4 shows that the estimated hazard ratio for comparing two people of the same age, with the same BMI, same systolic blood pressure, same smoking habit and same self-reported leisure activity level, but where one person has a cholesterol value one unit (1 mmol/l) higher than the other, is 1.331 (higher cholesterol compared to lower). We are 95% sure that the interval (1.195, 1.483) covers the true multiple-adjusted hazard ratio for a unit increase in cholesterol. Such one-unit hazard ratios (and confidence intervals) may (alternatively) be obtained from the standard SAS parameter estimates (the top part of Output 11.4) using (11.28) and (11.29) with $s = 1$.

The Wald tests in Output 11.4 suggest that some of the explanatory variables are unnecessary, at least in the presence of others, for predicting CHD. Certainly age and leisure activity seem likely to be redundant. We do not attempt a model building analysis here: see Example 10.15 for an example of a methodical approach.

*Example 11.11* We now use the SHHS data to investigate whether there is an interaction between sex and Bortner personality score in the determination of the coronary hazard for those free of CHD at baseline. Here we consider Bortner score represented by its quarters (as in Table 10.28), so that we shall be fitting an interaction between two categorical variables.

The four levels of Bortner score were fitted using the three dummy variables BORT2, BORT3 and BORT4 which all represent contrasts with the first quarter (that is, they are the variables X1, X2 and X3 in Table 10.29). Sex was fitted as the variable SEX1 which is unity for men and zero for women (X4 in Table 10.29). The interaction between them requires three more dummy variables which are most easily found by multiplying BORT2 by SEX1, BORT3 by SEX1 and BORT4 by SEX1 (to create X5–X7 in Table 10.30). The derived variables were called BOR2SEX1, BOR3SEX1 and BOR4SEX1 within the computer program.

Here there are four Cox models that may be fitted: Bortner score alone; sex alone; both variables; and the full model including both variables and their interaction. Results of model fitting appear in Table 11.4. From this we conclude that all effects are important.

Since there is a significant Bortner by sex interaction we cannot assess the two risk factors separately (see Section 4.9). Output 11.5 gives the results from fitting the full model (4).

**Table 11.4**   Likelihood ratio test results for Example 11.11

| Model | Δ versus null (d.f.) | Test details | | | |
|---|---|---|---|---|---|
| | | Δ | d.f. | p value | Effect |
| 1 Bortner (BORT2 + BORT3 + BORT4) | 14.61 (3) | 14.61 | 3 | 0.002 | Bortner |
| 2 Sex (SEX1) | 65.46 (1) | 65.46 | 1 | < 0.0001 | sex |
| 3 Bortner + Sex (BORT2 + BORT3 + BORT4 + SEX1) | 79.29 (4) | 64.68[a] 13.83[b] | 1 3 | < 0.0001 0.003 | sex\|Bortner Bortner\|sex |
| 4 Bortner*Sex (all variables) | 87.44 (7) | 8.15[c] | 3 | 0.043 | interaction\| Bortner, sex |

Note that the final model (4) includes the main effects (as all interaction models should). [a]Relative to model 1. [b]Relative to model 2. [c]Relative to model 3.

**Output 11.5**   SAS Results for Example 11.11, model 4

The PHREG Procedure

Analysis of Maximum Likelihood Estimates

| Variable | DF | Parameter Estimate | Standard Error | Wald Chi-Square | Pr > Chi-Square |
|---|---|---|---|---|---|
| BORT2 | 1 | −0.576319 | 0.28868 | 3.98567 | 0.0459 |
| BORT3 | 1 | −1.244067 | 0.36515 | 11.60763 | 0.0007 |
| BORT4 | 1 | −1.112305 | 0.36515 | 9.27909 | 0.0023 |
| SEX1 | 1 | 0.524491 | 0.22556 | 5.40687 | 0.0201 |
| BOR2SEX1 | 1 | 0.667988 | 0.34458 | 3.75794 | 0.0526 |
| BOR3SEX1 | 1 | 0.952828 | 0.42014 | 5.14326 | 0.0233 |
| BOR4SEX1 | 1 | 0.888172 | 0.41547 | 4.56992 | 0.0325 |

From Output 11.5 we can easily determine hazard ratios for Bortner score, comparing each other quarter with the first, for each sex group separately. All we need do is to pick out the BORT and interaction terms that are non-zero for the particular Bortner–sex combination that we wish to compare with the first Bortner quarter of the same sex group, just as in Example 10.21. For instance, the male hazard ratio for Bortner quarter 4 versus Bortner quarter 1 is

$$\exp(-1.112305 + 0.888172) = 0.80,$$

whilst the corresponding female hazard ratio is

$$\exp(-1.112305) = 0.33.$$

The female hazard ratio does not require the BOR4SEX1 interaction term because the corresponding $x$ variable is defined to be zero when SEX1 $= 0$ (that is, for females).

Because they involve only one term, confidence intervals for female hazard ratios are easy to compute from Output 11.5. Thus the female hazard ratio comparing Bortner quarter 4 with quarter 1 has 95% confidence interval

$$\exp(-1.112305 \pm 1.96 \times 0.36515)$$

or (0.16, 0.67). Similar calculations give the other two female hazard ratios with Bortner quarter 1 as base.

For men, since the log hazard ratio estimates are the sum of two terms, each corresponding variance is the sum of two variances plus twice the covariance (as in the example given in Section 10.6). Output 11.5 does not include the covariances, since these are not produced by default within SAS (but see Example 11.12). Rather than asking for them and carrying out computations with covariances, a short-cut procedure was adopted just as in Example 10.22. Sex was fitted as SEX2, which is unity for women and zero for men, rather than as SEX1 as previously defined. The interaction terms were then recalculated, as BOR2SEX2 $=$ BORT2×SEX2 etc., and model 4 in Table 11.4 was refitted. Results appear as Output 11.6. In this, the terms involving sex (main effect and interaction) must have the same magnitude but opposite sign compared with Output 11.5. The estimates of hazard ratios from this output will turn out to be exactly as before; for instance, the Bortner 4 versus 1 ratio for men is

$$\exp(-0.224133) = 0.80,$$

and for women is

$$\exp(-0.224133 - 0.888172) = 0.33,$$

as before. For men (but not women), 95% confidence intervals are easy to derive directly from Output 11.6. For instance, the male Bortner 4 versus 1 confidence interval is

$$\exp(-0.224133 \pm 1.96 \times 0.19820)$$

or (0.54, 1.18). The full set of hazard ratios and confidence intervals is given in Table 11.5. The numerical results are very similar to those in Table 10.34 and the inferences are thus identical: Bortner score has little effect on the risk of CHD for men, but has an inverse relation for women.

**Output 11.6**    Further SAS results for Example 11.11, model 4, using a different variable to represent sex compared to that used in Output 11.5

The PHREG Procedure

Analysis of Maximum Likelihood Estimates

| Variable | DF | Parameter Estimate | Standard Error | Wald Chi-Square | Pr > Chi-Square |
|---|---|---|---|---|---|
| BORT2 | 1 | 0.091669 | 0.18815 | 0.23737 | 0.6261 |
| BORT3 | 1 | −0.291239 | 0.20782 | 1.96396 | 0.1611 |
| BORT4 | 1 | −0.224133 | 0.19820 | 1.27878 | 0.2581 |
| SEX2 | 1 | −0.524491 | 0.22556 | 5.40687 | 0.0201 |
| BOR2SEX2 | 1 | −0.667988 | 0.34458 | 3.75794 | 0.0526 |
| BOR3SEX2 | 1 | −0.952830 | 0.42014 | 5.14327 | 0.0233 |
| BOR4SEX2 | 1 | −0.888172 | 0.41547 | 4.56992 | 0.0325 |

**Table 11.5**    Hazard ratios (95% confidence intervals) by sex and Bortner quarter for SHHS subjects who were free of CHD at baseline

| Quarter of Bortner score | Sex | |
|---|---|---|
| | Male | Female |
| 1 | 1 | 1 |
| 2 | 1.10 (0.76, 1.59) | 0.56 (0.32, 0.99) |
| 3 | 0.75 (0.50, 1.12) | 0.29 (0.14, 0.59) |
| 4 | 0.80 (0.54, 1.18) | 0.33 (0.16, 0.67) |

*Example 11.12*    Bortner score is measured as a quantitative variable in the SHHS and so it is possible to repeat Example 11.11 using the raw, ungrouped, form of Bortner score. Taking BORTNER as the variable which measures Bortner score and SEX1, as in Example 11.11, to be the dummy variable for sex, the interaction between the quantitative and categorical variables is modelled as BORTSEX1 = BORTNER×SEX1. That is, the interaction is represented by a single explanatory variable which takes the value of the Bortner score for men and zero for women. As in Example 11.11, four models for the hazard ratio are possible, one of which is the 'sex only' model which is exactly as in Example 11.11. Table 11.6 gives results of model fitting: model 4 is required to predict the hazard ratio for a coronary event, and parameter estimates from fitting it with PROC PHREG are shown in Output 11.7. This time the variance-covariance matrix is included.

The estimated hazard ratio and 95% confidence interval for an increase of one unit in the Bortner score is easily found for women as 0.987 (0.981, 0.993). For men the estimate is easy to produce as $\exp(-0.012928 + 0.010473) = 0.998$. The corresponding estimated standard error is

$$\sqrt{0.0000098761 + 0.0000128513 + 2(-0.0000098760)} = 0.0017248,$$

giving a 95% confidence interval for the hazard ratio of

$$\exp\{(-0.012928 + 0.010473) \pm 1.96 \times 0.0017248)\}$$

or (0.994, 1.001). Hence the hazard for CHD comes down slightly as Bortner score goes up for each sex, but the effect for men is explainable by chance variation (since unity is in the 95% confidence interval).

**Table 11.6**  Likelihood ratio test results for Example 11.12

| Model | $\Delta$ vs. null (d.f.) | Test details | | | Effect |
|---|---|---|---|---|---|
| | | $\Delta$ | d.f. | p value | |
| 1 Bortner (BORTNER) | 10.81 (1) | 10.81 | 1 | 0.001 | Bortner |
| 2 sex (SEX1) | 65.46 (1) | 65.46 | 1 | < 0.0001 | sex |
| 3 Bortner + sex (BORTNER + SEX1) | 75.58 (2) | 64.77[a] | 1 | < 0.0001 | sex\|Bortner |
| | | 10.12[b] | 1 | 0.002 | Bortner\|sex |
| 4 Bortner*sex (BORTNER + SEX1 + BORTSEX1) | 84.02 (3) | 8.44[c] | 1 | 0.004 | interaction\| Bortner, sex |

Note that the final model, 4, includes the main effects (as all interaction models should).
[a] Relative to model 1. [b] Relative to model 2. [c] Relative to model 3.

**Output 11.7**   SAS results for Example 11.12, model 4

The PHREG Procedure

Analysis of Maximum Likelihood Estimates

| Variable | DF | Parameter Estimate | Standard Error | Wald Chi-Square | Pr > Chi-Square |
|---|---|---|---|---|---|
| BORTNER | 1 | −0.012928 | 0.00314 | 16.92403 | 0.0001 |
| SEX1 | 1 | −0.613311 | 0.57226 | 1.14862 | 0.2838 |
| BORTSEX1 | 1 | 0.010473 | 0.00358 | 8.53414 | 0.0035 |

Estimated Covariance Matrix

| | BORTNER | SEX1 | BORTSEX1 |
|---|---|---|---|
| BORTNER | 0.0000098761 | 0.0014969151 | −.0000098760 |
| SEX1 | 0.0014969151 | 0.3274817434 | −.0019886082 |
| BORTSEX1 | −.0000098760 | −.0019886082 | 0.0000128513 |

### 11.6.1   Time-dependent covariates

In all the examples so far we have assumed that the explanatory variables, or **covariates**, are fixed at baseline. In some situations we may have updates on the values of these variables, or perhaps just a subset of them, as the study progresses. This situation is quite common in clinical trials where subjects are invited to attend clinics every few months. At each clinic a number of health checks may be carried out – for example, the current size of a tumour may be measured. In cohort studies the initial study questionnaire may be readministered every few years to discover the latest smoking habit, diet, activity level, etc. of each study participant. In occupational cohort studies the current exposure to suspected toxic substances, and other information, could be recorded regularly. In survival analysis, explanatory variables with such updated information are called **time-dependent covariates**.

Cox (1972) showed that such variables may be included in his regression model. The most recent value of a time-dependent covariate is used at each specific time in the model. This is not necessarily a directly observed value; it could, for example, be the maximum value of a variable observed so far, or the difference between the current maximum and minimum values.

Consider a time-dependent covariate $x(t)$ which takes the value 1 if the risk factor is present, and 0 if absent, at time $t$. For example, $x(t)$ might record whether a subject is a smoker at time $t$. The Cox regression model for the log hazard ratio then assumes

$$\log_e \hat{\phi} = b_1 x_1 + b_2 x_2 + \cdots + b_k x_k + b x(t), \tag{11.33}$$

where $x_1, x_2, \ldots, x_k$ are a set of fixed covariates, as in (11.30). The hazard ratio for someone who smokes at time $t$ compared with someone who does not, with all other variables fixed, is then estimated to be

$$\hat{\phi} = \exp(b),$$

just as in the case where $x$ represents a fixed covariate. Similarly, when $x$ is a quantitative variable, such as blood pressure,

$$\hat{\phi} = \exp(bs)$$

will estimate the hazard ratio for an increase in $s$ units of blood pressure, as in (11.28). We can test for the significance of $x(t)$ by comparing minus twice log likelihoods for the models with and without this term, just as when all the covariates are fixed at baseline.

Since (11.33) depends upon $t$, the hazard ratio is allowed to vary over time whenever time-dependent covariates are included in a model. For this, and other reasons (see Altman and De Stavola, 1994) time-dependent proportional hazards models can be difficult to interpret. A simple example of their use is provided by Collett (1994).

## 11.7   The Weibull proportional hazards model

The Weibull proportional hazards model assumes that the survival times in the base group follow a Weibull distribution. That is, the baseline hazard is, from (11.14),

$$h_0(t) = \lambda\gamma(t^{\gamma-1}), \tag{11.34}$$

for some value of $\lambda$ and $\gamma$. Unlike the Cox model, we will estimate the Weibull parameters $\lambda$ and $\gamma$ from observed data, and thus estimate the baseline hazard. Under the PH assumption, (11.18), when two groups are compared the hazard in the numerator (comparison) group is

$$h_1(t) = \phi h_0(t),$$

where $\phi$ is the hazard ratio. Hence

$$h_1(t) = \phi\lambda\gamma(t^{\gamma-1}). \tag{11.35}$$

By reference to (11.14), we can see that (11.35) is in the form of a Weibull hazard with scale parameter $\phi\lambda$ and shape parameter $\gamma$. Hence, if $h_0(t)$ has a Weibull form and the hazards are proportional (that is, time-homogeneous) then $h_1(t)$ also has a Weibull form with the same shape parameter.

Generalizations from this two-group comparison to the other situations covered by Section 11.5 show that all hazards will have the Weibull form with the same shape parameter throughout. Figure 11.11 actually shows log hazards from four Weibull distributions, each of which has $\gamma = 3$ but a different $\lambda$. In Example 11.6, when a Weibull PH model is used, the hazard for 50-year-old heavy drinkers with a BMI of 28.2 is estimated as

$$\exp\left(b_1^{(2)} + 50b_2 + 28.2b_3\right)\lambda\gamma\left(t^{\gamma-1}\right).$$

When a Weibull PH model is used we estimate $\lambda$ and $\gamma$ as well as all the $\beta$ regression ('slope') parameters. Maximum likelihood estimation requires iterative calculation, and so a statistical computer package is required.

We shall view results from the SAS routine PROC LIFEREG. This fits a range of probability models (including the exponential), although the Weibull PH model is the default. Exponential models are dealt with similarly to Weibull models, and so only Weibull models (with greater applicability) are described here. One snag with PROC LIFEREG is the log-linear representation used, as mentioned in Section 11.4.4. Due to this, the regression parameters produced by SAS, which we shall call $\{B_i\}$, must be transformed to produce the regression parameters $\{b_i\}$ introduced in Section 11.5. This is achieved through the general result

$$b_i = -B_i/\xi, \tag{11.36}$$

where $\xi$ is the SAS PROC LIFEREG scale parameter. The standard error of $b_i$ is estimated by

$$\hat{\text{se}}(b_i) = \frac{1}{\xi^2}\sqrt{\xi^2 V(B_i) + B_i^2\, V(\xi) - 2\xi B_i\, C(\xi,\, B_i)}, \tag{11.37}$$

as shown by Collett (1994).

We shall now illustrate the use of Weibull PH models through some of the same examples that were used for Cox regression in Section 11.6. Since model selection and hazard ratio interpretation follow in an identical way to the Cox model, only the first two examples from Section 11.6 (Examples 11.7 and 11.8) will be reanalysed. All results will be found to be very similar to those from the analogous Cox analysis; however, this is not the case in general as the imposition of the Weibull form may produce different inferences. In Section 11.8 we shall consider how to check whether the Weibull PH form is appropriate; if it is, we would anticipate similar estimates to when the Cox model is used.

*Example 11.13*  A Weibull PH regression model was fitted to the cellularity group data of Example 11.7 using SAS PROC LIFEREG. Cellularity was represented by the variable CELLULAR, declared as a categorical variable (a CLASS variable in SAS terminology) with value 1 for high and 2 for low cellularity. Output 11.8 gives the results.

By the standard SAS rules (Section 9.2.7) the $B$ parameter representing the last level of any CLASS variable is automatically set to zero; hence, CELLULAR = 2 has parameter zero here. According to the result in Section 11.5.2, this makes the baseline hazard in the PH model the hazard for low cellularity (CELLULAR = 2). The model fitted is

$$\log_e \hat{\phi} = bx,$$

where

$$x = \begin{cases} 1 & \text{for high cellularity} \\ 0 & \text{for low cellularity.} \end{cases}$$

We pick out the SAS regression parameter, $B$, as the coefficient for high cellularity (CELLULAR = 1) in Output 11.8. From this output:

$$\hat{\alpha} = 4.00395209 \qquad V(\hat{\alpha}) = 0.018755$$
$$\hat{\xi} = 0.57448463 \qquad V(\hat{\xi}) = 0.007316$$
$$B = -0.3635417 \qquad V(B) = 0.058634$$

$$\hat{C}(\hat{\xi}, B) = -0.000272$$

**Output 11.8**   SAS results for Example 11.13

Lifereg Procedure

| Variable | DF | Estimate | Std Err | ChiSquare | Pr > Chi | Label/Value |
|----------|-----|----------|---------|-----------|----------|-------------|
| INTERCPT | 1 | 4.00395209 | 0.136948 | 854.8025 | 0.0001 | Intercept |
| CELLULAR | 1 | | | 2.254014 | 0.1333 | |
| | 1 | −0.3635417 | 0.242145 | 2.254014 | 0.1333 | 1 |
| | 0 | 0 | 0 | . | . | 2 |
| SCALE | 1 | 0.57448463 | 0.085534 | | | |

Estimated Covariance Matrix

| | INTERCPT | CELLULAR.1 | SCALE |
|----------|----------|------------|-------|
| INTERCPT | 0.018755 | −0.017252 | −0.003183 |
| CELLULAR.1 | −0.017252 | 0.058634 | −0.000272 |
| SCALE | −0.003183 | −0.000272 | 0.007316 |

By (11.17),

$$\hat{\lambda} = \exp(-4.00395209/0.57448463) = 0.0009400$$
$$\hat{\gamma} = 1/0.57448463 = 1.7407.$$

By (11.36),

$$b = -(-0.3635417)/0.57448463 = 0.6328.$$

By (11.37),

$$\hat{se}(b) = \left( \sqrt{0.01935113 + 0.00096690 - 0.00011361} \right)/0.33003259 = 0.4307.$$

Then, by (11.25) and (11.26), the estimated hazard ratio (high versus low cellularity) is $\hat{\phi} = \exp(0.6328) = 1.88$, with 95% confidence interval

$$\exp(0.6328 \pm 1.96 \times 0.4307)$$

or (0.81, 4.38). The estimated hazard function for those with low cellularity is the estimated baseline hazard, (11.34),

$$0.0009400 \times 1.7407 t^{0.7407} = 0.001636 t^{0.7407},$$

and the estimated hazard function for high cellularity is, from (11.35),

$$\hat{\phi} \times 0.001636 t^{0.7407} = 0.003081 t^{0.7407}.$$

If we wish, we can also specify the fitted survival functions for each group from (11.13). For low and high cellularity, respectively, these are

$$\exp\left\{ -\hat{\lambda}(t^{\hat{\gamma}}) \right\} = \exp(-0.0009400 t^{1.7407})$$

and

$$\exp\left\{ -\hat{\phi}\hat{\lambda}(t^{\hat{\gamma}}) \right\} = \exp(-0.0017699 t^{1.7407}).$$

So that these can be compared with the observed survival functions, Kaplan–Meier estimates of the two survival functions were calculated and plotted together with these fitted functions. The results are shown in Figure 11.12. Agreement is quite good, suggesting that the Weibull model is reasonable. However, a curve and step function are hard to compare by eye; an easier graphical test may be found in Section 11.8.1.

As with Cox models, nested Weibull PH regression models are best compared through $\Delta$ as defined by (11.31). We can test the effect of cellularity in Example 11.13 by finding the difference in minus twice log likelihoods of the Weibull model with cellularity as the explanatory variable and the Weibull model with no explanatory variables (the null model). The latter has already been described in Example 11.5, since this is the model of a single Weibull form for the entire glioblastoma multiforme data set. In this example $\Delta = 1.977$ (from computer output not shown); comparing this to $\chi_1^2$ leads to the conclusion that cellularity has no significant effect ($p > 0.1$). This is consistent with the chi-square test for CELLULAR given in Output 11.8 ($p = 0.1333$) and with the finding in Example 11.7.

As the foregoing shows, provided that we do not wish to use the model to estimate the baseline hazard, and are content with comparative measures of chance, there is little difference in the way Cox and Weibull PH regression

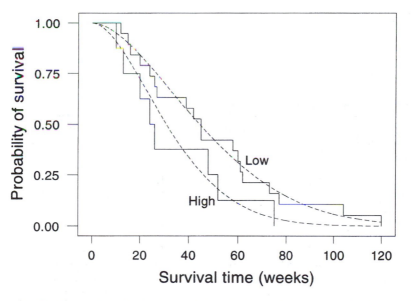

**Figure 11.12** Observed (solid line) and Weibull (dashed line) survival functions by cellularity, glioblastoma multiforme data.

models are interpreted. An example of a multiple regression model with quantitative variables will suffice to confirm this.

*Example 11.14*   Output 11.9 shows the results of fitting a Weibull PH model to the problem of Example 11.10 using PROC LIFEREG. Table 11.7 copies the $B$ coefficients from Output 11.9 and uses (11.36) and then either (11.25) or (11.28) to produce the remaining columns. A complete analysis accounts for sample-to-sample variation, through (11.37) and (11.26) or (11.29); nested models are compared using (11.31). However, the inferences obtained turn out to be very similar to those in Example 11.10 and, in general terms, Examples 10.12 and 10.15.

**Output 11.9**   SAS results for Example 11.14

Lifereg Procedure

| Variable | DF | Estimate | Std Err | ChiSquare | Pr > Chi | Label/Value |
|---|---|---|---|---|---|---|
| INTERCPT | 1 | 15.7827055 | 0.924108 | 291.6875 | 0.0001 | Intercept |
| AGE | 1 | −0.0141529 | 0.010503 | 1.815878 | 0.1778 | |
| TOTCHOL | 1 | −0.2272931 | 0.046374 | 24.02299 | 0.0001 | |
| BMI | 1 | −0.0304403 | 0.016428 | 3.433401 | 0.0639 | |
| SYSTOL | 1 | −0.0159883 | 0.003079 | 26.9596 | 0.0001 | |
| SMOKING | 2 | | | 12.19109 | 0.0023 | |
| | 1 | −0.2489507 | 0.194424 | 1.639552 | 0.2004 | 2 |
| | 1 | −0.5545938 | 0.173707 | 10.19331 | 0.0014 | 3 |
| | 0 | 0 | 0 | . | . | 4 |
| ACTIVITY | 2 | | | 1.228051 | 0.5412 | |
| | 1 | 0.15192498 | 0.137743 | 1.216526 | 0.2700 | 2 |
| | 1 | 0.09164109 | 0.177934 | 0.265253 | 0.6065 | 3 |
| | 0 | 0 | 0 | . | . | 4 |
| SCALE | 1 | 0.79352151 | 0.055601 | | | |

**Table 11.7**   Interpretation of parameter estimates in Output 11.9

| Explanatory variable | Regression coefficients | | Estimated hazard ratio | |
|---|---|---|---|---|
| | $B$ | $b$ | $\hat{\phi}$ | Effect[a] |
| age | −0.014 152 9 | 0.017 84 | 1.02 | increase of 1 year |
| total cholesterol | −0.227 293 1 | 0.286 44 | 1.33 | increase of 1 mmol/l |
| body mass index | −0.030 440 3 | 0.038 36 | 1.04 | increase of 1 kg/$m^2$ |
| systolic blood pressure | −0.015 988 3 | 0.020 15 | 1.02 | increase of 1 mmHg |
| smoking | −0.248 950 7 | 0.313 73 | 1.37 | ex versus never smoker |
| | −0.554 593 8 | 0.698 90 | 2.01 | current versus never smoker |
| leisure activity | 0.151 925 0 | −0.191 46 | 0.83 | average versus active |
| | 0.091 641 1 | −0.115 49 | 0.89 | inactive versus active |

[a]Adjusted for all other explanatory variables.

## 11.8    Model checking

In the last few sections we have assumed proportional hazards and/or a Weibull (or exponential) form for the survival data. We now consider some procedures that enable these assumptions to be checked. Such procedures should always be carried out before a particular model is accepted.

### 11.8.1    Log cumulative hazard plots

The **log cumulative hazard** (LCH) function (sometimes called the **integrated hazard function**) is

$$H(t) = \log_e\{-\log_e S(t)\}. \tag{11.38}$$

A plot of the estimated LCH function against the logarithm of survival time (the **LCH plot**) may be used to check both the proportional hazards assumption and the assumption of a Weibull (or exponential) distribution for survival data, as required.

Consider, first, the following one-sample problem: a set of survival data is available and we wish to check whether the Weibull distribution provides an appropriate probability model. Substituting the Weibull survival function, (11.13), into (11.38) gives

$$H(t) = \log_e \lambda + \gamma \log_e t, \tag{11.39}$$

which is the equation of a straight line. Hence if we obtain observed values of the LCH and plot these against the logarithm of survival time, we expect to find a straight line if the Weibull assumption is correct. Moreover, (11.39) shows that the slope of this line will provide an estimate of $\gamma$ and the intercept will provide an estimate of $\log_e \lambda$. In general, these will only be rough estimates, and the maximum likelihood estimates are much preferred. Nevertheless, if the slope of the line is around unity we can conclude that an exponential model will suffice (since a Weibull with $\gamma = 1$ is an exponential).

*Example 11.15*  In Example 11.5 we fitted a Weibull distribution to the glioblastoma multiforme data. Now we shall use the LCH plot to check the assumption that the Weibull is appropriate. First we need to calculate the observed LCH values using (11.38) with the observed survival probabilities in the right-hand side. In Table 11.1 we have the Kaplan–Meier estimates of $S(t)$; these are reproduced in Table 11.8, together with the estimated LCH function from substituting these into (11.38). Since there are 23 distinct survival times, Table 11.8 has 23 rows. However since $\log 0$ is undefined the LCH function cannot be evaluated at the final survival time (120 weeks). The remaining 22 pairs of LCH and log time values are plotted in Figure 11.13.

Figure 11.13 shows a reasonable approximation to a straight line, and so the Weibull model seems acceptable. To consider whether the simpler exponential model is sufficient we

**Table 11.8**  LCH plot calculations for Example 11.15

| Time (weeks) | log (time) | Estimates P(survival) | LCH |
|---|---|---|---|
| 10 | 2.30 | 0.9630 | −3.277 |
| 12 | 2.48 | 0.9259 | −2.565 |
| 13 | 2.56 | 0.8889 | −2.139 |
| 15 | 2.71 | 0.8519 | −1.830 |
| 16 | 2.77 | 0.8148 | −1.586 |
| 20 | 3.00 | 0.7407 | −1.204 |
| 24 | 3.18 | 0.6667 | −0.903 |
| 26 | 3.26 | 0.5926 | −0.648 |
| 27 | 3.30 | 0.5556 | −0.531 |
| 39 | 3.66 | 0.5185 | −0.420 |
| 42 | 3.74 | 0.4815 | −0.313 |
| 45 | 3.81 | 0.4074 | −0.108 |
| 48 | 3.87 | 0.3704 | −0.007 |
| 52 | 3.95 | 0.3333 | 0.094 |
| 58 | 4.06 | 0.2963 | 0.196 |
| 60 | 4.09 | 0.2593 | 0.300 |
| 61 | 4.11 | 0.2222 | 0.408 |
| 62 | 4.13 | 0.1852 | 0.523 |
| 73 | 4.29 | 0.1481 | 0.467 |
| 75 | 4.32 | 0.1111 | 0.787 |
| 77 | 4.34 | 0.0741 | 0.957 |
| 104 | 4.64 | 0.0370 | 1.193 |
| 120 | 4.79 | 0.0000 | − |

need to judge whether the slope of the approximating line is around unity. This may be done by eye or by fitting a least-squares linear regression line to the data (as enumerated in Table 11.8). The latter, using (9.13), produced a slope of 1.69, well above 1.0. Hence there is evidence to reject the exponential model. Notice that the estimate of $\gamma$ is not dissimilar to the maximum likelihood estimate of 1.674 found in Example 11.5. The intercept of −6.52 from the simple linear regression fit (using (9.14)) leads to an estimate of $\log_e(-6.52) = 0.00147$ for $\lambda$. This is also in good agreement with the result in Example 11.5.

Consider, now, the two-sample problem in which we wish to assume that the hazards are proportional. If we let $H_1(t)$ be the LCH function for the comparison group and $H_0(t)$ be the LCH function for the base group (that is, the baseline LCH) then under the PH assumption, (11.18),

$$H_1(t) = \phi H_0(t),$$

from which it may be shown that

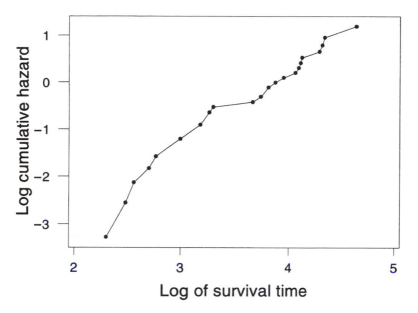

**Figure 11.13**    LCH plot for the glioblastoma multiforme data (note that time was measured in weeks).

$$H_1(t) = \log_e \phi + H_0(t), \tag{11.40}$$

for any survival time $t$. Hence a joint plot of the two estimated LCH functions against log time should produce parallel curves if the PH assumption is valid. By (11.40), the vertical separation of the two curves in the LCH plot will provide an estimate of $\log \phi$, although the maximum likelihood estimate from fitting the PH model is likely to be much more accurate.

If the baseline hazard has the Weibull form then (11.39) shows that the two-group LCH plot will produce parallel *lines*. Hence parallel relationships suggest that a Cox PH regression model may be used; if the relationships are straight lines then a Weibull PH regression model may be used instead. Furthermore, if the parallel straight lines have slope unity then the exponential PH model will suffice.

*Example 11.16*    In Examples 11.7 and 11.13 we used PH regression models to compare low- and high-cellularity groups. To check the PH assumption for this problem Kaplan–Meier estimates (Section 5.4) are first obtained for each cellularity group. These are then used to calculate the corresponding estimated LCHs as in Table 11.8, but now separately by cellularity group. Logarithms need to be calculated for each observed survival time, again as in Table 11.8, again for each group separately.

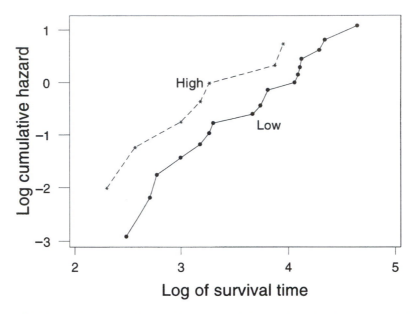

**Figure 11.14**  LCH plot for the glioblastoma multiforme data showing low- and high-cellularity groups separately (note that time was measured in weeks).

These steps were carried out; Figure 11.14 shows the results. This LCH plot gives a good approximation to two parallel lines and hence a Weibull PH regression model is acceptable. Since the condition for a Cox model is less strenuous, this model is a possible alternative.

When there are several groups the PH assumption requires a set of parallel relationships; again the Weibull and PH assumptions together require parallel lines. Calculations are straightforward as a generalization of the two-sample problem. Quantitative variables would need to be grouped at the outset.

*Example 11.17*  Figure 11.15 gives the LCH plot for cholesterol fifths in the SHHS, as used in Example 11.8 (that is, for men with no CHD symptoms at baseline). A particular feature of this plot is the long line from the left for the 3rd fifth. However, this is caused by the sole individual who had a CHD event on the first day of follow-up (so that log time $= \log 1 = 0$). The remaining values produce reasonably parallel lines, except that the bottom two fifths seem to intertwine. Hence there is no strong reason to reject a Cox or Weibull PH model for comparing cholesterol fifths, although we would expect similar hazards in the two lowest fifths, as indeed we found in Example 11.8 (there after adjustment for blood pressure). The rank order of the LCH values in Figure 11.15 will correspond with the rank order of the hazards themselves.

In general we should be concerned about the PH assumption whenever the lines (or curves) run at different angles – particularly when they cross. However,

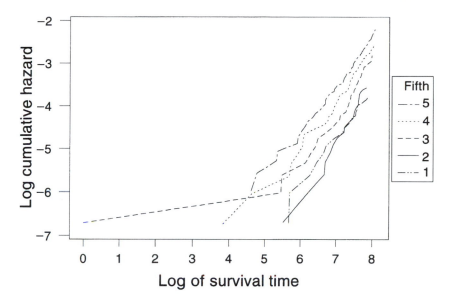

**Figure 11.15**  LCH plot for cholesterol fifths for SHHS men free of CHD at baseline (note that time was measured in years).

as Example 11.17 shows, lines can cross due to unusual values, particularly early event outliers, or due to similar hazards, where the hazard ratio stays near unity but moves slightly above or below unity as time increases. Sampling variation can produce more subtle perturbations from parallel relationships. Hence the LCH plot has its limitations as a diagnostic tool; it would be better to combine it with at least one of the objective methods that follow.

### 11.8.2  *An objective test of proportional hazards for the Cox model*

An objective test of the PH assumption for the Cox model may be obtained by introducing a time-dependent covariate. This follows from our observation, in Section 11.6.1, that the hazard may vary over time (thus violating the PH assumption) when a time-dependent covariate is included in the Cox model.

Consider an explanatory variable $x_1$ which we wish to test for PH within the Cox model. Define a new variable, $x_2$, as the product of $x_1$ and time, $x_2 = x_1 t$. Then fit the time-dependent Cox regression model

$$\log_e \phi = \beta_1 x_1 + \beta_2 x_2(t), \tag{11.41}$$

where $x_2$ is written as $x_2(t)$ to show that it varies with time. We then compare the fits of (11.41) and the model with the fixed covariate $x_1$ alone. A significant difference implies that the hazards associated with $x_1$ are not proportional. Values of $\beta_2$ larger than zero imply that the hazard ratio increases with time, $\beta_2 < 0$ implies that the hazard ratio decreases with time and $\beta_2 = 0$ is consistent with PH.

*Example 11.18* In Example 11.7 we assumed that the hazards for cellularity were proportional when a Cox model was used. To test this, the variable representing cellularity (coded 1 for low and 2 for high) was multiplied by time. Calling this product $x_2$ and calling the cellularity variable $x_1$, the Cox model (11.41) was fitted in SAS. The value of minus twice the log likelihood was returned as 128.019. This is to be compared with the equivalent value when $x_1$ is fitted alone, 128.064 from Output 11.1. The difference, $\Delta = 0.045$, is not significant $(p > 0.10)$ on comparison with $\chi_1^2$. The estimated value of $\beta_2$ is $-0.0047$, so that the hazard ratio (high versus low) appears to decrease slightly with time, but not in any important way.

One drawback with the test introduced here is that it is, as with all models involving time-dependent covariates, computationally demanding. Matters can be improved by taking $x_2 = x_1(t - t_\mathrm{m})$ where $t_\mathrm{m}$ is the median survival time, or $x_2 = x_1 \log t$. Even then, data sets with a large number of observations, such as the SHHS, require a powerful computer to fit (11.41) within a reasonable amount of time.

### 11.8.3    An objective test of proportional hazards for the Weibull model

As we saw in Section 11.7, the Weibull PH model requires the Weibull hazards to have the same shape parameter. Hence, a test for a common shape parameter will provide a test of the PH assumption.

Consider an explanatory variable with $\ell$ groups. We fit separate Weibull models to the data for each separate group. The sum of the minus twice log likelihoods for these individual fits gives the measure of fit for the overall model with distinct shape parameters for each group. This is to be subtracted from the value of minus twice log likelihood for the Weibull PH regression model for the entire data (that is, using a common shape parameter for each group). The difference is compared to chi-square with $\ell - 1$ d.f.

*Example 11.19* In Example 11.13 we assumed that the hazards for cellularity were proportional when a Weibull model was used. To test this, Weibull models were fitted to the low- and high-cellularity data separately. The values of minus twice log likelihood derived from SAS PROC LIFEREG output were 37.50 and 16.46, respectively. The value of minus twice log likelihood from fitting the PH model for cellularity to the entire data set (as in Example 11.13) was 53.98. Hence we compare $53.98 - (37.50 + 16.46) = 0.02$ with $\chi_1^2$. As the result is clearly non-significant we can conclude that there is no evidence that a different shape parameter is required for each group. Hence there is no evidence against PH.

### 11.8.4   Residuals and influence

As with other modelling procedures, model checking should include consideration of residuals and influential values. Various types of residual have been suggested for the Cox and Weibull models, and most computer packages that fit such models will produce residuals. However, interpretation is not easy, particularly because certain residuals may still have a pattern even when the fitted model is 'correct' and because censored and uncensored observations often cluster separately. An added problem with residuals from the Cox model is that they may depend upon the method used to approximate the baseline hazard (Section 11.3).

The interested reader is referred to the specialist textbooks by Kalbfleisch and Prentice (1980), Fleming and Harrington (1991) and Collett (1994). The latter gives a particularly good account of influential observations. Reviews of lack of fit methods for the Cox model are given by Kay (1984) and Le and Zelterman (1992).

### 11.8.5   Non-proportional hazards

When the PH assumption fails, more complex models, beyond our current scope, may be necessary. See the textbooks just referenced for details. Heterogeneity (Section 10.10.3) in survival analysis is generally referred to as a **frailty** effect. Methods for dealing with it are suggested by Clayton and Cuzick (1985).

One situation where hazards are non-proportional that is very easy to deal with, using the Cox approach, deserves mention. This is where there is lack of proportionality for one explanatory variable and yet all other explanatory variables act proportionately and in the same way within each of the strata formed by the 'problem' variable. The solution, which is easily applied using standard software for the Cox model, is to fit a **stratified Cox model**. A separate (unknown) baseline hazard function is assumed here for each stratum of the 'problem' variable. Interpretation of the regression coefficients (the $b$ parameters) follows just as for the standard Cox model.

## 11.9   Poisson regression

Suppose, now, that follow-up data are recorded in the form of the number of events and the number of person-years, as in Section 5.6, possibly disaggregated in some way (for example, by age group). A reasonable assumption is that the number of events follows a **Poisson** distribution, since the Poisson is the appropriate probability model for counts of rare, independent events of any sort (see Clarke and Cooke, 1992). With this assumption we shall define regression models for person-years data. Subsequently, in Section 11.9.4, we will see how the same models may be used with a different type of data.

### 11.9.1    Simple regression

Consider, first, the situation where person-years analysis is to be used to compare two groups: say the 'unexposed' (group 1) and 'exposed' (group 2). Let the dummy explanatory variable $x$ denote group membership:

$$x = \begin{cases} 1 & \text{for members of group 2} \\ 0 & \text{for members of group 1.} \end{cases} \qquad (11.42)$$

Then we shall adopt the following linear model for the logarithm of the estimated person-years rate, $\hat{\rho}$:

$$\log_e \hat{\rho} = b_0 + b_1 x, \qquad (11.43)$$

where $b_0$ and $b_1$ are some constants estimated from the observed data.

This is entirely analogous to the procedure in logistic regression where some transformation of the estimated risk, $\hat{r}$, is assumed to have a linear relationship with the explanatory variable: see (10.3). We can use a statistical computer package to fit (11.43), taking account of the Poisson variation in the observed data, just as we fit the linear model for the transformed $\hat{r}$, accounting for the appropriate binomial variation, in Chapter 10.

A further step is required to get (11.43) into the form of a generalized linear model, for which computer routines are widely available. Since, by (5.18), $\hat{\rho} = e/y$, where $e$ is the number of events and $y$ is the number of person-years, then

$$\log_e \hat{\rho} = \log_e e - \log_e y,$$

so that (11.43) gives

$$\log_e e = \log_e y + b_0 + b_1 x. \qquad (11.44)$$

Note that the e subscript in (11.44) refers to the base of the logarithm (as usual) and should not be confused with $e$ standing for the number of events.

In (11.44) the term $\log_e y$ is called the **offset**. In general, an offset is an explanatory variable with a known regression parameter (here unity, since the variable $\log_e y$ is multiplied by 1), which consequently does not need to be estimated. In (11.44) the offset is the amount which must be added to the regression equation, $b_0 + b_1 x$, in order to estimate $e$ for any given $x$. So the regression prediction must be 'offset' by this amount. The offset will need to be declared to the computer package chosen to fit the Poisson regression model.

Usually $b_0$ and $b_1$ in (11.44) are taken to be the maximum likelihood estimates for their population equivalents, as calculated by commercial software. Once we know $b_0$ and $b_1$ we would normally be most interested in estimating rates and relative rates. For the exposed group, (11.42) and (11.43) give

$$\log_e \hat{\rho}_2 = b_0 + b_1 \times 1 = b_0 + b_1, \tag{11.45}$$

whilst for the unexposed

$$\log_e \hat{\rho}_1 = b_0 + b_1 \times 0 = b_0, \tag{11.46}$$

where $\hat{\rho}_2$ and $\hat{\rho}_1$ are the estimated event rates in the two groups. Hence,

$$\log_e \hat{\rho}_2 - \log_e \hat{\rho}_1 = b_1,$$

so that

$$\hat{\omega} = \hat{\rho}_2/\hat{\rho}_1 = \exp(b_1) \tag{11.47}$$

is the estimated relative rate. So we can find the rates and relative rate from the fitted regression parameters. Notice the similarity with the way the odds and odds ratio were found from logistic regression models in Section 10.4.1.

From (11.46), a 95% confidence interval for the unexposed rate is given by

$$\exp\{b_0 \pm 1.96\hat{se}(b_0)\} \tag{11.48}$$

and, from (11.47), a 95% confidence interval for the relative rate is given by

$$\exp\{b_1 \pm 1.96\hat{se}(b_1)\}, \tag{11.49}$$

both of which are easily found from standard computer output. Slightly more work is needed to find a confidence interval for the rate in the exposed group. From (11.45),

$$se(\log_e \hat{\rho}_2) = \sqrt{V(b_0) + V(b_1) + 2C(b_0, b_1)}, \tag{11.50}$$

leading to the 95% confidence interval for $\rho_2$ of

$$\exp\{(b_0 + b_1) \pm 1.96\hat{se}(\log_e \hat{\rho}_2)\}. \tag{11.51}$$

We thus need the variance-covariance matrix of the regression parameters in order to evaluate (11.51).

*Example 11.20*  Consider the problem of comparing rates for coronary events by housing tenure status in the SHHS. Tenure status (owner-occupiers = 2, renters = 1), the number of events and the number of person-years, as specified in the 'Total' segment of Table 5.13, were read into PROC GENMOD in SAS. Logarithms of the person-years, by tenure status, were calculated and declared as an offset. Poisson variation was also specified and the variance-covariance matrix was requested. See the program in Appendix A.

**Output 11.10**   SAS results for Example 11.19

The GENMOD Procedure

Analysis of Parameter Estimates

| Parameter | | DF | Estimate | Std Err | ChiSquare | Pr > Chi |
|---|---|---|---|---|---|---|
| INTERCEPT | | 1 | −5.1866 | 0.0981 | 2797.6904 | 0.0000 |
| TENURE | 1 | 1 | 0.3705 | 0.1353 | 7.4955 | 0.0062 |
| TENURE | 2 | 0 | 0.0000 | 0.0000 | . | . |

Estimated Covariance Matrix

| Parameter Number | PRM1 | PRM2 |
|---|---|---|
| 1 | 0.00961538 | −0.00961538 |
| 2 | −0.00961538 | 0.01831104 |

Parameter Information

| Parameter | Effect | TENURE |
|---|---|---|
| 1 | INTERCEPT | |
| 2 | TENURE | 1 |
| 3 | TENURE | 2 |

Output 11.10 is an extract from SAS. Here the SAS terms 'INTERCEPT', 'PRM1' and 'Parameter Number 1' all refer to $b_0$ and 'TENURE 1', 'PRM2' and 'Parameter Number 2' all refer to $b_1$. By its standard rules (Section 9.2.7) SAS automatically fixes 'TENURE 2' to be zero. We now substitute values from this output into the equations specified earlier.

From (11.47), $\hat{\omega} = \exp(b_1) = \exp(0.3705) = 1.45$. From (11.46), $\hat{\rho}_1 = \exp(-5.1866) = 0.00559 = 5.59$ per thousand per year, and from (11.45), $\hat{\rho}_2 = \exp(-5.1866 + 0.3705) = 8.10$ per thousand per year. Of course $8.10/5.59 = 1.45$, as already found. Notice that the three estimates agree with the values obtained by simple arithmetic, using (5.18) as the standard definition, as given in the 'Total' segment of Table 5.13.

We can go further and calculate confidence intervals corresponding to the three estimates. From (11.49) the 95% confidence interval for $\omega$, the relative coronary event rate (renters versus owner-occupiers), is

$$\exp(0.3705 \pm 1.96 \times 0.1353)$$

or (1.11, 1.89). Since unity is outside this interval we reject the null hypothesis that there is no effect of housing tenure status on CHD at the 5% level of significance. Indeed, the $p$ value for this test is $p = 0.0062$ from the right-hand column of Output 11.10 (but see Section 10.7.4).

From (11.48) the 95% confidence interval for $\rho_1$, the coronary event rate for owner-occupiers, is

$$\exp(-5.1866 \pm 1.96 \times 0.0981)$$

or (4.61, 6.78) per thousand per year. From (11.50),

$$\hat{se}(\log_e \hat{\rho}_2) = \sqrt{0.00961538 + 0.01831104 + 2(-0.00961538)} = 0.093251.$$

Thus (11.51) gives the 95% confidence interval for $\rho_2$, the coronary event rate for renters, as

$$\exp\{(-5.1866 + 0.3705) \pm 1.96 \times 0.093251\}$$

or (6.75, 9.72) per thousand per year.

When there are several (more than 2) groups to compare, we replace $x$ in (11.43) and (11.44) by a set of dummy variables. Results are then usually summarized by the set of relative rates (with confidence intervals), taking one group to be the base against which all others are compared. This requires repeated use of (11.47) and (11.49). The procedure is an exact analogue of that used to create a set of odds ratios in Section 10.4.3. Where appropriate, trends across the relative rates may be fitted by analogy with Section 10.4.4. In Example 11.23 we shall see a worked example of how to deal with a categorical variable, with four levels, in a Poisson regression analysis.

### 11.9.2   Multiple regression

The simple regression model may be easily extended to the situation of several explanatory variables, all assumed to be categorical in what follows. The basic form of the multiple Poisson regression model, by extending (11.43), is

$$\log_e \hat{\rho} = b_0 + b_1 x_1 + b_2 x_2 + \cdots + b_k x_k,$$

where $x_1, x_2 \ldots x_k$ are the $k$ explanatory variables. Just as in other multiple regression models, each 'slope' parameter ($b_i$, for $i > 0$) represents the effect of its corresponding $x$ variable upon the dependent variable ($\log_e \hat{\rho}$), keeping all other $x$ variables fixed.

In particular, suppose two groups are to be compared, and let $x_k$ denote group membership just as in (11.42). That is,

$$x_k = \begin{cases} 1 & \text{for members of group 2 (exposed)} \\ 0 & \text{for members of group 1 (unexposed).} \end{cases}$$

Suppose that all other $x$ variables are confounding variables. Then, by reference to (11.47), the estimated relative rate for those exposed compared to those unexposed, adjusting for the confounders, is

$$\hat{\omega} = \exp(b_k) \tag{11.52}$$

with 95% confidence interval

$$\exp\{b_k \pm 1.96\hat{\text{se}}(b_k)\}, \tag{11.53}$$

as in (11.49). To allow for interactions we simply let some of the $x$s be interaction terms, as in Sections 10.9 and 11.6. This inevitably complicates the estimation procedure.

Comparison of two nested Poisson regression models is achieved by comparing the difference in deviance between models to chi-square with d.f. given by the difference in d.f. of the two models, in the same way as for logistic regression (Section 10.7).

*Example 11.21*   We have seen how to compare renters and owner-occupiers in the SHHS in Example 11.20. Now we consider the possible confounding effect of age, just as in the analysis of Example 5.14 where a Mantel–Haenszel analysis was used.

Data on age group (six in all), tenure status (renters, owner-occupiers), coronary events and person-years were input to SAS PROC GENMOD from Table 5.13 (this time omitting the 'Total' segment). The log of the person-years (in each age/tenure group) was calculated as an offset. An analysis of deviance was performed, each time adding one new term to those in the existing model, and results are given in Table 11.9.

We conclude that age has an effect on the coronary rate; tenure status has an effect over and above that of age; there is no difference in the effect of tenure across the age groups. This leads to adoption of the model

$$\log_e \hat{\rho} = b_0 + b_1 \times \text{age} + b_2 \times \text{tenure}.$$

When this was fitted, SAS PROC GENMOD gave the results in Output 11.11. In the data input TENURE = 1 denoted renters, TENURE = 2 denoted owner-occupiers and AGE took values from 1 to 6 according to the age group.

By (11.52), the estimated age-adjusted relative rate (renters compared to owner-occupiers) is $\exp(0.3439) = 1.41$. This is, to two decimal places, the same as the Mantel–Haenszel estimate found in Example 5.14.

By (11.53), the 95% confidence interval for the age-adjusted relative rate is

$$\exp(0.3439 \pm 1.96 \times 0.1356)$$

or (1.08, 1.84), which again happens to agree precisely with the results in Example 5.14. Note also that the $p$ value of 0.0112 for TENURE 1 in the right-hand column of Output 11.11 agrees with that found for tenure adjusted for age ($p = 0.011$) in Table 11.9 (see Section 10.7.4 for a discussion of this type of test).

As with simple regression models, the above methodology is easily extended to cope with a variable representing exposure at several levels. See Example 11.23.

**Table 11.9**   Analysis of deviance table for Example 11.21; each term adds to those in the previous row

| Terms in model | D | d.f. | ΔD | Δd.f. | p value |
|---|---|---|---|---|---|
| constant | 35.08 | 11 | – | – | – |
| + age | 10.10 | 6 | 24.98 | 5 | 0.0001 |
| + tenure | 3.66 | 5 | 6.44 | 1 | 0.011 |
| + age*tenure | 0 | 0 | 3.66 | 5 | 0.60 |

Note: As usual, * denotes interaction; Δ denotes 'difference in'; $D$ denotes deviance.

**Output 11.11**   SAS results for Example 11.21

The GENMOD Procedure

Analysis of Parameter Estimates

| Parameter | | DF | Estimate | Std Err | ChiSquare | Pr > Chi |
|-----------|---|----|----------|---------|-----------|----------|
| INTERCEPT |   | 1 | −4.9564 | 0.4158 | 142.0896 | 0.0000 |
| AGE | 1 | 1 | −1.4992 | 0.6057 | 6.1276 | 0.0133 |
| AGE | 2 | 1 | −0.3723 | 0.4360 | 0.7290 | 0.3932 |
| AGE | 3 | 1 | −0.2088 | 0.4297 | 0.2361 | 0.6270 |
| AGE | 4 | 1 | −0.2300 | 0.4300 | 0.2862 | 0.5927 |
| AGE | 5 | 1 | 0.2304 | 0.4303 | 0.2865 | 0.5924 |
| AGE | 6 | 0 | 0.0000 | 0.0000 | . | . |
| TENURE | 1 | 1 | 0.3439 | 0.1356 | 6.4376 | 0.0112 |
| TENURE | 2 | 0 | 0.0000 | 0.0000 | . | . |

### 11.9.3   Comparison of standardized event ratios

Poisson regression may also be used to compare standardized event ratios (SERs), providing an alternative to the approach adopted in Section 5.6.3.

Taking the variable $x$ as in (11.42), consider the model

$$\log_e(\text{SER}) = b_0 + b_1 x, \tag{11.54}$$

where, as introduced in Section 4.5.2, $SER = e/E$, in which $e$ is the observed and $E$ is the expected number of events ($E$ having been calculated using some suitable standard population). Hence,

$$\log_e(\text{SER}) = \log_e e - \log_e E,$$

and thus (11.54) gives

$$\log_e e = \log_e E + b_0 + b_1 x. \tag{11.55}$$

Note that (11.54) and (11.55) are the same as (11.43) and (11.44) except that $\hat{\rho}$ has been replaced by SER in (11.54) and $y$ has been replaced by $E$ in (11.55). Provided that these changes are made, all other formulae in Sections 11.9.1 and 11.9.2 transfer over. In particular, (11.47) and (11.49) suggest that an estimate for the relative SER is given by

$$\hat{\omega}_s = \exp(b_1), \tag{11.56}$$

with corresponding 95% confidence interval

$$\exp\{b_1 \pm 1.96\hat{se}(b_1)\}. \tag{11.57}$$

Note that the Poisson multiple regression model now provides a means of adjusting standardized event ratios. Since standardization is itself a form of adjustment, this produces hybrid adjustment. For instance, age-standardized mortality ratios might be further adjusted, through modelling, for smoking status, if suitable data were available.

*Example 11.22*  SAS PROC GENMOD was used to analyse the hypothetical chemical company data of Example 5.13. Observed and expected numbers of deaths were entered for each company, and the log of the expected number was declared as an offset. Codes for company were chosen so as to make the original company (of Example 5.10) the base group. Output 11.12 gives the results.

From (11.56), the estimated relative standardized mortality rate is $\exp(-0.8849) = 0.413$ which agrees, as it should, with the value calculated from first principles in Example 5.13. From (11.57) the 95% confidence interval for the standardized event ratio is

$$\exp(-0.8849 \pm 1.96 \times 0.5227)$$

or (0.148, 1.150). This is considerably narrower than the exact interval given in Example 5.13, the upper limit here being considerably smaller. This is explained by the small number of observed deaths (four) in the original chemical company, which compromises the approximation.

## 11.9.4  Routine or registration data

Although not concerned with follow-up data, this is the appropriate place to consider models for event rates which arise from routine or registration data. This is where the estimated event rate is

$$\hat{\rho} = e/p,$$

where $p$ is (typically) a mid-year population estimate, as in Section 3.8. Such rates may be modelled using Poisson regression. The rates are treated just as for follow-up (person-years) event rates except that $p$ replaces $y$ in (11.44) and all that follows in Sections 11.9.1 and 11.9.2. To show this, an example will suffice.

*Example 11.23*  We shall now use the Poisson regression model to compare coronary event rates between the deprivation groups in north Glasgow using the MONICA data given in Table 4.9. For each of the 32 age/deprivation groups defined by Table 4.9, codes for age (1–8 in rank order) and deprivation group, mid-year population size and number of events were

**Output 11.12**  SAS results for Example 11.22

The GENMOD Procedure

Analysis of Parameter Estimates

| Parameter | | DF | Estimate | Std Err | ChiSquare | Pr > Chi |
|-----------|---|----|----------|---------|-----------|----------|
| INTERCEPT | | 1 | 0.9889 | 0.5000 | 3.9114 | 0.0480 |
| COMPANY | 0 | 1 | −0.8849 | 0.5227 | 2.8658 | 0.0905 |
| COMPANY | 1 | 0 | 0.0000 | 0.0000 | . | . |

read into SAS. Deprivation group was coded so as to ensure that all slope parameters in the Poisson regression model represent comparisons with deprivation group I. As explained in Section 10.4.3, this may be achieved in SAS by coding group II as 2, III as 3, IV as 4 and I as 5.

As in Example 11.21, various models were fitted using PROC GENMOD. Each fit used the log of the mid-year population as an offset. This time the unadjusted effect of deprivation group ('depgp') was tested as well as the age-adjusted effect. Table 11.10 gives the results.

From Table 11.10 we conclude that age has a massive effect on the coronary rate; deprivation group has an effect both with and without taking account of age; age does not modify the effect of deprivation on the coronary rate. This leads to adopting model 4,

$$\log_e \hat{\rho} = b_0 + b_1 \times \text{age} + b_2 \times \text{depgp}$$

When fitted, this produced Output 11.13 from PROC GENMOD. Note the huge estimated standard error for age group 1. This is due to there being no events in age group 1 (25–29 years): see Table 4.9. Not surprisingly, SAS PROC GENMOD has not been able to estimate the effect for this group with reasonable precision. When large standard errors are found there is usually some problem with model fitting. Such problems may be avoided by combining groups – for instance, age groups 1 and 2 in this example. For the effects that we are interested in, those for the deprivation groups, and for Table 11.10 this modification makes very little difference, so we shall proceed with the model as fitted above.

By reference to (11.52), the age-adjusted relative rate for deprivation group II versus group I is $\exp(0.2599) = 1.30$. By reference to (11.53), the corresponding 95% confidence interval is

$$\exp(0.2599 \pm 1.96 \times 0.1526)$$

or (0.96, 1.75). The full set of estimated relative rates and confidence intervals is given in Table 11.11. Also shown are the relative SERs and corresponding 95% confidence intervals, each calculated from (5.22) and (5.23). Results by the two methods are in excellent agreement, despite the use of two different approaches to adjust for age. Notice that, since a relative SER is a relative indirect standardized rate, the estimates of the relative SER in Table 11.11 are exactly as plotted for indirect standardization in Figure 4.6.

Finally, rather than treating deprivation group as a categorical variable we can take it as ordinal and consider dose-response effects. This is appropriate here since the deprivation group numbers indicate increasing relative deprivation. Through the Poisson regression model it is straightforward to fit a trend in the log relative rate.

**Table 11.10**  Analysis of deviance table for Example 11.22

| Terms in model | D | d.f. | $\Delta D$ | $\Delta d.f.$ | p value |
|---|---|---|---|---|---|
| 1 constant | 697.79 | 31 | – | – | – |
| 2 age | 33.07 | 24 | 664.72 | 7 | < 0.0001 |
| 3 depgp | 662.87 | 28 | 34.92[a] | 3 | < 0.0001 |
| 4 age + depgp | 13.46 | 21 | 19.61[b] | 3 | 0.0002 |
| 5 age*depgp | 0 | 0 | 13.46[c] | 21 | 0.89 |

Note: the final model contains the two constituent main effects (as all interaction models should).
[a]Compared to model 1. [b]Compared to model 2. [c]Compared to model 4.

**Output 11.13**    SAS results for Example 11.23, model 4

The GENMOD Procedure

Analysis of Parameter Estimates

| Parameter | | DF | Estimate | Std Err | ChiSquare | Pr > Chi |
|---|---|---|---|---|---|---|
| INTERCEPT | | 1 | − 4.3850 | 0.1331 | 1084.6739 | 0.0000 |
| AGE | 1 | 1 | −25.9977 | 24469.4450 | 0.0000 | 0.9992 |
| AGE | 2 | 1 | − 5.5785 | 1.0028 | 30.9433 | 0.0000 |
| AGE | 3 | 1 | − 2.9358 | 0.3108 | 89.1975 | 0.0000 |
| AGE | 4 | 1 | − 1.7787 | 0.1923 | 85.5451 | 0.0000 |
| AGE | 5 | 1 | − 1.1739 | 0.1577 | 55.3889 | 0.0000 |
| AGE | 6 | 1 | − 0.9280 | 0.1411 | 43.2456 | 0.0000 |
| AGE | 7 | 1 | − 0.4503 | 0.1193 | 14.2381 | 0.0002 |
| AGE | 8 | 0 | 0.0000 | 0.0000 | . | . |
| DEPGP | 2 | 1 | 0.2599 | 0.1526 | 2.9003 | 0.0886 |
| DEPGP | 3 | 1 | 0.4852 | 0.1450 | 11.1946 | 0.0008 |
| DEPGP | 4 | 1 | 0.5724 | 0.1453 | 15.5249 | 0.0001 |
| DEPGP | 5 | 0 | 0.0000 | 0.0000 | . | . |

**Table 11.11**    Relative rates (with 95% confidence intervals) for coronary events for men in north Glasgow in 1991

| Deprivation group | Poisson regression method | Relative SERs method |
|---|---|---|
| I | 1 | 1 |
| II | 1.30 (0.96, 1.75) | 1.29 (0.95, 1.77) |
| III | 1.62 (1.22, 2.16) | 1.62 (1.21, 2.18) |
| IV | 1.77 (1.33, 2.36) | 1.77 (1.32, 2.39) |

As explained in Sections 10.4.4 and 10.7.3, we fit the linear trend by defining a quantitative variable which takes the values 1, 2, 3, 4 for successive deprivation groups I, II, III, IV. Retaining the confounding variable (age) throughout, Table 11.12 gives the appropriate analysis of deviance table. From this we conclude that there is a linear trend in the log relative rate, having allowed for age effects, and there is no evidence of any non-linearity. Thus increasing deprivation has a constant additive effect on the log relative rate, and thus a constant multiplicative effect on the relative rate, for coronary events.

When the linear trend model (model 3 in Table 11.12) was fitted in PROC GENMOD the parameter estimate (with estimated standard error) for the age-adjusted trend was found to be 0.1868 (0.0436). The age-adjusted relative rate for any deprivation group compared to the next most advantaged is thus $e^{0.1868} = 1.21$, with 95% confidence interval

$$\exp(0.1868 \pm 1.96 \times 0.0436)$$

or (1.11, 1.31).

**Table 11.12**  Analysis of deviance table for a dose-response analysis (age-adjusted). The terms in the model, besides age, refer to the assumed form of the deprivation group effect

| Model | D | d.f. | ΔD | Δd.f. | p value |
|---|---|---|---|---|---|
| 1 age | 33.07 | 24 | – | – | – |
| 2 age + categorical | 13.46 | 21 | 19.61[a] | 3 | 0.0002 |
| 3 age + linear | 14.42 | 23 | 18.65[a] | 1 | < 0.0001 |
| 4 age + quadratic | 13.52 | 22 | 0.90[b] | 1 | 0.34 |
| 5 age + cubic | 13.46 | 21 | 0.06[c] | 1 | 0.81 |

Note: The deviance and d.f. for the second and final models must be the same.
[a]Relative to model 1. [b]Relative to model 3. [c]Relative to model 4.

### 11.9.5   Generic data

The examples using Poisson regression described above all involve grouped data. As with logistic regression (Section 10.5), generic data may also be used as input and will give the same parameter estimates but different measures of fit (deviances). See McNeil (1996) for a worked example.

Generic data input will be necessary when we wish to model a continuous variable without first grouping it. When the model includes variables that alter during follow-up, multiple records would be necessary for each subject. For example, if we require relative rates by age group from generic data we must define separate observations (for entry into the computer package) for each age group for each person.

### 11.9.6   Model checking

Since Poisson regression is another member of the family of generalized linear models, not surprisingly the methods of model checking for logistic regression described in Section 10.10 may be adapted to the present context. In particular, with grouped data the model deviance compared to chi-square with the model d.f. gives an indication of overall lack of fit (Section 10.7.1). Heterogeneity (Section 10.10.3) is termed **extra-Poisson variation** in this context. Procedures for residuals and identifying influential observations follow similarly to logistic regression (Sections 10.10.1 and 10.10.2). Although formulae may vary, the results are used in precisely the same way. For example, SAS PROC GENMOD produces raw and deviance residuals for Poisson regression which are analogous to those described in Section 10.10.1.

## Exercises

(Most of these require the use of a computer package with appropriate procedures.)

11.1 Find the two sets of actuarial estimates of the hazard function for the Norwegian Multicentre Study data of Table C.8. Plot them on the same graph and comment on the results.

11.2 For the brain metastases data of Table C.4, treating anyone who did not die due to their tumour as censored,

(i) Using the life table computed in Exercise 5.2(i), estimate and plot the hazard function using both the person-time and actuarial methods.

(ii) Find the Kaplan–Meier estimates of the hazard function and plot them. Compare your result with that of (i).

(iii) Fit an exponential distribution to the survival times. Record and plot the fitted hazard function.

(iv) Fit a Weibull distribution to the survival times. Record and plot the fitted hazard function.

(v) Use an LCH plot to test the exponential and Weibull assumptions.

(vi) Compare survival experiences for those who have, and have not, received prior treatment using both the Weibull and Cox proportional hazards regression models. For both approaches, find the hazard ratio for prior versus no prior treatment and test for an effect of prior treatment, unadjusted and adjusted for age. Compare results with those of Exercise 5.2.

(vii) Use an LCH plot to check the proportional hazards assumption. Use the same plot to assess the assumption of separate Weibull distributions for the two prior treatment groups.

11.3 An epidemiological investigation considered the effect of abnormal platelets on survival for 100 patients with multiple myeloma. Since age and sex were thought to be potential confounding variables, these were recorded. The following variables from the study were entered into the SAS package: survival time (in months) from time of diagnosis; survival status ($0 =$ alive, $1 =$ dead) at end of the study; platelets ($0 =$ abnormal, $1 =$ normal) at diagnosis; age (in years) at diagnosis; sex ($1 =$ male, $2 =$ female).

(i) PROC PHREG (Cox regression) was used to analyse the data. All explanatory variables were treated as quantitative variables. An extract from the output produced by SAS is given in Output 11.14.

Estimate the hazard ratio for platelets adjusted for age and sex, together with the corresponding 99% confidence interval. Interpret your result. From the model fitted, would the estimated hazard ratios for platelets be different for 40-year-old men and 50-year-old women? If so, by how much?

(ii) A further seven models were fitted to the data. The deviance for each model is shown underneath Output 11.14.

Stating the effect controlled for in each case, determine the role of age and sex as effect modifiers of the platelet–myeloma relationship and determine the effect of platelets on myeloma. Would you consider the model used in (i) the 'best'?

**Output 11.14**    SAS output for Exercise 11.3(i)

The PHREG Procedure

Testing Global Null Hypothesis: BETA = 0

| Criterion | Without Covariates | With Covariates | Model Chi-Square |
|---|---|---|---|
| −2 LOG L | 327.114 | 306.005 | 21.106 with 3 DF |

Analysis of Maximum Likelihood Estimates

| Variable | DF | Parameter Estimate | Standard Error |
|---|---|---|---|
| PLATELETS | 1 | −0.720 | 0.197 |
| AGE | 1 | −0.003 | 0.015 |
| SEX | 1 | −0.307 | 0.083 |

| Terms fitted | Deviance |
|---|---|
| Platelets | 320.073 |
| Sex | 311.747 |
| Age | 321.814 |
| Platelets + sex | 307.825 |
| Platelets + age | 315.537 |
| Platelets + sex + age + sex*platelets | 304.611 |
| Platelets + sex + age + age*platelets | 306.000 |

Note: * denotes an interaction.

11.4 Refer to the lung cancer data of Table C.1, and use Cox regression models in the following.
   (i) Fit the model that relates survival to education only, testing for the effect of education. Compare your result to that of Exercise 5.3(iv). Add a time-dependent covariate, education multiplied by time, to test the basic assumption of this Cox model.
   (ii) Find estimated hazard ratios (with 95% confidence limits) to assess the effect of each of the six explanatory variables (including education) when considered individually. Take the group labelled '1' as the base group for each categorical variable.
   (iii) Continue to find the most appropriate Cox multiple regression model to predict survival time.
11.5 Reanalyse the data given in Exercise 5.5 using Poisson regression: find relative rates with 95% confidence intervals, taking the lowest exposure group as base. Test for linear trend, and for non-linear polynomial relationships, across the exposure groups, taking the mid-points of each exposure group as the 'scores' for the groups. You should assume a maximum dust exposure of 1200, so as to produce verifiable results.

11.6 For the smelter workers data in Table C.5, fit the appropriate Poisson regression model so as to determine the $p$ value for the effect of exposure to arsenic, adjusting for age group and calendar period. Also find the adjusted relative rate for high versus low exposure, together with a 95% confidence interval. Compare your results with those of Exercises 5.8(ii) and 5.8(iii).

11.7 Reanalyse the data given in Exercise 5.7: find a set of estimated relative rates with 95% confidence intervals using Poisson regression models for each vitamin (low intake = base), and compare with the results found in Exercise 5.7. Carry out tests for linear trend in the rates.

11.8 Berry (1983) gives the following observed and expected numbers of deaths due to lung cancer in men suffering from asbestosis. The data are disaggregated by the Pneumoconiosis Medical Panel at which the men were certified and the disability benefit awarded when first certified (the relative amount of compensation).

|  | Number | |
| --- | --- | --- |
| Compensation | Observed | Expected |
| London Panel | | |
| Low | 51 | 5.03 |
| Medium | 17 | 1.29 |
| High | 10 | 0.38 |
| Cardiff Panel | | |
| Low | 12 | 4.05 |
| Medium | 14 | 0.98 |
| High | 5 | 0.29 |

Fit all possible Poisson regression models, fitting (where appropriate) Compensation and Panel as categorical variables. Hence, test for all possible effects. Use your results to decide which (if any) of Compensation, Panel and their interaction are related to lung cancer death. Give a suitable set of standardized mortality ratios, together with 95% confidence intervals, to summarize your findings. Express these graphically.

11.9 Refer to the nasal cancer data of Table C.15, taking each explanatory variable as categorical.
   (i) Use Poisson regression to test the effect of age, year of first employment and duration of exposure.
   (ii) Decide whether each of the three explanatory variables is important in the presence of the other two.
   (iii) Give estimates and 95% confidence intervals for the adjusted relative rates.

# Appendix A
# SAS Programs

Here a selection of SAS programs is presented. These were used to generate results given in Chapters 9–11. All programs were run under version 6.11 of SAS. In each case the exercise that used the corresponding analysis is specified, together with a brief description of the analysis. Underneath (in parentheses), any particular displays in the text that were constructed from the program are listed. The sections between a /* and a */ are comments which may be omitted.

In all cases the data step is included. Since data are usually read in with a new line for each case, this format is assumed here. Where data are read in as part of the program, the display has often been contracted (indicated by three dots) to save space. The full data are given in the text of this book. Where data are read in from a file, the user would need to replace the file specification given here (e.g. \woodward\sugar.dat) with one of his or her own. All the data sets that are read from files are available electronically: see Appendix C.

**Example 9.1 One-way ANOVA (creates Output 9.1)**

```
data dietary;
/* read in the data */
input diet cholest;
cards;
1 6.35
1 6.47
...
3 5.62
;
/* fit an ANOVA model with categorical variable DIET */
proc glm;
class diet;
model cholest = diet/solution;
run;
```

**Example 9.5 Simple linear regression (creates Output 9.2)**

```
data sugdmft;
/* read in the data from a file */
infile '\woodward\sugar.dat';
```

```
input type sugar dmft;
/* select out only developing countries (TYPE = 2) */
if type = 2;
/* fit an SLR model with SUGAR as the x variable */
proc glm;
model dmft = sugar;
run;
```

**Example 9.7  Two-way ANOVA (creates Outputs 9.3 and 9.5 and Table 9.13)**

```
data dietary;
/* read in the data */
input diet cholest sex;
cards;
1 6.35 1
1 6.47 1
...
3 5.62 2
;
/* fit an ANOVA model with categorical variables DIET and
   SEX */
proc glm;
class diet sex;
model cholest = diet sex/solution;
/* find least-squares means (standard errors) & test
   differences */
lsmeans diet/stderr pdiff;
run;
```

**Example 9.9  Two-way ANOVA with interaction (creates Output 9.6)**

```
data dietary;
/* read in the data */
input diet cholest sex;
cards;
1 6.35 1
1 6.47 1
...
3 5.62 2
;
/* fit a two-way ANOVA model with interaction */
proc glm;
class diet sex;
model cholest = diet sex diet*sex/solution;
run;
```

**Example 9.11 General linear model selection with transformed *y* variable (creates Outputs 9.12–9.15)**

```
data sugdmft;
/* read in the data from a file */
infile '\woodward\sugar.dat';
input type sugar dmft;
/* transform the y variable */
logdmft = log(dmft);
/* single line (SLR) model */
proc glm;
model logdmft = sugar;
/* step (one-way ANOVA) model */
proc glm;
class type;
model logdmft = type/solution;
/* parallel lines model */
proc glm;
class type;
model logdmft = sugar type/solution;
/* separate lines model */
proc glm;
class type;
model logdmft = sugar type sugar*type/solution;
run;
```

**Example 9.12 Multiple regression selection (creates Tables 9.19–9.21)**

```
data SHHS;
/* read in the data from a file */
infile '\woodward\hdl.dat';
input hdl age alcohol cholest fibre;
/* find all correlations */
proc corr;
var hdl age alcohol cholest fibre;
/* fit all possible regression models for HDL */
proc glm;
model hdl = age;
proc glm;
model hdl = alcohol;
proc glm;
model hdl = cholest;
proc glm;
model hdl = fibre;
```

```
proc glm;
model hdl = age alcohol;
proc glm;
model hdl = age cholest;
proc glm;
model hdl = age fibre;
proc glm;
model hdl = alcohol cholest;
proc glm;
model hdl = alcohol fibre;
proc glm;
model hdl = cholest fibre;
proc glm;
model hdl = age alcohol cholest;
proc glm;
model hdl = age alcohol fibre;
proc glm;
model hdl = age cholest fibre;
proc glm;
model hdl = alcohol cholest fibre;
proc glm;
model hdl = age alcohol cholest fibre;
/* re-fit 'best' model with alcohol entered first */
proc glm;
model hdl = alcohol age;
run;
```

**Example 9.13  Residual plot (creates a similar plot to Figure 9.11)**

```
data sugdmft;
/* read in the data from a file */
infile '\woodward\sugar.dat';
input type sugar dmft;
/* select out only developing countries (TYPE = 2) */
if type = 2;
/* fit a SLR model with SUGAR as the x variable */
proc glm;
model dmft = sugar;
/* save derived values in a new file (left-hand side is SAS
   name in both cases) */
output out = newfile predicted=fitted student=stresid;
/* plot standardized residuals against fitted values */
proc plot;
plot stresid*fitted;
run;
```

**Example 10.4  Logistic regression with a binary variable (creates Tables 10.5 and 10.6)**

```
data pooling;
/* read in the data */
input smoking r n;
cards;
1 166 1342
0  50   563
;
/* fit a logistic regression model with explanatory
   variable SMOKING */
proc genmod;
/* include variance-covariance matrix using COVB */
model r/n = smoking/dist = binomial link = logit covb;
run;
```

**Examples 10.6, 10.7 and 10.13  Logistic regression with a categorical variable (creates Tables 10.8, 10.9 and 10.11 and used in Figure 10.5)**

```
data monica;
/* read in the data */
input rank r n;
cards;
1 10 38
2 40 86
3 36 57
4 226 300
5 83 108
6 60 73
;
/* fit a logistic regression model with categorical
   variable RANK */
proc genmod;
class rank;
/* include variance-covariance matrix using COVB */
model r/n = rank/dist = bin link = logit covb;
/* refit the model using SOCLASS which has the first level
   of rank as its last level, as in Table 10.10 */
data two;
/* first, reset the data */
set monica;
soclass = rank;
/* compute the new explanatory variable */
```

```
if rank = 1 then soclass = 7;
/* fit a logistic regression model with categorical
   variable SOCLASS */
proc genmod;
class soclass;
/* this time use the MAKE command to save the estimates and
   standard errors which will be kept in a new file: this
   makes ESTIMATE the estimated logit with STDERR its
   standard error */
make 'parmest' out = newfile;
model r/n = soclass/dist = bin link = logit;
/* read in the new file */
data three;
set newfile;
/* make ODDSRAT the odds ratio, LOWER and UPPER the
   confidence limits */
oddsrat = exp(estimate);
lower = exp(estimate-1.96*stderr);
upper = exp(estimate+1.96*stderr);
/* print out the results */
proc print;
var parm oddsrat lower upper;
run;
```

**Example 10.8  Logistic regression using dummy variables (creates Table 10.13)**

```
data monica;
/* read in the data and set up the dummy variables; note
   that x = (y) gives x the value 1 if y is true and 0 other-
   wise */
input rank r n;
x2 = (rank = 2);
x3 = (rank = 3);
x4 = (rank = 4);
x5 = (rank = 5);
x6 = (rank = 6);
/* here come the data */
cards;
1 10 38
2 40 86
3 36 57
4 226 300
5 83 108
6 60 73
;
```

```
/* fit a logistic regression model to the set of dummy
   variables */
proc genmod;
model r/n = x2 x3 x4 x5 x6/dist = bin link = logit;
run;
```

**Example 10.10  Logistic regression with generic data (creates Output 10.1)**

```
data shhs;
/* read in the data from a file */
infile '\woodward\agedeath.dat';
input age death;
/* compute the risk denominator as one for each person */
n = 1;
/* fit a logistic regression model with the explanatory
   variable AGE */
proc genmod;
model death/n = age/ dist = bin link = logit;
run;
```

**Examples 10.11, 10.14 and 10.20  Logistic regression selection (creates Tables 10.15 and 10.20, and is used to make Table 10.27)**

```
data shhs;
/* read in the data */
input sbp5th chol5th chd n;
/* reset the first level of each categorical variable to be
   its last */
if sbp5th = 1 then sbp5th = 6;
if chol5th = 1 then chol5th = 6;
/* here come the data */
cards;
1 1 1 190
1 2 0 183
1 3 4 178
1 4 8 157
1 5 4 132
2 1 2 203
2 2 2 175
. . .
5 5 23 180
;
/* fit empty model */
```

```
proc genmod;
model chd/n =  /dist = bin link = logit;
/* fit categorical variable SBP5TH */
proc genmod;
class sbp5th;
model chd/n = sbp5th/dist = bin link = logit;
/* fit categorical variable CHOL5TH */
proc genmod;
class chol5th;
model chd/n = chol5th/dist = bin link = logit;
/* fit bivariate model: as this turns out to be 'best', this
   time the estimates are stored in a new file using the
   MAKE command */
proc genmod;
class sbp5th chol5th;
make 'parmest' out = newfile;
model chd/n = sbp5th chol5th/dist = bin link = logit;
/* read in the new file */
data results;
set newfile;
/* make ODDSRAT the odds ratio, LOWER and UPPER the confi-
   dence limits */
oddsrat = exp(estimate);
lower = exp(estimate-1.96*stderr);
upper = exp(estimate+1.96*stderr);
/* print out the results */
proc print;
var parm oddsrat lower upper;
run;
```

**Examples 10.12 and 10.15 Logistic regression selection with generic data (used in Tables 10.16 and 10.22–10.24)**

```
data shhs;
/* read in the data from a file (includes DAYS which is not
   used here) */
infile '\woodward\multshhs.dat';
input age totchol bmi systol smoking activity chd days;
/* compute the risk denominator as one for each person */
one = 1;
/* reset the first level of each categorical variable to be
   its last */
if activity = 1 then activity = 4;
if smoking = 1 then smoking = 4;
```

```
/* fit model with all explanatory variables, for Table
   10.16 */
proc genmod;
class smoking activity;
model chd/one = age totchol bmi systol smoking activity/
 dist = bin link = logit;
/* fit the logistic regression models listed in Example
   10.15, in order */
proc genmod;
model chd/one =  /dist = bin link = logit;
proc genmod;
model chd/one = age/dist = bin link = logit;
proc genmod;
model chd/one = totchol/dist = bin link = logit;
proc genmod;
model chd/one = bmi/dist = bin link = logit;
proc genmod;
model chd/one = systol/dist = bin link = logit;
proc genmod;
class smoking;
model chd/one = smoking/dist = bin link = logit;
proc genmod;
class activity;
model chd/one = activity/dist = bin link = logit;
proc genmod;
class smoking;
model chd/one = age totchol bmi systol smoking/dist = bin
   link = logit;
proc genmod;
class smoking;
model chd/one = totchol bmi systol smoking/dist = bin
   link = logit;
proc genmod;
class smoking;
model chd/one = age bmi systol smoking/dist = bin link =
   logit;
proc genmod;
class smoking;
model chd/one = age totchol systol smoking/dist = bin
   link = logit;
proc genmod;
class smoking;
model chd/one = age totchol bmi smoking/dist = bin
   link = logit;
proc genmod;
```

```
model chd/one = age totchol bmi systol/dist = bin
   link = logit;
proc genmod;
class smoking;
model chd/one = bmi systol smoking/dist = bin
   link = logit;
proc genmod;
class smoking;
model chd/one = totchol systol smoking/dist = bin
   link =logit;
proc genmod;
class smoking;
model chd/one = totchol bmi smoking/dist = bin
   link = logit;
proc genmod;
model chd/one = totchol bmi systol/dist = bin
   link = logit;
proc genmod;
class smoking activity;
model chd/one = totchol bmi systol smoking activity/
   dist = bin link = logit;
run;
```

**Examples 10.16 and 10.17 Logistic regression with an ordered categorical $x$ variable (creates Tables 10.25 and 10.26 and is used to make Figure 10.7)**

```
data monica;
/* read in the data and set up polynomial terms */
input rank r n;
rank2 = rank**2;
rank3 = rank**3;
rank4 = rank**4;
rank5 = rank**5;
cards;
1    10    38
2    40    86
3    36    57
4   226   300
5    83   108
6    60    73
;
/* fit null model */
proc genmod;
model r/n = /dist = bin link = logit;
```

```
/* fit categorical variable RANK */
proc genmod;
class rank;
model r/n = rank/dist = bin link = logit;
/* fit ordinal variable RANK */
proc genmod;
model r/n = rank/dist = bin link = logit;
/* fit remaining polynomial models */
proc genmod;
model r/n = rank rank2/dist = bin link = logit;
proc genmod;
model r/n = rank rank2 rank3/dist = bin link = logit;
proc genmod;
model r/n = rank rank2 rank3 rank4/dist = bin link = logit;
proc genmod;
model r/n = rank rank2 rank3 rank4 rank5/dist = bin
   link = logit;
run;
```

**Example 10.21 Logistic regression with categorical–categorical interaction (creates Tables 10.32 and 10.33 and Output 10.3)**

```
data shhs;
/* read in the data */
input bort sex x1 x2 x3 x4 x5 x6 x7 chd n;
/* reset first level of BORT to be its last */
if bort = 1 then bort = 5;
/* here come the data: see Table 10.31 */
cards;
1 1 0 0 0 1 0 0 0 57 1079
1 2 0 0 0 0 0 0 0 30  945
2 1 1 0 0 1 1 0 0 56  974
2 2 1 0 0 0 0 0 0 20 1101
3 1 0 1 0 1 0 1 0 39  966
3 2 0 1 0 0 0 0 0 10 1076
4 1 0 0 1 1 0 0 1 46 1068
4 2 0 0 1 0 0 0 0 10  948
;
/* start with the null model */
proc genmod;
model chd/n = /dist = bin link = logit;
/* first analysis uses the dummy variables */
/* fit Bortner quarter */
proc genmod;
```

```
model chd/n = x1 x2 x3/dist = bin link = logit;
/* fit sex */
proc genmod;
model chd/n = x4/dist = bin link = logit;
/* fit Bortner and sex */
proc genmod;
model chd/n = x1 x2 x3 x4/dist = bin link = logit;
/* fit interaction */
proc genmod;
model chd/n = x1 x2 x3 x4 x5 x6 x7/dist = bin link = logit;
/* second (equivalent) analysis uses CLASS statements */
/* fit Bortner quarter */
proc genmod;
class bort;
model chd/n = bort/dist = bin link = logit;
/* fit sex */
proc genmod;
class sex;
model chd/n = sex/dist = bin link = logit;
/* fit Bortner and sex */
proc genmod;
class bort sex;
model chd/n = bort sex/dist = bin link = logit;
/* fit interaction */
proc genmod;
class bort sex;
model chd/n = bort sex bort*sex/dist = bin link = logit;
run;
```

**Example 10.22 Logistic regression with categorical–quantitative interaction (creates Table 10.35 (model 5) and Outputs 10.4 and 10.5)**

```
data shhs;
/* read in the data from a file, includes BORT4TH and DAYS
   which are not used here */
infile '\woodward\bortner.dat';
input sex bortner bort4th chd days;
/* compute the risk denominator as one for each person */
one = 1;
/* fit model 5 of Table 10.35 */
proc genmod;
class sex;
/* save estimates etc. as in Example 10.11 */
make 'parmest' out = newfile;
```

```
model chd/one = sex bortner sex*bortner/dist = bin
   link = logit;
data results;
set newfile;
oddsrat = exp(estimate);
lower = exp(estimate-1.96*stderr);
upper = exp(estimate+1.96*stderr);
/* print estimates etc. */
proc print;
var parm oddsrat lower upper;
/* reverse levels for SEX and refit model etc.*/
data two;
set shhs;
sex2 = 3-sex;
proc genmod;
class sex2;
make 'parmest' out = nextfile;
model chd/one = sex2 bortner sex2*bortner/dist = bin
   link = logit;
data neworder;
set nextfile;
oddsrat = exp(estimate);
lower = exp(estimate-1.96*stderr);
upper = exp(estimate+1.96*stderr);
proc print;
var parm oddsrat lower upper;
run;
```

**Example 10.23 Logistic regression with residual analysis (creates Table 10.36)**

```
data shhs;
/* read in the data */
input age e n;
cards;
40   1 251
41 12 317
...
59 49 302
;
/* fit the explanatory variable AGE */
proc genmod;
/* use the MAKE command to store residuals etc. in a new
   file: this makes RESRAW the raw residual, RESDEV the
   deviance residual and PRED the predicted value with
   standard deviation STD */
```

```
make 'obstats' out = newfile;
model e/n = age/link = logit dist = bin obstats;
/* combine data and residuals in another file */
data diagnose;
set shhs;
set newfile;
/* compute the leverage */
h = n*pred*(1-pred)*std*std;
/* compute the standardized residuals */
resstand = resdev/sqrt(1-h);
/* compute the expected number of deaths */
expected = n*pred;
/* print out Table 10.36 */
proc print;
var age e expected resraw resdev resstand;
run;
```

**Example 10.25  Logistic regression for an unmatched case–control study**

```
data autier;
/* read in the data */
input protect cases n;
cards;
1   99 231
0 303 593
;
/* fit empty model */
proc genmod;
model cases/n = /dist = bin link = logit;

/* fit explanatory variable PROTECT and save estimates
    etc. */
proc genmod;
make 'parmest' out = newfile;
model cases/n = protect/dist = bin link = logit;
data results;
set newfile;
oddsrat = exp(estimate);
lower = exp(estimate-1.96*stderr);
upper = exp(estimate+1.96*stderr);
proc print;
var parm oddsrat lower upper;
run;
```

**Example 10.27  Logistic regression for a matched case–control study**

```
data ddimer;
/* read in the data from a file */
infile '\woodward\ddimer.dat';
input setno cc ddimer SBP;
/* set up SWITCH as 2 for controls, 1 for cases */
switch = 2;
if cc = 1 then switch = 1;
/* fit stratified Cox regression models with TIES = DIS-
   CRETE option: here SETNO defines the strata, SWITCH
   takes the place of the survival time and CC becomes the
   censoring variable, with a control outcome as censored
   */
/* fit DDIMER, printing estimates etc. using the risk
   limits (RL) subcommand */
proc phreg;
model switch*cc(0) = ddimer/ties = discrete rl;
strata setno;
/* fit SBP */
proc phreg;
model switch*cc(0) = SBP/ties = discrete;
strata setno;
/* fit SBP and DDIMER, printing estimates etc. */
proc phreg;
model switch*cc(0) = SBP ddimer/ties = discrete rl;
strata setno;
run;
```

**Example 10.29  Proportional odds model with a binary explanatory variable (creates Output 10.6)**

```
data shhs;
/* read in the data */
input parnts chdgrade count;
cards;
1 1  104
1 2   17
1 3   45
1 4  830
0 1  192
0 2   30
0 3  122
0 4 3376
;
```

```
/* fit proportional odds regression model */
proc logistic;
weight count;
model chdgrade = parnts;
run;
```

**Example 11.1  Kaplan–Meier estimation and survival plot (creates a similar plot to Figure 11.2)**

```
data karkavel;
/* read in the data */
input weeks;
cards;
120
104
...
10
;
/* find KM estimates and plot them */
proc lifetest plots = (s);
time weeks;
run;
```

**Example 11.5  Fitting a Weibull distribution**

```
data karkavel;
/* read in the data */
input weeks;
cards;
120
104
...
10
;
/* fit a Weibull distribution (a regression with no ex-
   planatory variables) */
proc lifereg;
model weeks = ;
run;
```

**Example 11.7  Cox regression with a binary explanatory variable (creates Output 11.1)**

```
data karkavel;
/* read in the data */
input weeks cellular;
cards;
120 1
104 1
...
10 2
;
/* fit Cox model and print hazard ratios etc. using the risk
   limits (RL) subcommand */
proc phreg;
model weeks = cellular/rl;
run;
```

**Example 11.8  Cox multiple regression selection (creates Table 11.2 and Output 11.2)**

```
data shhs;
/* read in the data from a file */
infile '\woodward\sbpchol.dat';
input chol5th sbp5th chd days;
/* set up two sets of dummy variables */
chol2 = (chol5th = 2);
chol3 = (chol5th = 3);
chol4 = (chol5th = 4);
chol5 = (chol5th = 5);
sbp2 = (sbp5th = 2);
sbp3 = (sbp5th = 3);
sbp4 = (sbp5th = 4);
sbp5 = (sbp5th = 5);
/* fit all possible (non-empty) regression models where
   censoring occurs when CHD = 0 */
proc phreg;
model days*CHD(0) = sbp2 sbp3 sbp4 sbp5;
proc phreg;
model days*CHD(0) = chol2 chol3 chol4 chol5;
/* print estimates of hazard ratio etc. for best model */
proc phreg;
model days*CHD(0) = sbp2 sbp3 sbp4 sbp5 chol2 chol3 chol4
   chol5/rl;
run;
```

**Example 11.9 Cox regression with an ordinal explanatory variable (creates Output 11.3)**

```
data shhs;
/* read in the data from a file (includes CHOL5TH which is
   not used here) */
infile '\woodward\sbpchol.dat';
input chol5th sbp5th chd days;
/* fit model for linear effect where censoring occurs when
   CHD = 0 */
proc phreg;
model days*chd(0) = sbp5th/rl;
run;
```

**Example 11.11 Cox regression with categorical–categorical interaction (creates Outputs 11.5 and 11.6 and is used in Table 11.4 (model 4) and Table 11.5)**

```
data shhs;
/* read in the data from a file (includes BORTNER which is
   not used here) */
infile '\woodward\bortner.dat';
input sex bortner bort4th chd days;
/* define dummy variables for Bortner quarter */
bort2 = (bort4th = 2);
bort3 = (bort4th = 3);
bort4 = (bort4th = 4);
/* define dummy variable for sex */
sex1 = (sex = 1);
/* define interaction terms */
bor2sex1 = bort2*sex1;
bor3sex1 = bort3*sex1;
bor4sex1 = bort4*sex1;
/* fit model with interaction where censoring occurs when
   CHD = 0 */
proc phreg;
model days*chd(0) = bort2 bort3 bort4 sex1 bor2sex1
   bor3sex1 bor4sex1/rl;
/* refit the model with the sex term reversed */
data two;
set shhs;
/* define reversed terms */
sex2 = 1-sex1;
bor2sex2 = bort2*sex2;
bor3sex2 = bort3*sex2;
```

```
bor4sex2 = bort4*sex2;
/* fit model with interaction where censoring occurs when
   CHD = 0 */
proc phreg;
model days*chd(0) = bort2 bort3 bort4 sex2 bor2sex2
   bor3sex2 bor4sex2/rl;
run;
```

**Example 11.12 Cox regression with categorical–quantitative interaction (creates Output 11.7 and is used in Table 11.6 model 4)**

```
data shhs;
/* read in the data from a file (includes BORT4TH which is
   not used here) */
infile '\woodward\bortner.dat';
input sex bortner bort4th chd days;
/* define a dummy variable for sex and the interaction term
   */
sex1 = (sex = 1);
bortsex1 = bortner*sex1;
/* fit model with interaction where censoring occcurs when
   CHD = 0 */
proc phreg;
/* include variance-covariance matrix using COVB */
model days*chd(0) = bortner sex1 bortsex1 /rl covb;
run;
```

**Example 11.13 Weibull regression with a categorical explanatory variable (creates Output 11.8 and is used to produce Figure 11.12)**

```
data karkavel;
*\ read in the data: note that CELLULAR is read with
   reversed codes here compared with Example 11.7 because
   a CLASS statement is used in the subsequent data analy-
   sis */
input weeks cellular;
cards;
120 2
104 2
...
10 1
;
```

```
/* fit Weibull model with categorical variable CELLULAR */
proc lifereg;
class cellular;
/* include variance-covariance matrix using COVB */
model weeks = cellular/covb;
run;
```

**Example 11.14  Weibull multiple regression (creates Output 11.9)**

```
data shhs;
/* read in the data from a file */
infile '\woodward\multshhs.dat';
input age totchol bmi systol smoking activity chd days;
/* reset the first level of each categorical variable to be
   the last */
if activity = 1 then activity = 4;
if smoking = 1 then smoking = 4;
/* fit Weibull regression where censoring occurs when
   CHD = 0 */
proc lifereg;
class activity smoking;
model days*chd(0) = age totchol bmi systol smoking
   activity;
run;
```

**Example 11.16  Log cumulative hazard plot (creates a similar plot to Figure 11.14)**

```
data karkavel;
*\ read in the data */
input weeks cellular;
cards;
120 1
104 1
...
10 2
;
/* find K-M estimates and produce LCH plot: note that log-
   rank and generalized Wilcoxon tests will also be
   applied */
proc lifetest plots = (lls);
time weeks;
strata cellular;
run;
```

**Example 11.18  Cox regression with a time-dependent covariate**

```
data karkavel;
*\ read in the data */
input weeks cellular;
cards;
120 1
104 1
...
10 2
;
/* fit Cox model without the time-dependent covariate */
proc phreg;
model weeks = cellular;
/* fit Cox model with the time-dependent covariate,
   computed as TIMEDEP */
proc phreg;
timedep = cellular*weeks;
model weeks = cellular timedep;
run;
```

**Example 11.20  Poisson regression with a binary variable (creates Output 11.10)**

```
data shhs;
/* read in the data and compute logs of person-years */
input tenure events py;
logpy = log(py);
cards;
1 115 14200.945
2 104 18601.467
;
/* fit Poisson regression model with categorical variable
   TENURE */
proc genmod;
class tenure;
/* also print variance-covariance matrix using COVB */
model events = tenure/dist = poisson link = log
   offset = logpy covb;
run;
```

**Example 11.21  Poisson regression including confounding and interaction (creates Output 11.11)**

```
data shhs;
/* read in the data and compute logs of person-years */
```

```
input age tenure events py;
logpy = log(py);
cards;
1 1 2 1107.447
1 2 3 1619.328
. . .
6 2 4 356.394
;
/* fit Poisson regression models, adding terms one at a
   time */
proc genmod;
model events = /dist = poisson link = log offset = logpy;
proc genmod;
class age;
model events = age/dist = poisson link = log
   offset = logpy;
proc genmod;
class age tenure;
model events = age tenure/dist = poisson link = log
   offset = logpy;
proc genmod;
class age tenure;
model events = age tenure age*tenure/dist = poisson
   link = log offset = logpy;
/* after deciding on the best model, refit it and get SAS to
   compute the relative rates and 95% confidence intervals
   using the MAKE command, putting results to a new file */
proc genmod;
class age tenure;
make 'parmest' out = newfile;
model events = age tenure/dist = poisson link = log
   offset = logpy;
/* read in the new file */
data results;
set newfile;
/* make RELRATE the relative rate, LOWER and UPPER the
   confidence limits */
relrate = exp(estimate);
lower = exp(estimate-1.96*stderr);
upper = exp(estimate+1.96*stderr);
/* print out results */
proc print;
var parm relrate lower upper;
run;
```

**Example 11.22  Poisson regression to compare standardized event ratios (creates Output 11.12)**

```
data chemical;
/* read in the data and compute logs of the expected numbers
    */
input company observed expected;
logE = log(expected);
cards;
0 43 38.755
1  4  1.488
;
/* fit the empty and full models */
proc genmod;
model observed = /dist = poisson link = log offset = logE;
proc genmod;
class company;
/* use MAKE as in last example */
make 'parmest' out = newfile;
model observed = company/dist = poisson link = log
    offset = logE;
/* read in the new file */
data results;
set newfile;
/* make RELRATE the relative rate, LOWER and UPPER the
    confidence limits */
relrate = exp(estimate);
lower = exp(estimate-1.96*stderr);
upper = exp(estimate+1.96*stderr);
/* print out results */
proc print;
var parm relrate lower upper;
run;
```

**Example 11.23  Poisson regression selection with registration data (creates Output 11.13 and Tables 11.10, 11.11 (left) and 11.12)**

```
data monica;
/* read in the data and compute the logs of the population
    sizes */
input age dep pop events;
logpop = log(pop);
/* define DEPGP to have the first level of DEPGP as its last
    level */
```

```
depgp = dep;
if dep = 1 then depgp = 5;
/* define polynomial terms */
dep2 = dep**2;
dep3 = dep**3;
/* here come the data */
cards;
1 1 47840
1 2 49720
1 3 43510
1 4 44400
2 1 42100
2 2 40450
...
8 4 2380 56
;
/* fit null model */
proc genmod;
model events = /dist = Poisson link = log offset = logpop;
/* fit the risk factor only */
proc genmod;
class depgp;
model events = depgp/dist = Poisson link = log
    offset = logpop;
/* fit the confounder only */
proc genmod;
class age;
model events = age/dist = Poisson link = log
    offset = logpop;
/* fit the confounder plus the risk factor: MAKE is used to
    produce the left-hand side of Table 11.11 */
proc genmod;
class age depgp;
make 'parmest' out = newfile;
model events = age depgp/dist = Poisson link = log
    offset = logpop;
/* read in the new file */
data results;
set newfile;
/* make RELRATE the relative rate, LOWER and UPPER the
    confidence limits */
relrate = exp(estimate);
lower = exp(estimate-1.96*stderr);
upper = exp(estimate+1.96*stderr);
/* print out results */
proc print;
```

```
var parm relrate lower upper;
/* explore the polynomial effects of DEP, adjusted for
   AGE: note that the DATA = statement refers back to the
   'old' file */
proc genmod data = monica;
class age;
model events = age dep/dist = Poisson link = log
   offset = logpop;
proc genmod data = monica;
class age;
model events = age dep dep2/dist = Poisson link = log
   offset = logpop;
proc genmod data = monica;
class age;
model events = age dep dep2 dep3/ dist = Poisson link = log
   offset = logpop;
run;
```

# Appendix B
# Statistical tables

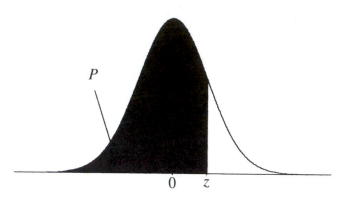

**Table B.1**  The standard normal distribution
The normal distribution with mean 0 and standard deviation 1 is tabulated below. For each value $z$, the quantity given is the proportion $P$ of the distribution less than $z$. For a normal distribution, with mean $\mu$ and variance $\sigma^2$, the proportion of the distribution less than some value $x$, is obtained by calculating $z = (x - \mu)/\sigma$ and reading off the proportion corresponding to this value of $z$.

| $z$ | $P$ | $z$ | $P$ | $z$ | $P$ | $z$ | $P$ | $z$ | $P$ | $z$ | $P$ |
|---|---|---|---|---|---|---|---|---|---|---|---|
| −4.00 | 0.00003 | −2.05 | 0.0202 | −1.00 | 0.1587 | 0.00 | 0.5000 | 1.05 | 0.8531 | 2.10 | 0.9821 |
| −3.50 | 0.00023 | −2.00 | 0.0228 | −0.95 | 0.1711 | 0.05 | 0.5199 | 1.10 | 0.8643 | 2.15 | 0.9842 |
| −3.00 | 0.0013 | −1.95 | 0.0256 | −0.90 | 0.1841 | 0.10 | 0.5398 | 1.15 | 0.8749 | 2.20 | 0.9861 |
| −2.95 | 0.0016 | −1.90 | 0.0287 | −0.85 | 0.1977 | 0.15 | 0.5596 | 1.20 | 0.8849 | 2.25 | 0.9878 |
| −2.90 | 0.0019 | −1.85 | 0.0322 | −0.80 | 0.2119 | 0.20 | 0.5793 | 1.25 | 0.8944 | 2.30 | 0.9893 |
| −2.85 | 0.0022 | −1.80 | 0.0359 | −0.75 | 0.2266 | 0.25 | 0.5987 | 1.30 | 0.9032 | 2.35 | 0.9906 |
| −2.80 | 0.0026 | −1.75 | 0.0401 | −0.70 | 0.2420 | 0.30 | 0.6179 | 1.35 | 0.9115 | 2.40 | 0.9918 |
| −2.75 | 0.0030 | −1.70 | 0.0446 | −0.65 | 0.2578 | 0.35 | 0.6368 | 1.40 | 0.9192 | 2.45 | 0.9929 |
| −2.70 | 0.0035 | −1.65 | 0.0495 | −0.60 | 0.2743 | 0.40 | 0.6554 | 1.45 | 0.9265 | 2.50 | 0.9938 |
| −2.65 | 0.0040 | −1.60 | 0.0548 | −0.55 | 0.2912 | 0.45 | 0.6736 | 1.50 | 0.9332 | 2.55 | 0.9946 |
| −2.60 | 0.0047 | −1.55 | 0.0606 | −0.50 | 0.3085 | 0.50 | 0.6915 | 1.55 | 0.9394 | 2.60 | 0.9953 |
| −2.55 | 0.0054 | −1.50 | 0.0668 | −0.45 | 0.3264 | 0.55 | 0.7088 | 1.60 | 0.9452 | 2.65 | 0.9960 |
| −2.50 | 0.0062 | −1.45 | 0.0735 | −0.40 | 0.3446 | 0.60 | 0.7257 | 1.65 | 0.9505 | 2.70 | 0.9965 |
| −2.45 | 0.0071 | −1.40 | 0.0808 | −0.35 | 0.3632 | 0.65 | 0.7422 | 1.70 | 0.9554 | 2.75 | 0.9970 |
| −2.40 | 0.0082 | −1.35 | 0.0885 | −0.30 | 0.3821 | 0.70 | 0.7580 | 1.75 | 0.9599 | 2.80 | 0.9974 |
| −2.35 | 0.0094 | −1.30 | 0.0968 | −0.25 | 0.4013 | 0.75 | 0.7734 | 1.80 | 0.9641 | 2.85 | 0.9978 |
| −2.30 | 0.0107 | −1.25 | 0.1056 | −0.20 | 0.4207 | 0.80 | 0.7881 | 1.85 | 0.9678 | 2.90 | 0.9981 |
| −2.25 | 0.0122 | −1.20 | 0.1151 | −0.15 | 0.4404 | 0.85 | 0.8023 | 1.90 | 0.9713 | 2.95 | 0.9984 |
| −2.20 | 0.0139 | −1.15 | 0.1251 | −0.10 | 0.4602 | 0.90 | 0.8159 | 1.95 | 0.9744 | 3.00 | 0.9987 |
| −2.15 | 0.0158 | −1.10 | 0.1357 | −0.05 | 0.4801 | 0.95 | 0.8289 | 2.00 | 0.9772 | 3.50 | 0.99977 |
| −2.10 | 0.0179 | −1.05 | 0.1469 | 0.00 | 0.5000 | 1.00 | 0.8413 | 2.05 | 0.9798 | 4.00 | 0.99997 |

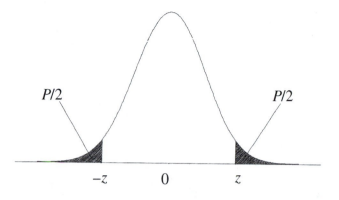

**Table B.2**  Critical values for the standard normal distribution.
This table gives (two-sided) critical values for the standard normal distribution. These are the values of $z$ for which a given percentage, $P$, of the standard normal distribution lies outside the range from $-z$ to $+z$

| $P$ | $z$ |
|---|---|
| 90 | 0.1257 |
| 80 | 0.2533 |
| 70 | 0.3853 |
| 60 | 0.5244 |
| 50 | 0.6745 |
| 40 | 0.8416 |
| 30 | 1.0364 |
| 20 | 1.2816 |
| 15 | 1.4395 |
| 10 | 1.6449 |
| 5 | 1.9600 |
| 2 | 2.3263 |
| 1 | 2.5758 |
| 0.2 | 3.0902 |
| 0.1 | 3.2905 |
| 0.02 | 3.7190 |
| 0.01 | 3.8906 |

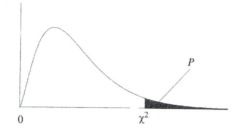

**Table B.3**  Critical values for the chi-square distribution
This table gives (one-sided) critical values for the chi-square distribution with $v$ degrees of freedom. These are the values of $\chi^2$ for which a given percentage, $P$, of the chi-square distribution is greater than $\chi^2$.

| P | 97.5 | 95 | 50 | 10 | 5 | 2.5 | 1 | 0.1 |
|---|------|------|------|------|------|------|------|------|
| $v = 1$ | 0.000982 | 0.00393 | 0.45 | 2.71 | 3.84 | 5.02 | 6.64 | 10.8 |
| 2 | 0.0506 | 0.103 | 1.39 | 4.61 | 5.99 | 7.38 | 9.21 | 13.8 |
| 3 | 0.216 | 0.352 | 2.37 | 6.25 | 7.81 | 9.35 | 11.3 | 16.3 |
| 4 | 0.484 | 0.711 | 3.36 | 7.78 | 9.49 | 11.1 | 13.3 | 18.5 |
| 5 | 0.831 | 1.15 | 4.35 | 9.24 | 11.1 | 12.8 | 15.1 | 20.5 |
| 6 | 1.24 | 1.64 | 5.35 | 10.6 | 12.6 | 14.5 | 16.8 | 22.5 |
| 7 | 1.69 | 2.17 | 6.35 | 12.0 | 14.1 | 16.0 | 18.5 | 24.3 |
| 8 | 2.18 | 2.73 | 7.34 | 13.4 | 15.5 | 17.5 | 20.1 | 26.1 |
| 9 | 2.70 | 3.33 | 8.34 | 14.7 | 16.9 | 19.0 | 21.7 | 27.9 |
| 10 | 3.25 | 3.94 | 9.34 | 16.0 | 18.3 | 20.5 | 23.2 | 29.6 |
| 11 | 3.82 | 4.57 | 10.3 | 17.3 | 19.7 | 21.9 | 24.7 | 31.3 |
| 12 | 4.40 | 5.23 | 11.3 | 18.5 | 21.0 | 23.3 | 26.2 | 32.9 |
| 13 | 5.01 | 5.89 | 12.3 | 19.8 | 22.4 | 24.7 | 27.7 | 34.5 |
| 14 | 5.63 | 6.57 | 13.3 | 21.1 | 23.7 | 26.1 | 29.1 | 36.1 |
| 15 | 6.26 | 7.26 | 14.3 | 22.3 | 25.0 | 27.5 | 30.6 | 37.7 |
| 16 | 6.91 | 7.96 | 15.3 | 23.5 | 26.3 | 28.8 | 32.0 | 39.3 |
| 17 | 7.56 | 8.67 | 16.3 | 24.8 | 27.6 | 30.2 | 33.4 | 40.8 |
| 18 | 8.23 | 9.39 | 17.3 | 26.0 | 28.9 | 31.5 | 34.8 | 42.3 |
| 19 | 8.91 | 10.1 | 18.3 | 27.2 | 30.1 | 32.9 | 36.2 | 43.8 |
| 20 | 9.59 | 10.9 | 19.3 | 28.4 | 31.4 | 34.2 | 37.6 | 45.3 |
| 22 | 11.0 | 12.3 | 21.3 | 30.8 | 33.9 | 36.8 | 40.3 | 48.3 |
| 24 | 12.4 | 13.9 | 23.3 | 33.2 | 36.4 | 39.4 | 43.0 | 51.2 |
| 26 | 13.8 | 15.4 | 25.3 | 35.6 | 38.9 | 41.9 | 45.6 | 54.1 |
| 28 | 15.3 | 16.9 | 27.3 | 37.9 | 41.3 | 44.5 | 48.3 | 56.9 |
| 30 | 16.8 | 18.5 | 29.3 | 40.3 | 43.8 | 47.0 | 50.9 | 59.7 |
| 35 | 20.6 | 22.5 | 34.3 | 46.1 | 49.8 | 53.2 | 57.3 | 66.6 |
| 40 | 24.4 | 26.5 | 39.3 | 51.8 | 55.8 | 59.3 | 63.7 | 73.4 |
| 45 | 28.4 | 30.6 | 44.3 | 57.5 | 61.7 | 65.4 | 70.0 | 80.1 |
| 50 | 32.4 | 34.8 | 49.3 | 63.2 | 67.5 | 71.4 | 76.2 | 86.7 |
| 55 | 36.4 | 39.0 | 54.3 | 68.8 | 73.3 | 77.4 | 82.3 | 93.2 |
| 60 | 40.5 | 43.2 | 59.3 | 74.4 | 79.1 | 83.3 | 88.4 | 99.7 |

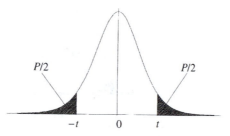

**Table B.4**   Critical values for Student's $t$ distribution
This table gives (two-sided) critical values for the $t$ distribution on $v$ degrees of freedom. These are the values of $t$ for which a given percentage, $P$, of the $t$ distribution lies outside the range $-t$ to $+t$. As the number of degrees of freedom increases, the distribution becomes closer to the standard normal distribution.

| $P$ | 50 | 20 | 10 | 5 | 2 | 1 | 0.2 | 0.1 |
|---|---|---|---|---|---|---|---|---|
| $v = 1$ | 1.00 | 3.08 | 6.31 | 12.7 | 31.8 | 63.7 | 318 | 637 |
| 2 | 0.82 | 1.89 | 2.92 | 4.30 | 6.96 | 9.92 | 22.3 | 31.6 |
| 3 | 0.76 | 1.64 | 2.35 | 3.18 | 4.54 | 5.84 | 10.2 | 12.9 |
| 4 | 0.74 | 1.53 | 2.13 | 2.78 | 3.75 | 4.60 | 7.17 | 8.61 |
| 5 | 0.73 | 1.48 | 2.02 | 2.57 | 3.36 | 4.03 | 5.89 | 6.87 |
| 6 | 0.72 | 1.44 | 1.94 | 2.45 | 3.14 | 3.71 | 5.21 | 5.96 |
| 7 | 0.71 | 1.42 | 1.89 | 2.36 | 3.00 | 3.50 | 4.79 | 5.41 |
| 8 | 0.71 | 1.40 | 1.86 | 2.31 | 2.90 | 3.36 | 4.50 | 5.04 |
| 9 | 0.70 | 1.38 | 1.83 | 2.26 | 2.82 | 3.25 | 4.30 | 4.78 |
| 10 | 0.70 | 1.37 | 1.81 | 2.23 | 2.76 | 3.17 | 4.14 | 4.59 |
| 11 | 0.70 | 1.36 | 1.80 | 2.20 | 2.72 | 3.11 | 4.03 | 4.44 |
| 12 | 0.70 | 1.36 | 1.78 | 2.18 | 2.68 | 3.05 | 3.93 | 4.32 |
| 13 | 0.69 | 1.35 | 1.77 | 2.16 | 2.65 | 3.01 | 3.85 | 4.22 |
| 14 | 0.69 | 1.35 | 1.76 | 2.14 | 2.62 | 2.98 | 3.79 | 4.14 |
| 15 | 0.69 | 1.34 | 1.75 | 2.13 | 2.60 | 2.95 | 3.73 | 4.07 |
| 16 | 0.69 | 1.34 | 1.75 | 2.12 | 2.58 | 2.92 | 3.69 | 4.01 |
| 17 | 0.69 | 1.33 | 1.74 | 2.11 | 2.57 | 2.90 | 3.65 | 3.96 |
| 18 | 0.69 | 1.33 | 1.73 | 2.10 | 2.55 | 2.88 | 3.61 | 3.92 |
| 19 | 0.69 | 1.33 | 1.73 | 2.09 | 2.54 | 2.86 | 3.58 | 3.88 |
| 20 | 0.69 | 1.32 | 1.72 | 2.09 | 2.53 | 2.85 | 3.55 | 3.85 |
| 22 | 0.69 | 1.32 | 1.72 | 2.07 | 2.51 | 2.82 | 3.51 | 3.79 |
| 24 | 0.68 | 1.32 | 1.71 | 2.06 | 2.49 | 2.80 | 3.47 | 3.75 |
| 26 | 0.68 | 1.32 | 1.71 | 2.06 | 2.48 | 2.78 | 3.44 | 3.71 |
| 28 | 0.68 | 1.31 | 1.70 | 2.05 | 2.47 | 2.76 | 3.41 | 3.67 |
| 30 | 0.68 | 1.31 | 1.70 | 2.04 | 2.46 | 2.75 | 3.39 | 3.65 |
| 35 | 0.68 | 1.31 | 1.69 | 2.03 | 2.44 | 2.72 | 3.34 | 3.59 |
| 40 | 0.68 | 1.30 | 1.68 | 2.02 | 2.42 | 2.70 | 3.31 | 3.55 |
| 45 | 0.68 | 1.30 | 1.68 | 2.01 | 2.41 | 2.69 | 3.28 | 3.52 |
| 50 | 0.68 | 1.30 | 1.68 | 2.01 | 2.40 | 2.68 | 3.26 | 3.50 |
| 55 | 0.68 | 1.30 | 1.67 | 2.00 | 2.40 | 2.67 | 3.25 | 3.48 |
| 60 | 0.68 | 1.30 | 1.67 | 2.00 | 2.39 | 2.66 | 3.23 | 3.46 |
| $\infty$ | 0.67 | 1.28 | 1.64 | 1.96 | 2.33 | 2.58 | 3.09 | 3.29 |

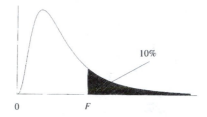

**Table B.5**   Critical values for the $F$ distribution
These tables give (one-sided) critical values of the $F$ distribution. In each sub-table, the percentage
of the $F$ distribution in the title is above the tabulated $F$ value.
   The $F$ distribution arises from the ratio of two independent estimates of variance; $v_1$ and $v_2$ are
(respectively) the degrees of freedom of the estimates in the numerator and denominator.
(a) 10% critical values

| $v_1$ | 1 | 2 | 3 | 4 | 5 | 6 | 7 | 8 | 10 | 12 | 24 |
|---|---|---|---|---|---|---|---|---|---|---|---|
| $v_2 = 2$ | 8.53 | 9.00 | 9.16 | 9.24 | 9.29 | 9.33 | 9.35 | 9.37 | 9.39 | 9.41 | 9.45 |
| 3 | 5.54 | 5.46 | 5.39 | 5.34 | 5.31 | 5.28 | 5.27 | 5.25 | 5.23 | 5.22 | 5.18 |
| 4 | 4.54 | 4.32 | 4.19 | 4.11 | 4.05 | 4.01 | 3.98 | 3.95 | 3.92 | 3.90 | 3.83 |
| 5 | 4.06 | 3.78 | 3.62 | 3.52 | 3.45 | 3.40 | 3.37 | 3.34 | 3.30 | 3.27 | 3.19 |
| 6 | 3.78 | 3.46 | 3.29 | 3.18 | 3.11 | 3.05 | 3.01 | 2.98 | 2.94 | 2.90 | 2.82 |
| 7 | 3.59 | 3.26 | 3.07 | 2.96 | 2.88 | 2.83 | 2.78 | 2.75 | 2.70 | 2.67 | 2.58 |
| 8 | 3.46 | 3.11 | 2.92 | 2.81 | 2.73 | 2.67 | 2.62 | 2.59 | 2.54 | 2.50 | 2.40 |
| 9 | 3.36 | 3.01 | 2.81 | 2.69 | 2.61 | 2.55 | 2.51 | 2.47 | 2.42 | 2.38 | 2.28 |
| 10 | 3.28 | 2.92 | 2.73 | 2.61 | 2.52 | 2.46 | 2.41 | 2.38 | 2.32 | 2.28 | 2.18 |
| 11 | 3.23 | 2.86 | 2.66 | 2.54 | 2.45 | 2.39 | 2.34 | 2.30 | 2.25 | 2.21 | 2.10 |
| 12 | 3.18 | 2.81 | 2.61 | 2.48 | 2.39 | 2.33 | 2.28 | 2.24 | 2.19 | 2.15 | 2.04 |
| 13 | 3.14 | 2.76 | 2.56 | 2.43 | 2.35 | 2.28 | 2.23 | 2.20 | 2.14 | 2.10 | 1.98 |
| 14 | 3.10 | 2.73 | 2.52 | 2.39 | 2.31 | 2.24 | 2.19 | 2.15 | 2.10 | 2.05 | 1.94 |
| 15 | 3.07 | 2.70 | 2.49 | 2.36 | 2.27 | 2.21 | 2.16 | 2.12 | 2.06 | 2.02 | 1.90 |
| 16 | 3.05 | 2.67 | 2.46 | 2.33 | 2.24 | 2.18 | 2.13 | 2.09 | 2.03 | 1.99 | 1.87 |
| 17 | 3.03 | 2.64 | 2.44 | 2.31 | 2.22 | 2.15 | 2.10 | 2.06 | 2.00 | 1.96 | 1.84 |
| 18 | 3.01 | 2.62 | 2.42 | 2.29 | 2.20 | 2.13 | 2.08 | 2.04 | 1.98 | 1.93 | 1.81 |
| 19 | 2.99 | 2.61 | 2.40 | 2.27 | 2.18 | 2.11 | 2.06 | 2.02 | 1.96 | 1.91 | 1.79 |
| 20 | 2.97 | 2.59 | 2.38 | 2.25 | 2.16 | 2.09 | 2.04 | 2.00 | 1.94 | 1.89 | 1.77 |
| 22 | 2.95 | 2.56 | 2.35 | 2.22 | 2.13 | 2.06 | 2.01 | 1.97 | 1.90 | 1.86 | 1.73 |
| 24 | 2.93 | 2.54 | 2.33 | 2.19 | 2.10 | 2.04 | 1.98 | 1.94 | 1.88 | 1.83 | 1.70 |
| 26 | 2.91 | 2.52 | 2.31 | 2.17 | 2.08 | 2.01 | 1.96 | 1.92 | 1.86 | 1.81 | 1.68 |
| 28 | 2.89 | 2.50 | 2.29 | 2.16 | 2.06 | 2.00 | 1.94 | 1.90 | 1.84 | 1.79 | 1.66 |
| 30 | 2.88 | 2.49 | 2.28 | 2.14 | 2.05 | 1.98 | 1.93 | 1.88 | 1.82 | 1.77 | 1.64 |
| 35 | 2.85 | 2.46 | 2.25 | 2.11 | 2.02 | 1.95 | 1.90 | 1.85 | 1.79 | 1.74 | 1.60 |
| 40 | 2.84 | 2.44 | 2.23 | 2.09 | 2.00 | 1.93 | 1.87 | 1.83 | 1.76 | 1.71 | 1.57 |
| 45 | 2.82 | 2.42 | 2.21 | 2.07 | 1.98 | 1.91 | 1.85 | 1.81 | 1.74 | 1.70 | 1.55 |
| 50 | 2.81 | 2.41 | 2.20 | 2.06 | 1.97 | 1.90 | 1.84 | 1.80 | 1.73 | 1.68 | 1.54 |
| 55 | 2.80 | 2.40 | 2.19 | 2.05 | 1.95 | 1.88 | 1.83 | 1.78 | 1.72 | 1.67 | 1.52 |
| 60 | 2.79 | 2.39 | 2.18 | 2.04 | 1.95 | 1.87 | 1.82 | 1.77 | 1.71 | 1.66 | 1.51 |

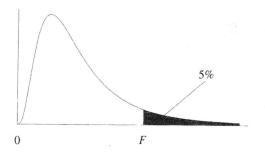

0    F

5%

(b) 5% critical values

| $v_1$ | 1 | 2 | 3 | 4 | 5 | 6 | 7 | 8 | 10 | 12 | 24 |
|---|---|---|---|---|---|---|---|---|---|---|---|
| $v_2 = 2$ | 18.5 | 19.0 | 19.2 | 19.2 | 19.3 | 19.3 | 19.4 | 19.4 | 19.4 | 19.4 | 19.5 |
| 3 | 10.1 | 9.55 | 9.28 | 9.12 | 9.01 | 8.94 | 8.89 | 8.85 | 8.79 | 8.74 | 8.64 |
| 4 | 7.71 | 6.94 | 6.59 | 6.39 | 6.26 | 6.16 | 6.09 | 6.04 | 5.96 | 5.91 | 5.77 |
| 5 | 6.61 | 5.79 | 5.41 | 5.19 | 5.05 | 4.95 | 4.88 | 4.82 | 4.74 | 4.68 | 4.53 |
| 6 | 5.99 | 5.14 | 4.76 | 4.53 | 4.39 | 4.28 | 4.21 | 4.15 | 4.06 | 4.00 | 3.84 |
| 7 | 5.59 | 4.74 | 4.35 | 4.12 | 3.97 | 3.87 | 3.79 | 3.73 | 3.64 | 3.57 | 3.41 |
| 8 | 5.32 | 4.46 | 4.07 | 3.84 | 3.69 | 3.58 | 3.50 | 3.44 | 3.35 | 3.28 | 3.12 |
| 9 | 5.12 | 4.26 | 3.86 | 3.63 | 3.48 | 3.37 | 3.29 | 3.23 | 3.14 | 3.07 | 2.90 |
| 10 | 4.96 | 4.10 | 3.71 | 3.48 | 3.33 | 3.22 | 3.14 | 3.07 | 2.98 | 2.91 | 2.74 |
| 11 | 4.84 | 3.98 | 3.59 | 3.36 | 3.20 | 3.09 | 3.01 | 2.95 | 2.85 | 2.79 | 2.61 |
| 12 | 4.75 | 3.89 | 3.49 | 3.26 | 3.11 | 3.00 | 2.91 | 2.85 | 2.75 | 2.69 | 2.51 |
| 13 | 4.67 | 3.81 | 3.41 | 3.18 | 3.03 | 2.92 | 2.83 | 2.77 | 2.67 | 2.60 | 2.42 |
| 14 | 4.60 | 3.74 | 3.34 | 3.11 | 2.96 | 2.85 | 2.76 | 2.70 | 2.60 | 2.53 | 2.35 |
| 15 | 4.54 | 3.68 | 3.29 | 3.06 | 2.90 | 2.79 | 2.71 | 2.64 | 2.54 | 2.48 | 2.29 |
| 16 | 4.49 | 3.63 | 3.24 | 3.01 | 2.85 | 2.74 | 2.66 | 2.59 | 2.49 | 2.42 | 2.24 |
| 17 | 4.45 | 3.59 | 3.20 | 2.96 | 2.81 | 2.70 | 2.61 | 2.55 | 2.45 | 2.38 | 2.19 |
| 18 | 4.41 | 3.55 | 3.16 | 2.93 | 2.77 | 2.66 | 2.58 | 2.51 | 2.41 | 2.34 | 2.15 |
| 19 | 4.38 | 3.52 | 3.13 | 2.90 | 2.74 | 2.63 | 2.54 | 2.48 | 2.38 | 2.31 | 2.11 |
| 20 | 4.35 | 3.49 | 3.10 | 2.87 | 2.71 | 2.60 | 2.51 | 2.45 | 2.35 | 2.28 | 2.08 |
| 22 | 4.30 | 3.44 | 3.05 | 2.82 | 2.66 | 2.55 | 2.46 | 2.40 | 2.30 | 2.23 | 2.03 |
| 24 | 4.26 | 3.40 | 3.01 | 2.78 | 2.62 | 2.51 | 2.42 | 2.36 | 2.25 | 2.18 | 1.98 |
| 26 | 4.23 | 3.37 | 2.98 | 2.74 | 2.59 | 2.47 | 2.39 | 2.32 | 2.22 | 2.15 | 1.95 |
| 28 | 4.20 | 3.34 | 2.95 | 2.71 | 2.56 | 2.45 | 2.36 | 2.29 | 2.19 | 2.12 | 1.91 |
| 30 | 4.17 | 3.32 | 2.92 | 2.69 | 2.53 | 2.42 | 2.33 | 2.27 | 2.16 | 2.09 | 1.89 |
| 35 | 4.12 | 3.27 | 2.87 | 2.64 | 2.49 | 2.37 | 2.29 | 2.22 | 2.11 | 2.04 | 1.83 |
| 40 | 4.08 | 3.23 | 2.84 | 2.61 | 2.45 | 2.34 | 2.25 | 2.18 | 2.08 | 2.00 | 1.79 |
| 45 | 4.06 | 3.20 | 2.81 | 2.58 | 2.42 | 2.31 | 2.22 | 2.15 | 2.05 | 1.97 | 1.76 |
| 50 | 4.03 | 3.18 | 2.79 | 2.56 | 2.40 | 2.29 | 2.20 | 2.13 | 2.03 | 1.95 | 1.74 |
| 55 | 4.02 | 3.16 | 2.77 | 2.54 | 2.38 | 2.27 | 2.18 | 2.11 | 2.01 | 1.93 | 1.72 |
| 60 | 4.00 | 3.15 | 2.76 | 2.53 | 2.37 | 2.25 | 2.17 | 2.10 | 1.99 | 1.92 | 1.70 |

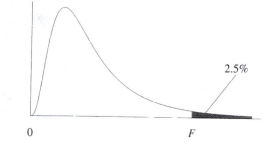

(c) 2.5% critical values

| $v_1$ | 1 | 2 | 3 | 4 | 5 | 6 | 7 | 8 | 10 | 12 | 24 |
|---|---|---|---|---|---|---|---|---|---|---|---|
| $v_2 = 2$ | 38.5 | 39.0 | 39.2 | 39.3 | 39.3 | 39.3 | 39.4 | 39.4 | 39.4 | 39.4 | 39.5 |
| 3 | 17.4 | 16.0 | 15.4 | 15.1 | 14.9 | 14.7 | 14.6 | 14.5 | 14.4 | 14.3 | 14.1 |
| 4 | 12.2 | 10.7 | 9.98 | 9.60 | 9.36 | 9.20 | 9.07 | 8.98 | 8.84 | 8.75 | 8.51 |
| 5 | 10.0 | 8.43 | 7.76 | 7.39 | 7.15 | 6.98 | 6.85 | 6.76 | 6.62 | 6.52 | 6.28 |
| 6 | 8.81 | 7.26 | 6.60 | 6.23 | 5.99 | 5.82 | 5.70 | 5.60 | 5.46 | 5.37 | 5.12 |
| 7 | 8.07 | 6.54 | 5.89 | 5.52 | 5.29 | 5.12 | 4.99 | 4.90 | 4.76 | 4.67 | 4.41 |
| 8 | 7.57 | 6.06 | 5.42 | 5.05 | 4.82 | 4.65 | 4.53 | 4.43 | 4.30 | 4.20 | 3.95 |
| 9 | 7.21 | 5.71 | 5.08 | 4.72 | 4.48 | 4.32 | 4.20 | 4.10 | 3.96 | 3.87 | 3.61 |
| 10 | 6.94 | 5.46 | 4.83 | 4.47 | 4.24 | 4.07 | 3.95 | 3.85 | 3.72 | 3.62 | 3.37 |
| 11 | 6.72 | 5.26 | 4.63 | 4.28 | 4.04 | 3.88 | 3.76 | 3.66 | 3.53 | 3.43 | 3.17 |
| 12 | 6.55 | 5.10 | 4.47 | 4.12 | 3.89 | 3.73 | 3.61 | 3.51 | 3.37 | 3.28 | 3.02 |
| 13 | 6.41 | 4.97 | 4.35 | 4.00 | 3.77 | 3.60 | 3.48 | 3.39 | 3.25 | 3.15 | 2.89 |
| 14 | 6.30 | 4.86 | 4.24 | 3.89 | 3.66 | 3.50 | 3.38 | 3.29 | 3.15 | 3.05 | 2.79 |
| 15 | 6.20 | 4.77 | 4.15 | 3.80 | 3.58 | 3.41 | 3.29 | 3.20 | 3.06 | 2.96 | 2.70 |
| 16 | 6.12 | 4.69 | 4.08 | 3.73 | 3.50 | 3.34 | 3.22 | 3.12 | 2.99 | 2.89 | 2.63 |
| 17 | 6.04 | 4.62 | 4.01 | 3.66 | 3.44 | 3.28 | 3.16 | 3.06 | 2.92 | 2.82 | 2.56 |
| 18 | 5.98 | 4.56 | 3.95 | 3.61 | 3.38 | 3.22 | 3.10 | 3.01 | 2.87 | 2.77 | 2.50 |
| 19 | 5.92 | 4.51 | 3.90 | 3.56 | 3.33 | 3.17 | 3.05 | 2.96 | 2.82 | 2.72 | 2.45 |
| 20 | 5.87 | 4.46 | 3.86 | 3.51 | 3.29 | 3.13 | 3.01 | 2.91 | 2.77 | 2.68 | 2.41 |
| 22 | 5.79 | 4.38 | 3.78 | 3.44 | 3.22 | 3.05 | 2.93 | 2.84 | 2.70 | 2.60 | 2.33 |
| 24 | 5.72 | 4.32 | 3.72 | 3.38 | 3.15 | 2.99 | 2.87 | 2.78 | 2.64 | 2.54 | 2.27 |
| 26 | 5.66 | 4.27 | 3.67 | 3.33 | 3.10 | 2.94 | 2.82 | 2.73 | 2.59 | 2.49 | 2.22 |
| 28 | 5.61 | 4.22 | 3.63 | 3.29 | 3.06 | 2.90 | 2.78 | 2.69 | 2.55 | 2.45 | 2.17 |
| 30 | 5.57 | 4.18 | 3.59 | 3.25 | 3.03 | 2.87 | 2.75 | 2.65 | 2.51 | 2.41 | 2.14 |
| 35 | 5.48 | 4.11 | 3.52 | 3.18 | 2.96 | 2.80 | 2.68 | 2.58 | 2.44 | 2.34 | 2.06 |
| 40 | 5.42 | 4.05 | 3.46 | 3.13 | 2.90 | 2.74 | 2.62 | 2.53 | 2.39 | 2.29 | 2.01 |
| 45 | 5.38 | 4.01 | 3.42 | 3.09 | 2.86 | 2.70 | 2.58 | 2.49 | 2.35 | 2.25 | 1.96 |
| 50 | 5.34 | 3.97 | 3.39 | 3.05 | 2.83 | 2.67 | 2.55 | 2.46 | 2.32 | 2.22 | 1.93 |
| 55 | 5.31 | 3.95 | 3.36 | 3.03 | 2.81 | 2.65 | 2.53 | 2.43 | 2.29 | 2.19 | 1.90 |
| 60 | 5.29 | 3.93 | 3.34 | 3.01 | 2.79 | 2.63 | 2.51 | 2.41 | 2.27 | 2.17 | 1.88 |

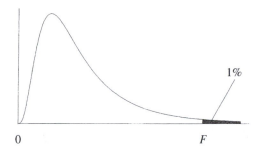

1%

0                                          F

(d) 1% critical values

| $v_1$ | 1 | 2 | 3 | 4 | 5 | 6 | 7 | 8 | 10 | 12 | 24 |
|---|---|---|---|---|---|---|---|---|---|---|---|
| $v_2 = 2$ | 98.5 | 99.0 | 99.2 | 99.3 | 99.3 | 99.3 | 99.4 | 99.4 | 99.4 | 99.4 | 99.5 |
| 3 | 34.1 | 30.8 | 29.5 | 28.7 | 28.2 | 27.9 | 27.7 | 27.5 | 27.2 | 27.1 | 26.6 |
| 4 | 21.2 | 18.0 | 16.7 | 16.0 | 15.5 | 15.2 | 15.0 | 14.8 | 14.6 | 14.4 | 13.9 |
| 5 | 16.3 | 13.3 | 12.1 | 11.4 | 11.0 | 10.7 | 10.5 | 10.3 | 10.1 | 9.89 | 9.47 |
| 6 | 13.8 | 10.9 | 9.78 | 9.15 | 8.75 | 8.47 | 8.26 | 8.10 | 7.87 | 7.72 | 7.31 |
| 7 | 12.3 | 9.55 | 8.45 | 7.85 | 7.46 | 7.19 | 6.99 | 6.84 | 6.62 | 6.47 | 6.07 |
| 8 | 11.3 | 8.65 | 7.59 | 7.01 | 6.63 | 6.37 | 6.18 | 6.03 | 5.81 | 5.67 | 5.28 |
| 9 | 10.6 | 8.02 | 6.99 | 6.42 | 6.06 | 5.80 | 5.61 | 5.47 | 5.26 | 5.11 | 4.73 |
| 10 | 10.0 | 7.56 | 6.55 | 5.99 | 5.64 | 5.39 | 5.20 | 5.06 | 4.85 | 4.71 | 4.33 |
| 11 | 9.65 | 7.21 | 6.22 | 5.67 | 5.32 | 5.07 | 4.89 | 4.74 | 4.54 | 4.40 | 4.02 |
| 12 | 9.33 | 6.93 | 5.95 | 5.41 | 5.06 | 4.82 | 4.64 | 4.50 | 4.30 | 4.16 | 3.78 |
| 13 | 9.07 | 6.70 | 5.74 | 5.21 | 4.86 | 4.62 | 4.44 | 4.30 | 4.10 | 3.96 | 3.59 |
| 14 | 8.86 | 6.51 | 5.56 | 5.04 | 4.69 | 4.46 | 4.28 | 4.14 | 3.94 | 3.80 | 3.43 |
| 15 | 8.68 | 6.36 | 5.42 | 4.89 | 4.56 | 4.32 | 4.14 | 4.00 | 3.80 | 3.67 | 3.29 |
| 16 | 8.53 | 6.23 | 5.29 | 4.77 | 4.44 | 4.20 | 4.03 | 3.89 | 3.69 | 3.55 | 3.18 |
| 17 | 8.40 | 6.11 | 5.18 | 4.67 | 4.34 | 4.10 | 3.93 | 3.79 | 3.59 | 3.46 | 3.08 |
| 18 | 8.29 | 6.01 | 5.09 | 4.58 | 4.25 | 4.01 | 3.84 | 3.71 | 3.51 | 3.37 | 3.00 |
| 19 | 8.18 | 5.93 | 5.01 | 4.50 | 4.17 | 3.94 | 3.77 | 3.63 | 3.43 | 3.30 | 2.92 |
| 20 | 8.10 | 5.85 | 4.94 | 4.43 | 4.10 | 3.87 | 3.70 | 3.56 | 3.37 | 3.23 | 2.86 |
| 22 | 7.95 | 5.72 | 4.82 | 4.31 | 3.99 | 3.76 | 3.59 | 3.45 | 3.26 | 3.12 | 2.75 |
| 24 | 7.82 | 5.61 | 4.72 | 4.22 | 3.90 | 3.67 | 3.50 | 3.36 | 3.17 | 3.03 | 2.66 |
| 26 | 7.72 | 5.53 | 4.64 | 4.14 | 3.82 | 3.59 | 3.42 | 3.29 | 3.09 | 2.96 | 2.58 |
| 28 | 7.64 | 5.45 | 4.57 | 4.07 | 3.75 | 3.53 | 3.36 | 3.23 | 3.03 | 2.90 | 2.52 |
| 30 | 7.56 | 5.39 | 4.51 | 4.02 | 3.70 | 3.47 | 3.30 | 3.17 | 2.98 | 2.84 | 2.47 |
| 35 | 7.42 | 5.27 | 4.40 | 3.91 | 3.59 | 3.37 | 3.20 | 3.07 | 2.88 | 2.74 | 2.36 |
| 40 | 7.31 | 5.18 | 4.31 | 3.83 | 3.51 | 3.29 | 3.12 | 2.99 | 2.80 | 2.66 | 2.29 |
| 45 | 7.23 | 5.11 | 4.25 | 3.77 | 3.45 | 3.23 | 3.07 | 2.94 | 2.74 | 2.61 | 2.23 |
| 50 | 7.17 | 5.06 | 4.20 | 3.72 | 3.41 | 3.19 | 3.02 | 2.89 | 2.70 | 2.56 | 2.18 |
| 55 | 7.12 | 5.01 | 4.16 | 3.68 | 3.37 | 3.15 | 2.98 | 2.85 | 2.66 | 2.53 | 2.15 |
| 60 | 7.08 | 4.98 | 4.13 | 3.65 | 3.34 | 3.12 | 2.95 | 2.82 | 2.63 | 2.50 | 2.12 |

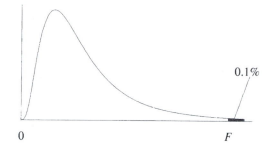

0                                                    F

(e) 0.1% critical values

| $v_1$ | 1 | 2 | 3 | 4 | 5 | 6 | 7 | 8 | 10 | 12 | 24 |
|---|---|---|---|---|---|---|---|---|---|---|---|
| $v_2 = 2$ | 998.5 | 999.0 | 999.2 | 999.3 | 999.3 | 999.3 | 999.4 | 999.4 | 999.4 | 999.4 | 999.5 |
| 3 | 167.0 | 148.5 | 141.1 | 137.1 | 134.6 | 132.9 | 131.6 | 130.6 | 129.3 | 128.3 | 125.9 |
| 4 | 74.1 | 61.3 | 56.2 | 53.4 | 51.7 | 50.5 | 49.7 | 49.0 | 48.1 | 47.4 | 45.8 |
| 5 | 47.2 | 37.1 | 33.2 | 31.1 | 29.8 | 28.8 | 28.2 | 27.7 | 26.9 | 26.4 | 25.1 |
| 6 | 35.5 | 27.0 | 23.7 | 21.9 | 20.8 | 20.0 | 19.5 | 19.0 | 18.4 | 18.0 | 16.9 |
| 7 | 29.3 | 21.7 | 18.8 | 17.2 | 16.2 | 15.5 | 15.0 | 14.6 | 14.1 | 13.7 | 12.7 |
| 8 | 25.4 | 18.5 | 15.8 | 14.4 | 13.5 | 12.9 | 12.4 | 12.1 | 11.5 | 11.2 | 10.3 |
| 9 | 22.9 | 16.4 | 13.9 | 12.6 | 11.7 | 11.1 | 10.7 | 10.4 | 9.89 | 9.57 | 8.72 |
| 10 | 21.0 | 14.9 | 12.6 | 11.3 | 10.5 | 9.93 | 9.52 | 9.20 | 8.75 | 8.45 | 7.64 |
| 11 | 19.7 | 13.8 | 11.6 | 10.4 | 9.58 | 9.05 | 8.66 | 8.35 | 7.92 | 7.63 | 6.85 |
| 12 | 18.6 | 13.0 | 10.8 | 9.63 | 8.89 | 8.38 | 8.00 | 7.71 | 7.29 | 7.00 | 6.25 |
| 13 | 17.8 | 12.3 | 10.2 | 9.07 | 8.35 | 7.86 | 7.49 | 7.21 | 6.80 | 6.52 | 5.78 |
| 14 | 17.1 | 11.8 | 9.73 | 8.62 | 7.92 | 7.44 | 7.08 | 6.80 | 6.40 | 6.13 | 5.41 |
| 15 | 16.6 | 11.3 | 9.34 | 8.25 | 7.57 | 7.09 | 6.74 | 6.47 | 6.08 | 5.81 | 5.10 |
| 16 | 16.1 | 11.0 | 9.01 | 7.94 | 7.27 | 6.80 | 6.46 | 6.19 | 5.81 | 5.55 | 4.85 |
| 17 | 15.7 | 10.7 | 8.73 | 7.68 | 7.02 | 6.56 | 6.22 | 5.96 | 5.58 | 5.32 | 4.63 |
| 18 | 15.4 | 10.4 | 8.49 | 7.46 | 6.81 | 6.35 | 6.02 | 5.76 | 5.39 | 5.13 | 4.45 |
| 19 | 15.1 | 10.2 | 8.28 | 7.27 | 6.62 | 6.18 | 5.85 | 5.59 | 5.22 | 4.97 | 4.29 |
| 20 | 14.8 | 9.95 | 8.10 | 7.10 | 6.46 | 6.02 | 5.69 | 5.44 | 5.08 | 4.82 | 4.15 |
| 22 | 14.4 | 9.61 | 7.80 | 6.81 | 6.19 | 5.76 | 5.44 | 5.19 | 4.83 | 4.58 | 3.92 |
| 24 | 14.0 | 9.34 | 7.55 | 6.59 | 5.98 | 5.55 | 5.23 | 4.99 | 4.64 | 4.39 | 3.74 |
| 26 | 13.7 | 9.12 | 7.36 | 6.41 | 5.80 | 5.38 | 5.07 | 4.83 | 4.48 | 4.24 | 3.59 |
| 28 | 13.5 | 8.93 | 7.19 | 6.25 | 5.66 | 5.24 | 4.93 | 4.69 | 4.35 | 4.11 | 3.46 |
| 30 | 13.3 | 8.77 | 7.05 | 6.12 | 5.53 | 5.12 | 4.82 | 4.58 | 4.24 | 4.00 | 3.36 |
| 35 | 12.9 | 8.47 | 6.79 | 5.88 | 5.30 | 4.89 | 4.59 | 4.36 | 4.03 | 3.79 | 3.16 |
| 40 | 12.6 | 8.25 | 6.59 | 5.70 | 5.13 | 4.73 | 4.44 | 4.21 | 3.87 | 3.64 | 3.01 |
| 45 | 12.4 | 8.09 | 6.45 | 5.56 | 5.00 | 4.61 | 4.32 | 4.09 | 3.76 | 3.53 | 2.90 |
| 50 | 12.2 | 7.96 | 6.34 | 5.46 | 4.90 | 4.51 | 4.22 | 4.00 | 3.67 | 3.44 | 2.82 |
| 55 | 12.1 | 7.85 | 6.25 | 5.38 | 4.82 | 4.43 | 4.15 | 3.92 | 3.60 | 3.37 | 2.75 |
| 60 | 12.0 | 7.77 | 6.17 | 5.31 | 4.76 | 4.37 | 4.09 | 3.86 | 3.54 | 3.32 | 2.69 |

**Table B.6** Random numbers
In generating this table the digits 0 to 9 were equally likely to occur in each place.

| | | | | | | | | | | | | | |
|---|---|---|---|---|---|---|---|---|---|---|---|---|---|
| 14 | 72 | 60 | 92 | 72 | 97 | 83 | 00 | 02 | 77 | 28 | 11 | 37 | 33 |
| 78 | 02 | 65 | 38 | 92 | 90 | 07 | 13 | 11 | 95 | 58 | 88 | 64 | 55 |
| 77 | 10 | 41 | 31 | 90 | 76 | 35 | 00 | 25 | 78 | 80 | 18 | 77 | 32 |
| 85 | 21 | 57 | 89 | 27 | 08 | 70 | 32 | 14 | 58 | 81 | 83 | 41 | 55 |
| 75 | 05 | 14 | 19 | 00 | 64 | 53 | 01 | 50 | 80 | 01 | 88 | 74 | 21 |
| | | | | | | | | | | | | | |
| 57 | 19 | 77 | 98 | 74 | 82 | 07 | 22 | 42 | 89 | 12 | 37 | 16 | 56 |
| 59 | 59 | 47 | 98 | 07 | 41 | 38 | 12 | 06 | 09 | 19 | 80 | 44 | 13 |
| 76 | 96 | 73 | 88 | 44 | 25 | 72 | 27 | 21 | 90 | 22 | 76 | 69 | 67 |
| 96 | 90 | 76 | 82 | 74 | 19 | 81 | 28 | 61 | 91 | 95 | 02 | 47 | 31 |
| 63 | 61 | 36 | 80 | 48 | 50 | 26 | 71 | 16 | 08 | 25 | 65 | 91 | 75 |
| | | | | | | | | | | | | | |
| 65 | 02 | 65 | 25 | 45 | 97 | 17 | 84 | 12 | 19 | 59 | 27 | 79 | 18 |
| 37 | 16 | 64 | 00 | 80 | 06 | 62 | 11 | 62 | 88 | 59 | 54 | 12 | 53 |
| 58 | 29 | 55 | 59 | 57 | 73 | 78 | 43 | 28 | 99 | 91 | 77 | 93 | 89 |
| 79 | 68 | 43 | 00 | 06 | 63 | 26 | 10 | 26 | 83 | 94 | 48 | 25 | 31 |
| 87 | 92 | 56 | 91 | 74 | 30 | 83 | 39 | 85 | 99 | 11 | 73 | 34 | 98 |
| | | | | | | | | | | | | | |
| 96 | 86 | 39 | 03 | 67 | 35 | 64 | 09 | 62 | 36 | 46 | 86 | 54 | 13 |
| 72 | 20 | 60 | 14 | 48 | 08 | 36 | 92 | 58 | 99 | 15 | 30 | 47 | 87 |
| 67 | 61 | 97 | 37 | 73 | 55 | 47 | 97 | 25 | 65 | 67 | 67 | 41 | 35 |
| 25 | 09 | 03 | 43 | 83 | 82 | 60 | 26 | 81 | 96 | 51 | 05 | 77 | 72 |
| 72 | 14 | 78 | 75 | 39 | 54 | 75 | 77 | 55 | 59 | 71 | 73 | 15 | 56 |
| | | | | | | | | | | | | | |
| 59 | 93 | 34 | 37 | 34 | 27 | 07 | 66 | 15 | 63 | 14 | 50 | 74 | 29 |
| 21 | 48 | 85 | 56 | 91 | 43 | 50 | 71 | 58 | 96 | 14 | 31 | 55 | 61 |
| 96 | 32 | 49 | 79 | 42 | 71 | 79 | 69 | 52 | 39 | 45 | 04 | 49 | 91 |
| 16 | 85 | 53 | 65 | 11 | 36 | 08 | 14 | 86 | 60 | 40 | 18 | 51 | 15 |
| 64 | 28 | 96 | 90 | 23 | 12 | 98 | 92 | 28 | 94 | 57 | 41 | 99 | 11 |
| | | | | | | | | | | | | | |
| 60 | 54 | 36 | 51 | 15 | 63 | 83 | 42 | 63 | 08 | 01 | 89 | 18 | 53 |
| 42 | 86 | 68 | 06 | 36 | 25 | 82 | 26 | 85 | 49 | 76 | 15 | 90 | 13 |
| 00 | 49 | 62 | 15 | 53 | 32 | 31 | 28 | 38 | 88 | 14 | 97 | 80 | 33 |
| 26 | 64 | 87 | 61 | 67 | 53 | 23 | 68 | 51 | 98 | 60 | 59 | 02 | 33 |
| 02 | 95 | 21 | 53 | 34 | 23 | 10 | 82 | 82 | 82 | 48 | 71 | 02 | 39 |
| | | | | | | | | | | | | | |
| 65 | 47 | 77 | 14 | 75 | 30 | 32 | 81 | 10 | 83 | 03 | 97 | 24 | 37 |
| 28 | 55 | 15 | 36 | 46 | 33 | 06 | 22 | 29 | 23 | 81 | 14 | 20 | 91 |
| 59 | 75 | 78 | 49 | 51 | 02 | 20 | 17 | 02 | 30 | 32 | 78 | 44 | 79 |
| 87 | 54 | 57 | 69 | 63 | 31 | 61 | 25 | 92 | 31 | 16 | 44 | 02 | 10 |
| 94 | 53 | 87 | 97 | 15 | 23 | 08 | 71 | 26 | 06 | 25 | 87 | 48 | 97 |
| | | | | | | | | | | | | | |
| 79 | 43 | 75 | 93 | 39 | 10 | 18 | 51 | 28 | 17 | 65 | 43 | 22 | 06 |
| 48 | 38 | 71 | 77 | 53 | 37 | 80 | 13 | 60 | 63 | 59 | 75 | 89 | 73 |
| 98 | 30 | 59 | 32 | 90 | 05 | 86 | 12 | 83 | 70 | 50 | 30 | 25 | 65 |
| 85 | 80 | 16 | 77 | 35 | 74 | 09 | 32 | 06 | 30 | 91 | 55 | 92 | 33 |
| 87 | 03 | 96 | 27 | 05 | 59 | 64 | 25 | 33 | 07 | 03 | 08 | 55 | 58 |

**Table B.7** Sample size requirements for testing the value of a single mean or the difference between two means.
The table gives requirements for testing a single mean with a one-sided test directly. For two-sided tests use the column corresponding to half the required significance level.

| S | 5% significance | | 2.5% significance | | 1% significance | |
|---|---|---|---|---|---|---|
| | *90% power* | *95% power* | *90% power* | *95% power* | *90% power* | *95% power* |
| 0.01 | 85 639 | 108 222 | 105 075 | 129 948 | 130 170 | 157 705 |
| 0.02 | 21 410 | 27 056 | 26 269 | 32 487 | 32 543 | 39 427 |
| 0.03 | 9 516 | 12 025 | 11 675 | 14 439 | 14 464 | 17 523 |
| 0.04 | 5 353 | 6 764 | 6 568 | 8 122 | 8 136 | 9 857 |
| 0.05 | 3 426 | 4 329 | 4 203 | 5 198 | 5 207 | 6 309 |
| 0.06 | 2 379 | 3 007 | 2 919 | 3 610 | 3 616 | 4 381 |
| 0.07 | 1 748 | 2 209 | 2 145 | 2 652 | 2 657 | 3 219 |
| 0.08 | 1 339 | 1 691 | 1 642 | 2 031 | 2 034 | 2 465 |
| 0.09 | 1 058 | 1 337 | 1 298 | 1 605 | 1 608 | 1 947 |
| 0.10 | 857 | 1 083 | 1 051 | 1 300 | 1 302 | 1 578 |
| 0.15 | 381 | 481 | 467 | 578 | 579 | 701 |
| 0.20 | 215 | 271 | 263 | 325 | 326 | 395 |
| 0.25 | 138 | 174 | 169 | 208 | 209 | 253 |
| 0.30 | 96 | 121 | 117 | 145 | 145 | 176 |
| 0.35 | 70 | 89 | 86 | 107 | 107 | 129 |
| 0.40 | 54 | 68 | 66 | 82 | 82 | 99 |
| 0.45 | 43 | 54 | 52 | 65 | 65 | 78 |
| 0.50 | 35 | 44 | 43 | 52 | 53 | 64 |
| 0.55 | 29 | 36 | 35 | 43 | 44 | 53 |
| 0.60 | 24 | 31 | 30 | 37 | 37 | 44 |
| 0.65 | 21 | 26 | 25 | 31 | 31 | 38 |
| 0.70 | 18 | 23 | 22 | 27 | 27 | 33 |
| 0.75 | 16 | 20 | 19 | 24 | 24 | 29 |
| 0.80 | 14 | 17 | 17 | 21 | 21 | 25 |
| 0.85 | 12 | 15 | 15 | 18 | 19 | 22 |
| 0.90 | 11 | 14 | 13 | 17 | 17 | 20 |
| 0.95 | 10 | 12 | 12 | 15 | 15 | 18 |
| 1.00 | 9 | 11 | 11 | 13 | 14 | 16 |
| 2.00 | 3 | 3 | 3 | 4 | 4 | 4 |

**Table B.7** *cont.*

For tests of the difference between two means the total sample size (for the two groups combined) is obtained by multiplying the requirement given below by 4 if the two sample sizes are equal or by $(r + 1)^2/r$ if the ratio of the first to the second is $r : 1$ (assuming equal variances). Note that $S = $ difference/standard deviation.

| 0.5% significance | | 0.1% significance | | 0.05% significance | | |
|---|---|---|---|---|---|---|
| 90% power | 95% power | 90% power | 95% power | 90% power | 95% power | S |
| 148 794 | 178 142 | 191 125 | 224 211 | 209 040 | 243 580 | 0.01 |
| 37 199 | 44 536 | 47 782 | 56 053 | 52 260 | 60 895 | 0.02 |
| 16 533 | 19 794 | 21 237 | 24 913 | 23 227 | 27 065 | 0.03 |
| 9 300 | 11 134 | 11 946 | 14 014 | 13 065 | 15 224 | 0.04 |
| 5 952 | 7 126 | 7 645 | 8 969 | 8 362 | 9 744 | 0.05 |
| 4 134 | 4 949 | 5 310 | 6 229 | 5 807 | 6 767 | 0.06 |
| 3 037 | 3 636 | 3 901 | 4 576 | 4 267 | 4 972 | 0.07 |
| 2 325 | 2 784 | 2 987 | 3 504 | 3 267 | 3 806 | 0.08 |
| 1 837 | 2 200 | 2 360 | 2 769 | 2 581 | 3 008 | 0.09 |
| 1 488 | 1 782 | 1 912 | 2 243 | 2 091 | 2 436 | 0.10 |
| 662 | 792 | 850 | 997 | 930 | 1 083 | 0.15 |
| 372 | 446 | 478 | 561 | 523 | 609 | 0.20 |
| 239 | 286 | 306 | 359 | 335 | 390 | 0.25 |
| 166 | 198 | 213 | 250 | 233 | 271 | 0.30 |
| 122 | 146 | 157 | 184 | 171 | 199 | 0.35 |
| 93 | 112 | 120 | 141 | 131 | 153 | 0.40 |
| 74 | 88 | 95 | 111 | 104 | 121 | 0.45 |
| 60 | 72 | 77 | 90 | 84 | 98 | 0.50 |
| 50 | 59 | 64 | 75 | 70 | 81 | 0.55 |
| 42 | 50 | 54 | 63 | 59 | 68 | 0.60 |
| 36 | 43 | 46 | 54 | 50 | 58 | 0.65 |
| 31 | 37 | 40 | 46 | 43 | 50 | 0.70 |
| 27 | 32 | 34 | 40 | 38 | 44 | 0.75 |
| 24 | 28 | 30 | 36 | 33 | 39 | 0.80 |
| 21 | 25 | 27 | 32 | 29 | 34 | 0.85 |
| 19 | 22 | 24 | 28 | 26 | 31 | 0.90 |
| 17 | 20 | 22 | 25 | 24 | 27 | 0.95 |
| 15 | 18 | 20 | 23 | 21 | 25 | 1.00 |
| 4 | 5 | 5 | 6 | 6 | 7 | 2.00 |

**Table B.8**  Sample size requirements for testing the value of a single proportion
These tables give requirements for a one-sided test directly. For two-sided tests use the table corresponding to half the required significance level. Note that $\pi_0$ is the hypothesized proportion (under $H_0$) and $d$ is the difference to be tested.
(a) 5% significance, 90% power

| $d$ | 0.01 | 0.10 | 0.20 | 0.30 | 0.40 | $\pi_0$ 0.50 | 0.60 | 0.70 | 0.80 | 0.90 | 0.95 |
|---|---|---|---|---|---|---|---|---|---|---|---|
| 0.01 | 1 178 | 8 001 | 13 923 | 18 130 | 20 625 | 21 406 | 20 475 | 17 830 | 13 473 | 7 400 | 3 717 |
| 0.02 | 366 | 2 070 | 3 534 | 4 567 | 5 172 | 5 349 | 5 097 | 4 417 | 3 308 | 1 769 | 833 |
| 0.03 | 192 | 950 | 1 593 | 2 045 | 2 305 | 2 376 | 2 255 | 1 944 | 1 443 | 748 | 322 |
| 0.04 | 123 | 551 | 908 | 1 158 | 1 300 | 1 335 | 1 262 | 1 083 | 795 | 398 | 148 |
| 0.05 | 88 | 362 | 589 | 746 | 834 | 853 | 804 | 686 | 498 | 239 | |
| 0.06 | 67 | 258 | 414 | 521 | 580 | 591 | 555 | 471 | 338 | 155 | |
| 0.07 | 54 | 194 | 308 | 385 | 427 | 434 | 405 | 342 | 242 | 104 | |
| 0.08 | 44 | 152 | 238 | 296 | 327 | 331 | 308 | 258 | 181 | 71 | |
| 0.09 | 38 | 123 | 190 | 235 | 259 | 261 | 242 | 201 | 139 | 48 | |
| 0.10 | 32 | 102 | 156 | 191 | 210 | 211 | 195 | 161 | 109 | | |
| 0.15 | 18 | 49 | 72 | 87 | 93 | 92 | 83 | 66 | 40 | | |
| 0.20 | 12 | 30 | 42 | 49 | 52 | 50 | 44 | 33 | | | |
| 0.25 | 9 | 20 | 27 | 31 | 33 | 31 | 26 | 18 | | | |
| 0.30 | 7 | 14 | 19 | 22 | 22 | 20 | 16 | | | | |
| 0.35 | 5 | 11 | 14 | 16 | 16 | 14 | 10 | | | | |
| 0.40 | 4 | 9 | 11 | 12 | 11 | 10 | | | | | |
| 0.45 | 4 | 7 | 8 | 9 | 8 | 6 | | | | | |
| 0.50 | 3 | 6 | 7 | 7 | 6 | | | | | | |

(b) 5% significance, 95% power

| $d$ | 0.01 | 0.10 | 0.20 | 0.30 | 0.40 | $\pi_0$ 0.50 | 0.60 | 0.70 | 0.80 | 0.90 | 0.95 |
|---|---|---|---|---|---|---|---|---|---|---|---|
| 0.01 | 1 552 | 10 163 | 17 634 | 22 938 | 26 076 | 27 051 | 25 860 | 22 505 | 16 984 | 9 297 | 4 636 |
| 0.02 | 494 | 2 642 | 4 485 | 5 784 | 6 542 | 6 759 | 6 434 | 5 568 | 4 160 | 2 208 | 1 022 |
| 0.03 | 263 | 1 218 | 2 026 | 2 592 | 2 917 | 3 001 | 2 845 | 2 448 | 1 809 | 927 | 386 |
| 0.04 | 171 | 708 | 1 157 | 1 469 | 1 645 | 1 686 | 1 591 | 1 361 | 994 | 489 | 171 |
| 0.05 | 123 | 468 | 751 | 947 | 1 056 | 1 077 | 1 012 | 860 | 621 | 291 | |
| 0.06 | 95 | 334 | 529 | 662 | 735 | 747 | 698 | 590 | 420 | 185 | |
| 0.07 | 76 | 253 | 394 | 489 | 541 | 547 | 509 | 427 | 300 | 123 | |
| 0.08 | 63 | 198 | 305 | 377 | 414 | 418 | 387 | 322 | 223 | 82 | |
| 0.09 | 54 | 161 | 244 | 299 | 328 | 329 | 303 | 251 | 170 | 54 | |
| 0.10 | 47 | 133 | 200 | 244 | 266 | 266 | 244 | 200 | 133 | | |
| 0.15 | 27 | 65 | 93 | 110 | 118 | 115 | 103 | 80 | 46 | | |
| 0.20 | 18 | 39 | 54 | 63 | 65 | 63 | 54 | 39 | | | |
| 0.25 | 13 | 27 | 35 | 40 | 41 | 38 | 32 | 20 | | | |
| 0.30 | 10 | 19 | 25 | 28 | 28 | 25 | 19 | | | | |
| 0.35 | 8 | 15 | 18 | 20 | 19 | 17 | 12 | | | | |
| 0.40 | 6 | 11 | 14 | 15 | 14 | 11 | | | | | |
| 0.45 | 5 | 9 | 11 | 11 | 10 | 7 | | | | | |
| 0.50 | 4 | 7 | 8 | 8 | 7 | | | | | | |

(c) 2.5% significance, 90% power

| d | 0.01 | 0.10 | 0.20 | 0.30 | 0.40 | $\pi_0$ 0.50 | 0.60 | 0.70 | 0.80 | 0.90 | 0.95 |
|---|---|---|---|---|---|---|---|---|---|---|---|
| 0.01 | 1 402 | 9 781 | 17 056 | 22 228 | 25 297 | 26 265 | 25 131 | 21 895 | 16 557 | 9 116 | 4 601 |
| 0.02 | 428 | 2 523 | 4 323 | 5 595 | 6 342 | 6 563 | 6 259 | 5 429 | 4 073 | 2 189 | 1 043 |
| 0.03 | 222 | 1 154 | 1 946 | 2 503 | 2 826 | 2 915 | 2 770 | 2 392 | 1 780 | 931 | 409 |
| 0.04 | 141 | 667 | 1 108 | 1 417 | 1 593 | 1 638 | 1 552 | 1 333 | 983 | 498 | 193 |
| 0.05 | 100 | 438 | 718 | 912 | 1 022 | 1 047 | 988 | 845 | 617 | 301 | |
| 0.06 | 76 | 311 | 504 | 637 | 711 | 726 | 683 | 581 | 420 | 196 | |
| 0.07 | 61 | 234 | 374 | 470 | 523 | 532 | 499 | 422 | 302 | 133 | |
| 0.08 | 50 | 183 | 289 | 362 | 401 | 407 | 380 | 320 | 226 | 93 | |
| 0.09 | 42 | 147 | 231 | 287 | 317 | 321 | 298 | 249 | 174 | 64 | |
| 0.10 | 36 | 122 | 189 | 233 | 257 | 259 | 240 | 200 | 137 | | |
| 0.15 | 20 | 59 | 87 | 105 | 114 | 113 | 103 | 82 | 51 | | |
| 0.20 | 13 | 35 | 50 | 60 | 64 | 62 | 55 | 42 | | | |
| 0.25 | 10 | 24 | 33 | 38 | 40 | 38 | 33 | 23 | | | |
| 0.30 | 7 | 17 | 23 | 26 | 27 | 25 | 21 | | | | |
| 0.35 | 6 | 13 | 17 | 19 | 19 | 17 | 13 | | | | |
| 0.40 | 5 | 10 | 13 | 14 | 14 | 12 | | | | | |
| 0.45 | 4 | 8 | 10 | 11 | 10 | 8 | | | | | |
| 0.50 | 3 | 6 | 8 | 8 | 8 | | | | | | |

(d) 2.5% significance, 95% power

| d | 0.01 | 0.10 | 0.20 | 0.30 | 0.40 | $\pi_0$ 0.50 | 0.60 | 0.70 | 0.80 | 0.90 | 0.95 |
|---|---|---|---|---|---|---|---|---|---|---|---|
| 0.01 | 1 809 | 12 159 | 21 140 | 27 520 | 31 300 | 32 481 | 31 063 | 27 046 | 20 428 | 11 209 | 5 618 |
| 0.02 | 566 | 3 151 | 5 369 | 6 935 | 7 851 | 8 116 | 7 732 | 6 698 | 5 013 | 2 675 | 1 253 |
| 0.03 | 298 | 1 447 | 2 422 | 3 105 | 3 499 | 3 604 | 3 420 | 2 947 | 2 184 | 1 129 | 481 |
| 0.04 | 192 | 840 | 1 382 | 1 759 | 1 973 | 2 025 | 1 914 | 1 640 | 1 203 | 599 | 219 |
| 0.05 | 138 | 553 | 896 | 1 133 | 1 266 | 1 294 | 1 218 | 1 038 | 753 | 359 | |
| 0.06 | 105 | 395 | 630 | 792 | 881 | 897 | 841 | 712 | 510 | 231 | |
| 0.07 | 84 | 297 | 468 | 585 | 648 | 658 | 614 | 517 | 365 | 154 | |
| 0.08 | 70 | 233 | 363 | 450 | 497 | 502 | 467 | 390 | 272 | 105 | |
| 0.09 | 59 | 188 | 290 | 357 | 393 | 396 | 366 | 304 | 209 | 70 | |
| 0.10 | 51 | 156 | 237 | 291 | 318 | 319 | 294 | 243 | 164 | | |
| 0.15 | 29 | 76 | 110 | 131 | 141 | 139 | 125 | 99 | 59 | | |
| 0.20 | 19 | 46 | 64 | 75 | 78 | 76 | 66 | 49 | | | |
| 0.25 | 14 | 31 | 42 | 48 | 49 | 46 | 39 | 26 | | | |
| 0.30 | 11 | 22 | 29 | 33 | 33 | 30 | 24 | | | | |
| 0.35 | 8 | 17 | 21 | 24 | 23 | 21 | 15 | | | | |
| 0.40 | 7 | 13 | 16 | 18 | 17 | 14 | | | | | |
| 0.45 | 6 | 10 | 13 | 13 | 12 | 9 | | | | | |
| 0.50 | 5 | 8 | 10 | 10 | 9 | | | | | | |

**Table B.9** Total sample size requirements (for the two groups combined) for testing the ratio of two proportions (relative risk) with equal numbers in each group
These tables give requirements for a one-sided test directly. For two-sided tests use the table corresponding to half the required significance level. Note that $\pi$ is the proportion for the reference group (the denominator) and $\lambda$ is the relative risk to be tested.
(a) 5% significance, 90% power

| $\lambda$ | $\pi$ 0.001 | 0.005 | 0.010 | 0.050 | 0.100 | 0.150 | 0.200 | 0.500 | 0.900 |
|---|---|---|---|---|---|---|---|---|---|
| 0.10 | 23 244 | 4 636 | 2 310 | 448 | 216 | 138 | 100 | 30 | 8 |
| 0.20 | 32 090 | 6 398 | 3 188 | 618 | 298 | 190 | 136 | 40 | 10 |
| 0.30 | 45 406 | 9 052 | 4 508 | 874 | 418 | 268 | 192 | 56 | 14 |
| 0.40 | 66 554 | 13 268 | 6 606 | 1 278 | 612 | 390 | 278 | 78 | 18 |
| 0.50 | 102 678 | 20 466 | 10 190 | 1 968 | 940 | 598 | 426 | 118 | 26 |
| 0.60 | 171 126 | 34 104 | 16 976 | 3 274 | 1 562 | 990 | 706 | 192 | 38 |
| 0.70 | 323 228 | 64 410 | 32 058 | 6 176 | 2 940 | 1 862 | 1 322 | 352 | 62 |
| 0.80 | 770 020 | 153 422 | 76 348 | 14 688 | 6 980 | 4 412 | 3 128 | 814 | 126 |
| 0.90 | 3 251 102 | 647 690 | 322 264 | 61 924 | 29 380 | 18 534 | 13 110 | 3 346 | 450 |
| 1.10 | 3 593 120 | 715 666 | 355 984 | 68 240 | 32 272 | 20 282 | 14 288 | 3 496 | 292 |
| 1.20 | 941 030 | 187 410 | 93 208 | 17 846 | 8 426 | 5 286 | 3 716 | 890 | |
| 1.30 | 437 234 | 87 068 | 43 298 | 8 280 | 3 904 | 2 444 | 1 714 | 402 | |
| 1.40 | 256 630 | 51 098 | 25 406 | 4 854 | 2 284 | 1 428 | 1 000 | 228 | |
| 1.50 | 171 082 | 34 062 | 16 934 | 3 232 | 1 518 | 948 | 662 | 148 | |
| 1.60 | 123 556 | 24 596 | 12 226 | 2 330 | 1 094 | 680 | 474 | 104 | |
| 1.80 | 74 842 | 14 896 | 7 402 | 1 408 | 658 | 408 | 284 | 58 | |
| 2.00 | 51 318 | 10 212 | 5 074 | 962 | 448 | 278 | 192 | | |
| 3.00 | 17 102 | 3 400 | 1 688 | 316 | 146 | 88 | 60 | | |
| 4.00 | 9 498 | 1 886 | 934 | 174 | 78 | 46 | 30 | | |
| 5.00 | 6 410 | 1 272 | 630 | 116 | 52 | 30 | | | |
| 10.00 | 2 318 | 458 | 226 | 40 | | | | | |
| 20.00 | 992 | 194 | 94 | | | | | | |

(b) 5% significance, 95% power

| λ | 0.001 | 0.005 | 0.010 | π 0.050 | 0.100 | 0.150 | 0.200 | 0.500 | 0.900 |
|---|---|---|---|---|---|---|---|---|---|
| 0.10 | 29 372 | 5 856 | 2 918 | 566 | 272 | 174 | 126 | 36 | 10 |
| 0.20 | 40 552 | 8 086 | 4 026 | 780 | 374 | 240 | 172 | 50 | 12 |
| 0.30 | 57 378 | 11 438 | 5 696 | 1 102 | 528 | 336 | 240 | 68 | 16 |
| 0.40 | 84 102 | 16 764 | 8 346 | 1 612 | 772 | 490 | 350 | 98 | 20 |
| 0.50 | 129 754 | 25 860 | 12 874 | 2 484 | 1 186 | 754 | 536 | 146 | 30 |
| 0.60 | 216 250 | 43 094 | 21 450 | 4 136 | 1 970 | 1 250 | 888 | 238 | 44 |
| 0.70 | 408 460 | 81 390 | 40 506 | 7 800 | 3 712 | 2 348 | 1 666 | 440 | 74 |
| 0.80 | 973 072 | 193 874 | 96 476 | 18 556 | 8 816 | 5 568 | 3 946 | 1 024 | 154 |
| 0.90 | 4 108 420 | 818 476 | 407 234 | 78 240 | 37 116 | 23 408 | 16 554 | 4 216 | 556 |
| 1.10 | 4 540 658 | 904 406 | 449 874 | 86 248 | 40 796 | 25 644 | 18 068 | 4 432 | 384 |
| 1.20 | 1 189 190 | 236 838 | 117 794 | 22 560 | 10 656 | 6 688 | 4 704 | 1 132 | |
| 1.30 | 552 540 | 110 034 | 54 720 | 10 470 | 4 938 | 3 094 | 2 172 | 512 | |
| 1.40 | 324 310 | 64 576 | 32 110 | 6 138 | 2 890 | 1 808 | 1 266 | 292 | |
| 1.50 | 216 202 | 43 046 | 21 402 | 4 086 | 1 922 | 1 200 | 840 | 190 | |
| 1.60 | 156 142 | 31 086 | 15 454 | 2 948 | 1 384 | 864 | 602 | 132 | |
| 1.80 | 94 582 | 18 826 | 9 356 | 1 782 | 834 | 518 | 360 | 76 | |
| 2.00 | 64 852 | 12 906 | 6 414 | 1 218 | 570 | 352 | 244 | | |
| 3.00 | 21 612 | 4 298 | 2 132 | 402 | 184 | 112 | 76 | | |
| 4.00 | 12 004 | 2 384 | 1 182 | 220 | 100 | 60 | 40 | | |
| 5.00 | 8 102 | 1 608 | 796 | 146 | 66 | 38 | | | |
| 10.00 | 2 930 | 580 | 286 | 50 | | | | | |
| 20.00 | 1 252 | 246 | 120 | | | | | | |

(c) 2.5% significance, 90% power

| $\lambda$ | 0.001 | 0.005 | 0.010 | $\pi$ 0.050 | 0.100 | 0.150 | 0.200 | 0.500 | 0.900 |
|---|---|---|---|---|---|---|---|---|---|
| 0.10 | 28 518 | 5 688 | 2 834 | 550 | 266 | 170 | 122 | 38 | 10 |
| 0.20 | 39 374 | 7 852 | 3 912 | 760 | 366 | 234 | 168 | 50 | 14 |
| 0.30 | 55 710 | 11 108 | 5 532 | 1 072 | 514 | 328 | 236 | 68 | 18 |
| 0.40 | 81 658 | 16 278 | 8 106 | 1 568 | 752 | 478 | 342 | 98 | 24 |
| 0.50 | 125 984 | 25 112 | 12 502 | 2 416 | 1 154 | 734 | 524 | 146 | 32 |
| 0.60 | 209 964 | 41 846 | 20 832 | 4 020 | 1 918 | 1 218 | 866 | 236 | 48 |
| 0.70 | 396 588 | 79 030 | 39 334 | 7 578 | 3 610 | 2 286 | 1 624 | 434 | 78 |
| 0.80 | 944 780 | 188 246 | 93 680 | 18 026 | 8 570 | 5 416 | 3 840 | 1 004 | 160 |
| 0.90 | 3 988 950 | 794 694 | 395 412 | 75 986 | 36 058 | 22 748 | 16 092 | 4 114 | 560 |
| 1.10 | 4 408 574 | 878 078 | 436 766 | 83 716 | 39 586 | 24 876 | 17 520 | 4 280 | 350 |
| 1.20 | 1 154 592 | 229 938 | 114 356 | 21 892 | 10 334 | 6 480 | 4 554 | 1 086 | |
| 1.30 | 536 462 | 106 824 | 53 120 | 10 156 | 4 786 | 2 996 | 2 100 | 488 | |
| 1.40 | 314 870 | 62 692 | 31 170 | 5 952 | 2 800 | 1 750 | 1 224 | 278 | |
| 1.50 | 209 908 | 41 788 | 20 774 | 3 962 | 1 860 | 1 160 | 810 | 178 | |
| 1.60 | 151 596 | 30 176 | 15 000 | 2 858 | 1 340 | 834 | 580 | 124 | |
| 1.80 | 91 826 | 18 274 | 9 080 | 1 726 | 806 | 500 | 346 | 70 | |
| 2.00 | 62 964 | 12 528 | 6 224 | 1 180 | 550 | 340 | 234 | | |
| 3.00 | 20 982 | 4 170 | 2 068 | 388 | 178 | 108 | 72 | | |
| 4.00 | 11 654 | 2 314 | 1 146 | 212 | 96 | 56 | 36 | | |
| 5.00 | 7 864 | 1 560 | 772 | 142 | 62 | 36 | | | |
| 10.00 | 2 844 | 562 | 276 | 48 | | | | | |
| 20.00 | 1 216 | 238 | 114 | | | | | | |

(d) 2.5% significance, 95% power

| λ | 0.001 | 0.005 | 0.010 | π 0.050 | 0.100 | 0.150 | 0.200 | 0.500 | 0.900 |
|---|---|---|---|---|---|---|---|---|---|
| 0.10 | 35 268 | 7 034 | 3 504 | 680 | 328 | 210 | 150 | 44 | 12 |
| 0.20 | 48 694 | 9 708 | 4 836 | 938 | 450 | 288 | 206 | 60 | 16 |
| 0.30 | 68 896 | 13 736 | 6 840 | 1 324 | 634 | 404 | 290 | 82 | 20 |
| 0.40 | 100 986 | 20 130 | 10 024 | 1 938 | 928 | 590 | 422 | 118 | 26 |
| 0.50 | 155 802 | 31 054 | 15 460 | 2 984 | 1 426 | 906 | 646 | 178 | 36 |
| 0.60 | 259 664 | 51 748 | 25 758 | 4 968 | 2 368 | 1 502 | 1 068 | 288 | 54 |
| 0.70 | 490 462 | 97 732 | 48 642 | 9 368 | 4 460 | 2 822 | 2 004 | 532 | 92 |
| 0.80 | 1 168 420 | 232 800 | 115 848 | 22 286 | 10 590 | 6 692 | 4 742 | 1 234 | 190 |
| 0.90 | 4 933 188 | 982 796 | 488 996 | 93 958 | 44 578 | 28 118 | 19 888 | 5 072 | 678 |
| 1.10 | 5 452 174 | 1 085 950 | 540 172 | 103 550 | 48 972 | 30 780 | 21 684 | 5 310 | 450 |
| 1.20 | 1 427 912 | 284 378 | 141 436 | 27 082 | 12 788 | 8 024 | 5 640 | 1 352 | |
| 1.30 | 663 456 | 132 118 | 65 700 | 12 566 | 5 924 | 3 710 | 2 604 | 610 | |
| 1.40 | 389 410 | 77 538 | 38 552 | 7 366 | 3 468 | 2 168 | 1 518 | 348 | |
| 1.50 | 259 600 | 51 684 | 25 696 | 4 904 | 2 304 | 1 438 | 1 004 | 224 | |
| 1.60 | 187 484 | 37 322 | 18 552 | 3 536 | 1 660 | 1 034 | 720 | 156 | |
| 1.80 | 113 566 | 22 604 | 11 232 | 2 136 | 1 000 | 620 | 430 | 88 | |
| 2.00 | 77 870 | 15 496 | 7 698 | 1 462 | 682 | 422 | 292 | | |
| 3.00 | 25 950 | 5 158 | 2 560 | 480 | 220 | 134 | 90 | | |
| 4.00 | 14 414 | 2 862 | 1 418 | 264 | 118 | 70 | 46 | | |
| 5.00 | 9 726 | 1 930 | 956 | 176 | 78 | 46 | | | |
| 10.00 | 3 518 | 694 | 342 | 60 | | | | | |
| 20.00 | 1 504 | 294 | 142 | | | | | | |

**Table B.10**   Total sample size requirements (for the two groups combined) for unmatched case–control studies with equal numbers of cases and controls
These tables give requirements for a one-sided test directly. For two-sided tests use the table corresponding to half the required significance level. Note that $P$ is the prevalence of the risk factor in the entire population and $\lambda$ is the approximate relative risk to be tested.
(a) 5% significance, 90% power

| $\lambda$ | 0.010 | 0.050 | 0.100 | 0.200 | 0.300 | 0.400 | 0.500 | 0.700 | 0.900 |
|---|---|---|---|---|---|---|---|---|---|
| | | | | | *P* | | | | |
| 0.10 | 2 318 | 456 | 224 | 108 | 70 | 50 | 40 | 30 | 38 |
| 0.20 | 3 206 | 638 | 316 | 158 | 104 | 80 | 66 | 56 | 88 |
| 0.30 | 4 546 | 912 | 458 | 232 | 160 | 124 | 106 | 98 | 176 |
| 0.40 | 6 676 | 1 348 | 684 | 356 | 248 | 200 | 176 | 172 | 330 |
| 0.50 | 10 318 | 2 098 | 1 074 | 566 | 404 | 332 | 296 | 306 | 616 |
| 0.60 | 17 220 | 3 522 | 1 816 | 974 | 706 | 588 | 536 | 576 | 1 206 |
| 0.70 | 32 570 | 6 698 | 3 476 | 1 890 | 1 390 | 1 174 | 1 088 | 1 206 | 2 612 |
| 0.80 | 77 686 | 16 052 | 8 382 | 4 614 | 3 438 | 2 944 | 2 764 | 3 146 | 7 012 |
| 0.90 | 328 374 | 68 156 | 35 786 | 19 922 | 15 020 | 13 006 | 12 354 | 14 400 | 32 892 |
| 1.10 | 363 666 | 76 090 | 40 352 | 22 918 | 17 630 | 15 574 | 15 096 | 18 316 | 43 550 |
| 1.20 | 95 332 | 20 020 | 10 664 | 6 112 | 4 744 | 4 228 | 4 134 | 5 102 | 12 340 |
| 1.30 | 44 334 | 9 342 | 4 998 | 2 888 | 2 260 | 2 032 | 2 002 | 2 510 | 6 166 |
| 1.40 | 26 044 | 5 506 | 2 958 | 1 722 | 1 358 | 1 230 | 1 222 | 1 554 | 3 870 |
| 1.50 | 17 376 | 3 684 | 1 986 | 1 166 | 926 | 846 | 846 | 1 090 | 2 748 |
| 1.60 | 12 558 | 2 672 | 1 446 | 854 | 684 | 628 | 632 | 826 | 2 106 |
| 1.80 | 7 618 | 1 630 | 888 | 532 | 432 | 400 | 408 | 546 | 1 420 |
| 2.00 | 5 230 | 1 124 | 616 | 374 | 306 | 288 | 296 | 404 | 1 074 |
| 3.00 | 1 754 | 386 | 218 | 138 | 120 | 118 | 126 | 184 | 522 |
| 4.00 | 978 | 220 | 126 | 84 | 74 | 76 | 84 | 130 | 380 |
| 5.00 | 664 | 150 | 88 | 60 | 56 | 58 | 66 | 104 | 316 |
| 10.00 | 244 | 60 | 38 | 30 | 30 | 34 | 40 | 70 | 224 |
| 20.00 | 108 | 30 | 20 | 18 | 20 | 24 | 30 | 56 | 190 |

(b) 5% significance, 95% power

| λ | 0.010 | 0.050 | 0.100 | 0.200 | P 0.300 | 0.400 | 0.500 | 0.700 | 0.900 |
|---|---|---|---|---|---|---|---|---|---|
| 0.10 | 2 928 | 576 | 282 | 136 | 86 | 64 | 50 | 36 | 46 |
| 0.20 | 4 052 | 804 | 400 | 198 | 132 | 100 | 82 | 70 | 110 |
| 0.30 | 5 744 | 1 152 | 578 | 294 | 200 | 156 | 134 | 124 | 220 |
| 0.40 | 8 436 | 1 704 | 864 | 448 | 314 | 252 | 220 | 218 | 414 |
| 0.50 | 13 036 | 2 650 | 1 356 | 716 | 510 | 418 | 374 | 386 | 778 |
| 0.60 | 21 760 | 4 450 | 2 294 | 1 230 | 892 | 742 | 678 | 726 | 1 524 |
| 0.70 | 41 158 | 8 462 | 4 392 | 2 386 | 1 756 | 1 484 | 1 374 | 1 522 | 3 300 |
| 0.80 | 98 172 | 20 284 | 10 590 | 5 828 | 4 344 | 3 718 | 3 492 | 3 974 | 8 858 |
| 0.90 | 414 966 | 86 130 | 45 222 | 25 174 | 18 980 | 16 434 | 15 612 | 18 196 | 41 566 |
| 1.10 | 459 566 | 96 154 | 50 994 | 28 962 | 22 278 | 19 682 | 19 076 | 23 144 | 55 034 |
| 1.20 | 120 472 | 25 298 | 13 476 | 7 722 | 5 994 | 5 342 | 5 222 | 6 448 | 15 592 |
| 1.30 | 56 024 | 11 804 | 6 316 | 3 650 | 2 856 | 2 566 | 2 530 | 3 172 | 7 790 |
| 1.40 | 32 910 | 6 956 | 3 736 | 2 176 | 1 716 | 1 554 | 1 544 | 1 964 | 4 890 |
| 1.50 | 21 958 | 4 656 | 2 510 | 1 472 | 1 170 | 1 066 | 1 066 | 1 376 | 3 472 |
| 1.60 | 15 870 | 3 374 | 1 826 | 1 080 | 864 | 792 | 798 | 1 042 | 2 660 |
| 1.80 | 9 626 | 2 058 | 1 122 | 672 | 544 | 506 | 516 | 688 | 1 794 |
| 2.00 | 6 610 | 1 420 | 778 | 472 | 386 | 364 | 374 | 510 | 1 356 |
| 3.00 | 2 214 | 486 | 274 | 174 | 150 | 148 | 158 | 232 | 658 |
| 4.00 | 1 236 | 276 | 158 | 104 | 94 | 94 | 104 | 162 | 480 |
| 5.00 | 838 | 190 | 110 | 76 | 70 | 72 | 82 | 132 | 400 |
| 10.00 | 308 | 74 | 46 | 36 | 36 | 40 | 50 | 86 | 282 |
| 20.00 | 136 | 36 | 26 | 22 | 24 | 30 | 38 | 70 | 238 |

(c) 2.5% significance, 90% power

| λ | 0.010 | 0.050 | 0.100 | 0.200 | P 0.300 | 0.400 | 0.500 | 0.700 | 0.900 |
|---|---|---|---|---|---|---|---|---|---|
| 0.10 | 2 844 | 560 | 274 | 132 | 86 | 62 | 48 | 36 | 46 |
| 0.20 | 3 934 | 782 | 390 | 194 | 128 | 98 | 80 | 68 | 108 |
| 0.30 | 5 578 | 1 120 | 562 | 286 | 196 | 154 | 132 | 122 | 216 |
| 0.40 | 8 192 | 1 656 | 840 | 436 | 306 | 246 | 216 | 212 | 404 |
| 0.50 | 12 658 | 2 574 | 1 318 | 696 | 496 | 406 | 364 | 376 | 756 |
| 0.60 | 21 128 | 4 322 | 2 228 | 1 194 | 866 | 722 | 658 | 706 | 1 480 |
| 0.70 | 39 962 | 8 218 | 4 264 | 2 318 | 1 706 | 1 442 | 1 336 | 1 480 | 3 206 |
| 0.80 | 95 318 | 19 696 | 10 284 | 5 660 | 4 220 | 3 612 | 3 390 | 3 860 | 8 602 |
| 0.90 | 402 898 | 83 626 | 43 908 | 24 442 | 18 430 | 15 958 | 15 160 | 17 668 | 40 358 |
| 1.10 | 446 202 | 93 358 | 49 512 | 28 120 | 21 632 | 19 110 | 18 522 | 22 472 | 53 434 |
| 1.20 | 116 970 | 24 562 | 13 086 | 7 500 | 5 820 | 5 188 | 5 072 | 6 260 | 15 140 |
| 1.30 | 54 396 | 11 462 | 6 132 | 3 544 | 2 774 | 2 492 | 2 456 | 3 080 | 7 564 |
| 1.40 | 31 954 | 6 756 | 3 628 | 2 114 | 1 668 | 1 510 | 1 500 | 1 908 | 4 750 |
| 1.50 | 21 320 | 4 522 | 2 438 | 1 432 | 1 138 | 1 038 | 1 038 | 1 338 | 3 372 |
| 1.60 | 15 410 | 3 278 | 1 774 | 1 048 | 840 | 770 | 776 | 1 012 | 2 584 |
| 1.80 | 9 348 | 2 000 | 1 090 | 652 | 530 | 492 | 502 | 670 | 1 744 |
| 2.00 | 6 418 | 1 380 | 756 | 460 | 376 | 354 | 364 | 496 | 1 318 |
| 3.00 | 2 152 | 472 | 266 | 170 | 146 | 144 | 154 | 226 | 640 |
| 4.00 | 1 200 | 268 | 154 | 104 | 92 | 94 | 104 | 158 | 466 |
| 5.00 | 814 | 186 | 108 | 74 | 68 | 72 | 80 | 128 | 390 |
| 10.00 | 300 | 74 | 46 | 36 | 36 | 40 | 48 | 86 | 274 |
| 20.00 | 134 | 36 | 26 | 22 | 26 | 30 | 38 | 70 | 232 |

(d) 2.5% significance, 95% power

| $\lambda$ | 0.010 | 0.050 | 0.100 | 0.200 | $P$ 0.300 | 0.400 | 0.500 | 0.700 | 0.900 |
|---|---|---|---|---|---|---|---|---|---|
| 0.10 | 3 516 | 692 | 338 | 162 | 104 | 76 | 60 | 44 | 56 |
| 0.20 | 4 864 | 966 | 480 | 238 | 158 | 120 | 98 | 84 | 134 |
| 0.30 | 6 898 | 1 382 | 694 | 352 | 242 | 188 | 162 | 150 | 266 |
| 0.40 | 10 130 | 2 046 | 1 038 | 538 | 376 | 302 | 266 | 262 | 498 |
| 0.50 | 15 654 | 3 182 | 1 628 | 860 | 614 | 502 | 450 | 464 | 936 |
| 0.60 | 26 130 | 5 344 | 2 754 | 1 476 | 1 072 | 892 | 814 | 874 | 1 830 |
| 0.70 | 49 420 | 10 162 | 5 274 | 2 866 | 2 110 | 1 782 | 1 652 | 1 828 | 3 964 |
| 0.80 | 117 880 | 24 358 | 12 716 | 7 000 | 5 218 | 4 466 | 4 192 | 4 772 | 10 638 |
| 0.90 | 498 270 | 103 420 | 54 300 | 30 228 | 22 790 | 19 734 | 18 746 | 21 850 | 49 910 |
| 1.10 | 551 824 | 115 458 | 61 230 | 34 776 | 26 752 | 23 632 | 22 904 | 27 790 | 66 082 |
| 1.20 | 144 656 | 30 376 | 16 182 | 9 274 | 7 198 | 6 414 | 6 272 | 7 742 | 18 724 |
| 1.30 | 67 272 | 14 174 | 7 584 | 4 382 | 3 430 | 3 082 | 3 038 | 3 808 | 9 354 |
| 1.40 | 39 518 | 8 354 | 4 486 | 2 614 | 2 062 | 1 866 | 1 854 | 2 358 | 5 874 |
| 1.50 | 26 366 | 5 590 | 3 014 | 1 768 | 1 406 | 1 282 | 1 282 | 1 652 | 4 170 |
| 1.60 | 19 056 | 4 052 | 2 192 | 1 296 | 1 036 | 952 | 958 | 1 252 | 3 194 |
| 1.80 | 11 560 | 2 472 | 1 346 | 806 | 654 | 608 | 618 | 826 | 2 156 |
| 2.00 | 7 936 | 1 706 | 936 | 566 | 464 | 436 | 450 | 614 | 1 628 |
| 3.00 | 2 660 | 584 | 328 | 210 | 180 | 176 | 190 | 280 | 790 |
| 4.00 | 1 484 | 332 | 190 | 126 | 112 | 114 | 126 | 196 | 576 |
| 5.00 | 1 006 | 228 | 134 | 92 | 84 | 88 | 98 | 158 | 480 |
| 10.00 | 370 | 90 | 56 | 44 | 44 | 50 | 60 | 104 | 338 |
| 20.00 | 164 | 44 | 30 | 28 | 29 | 35 | 45 | 84 | 286 |

**Table B.11**  Critical values for Pearson's correlation coefficient
The table shows the smallest value of the correlation coefficient that is significant at the particular significance level. These are to be used in two-sided significance tests where the null hypothesis is that the correlation is zero.

| Sample size | Significance level | | | |
|---|---|---|---|---|
| | 10% | 5% | 1% | 0.1% |
| 3 | 0.9877 | 0.9969 | 0.9999 | 0.9999 |
| 4 | 0.900 | 0.950 | 0.990 | 0.999 |
| 5 | 0.805 | 0.878 | 0.959 | 0.991 |
| 6 | 0.729 | 0.811 | 0.917 | 0.974 |
| 7 | 0.669 | 0.754 | 0.875 | 0.951 |
| 8 | 0.621 | 0.707 | 0.834 | 0.925 |
| 9 | 0.582 | 0.666 | 0.798 | 0.898 |
| 10 | 0.549 | 0.632 | 0.765 | 0.872 |
| 11 | 0.521 | 0.602 | 0.735 | 0.847 |
| 12 | 0.497 | 0.576 | 0.708 | 0.823 |
| 13 | 0.476 | 0.553 | 0.684 | 0.801 |
| 14 | 0.457 | 0.532 | 0.661 | 0.780 |
| 15 | 0.441 | 0.514 | 0.641 | 0.760 |
| 16 | 0.426 | 0.497 | 0.623 | 0.742 |
| 17 | 0.412 | 0.482 | 0.606 | 0.725 |
| 18 | 0.400 | 0.468 | 0.590 | 0.708 |
| 19 | 0.389 | 0.456 | 0.575 | 0.693 |
| 20 | 0.378 | 0.444 | 0.561 | 0.679 |
| 21 | 0.369 | 0.433 | 0.549 | 0.665 |
| 22 | 0.360 | 0.423 | 0.537 | 0.652 |
| 27 | 0.323 | 0.381 | 0.487 | 0.597 |
| 32 | 0.296 | 0.349 | 0.449 | 0.554 |
| 42 | 0.257 | 0.304 | 0.393 | 0.490 |
| 52 | 0.231 | 0.273 | 0.354 | 0.443 |
| 62 | 0.211 | 0.250 | 0.325 | 0.408 |
| 82 | 0.183 | 0.217 | 0.283 | 0.357 |
| 102 | 0.164 | 0.195 | 0.254 | 0.321 |

# Appendix C
# Example data sets

* These data sets are all available electronically at
  http://www.reading.ac.uk/AcaDepts/sn/wsn1/publications99.html

**Table C.1**   Lung cancer data

The Bombay Cancer Registry obtains data from all cancer patients registered in the 168 government and private hospitals and nursing homes in Bombay, and from death records maintained by the Bombay Municipal Corporation. The survival times of each subject with lung cancer from time of first diagnosis to death (or censoring) were recorded over the period from 1 January 1989 to 31 December 1991. Data from the 682 subjects concerned are given below. In order, the variables are:

SURVIVAL TIME (days)

| | | | |
|---|---|---|---|
| CENSORED? | 0 = no | 1 = yes | |
| SEX | 1 = male | 2 = female | |
| AGE (years) | | | |
| EDUCATION | 1 = literate | 2 = illiterate | |
| RELIGION | 1 = Hindu | 2 = Christian | 3 = Muslim |
| MARITAL STATUS | 1 = single | 2 = separated/divorced | 3 = married |
| TYPE OF TUMOUR | 1 = local | 2 = regional | 3 = advanced |

The data are arranged in four segments.

| | | | |
|---|---|---|---|
| 1 0 1 58 2 3 3 2 | 2 0 1 46 2 1 3 3 | 6 1 1 65 1 3 3 2 | 9 0 1 59 2 1 3 3 |
| 1 0 1 75 2 3 3 3 | 2 0 1 75 2 1 3 1 | 6 1 1 30 2 1 3 2 | 9 0 1 53 2 1 1 2 |
| 1 0 1 60 2 3 3 3 | 3 0 1 65 2 3 3 3 | 6 0 1 60 2 3 3 2 | 9 1 1 32 2 1 3 3 |
| 1 0 1 64 2 1 3 3 | 3 0 2 65 2 1 3 2 | 6 0 2 30 2 1 2 2 | 9 0 2 45 2 1 3 1 |
| 1 0 2 45 2 2 3 2 | 3 0 2 60 2 3 3 3 | 6 0 1 50 1 1 3 1 | 10 0 1 62 2 1 1 2 |
| 1 0 1 70 2 1 3 3 | 3 0 2 74 2 1 3 2 | 6 0 2 80 2 1 3 1 | 10 0 2 64 2 1 3 3 |
| 1 0 1 55 2 1 3 3 | 3 0 1 68 2 1 3 3 | 6 0 1 65 1 1 3 2 | 10 0 1 78 2 1 3 3 |
| 1 0 2 65 2 1 3 2 | 3 0 1 50 2 1 3 3 | 6 0 1 54 2 1 3 3 | 10 0 2 60 1 1 3 1 |
| 1 0 1 55 2 3 3 2 | 3 0 1 32 2 3 3 3 | 6 0 1 50 2 1 3 2 | 10 0 1 50 1 1 3 2 |
| 1 0 1 56 2 2 1 3 | 3 0 1 52 2 1 3 2 | 6 0 1 42 2 1 3 1 | 10 0 2 11 2 1 1 1 |
| 1 0 1 65 2 2 3 2 | 4 0 2 22 2 1 3 1 | 6 0 1 65 1 1 3 2 | 10 0 2 59 2 1 3 2 |
| 1 0 1 65 2 1 3 2 | 4 0 2 52 2 1 3 1 | 6 0 1 65 2 2 1 2 | 11 0 1 75 2 3 1 2 |
| 1 0 1 70 2 3 3 2 | 4 0 1 60 2 3 3 2 | 6 0 1 65 2 1 3 1 | 11 0 1 76 2 1 3 3 |
| 1 0 1 62 2 3 3 3 | 4 0 2 42 2 3 3 3 | 6 0 1 77 2 1 3 3 | 11 0 1 70 1 1 3 2 |
| 1 1 1 63 2 1 3 1 | 4 0 1 40 2 1 3 2 | 6 0 1 60 2 1 3 1 | 11 0 1 65 2 3 3 3 |
| 1 0 1 75 2 1 3 3 | 4 0 1 36 2 1 1 3 | 7 0 1 60 2 1 3 3 | 11 0 1 57 1 1 3 1 |
| 1 0 1 75 2 1 3 3 | 4 0 1 39 2 2 3 2 | 7 0 1 45 2 1 3 2 | 12 0 2 56 2 1 1 1 |
| 1 0 1 30 2 1 3 3 | 4 0 1 75 2 2 2 1 | 7 1 1 71 1 1 3 1 | 12 0 1 46 2 3 3 3 |
| 2 0 1 40 2 3 3 3 | 4 0 1 67 2 3 3 1 | 7 0 1 65 2 1 3 3 | 12 0 1 85 2 1 1 2 |
| 2 0 2 81 2 2 1 2 | 4 0 1 53 2 1 3 3 | 7 0 1 70 1 1 3 2 | 12 0 1 63 2 1 3 2 |
| 2 0 1 70 2 1 1 1 | 4 0 1 39 1 2 1 3 | 7 0 1 62 2 1 2 3 | 12 0 1 55 2 1 1 2 |
| 2 0 1 60 2 3 3 3 | 4 0 1 65 2 3 3 2 | 7 0 1 84 2 1 1 2 | 12 0 1 38 2 3 3 2 |
| 2 0 1 47 2 2 1 1 | 4 0 1 69 2 2 1 3 | 8 0 1 55 2 1 3 3 | 12 0 1 40 2 3 3 2 |
| 2 0 1 55 2 1 1 3 | 5 0 1 50 1 3 3 1 | 8 0 1 62 2 1 3 3 | 12 0 1 57 2 3 3 3 |
| 2 0 1 65 2 1 3 3 | 5 0 2 70 2 3 3 3 | 8 0 2 40 2 1 3 1 | 12 0 1 55 2 1 3 3 |
| 2 0 2 50 2 2 3 2 | 5 0 1 49 2 3 1 1 | 9 0 1 60 2 1 3 2 | 13 0 1 35 2 1 1 1 |
| 2 0 1 65 2 1 3 3 | 5 0 1 48 2 1 3 3 | 9 0 1 56 2 1 1 2 | 13 0 1 60 2 1 3 2 |
| 2 0 1 55 2 2 3 2 | 5 0 1 70 2 1 3 2 | 9 0 1 70 2 1 3 2 | 13 0 1 47 2 1 3 2 |

| | | | |
|---|---|---|---|
| 2 0 2 65 2 3 3 2 | 5 0 1 65 2 1 3 3 | 9 0 1 74 2 1 1 2 | 13 1 1 61 2 3 3 1 |
| 2 0 1 72 2 1 3 3 | 5 0 1 62 2 1 3 2 | 9 0 2 50 2 1 1 1 | 13 0 1 70 2 1 1 2 |
| 2 0 1 70 2 1 3 1 | 5 0 1 60 2 1 3 3 | 9 0 1 45 2 1 3 3 | 13 0 1 55 1 1 3 2 |
| 2 0 1 65 2 1 3 3 | 6 0 1 64 2 1 3 1 | 9 0 1 60 2 1 3 1 | 13 0 1 25 2 1 1 2 |
| 2 0 1 50 2 1 3 3 | 6 0 2 50 2 1 3 3 | 9 0 1 52 1 2 3 2 | 14 0 1 62 2 1 3 2 |
| 2 0 2 60 2 1 3 3 | 6 0 1 51 2 1 3 3 | 9 0 1 30 2 1 3 3 | 14 0 1 63 2 1 1 2 |
| 14 0 1 38 2 3 3 3 | 29 0 1 60 2 3 3 1 | 44 0 1 21 1 1 1 3 | 75 0 1 80 2 1 3 3 |
| 15 0 1 71 2 1 3 3 | 30 0 2 50 2 1 2 3 | 45 0 2 85 2 2 1 2 | 75 0 1 30 2 1 3 3 |
| 15 0 1 78 2 3 3 3 | 30 0 1 56 2 1 3 3 | 45 0 1 76 1 1 3 2 | 75 0 1 62 2 1 3 1 |
| 15 0 1 65 1 1 3 2 | 30 0 1 66 2 1 3 3 | 46 1 1 46 2 1 3 1 | 76 1 2 64 2 2 2 1 |
| 15 0 1 55 2 3 3 2 | 31 0 1 56 2 1 3 2 | 46 0 1 50 2 3 3 1 | 76 1 1 67 2 1 3 1 |
| 15 0 1 78 2 1 3 2 | 31 0 2 55 2 3 3 2 | 46 0 1 45 2 1 3 1 | 76 1 1 71 1 1 3 1 |
| 16 0 2 55 2 1 3 2 | 31 0 2 44 2 3 3 3 | 46 1 1 55 1 1 3 1 | 76 1 1 44 2 1 3 1 |
| 16 0 1 21 2 1 1 1 | 31 1 1 65 2 2 3 3 | 46 0 1 63 2 3 3 1 | 77 0 1 59 2 2 3 3 |
| 17 0 1 40 2 3 3 3 | 31 1 1 44 2 1 3 2 | 46 0 1 58 2 1 3 3 | 78 1 2 40 2 3 3 3 |
| 17 1 1 66 2 2 1 1 | 32 0 2 40 2 1 3 2 | 46 1 1 55 2 3 3 1 | 78 1 1 46 1 3 3 1 |
| 17 0 1 76 2 2 3 2 | 32 0 1 60 2 1 3 3 | 47 0 1 86 1 1 3 2 | 79 0 1 45 2 1 3 3 |
| 17 0 1 62 2 1 2 1 | 32 1 1 47 1 1 3 1 | 47 0 1 46 2 1 2 3 | 81 0 1 70 1 1 3 2 |
| 17 0 1 60 2 1 3 1 | 33 0 1 50 2 3 3 1 | 47 0 2 60 2 1 1 1 | 81 1 2 60 2 1 3 1 |
| 17 0 1 63 1 1 3 1 | 34 0 2 75 1 3 2 2 | 48 1 1 65 2 1 3 2 | 82 0 1 73 1 1 1 2 |
| 18 0 1 45 2 1 3 3 | 34 0 1 32 2 1 1 3 | 48 1 1 60 2 1 3 2 | 82 1 2 50 1 1 1 1 |
| 18 0 1 45 2 1 1 2 | 34 0 1 58 2 1 3 3 | 48 0 1 75 1 1 3 2 | 82 0 1 65 1 1 3 1 |
| 18 0 1 60 2 1 3 2 | 34 0 1 50 2 3 3 3 | 48 0 1 44 1 1 3 2 | 82 0 1 66 2 1 3 3 |
| 18 1 1 70 2 3 3 3 | 34 0 1 70 2 1 3 2 | 48 0 1 72 2 1 3 2 | 82 1 2 65 2 1 3 3 |
| 18 1 1 51 2 1 3 1 | 34 0 1 70 2 1 3 3 | 48 0 1 65 1 1 3 2 | 83 0 1 57 2 1 3 3 |
| 19 0 2 45 2 1 3 2 | 34 0 1 65 2 2 3 2 | 49 1 1 56 2 1 1 1 | 83 1 2 27 1 1 3 1 |
| 19 1 2 45 2 1 2 1 | 34 1 1 65 2 1 3 2 | 50 0 1 55 2 1 3 3 | 83 0 1 60 2 3 3 1 |
| 19 1 1 71 1 1 3 3 | 35 0 1 89 2 1 1 2 | 52 0 1 75 2 3 3 3 | 83 1 1 50 2 1 3 1 |
| 20 1 1 51 2 3 3 2 | 35 0 1 65 2 3 3 2 | 52 0 1 70 1 1 2 2 | 84 0 1 46 2 1 3 2 |
| 20 0 1 60 2 1 3 3 | 35 0 1 57 2 1 3 1 | 52 0 1 52 2 1 3 2 | 84 0 1 35 2 1 3 3 |
| 20 0 1 35 1 1 3 1 | 35 0 1 40 1 1 3 2 | 52 0 1 50 1 3 3 1 | 84 0 2 68 2 1 1 3 |
| 20 0 1 59 2 2 3 2 | 35 0 1 57 1 1 3 2 | 53 0 1 65 1 1 3 1 | 85 0 1 50 1 1 3 1 |
| 20 0 1 68 1 1 2 2 | 35 1 2 40 1 1 3 3 | 53 0 1 53 1 1 3 2 | 86 0 1 45 2 1 3 3 |
| 21 0 1 42 1 1 3 1 | 36 1 1 68 2 1 3 3 | 54 1 1 61 1 3 3 1 | 87 1 1 36 2 1 3 2 |
| 21 0 1 45 2 1 3 1 | 36 0 1 64 2 1 2 2 | 54 1 1 32 2 1 3 2 | 87 0 1 65 2 1 3 3 |
| 21 0 1 57 1 1 3 1 | 36 0 1 70 1 3 3 2 | 54 0 1 25 2 1 1 3 | 88 0 2 42 2 1 3 1 |
| 21 0 1 60 1 1 3 2 | 36 0 2 50 2 3 3 1 | 58 1 1 47 1 2 3 1 | 89 0 1 60 1 3 3 2 |
| 22 0 1 65 2 1 3 2 | 36 0 1 75 2 3 3 3 | 58 1 1 50 2 3 1 1 | 89 0 1 55 2 1 3 3 |
| 22 0 1 55 2 1 3 2 | 36 0 2 65 2 1 3 2 | 59 0 1 48 2 1 1 3 | 89 0 1 59 2 3 3 3 |
| 22 0 1 55 2 3 3 1 | 36 0 2 50 1 1 3 2 | 59 0 1 60 2 1 3 1 | 89 1 1 68 1 1 3 3 |
| 22 0 1 60 2 1 3 3 | 37 0 1 55 2 3 3 3 | 60 0 1 55 1 1 3 2 | 89 1 1 52 2 1 3 3 |
| 23 0 1 32 2 1 1 2 | 37 0 1 56 2 3 3 2 | 60 0 1 81 1 1 3 2 | 89 0 1 56 1 1 3 1 |
| 23 0 1 72 2 3 3 3 | 37 0 1 74 2 1 3 2 | 62 1 1 42 1 1 3 1 | 90 1 1 57 2 2 2 3 |
| 24 0 1 72 2 2 1 2 | 38 0 1 30 2 1 1 1 | 62 0 1 50 1 1 3 2 | 90 1 1 70 1 3 3 3 |

```
24 0 2 72 2 1 3 2      39 0 1 63 2 2 3 3      65 0 1 74 2 1 3 3      90 0 1 58 2 1 3 2
24 0 1 50 2 1 3 2      39 0 1 50 2 1 1 3      65 0 1 52 2 1 3 3      91 0 1 32 2 1 1 1
24 1 2 55 2 1 3 1      40 0 1 48 2 1 3 1      66 0 2 50 2 1 3 3      91 1 1 34 2 1 3 2
26 0 1 60 1 1 1 1      40 1 1 57 2 1 3 1      68 0 1 65 1 3 3 2      91 1 1 60 2 2 1 3
26 0 1 55 2 1 1 2      40 1 1 33 1 2 3 2      68 0 1 53 1 1 3 2      92 0 1 70 2 1 3 3
26 0 1 52 2 1 3 2      40 1 1 72 2 1 3 2      68 0 1 68 1 1 3 2      94 1 2 50 1 1 3 2
26 1 1 42 2 1 3 2      40 1 1 36 1 3 3 2      70 0 1 70 2 3 2 3      94 0 2 65 1 2 2 2
26 0 2 70 2 1 2 2      41 0 1 52 2 3 3 2      70 0 1 60 2 1 3 2      94 1 1 57 2 1 3 1
26 1 1 63 1 1 3 3      41 0 2 65 1 1 3 2      71 0 1 67 2 1 3 3      95 1 2 50 2 1 3 3
27 0 1 70 2 1 3 3      41 1 1 72 1 1 3 1      71 0 1 55 2 3 3 1      95 1 1 60 2 3 3 3
27 1 1 60 2 1 3 3      42 0 1 40 2 3 3 2      72 0 2 43 2 2 3 2      95 1 2 60 2 3 2 1
27 0 2 70 2 3 2 3      42 1 1 64 2 2 3 3      73 0 1 67 1 1 3 2      96 1 1 59 1 1 3 3
27 0 2 38 1 3 3 1      42 0 1 67 2 2 1 2      73 1 2 70 2 2 2 1      97 0 1 53 2 1 3 3
28 1 1 70 2 3 3 1      42 0 1 50 1 1 3 2      74 1 1 56 1 2 3 1      97 0 1 40 2 1 3 3
28 0 2 45 2 3 3 3      43 0 2 80 2 1 2 3      74 1 2 60 2 3 3 1      100 0 2 45 1 3 3 1
28 1 1 57 1 1 3 1      43 0 1 82 1 1 3 2      74 1 1 64 2 1 1 1      100 0 1 60 2 1 3 3
29 0 1 39 1 1 3 1      44 0 1 70 2 1 3 2      75 0 1 66 2 1 3 2      101 0 1 50 2 1 3 1
101 0 1 66 2 1 3 3     145 1 1 45 1 3 3 2     203 1 2 70 2 3 3 3     261 0 1 49 2 3 3 3
101 1 1 60 2 1 3 1     145 0 1 45 1 1 3 2     203 1 1 60 2 1 1 3     261 1 1 55 2 3 3 1
102 1 1 63 1 1 3 1     146 1 1 77 2 1 3 1     204 1 1 45 2 3 3 3     261 1 1 50 2 1 3 1
102 0 1 55 2 3 3 3     147 0 1 59 1 1 3 3     205 0 2 60 2 1 1 1     261 0 1 56 2 3 3 1
102 0 1 65 2 1 3 3     147 0 1 40 2 1 2 2     206 1 1 60 2 1 3 1     263 0 1 48 2 1 3 3
103 0 1 60 2 1 3 2     147 0 1 39 1 1 3 2     207 1 1 60 1 1 3 2     265 1 2 35 2 1 3 1
104 0 1 46 2 1 3 3     148 0 1 60 2 1 3 1     207 1 2 65 1 1 2 2     266 1 2 68 1 1 3 1
104 0 1 65 1 1 3 2     149 1 1 70 2 1 3 3     208 1 1 62 2 1 3 1     266 1 1 65 2 2 3 1
105 0 1 68 2 1 3 3     149 0 1 50 2 1 3 3     209 0 1 55 2 1 3 3     267 1 2 66 2 1 3 2
106 1 1 60 2 3 3 2     149 1 1 69 1 1 1 1     210 1 1 52 2 1 3 1     267 0 1 75 2 1 3 3
107 0 1 65 1 1 3 1     150 1 2 78 1 2 3 1     210 1 1 52 2 2 3 1     268 1 1 49 2 1 3 3
108 1 1 70 2 2 2 1     151 0 1 55 2 1 3 3     210 1 1 65 2 1 1 3     269 1 1 60 2 1 3 1
108 0 2 50 2 1 3 3     153 0 2 69 2 1 2 2     211 0 2 40 2 1 3 2     270 1 1 50 1 3 3 1
108 1 1 68 2 1 3 3     153 0 2 48 1 1 3 2     213 1 1 58 2 1 3 1     271 1 1 40 2 3 3 3
109 0 1 74 2 2 3 2     154 0 1 57 1 1 3 1     214 0 2 75 2 1 1 3     271 0 2 70 2 3 3 3
110 0 1 50 2 3 3 1     155 1 1 53 2 3 3 2     216 0 1 68 2 1 3 3     271 0 1 64 2 3 3 3
110 0 1 51 2 1 3 2     155 1 1 51 1 1 3 2     216 0 1 80 1 2 3 2     272 1 2 52 2 1 2 2
112 0 1 70 2 1 1 2     155 1 1 54 1 3 3 1     216 0 1 59 1 1 3 1     272 1 1 55 2 3 3 3
114 1 1 70 2 3 3 3     156 0 2 60 2 1 3 1     216 1 1 45 2 1 3 2     273 1 1 60 2 3 1 1
114 0 1 72 2 1 3 2     158 1 2 70 2 1 3 3     217 0 2 73 2 1 3 3     274 0 1 65 2 1 3 3
115 1 1 70 1 1 3 2     159 1 1 71 2 1 3 1     217 1 1 72 2 1 3 2     274 0 2 45 2 1 3 3
115 1 1 53 2 1 3 1     159 1 1 69 2 3 3 3     220 0 1 59 2 1 3 2     275 1 1 73 2 1 1 3
116 1 1 70 2 1 3 1     160 0 1 36 1 1 3 1     220 1 1 38 1 3 3 2     275 1 2 70 2 3 2 1
116 1 1 52 1 1 1 1     161 1 1 66 1 2 3 1     222 0 1 46 2 1 3 3     277 1 1 50 2 3 3 1
117 0 1 66 2 1 3 2     161 0 1 75 2 1 3 3     222 0 1 71 2 1 3 3     277 0 1 52 2 1 3 3
117 1 1 45 2 1 3 1     161 1 1 42 2 1 3 1     223 0 1 50 2 3 3 1     277 1 1 48 1 1 3 1
121 1 1 60 2 2 3 1     161 0 1 60 2 1 3 3     223 1 1 55 1 1 3 2     279 1 1 70 2 1 2 1
```

121 1 1 55 1 1 3 2
121 1 1 72 2 1 3 2
122 1 2 70 2 1 3 2
123 0 1 60 1 1 3 1
123 0 1 46 2 1 3 3
124 0 1 55 1 1 3 1
124 0 2 45 2 1 3 1
125 0 1 65 2 1 3 3
126 0 1 70 2 1 3 1
128 0 1 68 2 1 3 3
128 1 1 40 2 1 1 1
130 1 1 40 1 3 3 2
130 1 1 45 2 1 3 1
131 0 1 70 2 1 3 3
132 0 2 67 2 1 3 1
132 1 1 60 2 1 3 3
136 1 1 63 1 3 3 2
136 0 2 68 2 1 2 3
138 0 1 70 2 1 3 3
138 0 1 50 2 1 3 3
139 0 1 69 2 1 3 1
139 0 1 67 2 1 3 3
139 0 1 60 2 1 1 2
139 0 1 62 2 3 3 1
141 1 1 45 2 1 3 1
143 0 1 50 2 3 3 3
143 0 1 52 1 1 3 2
144 1 1 21 1 2 1 1
307 0 1 40 2 3 3 3
308 0 1 37 2 3 3 3
309 1 1 63 1 1 3 1
310 1 1 59 1 1 3 3
312 1 1 75 1 2 1 2
314 0 1 57 2 1 3 3
314 1 1 60 2 1 3 1
314 1 1 55 1 1 3 2
314 0 2 41 2 3 3 3
318 1 1 42 1 1 3 3
319 1 1 55 1 1 3 1
319 1 1 60 2 3 3 1
320 0 1 45 1 1 3 2
321 0 1 53 2 1 3 3
322 0 1 65 2 3 3 3
323 1 2 72 2 1 3 2

165 1 1 50 1 1 3 3
167 0 1 41 2 2 3 3
170 0 1 55 2 1 3 3
171 0 1 32 2 3 3 3
172 1 1 48 1 1 2 3
172 1 1 50 2 1 3 3
173 0 1 50 1 3 3 1
174 0 1 73 1 1 3 1
175 0 1 58 2 1 3 3
177 1 1 65 1 1 3 1
178 0 1 50 2 3 1 3
178 0 1 64 2 1 3 3
178 0 1 50 2 1 2 1
179 1 1 43 1 1 3 2
180 0 1 55 2 1 3 3
180 0 1 38 2 1 3 3
183 1 1 60 2 3 3 1
186 0 2 50 2 1 3 3
188 0 2 55 2 1 3 3
189 0 1 66 2 1 3 3
190 0 1 55 2 1 3 3
192 1 1 60 2 3 3 3
193 1 1 80 2 1 3 2
194 0 1 66 2 1 3 2
194 0 1 64 1 2 3 2
196 1 1 57 1 1 3 1
199 1 1 50 1 1 3 1
199 0 2 66 2 1 3 2
420 1 2 58 2 1 1 2
420 1 1 58 1 1 1 1
423 0 2 57 2 1 3 3
429 0 2 60 2 1 2 3
430 0 1 62 2 1 3 3
443 0 1 64 2 1 3 3
446 1 2 58 2 1 1 2
450 1 1 61 2 1 3 1
454 0 1 55 2 2 3 3
454 1 1 55 2 1 1 2
455 0 1 65 2 1 3 3
460 0 2 75 2 1 2 3
461 1 1 51 2 1 3 1
476 1 1 65 2 1 3 2
479 0 2 52 2 1 3 3
492 0 1 73 2 3 3 3

223 0 1 72 2 1 3 1
227 1 1 44 2 1 3 1
229 0 1 46 2 3 3 3
229 0 1 45 2 1 3 3
230 1 1 72 2 2 3 1
231 1 1 58 2 1 3 1
231 1 1 53 1 2 3 3
231 1 1 70 2 3 3 1
234 0 1 41 2 1 3 3
234 1 1 60 2 3 3 3
235 1 1 57 1 1 3 2
236 0 1 70 1 2 3 3
238 1 1 40 1 1 2 2
238 1 1 68 1 1 3 2
238 0 1 53 2 1 3 3
241 1 1 65 2 2 3 1
242 1 1 76 2 1 3 3
243 0 2 73 2 2 2 3
243 0 1 70 2 1 3 3
248 1 1 74 1 3 3 1
248 1 1 50 2 2 1 1
249 0 1 70 2 1 3 3
251 1 1 53 2 2 3 2
252 1 1 76 2 1 3 1
253 1 1 60 2 3 1 2
259 0 1 82 2 1 2 3
261 1 2 53 1 1 3 1
261 1 1 52 2 3 3 2
325 0 1 55 2 1 3 3
326 1 1 99 2 1 3 2
329 1 2 35 2 1 3 1
329 1 1 48 1 1 3 3
330 1 2 12 2 1 1 2
331 1 1 73 2 3 3 3
332 1 1 54 2 1 3 2
337 1 1 50 2 3 3 1
337 1 1 56 1 2 3 3
337 1 1 75 2 3 3 1
338 1 1 74 2 1 2 2
339 1 1 79 2 2 3 1
341 0 1 64 2 1 3 3
341 1 1 64 2 1 3 1
341 1 1 63 2 3 3 3
342 0 1 60 2 1 3 3

281 1 2 48 2 1 3 3
281 1 1 58 1 1 3 1
285 0 2 70 2 1 3 3
285 1 1 38 1 2 3 3
286 1 1 45 2 1 3 1
286 0 1 55 2 1 3 3
287 0 2 55 2 1 3 3
287 1 1 55 2 3 3 1
287 0 1 73 2 1 3 3
288 1 1 53 2 1 3 1
288 1 1 49 2 1 1 1
289 1 1 51 1 3 3 1
289 1 1 68 2 1 3 1
289 1 2 50 2 1 3 1
289 1 1 50 1 1 3 1
291 1 1 50 2 3 2 3
291 0 1 62 2 1 3 3
291 1 1 49 1 2 3 3
292 0 1 65 2 1 3 3
292 0 1 63 2 3 3 3
293 1 2 45 2 1 3 1
295 0 1 76 2 3 3 3
295 1 1 58 2 1 1 1
296 1 1 54 2 1 3 1
301 0 1 55 2 2 3 3
302 1 1 48 2 3 1 3
302 1 1 35 2 1 3 3
307 1 1 60 2 1 3 3
494 0 1 42 2 1 3 3
497 1 1 70 1 1 3 2
524 0 2 65 2 1 3 3
527 0 1 60 2 1 3 3
530 1 1 79 2 1 3 2
534 0 2 70 2 1 2 3
534 1 1 55 2 1 3 1
548 1 1 55 1 3 3 1
550 1 1 75 2 1 3 1
554 0 1 41 2 3 3 3
576 0 1 75 2 1 3 3
588 0 1 60 2 3 3 3
588 1 1 58 1 1 3 2
595 1 1 51 2 1 3 1
600 0 1 32 2 1 1 3
600 0 1 70 2 1 3 2

| | | | | | | | | | | | | | | | | | |
|---|---|---|---|---|---|---|---|---|---|---|---|---|---|---|---|---|---|
| 342 | 1 | 2 | 65 | 2 | 3 | 3 | 3 | | 408 | 0 | 1 | 56 | 2 | 1 | 3 | 3 |
| 343 | 1 | 2 | 35 | 2 | 1 | 3 | 1 | | 416 | 0 | 1 | 62 | 2 | 3 | 3 | 3 |
| 344 | 0 | 1 | 58 | 2 | 1 | 3 | 3 | | 618 | 1 | 1 | 67 | 1 | 1 | 3 | 2 |
| 344 | 0 | 2 | 44 | 2 | 1 | 3 | 3 | | 628 | 1 | 1 | 65 | 2 | 1 | 1 | 1 |
| 345 | 1 | 1 | 75 | 2 | 3 | 3 | 1 | | 632 | 0 | 1 | 52 | 2 | 1 | 3 | 3 |
| 348 | 1 | 1 | 47 | 2 | 1 | 3 | 1 | | 635 | 0 | 1 | 60 | 2 | 1 | 3 | 3 |
| 349 | 1 | 2 | 40 | 2 | 3 | 3 | 2 | | 639 | 1 | 2 | 62 | 1 | 1 | 2 | 2 |
| 350 | 1 | 2 | 38 | 2 | 1 | 3 | 1 | | 647 | 1 | 1 | 62 | 2 | 1 | 3 | 2 |
| 350 | 1 | 1 | 72 | 1 | 1 | 3 | 1 | | 653 | 1 | 1 | 70 | 2 | 1 | 3 | 2 |
| 350 | 1 | 1 | 55 | 1 | 1 | 3 | 3 | | 653 | 1 | 2 | 52 | 1 | 1 | 3 | 2 |
| 354 | 1 | 1 | 76 | 2 | 1 | 3 | 2 | | 656 | 0 | 1 | 37 | 2 | 1 | 3 | 3 |
| 355 | 1 | 1 | 41 | 1 | 1 | 3 | 1 | | 688 | 1 | 2 | 48 | 2 | 1 | 1 | 2 |
| 357 | 0 | 2 | 70 | 2 | 1 | 2 | 3 | | 692 | 1 | 1 | 52 | 2 | 1 | 3 | 2 |
| 368 | 0 | 1 | 50 | 2 | 1 | 1 | 3 | | 696 | 1 | 1 | 60 | 1 | 1 | 3 | 1 |
| 370 | 0 | 1 | 70 | 2 | 1 | 3 | 3 | | 700 | 0 | 1 | 54 | 2 | 3 | 3 | 3 |
| 375 | 0 | 1 | 57 | 2 | 1 | 3 | 3 | | 700 | 1 | 1 | 50 | 1 | 3 | 3 | 2 |
| 377 | 0 | 1 | 72 | 2 | 1 | 1 | 1 | | 705 | 0 | 1 | 50 | 2 | 3 | 3 | 3 |
| 380 | 0 | 1 | 70 | 2 | 1 | 3 | 3 | | 731 | 0 | 1 | 50 | 2 | 1 | 1 | 3 |
| 397 | 0 | 1 | 66 | 2 | 1 | 3 | 3 | | 812 | 0 | 2 | 52 | 2 | 1 | 3 | 3 |
| 397 | 0 | 1 | 69 | 2 | 1 | 3 | 3 | | 838 | 0 | 1 | 44 | 2 | 1 | 3 | 3 |
| 403 | 0 | 2 | 42 | 2 | 1 | 3 | 3 | | 852 | 0 | 1 | 62 | 2 | 3 | 3 | 3 |

**Table C.2**  A selected subset of data from the third Glasgow MONICA Survey
The MONICA Study is an international collaborative investigation into heart disease. Data from a random sample of 40 of the subjects in the third MONICA survey in north Glasgow are given below. The variables selected here are the subject's age and alcohol consumption in the past week, ascertained by questionnaire, and protein C and protein S measurements from blood samples. Alcohol consumption was classified using standard alcohol grades. See Lowe *et al.* (1997) for analysis of the full data set involving 1564 people.

In order, the variables shown below are:
AGE (years)
ALCOHOL GROUP 1 = non-drinker, 2 = occasional drinker (zero consumption in the past week), 3 = mild, 4 = medium,  5 = heavy
PROTEIN C (iu/dl)
PROTEIN S (% pool)


The data are arranged in three segments below.

| | | | | | | | | | | | |
|---|---|---|---|---|---|---|---|---|---|---|---|
| 67 | 1 | 143 | 66.40 | 46 | 2 | 181 | 125.33 | 36 | 4 | 80 | 107.90 |
| 71 | 2 | 172 | 136.95 | 35 | 3 | 110 | 107.07 | 62 | 1 | 111 | 101.26 |
| 35 | 5 | 99 | 102.92 | 34 | 3 | 96 | 99.60 | 46 | 4 | 92 | 85.49 |
| 74 | 4 | 104 | 136.12 | 25 | 3 | 93 | 64.74 | 59 | 4 | 126 | 142.76 |
| 58 | 5 | 114 | 115.37 | 63 | 3 | 83 | 87.98 | 53 | 2 | 188 | 102.09 |
| 39 | 5 | 150 | 117.86 | 58 | 4 | 81 | 92.96 | 39 | 3 | 94 | 87.98 |
| 67 | 5 | 82 | 124.50 | 56 | 2 | 90 | 105.41 | 55 | 3 | 153 | 104.58 |
| 67 | 2 | 115 | 63.91 | 28 | 4 | 106 | 100.43 | 72 | 3 | 108 | 131.97 |
| 65 | 1 | 151 | 131.97 | 48 | 4 | 88 | 92.13 | 28 | 4 | 106 | 89.64 |
| 66 | 1 | 162 | 97.94 | 65 | 2 | 92 | 93.79 | 71 | 2 | 105 | 99.60 |
| 43 | 4 | 87 | 116.20 | 39 | 5 | 181 | 109.56 | 56 | 2 | 179 | 122.84 |
| 25 | 2 | 92 | 78.02 | 37 | 4 | 128 | 123.67 | 73 | 1 | 120 | 107.07 |
| 47 | 3 | 102 | 99.60 | 51 | 4 | 144 | 117.86 | 37 | 3 | 135 | 94.62 |
| 64 | 3 | 122 | 110.39 | | | | | | | | |

**Table C.3** Summary data from the complete third Glasgow MONICA Survey

This table gives summary results, as analysed in more detail by Woodward *et al.* (1997), from the same survey that gave rise to Table C.2 but now using the complete data set. The variables tabulated are sex, 10-year age group, factor IX status (high = above sex-specific median, low = below) by prevalent cardiovascular disease (CVD) status.

| Factor IX status | Age group (years) | | | | | | | | | | | |
| | 25–34 | | 35–44 | | 45–54 | | 55–64 | | 65–74 | | Total | |
| | CVD | No CVD | CVD | No CVD | CVD | No CVD | CVD | No CVD | CVD | No CVD | CVD | No CVD |
| **Males** | | | | | | | | | | | | |
| Low | 6 | 75 | 12 | 56 | 24 | 40 | 35 | 39 | 34 | 33 | 111 | 243 |
| High | 4 | 20 | 15 | 56 | 29 | 52 | 36 | 54 | 38 | 52 | 122 | 234 |
| Total | 10 | 95 | 27 | 112 | 53 | 92 | 71 | 93 | 72 | 85 | 233 | 477 |
| **Females** | | | | | | | | | | | | |
| Low | 18 | 69 | 21 | 87 | 21 | 62 | 19 | 37 | 27 | 24 | 106 | 279 |
| High | 11 | 32 | 11 | 34 | 36 | 58 | 39 | 59 | 57 | 62 | 154 | 245 |
| Total | 29 | 101 | 32 | 121 | 57 | 120 | 58 | 96 | 84 | 86 | 260 | 524 |

**Table C.4**  Brain metastases data
The table below shows survival times for 17 consecutive patients with brain metastases from lung tumours who were treated with hyperthermia plus nitrosoureas, as reported by Pontiggia *et al.* (1995).

| Age (years) | Prior treatment | Outcome | Survival time (months) |
|---|---|---|---|
| 69 | No | Death | 20 |
| 52 | Yes | Drop-out | 13 |
| 62 | No | Drop-out | 19 |
| 49 | No | Death | 12 |
| 60 | Yes | Death | 5 |
| 61 | Yes | Death | 23 |
| 61 | Yes | Death | 5 |
| 60 | No | Other cause | 12 |
| 56 | No | Death | 2 |
| 59 | No | Death | 28 |
| 64 | Yes | Death | 12 |
| 51 | No | Death | 7 |
| 67 | No | Death | 16 |
| 62 | No | Death | 12 |
| 45 | No | Death | 5 |
| 62 | No | Alive | 11 |
| 39 | Yes | Alive | 8 |

Note: 'Other cause' means a non-tumour-related death. All other deaths are due to tumours.

**Table C.5**  Smelter workers data

Breslow and Day (1987) give the following data from the Montana smelter workers study. These data are for men employed before 1925, showing the number of deaths and man-years (PYs) of low and high arsenic exposure within age groups and calendar periods. Low exposure means less than 1 year, high exposure means 15 or more years, of work in areas which are known to have a considerable amount of arsenic trioxide in their atmosphere. The study concluded in September 1977.

| Age group (years) | Exposure | Calendar period | | | | | | | |
| | | 1938–49 | | 1950–59 | | 1960–69 | | 1970–77 | |
| | | Deaths | PYs | Deaths | PYs | Deaths | PYs | Deaths | PYs |
| --- | --- | --- | --- | --- | --- | --- | --- | --- | --- |
| 40–49 | High | 0 | 337.29 | 0 | 121.00 | | | | |
| | Low | 2 | 3075.27 | 0 | 936.75 | | | | |
| 50–59 | High | 4 | 626.72 | 3 | 349.53 | 1 | 142.33 | | |
| | Low | 2 | 2849.76 | 3 | 2195.59 | 3 | 747.77 | | |
| 60–69 | High | 9 | 672.09 | 7 | 441.10 | 3 | 244.82 | 1 | 100.64 |
| | Low | 2 | 2085.43 | 7 | 1675.91 | 10 | 1501.73 | 1 | 440.21 |
| 70–79 | High | 1 | 277.25 | 2 | 268.27 | 1 | 197.20 | 2 | 92.75 |
| | Low | 3 | 833.61 | 6 | 973.32 | 6 | 1027.12 | 6 | 674.44 |

**Table C.6**  Venous thromboembolism data

In a matched case–control study of venous thromboembolism (VTE) and use of hormone replacement therapy (HRT), Daly *et al.* (1996) screened women aged 45–64 years admitted to hospitals in the Oxford Regional Health Authority with a suspected diagnosis of VTE. From these, 103 cases of idiopathic VTE were recruited. Each case was individually matched with up to two hospital controls with diagnoses judged to be unrelated to HRT use, such as diseases of the eyes, ears or skin. Matching criteria were 5-year age group, district of admission and data of admission (between 2 weeks before and 4 months after the admission date of the corresponding case). Altogether there were 178 controls. The data are given below. In order, the four variables are:

SET NUMBER (identifying the matched groups)

| | | |
|---|---|---|
| CASE–CONTROL STATUS | 0 = control | 1 = case |
| HRT STATUS | 0 = not a current user | 1 = current user |

BODY MASS INDEX $(kg/m^2)$

An asterisk denotes a missing value. The data are arranged in four segments.

| | | | |
|---|---|---|---|
| 1 1 0 32.74 | 15 0 1 35.87 | 29 0 0 32.19 | 42 0 0 28.52 |
| 1 0 0 22.00 | 16 1 1 28.52 | 32 1 0 34.05 | 43 1 0 24.78 |
| 1 0 0 29.83 | 16 0 0 25.65 | 32 0 1 31.38 | 43 0 1 19.20 |
| 2 1 0 29.26 | 16 0 0 21.05 | 33 1 1 23.14 | 43 0 0 30.34 |
| 2 0 1 20.42 | 17 1 1 29.16 | 33 0 0 20.17 | 44 1 0 19.80 |
| 2 0 0 21.36 | 17 0 0 27.89 | 33 0 0 30.91 | 44 0 0 22.89 |
| 4 1 0 23.56 | 17 0 1 22.15 | 34 1 0 20.39 | 44 0 0 22.58 |
| 4 0 0 30.63 | 20 1 1 28.68 | 34 0 0 31.60 | 46 1 0 24.39 |
| 4 0 0 25.39 | 20 0 1 24.10 | 34 0 0 20.73 | 46 0 0 21.99 |
| 5 1 1 30.76 | 20 0 1 45.00 | 35 1 0 21.14 | 46 0 0 25.86 |
| 5 0 1 27.99 | 22 1 1 31.25 | 35 0 0 23.90 | 47 1 0 23.32 |
| 5 0 0 25.30 | 22 0 0 * | 35 0 0 24.76 | 47 0 0 31.37 |
| 6 1 0 21.01 | 23 1 0 27.55 | 36 1 1 20.27 | 47 0 0 20.32 |
| 6 0 0 28.00 | 23 0 0 24.43 | 36 0 0 23.04 | 48 1 0 19.81 |
| 6 0 0 21.43 | 23 0 0 19.46 | 36 0 0 26.43 | 48 0 0 26.05 |
| 7 1 1 27.30 | 24 1 0 45.00 | 37 1 0 22.70 | 48 0 0 29.65 |
| 7 0 0 23.21 | 24 0 0 22.50 | 37 0 0 22.50 | 49 1 1 23.36 |
| 7 0 0 20.32 | 24 0 0 24.39 | 37 0 1 25.03 | 49 0 0 23.65 |
| 9 1 0 46.20 | 25 1 1 20.61 | 38 1 1 23.36 | 49 0 1 30.77 |
| 9 0 0 * | 25 0 0 20.41 | 38 0 0 35.87 | 51 1 1 32.42 |
| 10 1 1 26.45 | 25 0 0 27.06 | 38 0 0 27.89 | 51 0 0 25.56 |
| 10 0 0 20.55 | 26 1 0 28.34 | 39 1 0 21.53 | 51 0 1 23.72 |
| 10 0 0 31.50 | 26 0 0 30.04 | 39 0 0 27.47 | 52 1 1 23.55 |
| 11 1 1 27.63 | 27 1 1 32.27 | 39 0 0 33.98 | 52 0 0 31.74 |
| 11 0 0 23.05 | 27 0 1 23.08 | 40 1 1 25.15 | 52 0 0 30.36 |
| 11 0 1 18.76 | 27 0 1 28.36 | 40 0 0 24.80 | 53 1 1 27.33 |
| 12 1 0 39.19 | 28 1 1 22.70 | 41 1 1 29.77 | 53 0 0 17.38 |
| 12 0 0 23.90 | 28 0 0 24.24 | 41 0 0 28.60 | 53 0 0 28.37 |
| 12 0 0 23.90 | 28 0 1 26.53 | 41 0 1 19.79 | 54 1 0 21.78 |

```
15 1 0 24.72        29 1 1 30.09        42 1 0 38.66        54 0 0 33.94
15 0 1 21.36        29 0 1 26.27        42 0 0 27.33        54 0 1 23.16
55 1 0 19.88        72 0 0 29.16        97 1 0 28.92        119 0 1 26.31
55 0 1 29.26        73 1 0 25.67        97 0 0 22.47        121 1 1 27.48
55 0 1 28.60        73 0 1 26.54        101 1 0 31.03       121 0 0 25.74
56 1 0 34.49        73 0 1 22.21        101 0 0 28.91       122 1 0 23.90
56 0 0 34.02        74 1 0 25.46        101 0 0 29.00       122 0 0 42.22
56 0 0 26.21        74 0 0 25.16        102 1 0 24.19       122 0 0 25.81
57 1 1 26.31        74 0 0 23.92        102 0 0 28.43       123 1 1 25.93
57 0 0 24.46        76 1 0 22.02        102 0 0 31.64       123 0 0 28.23
57 0 0 21.61        76 0 0 27.03        103 1 1 39.49       123 0 1 22.82
58 1 1 21.36        76 0 0 18.22        103 0 0 23.81       124 1 0 30.04
58 0 1 28.16        77 1 1 28.52        103 0 0 24.09       124 0 0 26.05
58 0 0 27.00        77 0 0 27.03        105 1 0 23.90       124 0 1 25.76
60 1 0 26.31        77 0 0 39.20        105 0 0 29.07       125 1 0 25.70
60 0 0 31.72        81 1 0 20.65        106 1 0 34.38       125 0 0 22.07
60 0 0 29.07        81 0 1 25.09        106 0 1 18.72       126 1 0 38.27
61 1 0 36.33        81 0 0 28.35        106 0 0 21.53       126 0 1 29.65
61 0 0 26.96        82 1 1 15.20        107 1 1 26.37       126 0 0 25.62
62 1 0 *            82 0 0 33.05        107 0 0 26.45       127 1 1 21.88
62 0 0 27.06        82 0 0 26.22        107 0 0 21.97       127 0 0 33.10
62 0 0 24.98        83 1 1 22.50        108 1 1 25.26       127 0 1 21.91
63 1 0 21.15        83 0 1 32.42        108 0 0 20.73       128 1 1 33.98
63 0 0 23.84        83 0 1 20.90        109 1 0 27.30       128 0 1 22.50
64 1 1 24.51        84 1 0 36.70        109 0 0 33.27       128 0 0 23.37
64 0 1 22.70        84 0 0 23.80        110 1 0 31.86       129 1 0 29.88
64 0 0 24.09        84 0 1 28.30        110 0 0 21.30       129 0 0 27.55
65 1 0 31.72        86 1 1 21.42        112 1 1 28.68       130 1 0 23.37
65 0 0 19.49        86 0 0 21.88        112 0 1 27.85       130 0 0 26.10
65 0 0 23.63        87 1 1 23.37        112 0 0 24.10       130 0 0 31.03
66 1 0 23.91        87 0 0 22.32        114 1 1 32.42       131 1 0 31.99
66 0 0 24.61        87 0 0 21.86        114 0 0 28.13       131 0 0 21.97
67 1 1 34.38        88 1 0 34.58        115 1 0 29.65       133 1 0 38.44
67 0 0 34.58        88 0 0 20.76        115 0 0 24.19       133 0 0 22.23
67 0 1 34.37        93 1 1 27.41        115 0 0 21.05       133 0 1 39.36
70 1 1 25.44        93 0 1 24.09        116 1 0 23.96       134 1 1 21.91
70 0 1 23.11        94 1 1 30.04        116 0 0 25.76       134 0 1 28.72
70 0 1 21.88        94 0 0 23.82        116 0 1 20.32       135 1 0 29.16
71 1 0 25.76        95 1 0 20.73        117 1 0 40.75       135 0 0 24.46
71 0 0 24.86        95 0 0 25.12        117 0 0 29.96
72 1 0 26.31        96 1 0 30.36        117 0 0 21.97
72 0 0 23.63        96 0 0 30.36        119 1 1 27.53
```

**Table C.7**   Cerebral palsy data

In a randomized controlled single-blind parallel group study lumbo-sacral selective posterior rhizotomy (SPR) followed by intensive physiotherapy was compared with physiotherapy alone in improving motor function in children with diplegic cerebral palsy (Steinbok *et al.*, 1997). The table below shows the Gross Motor Function Measure before and after therapy (lasting for 9 months) for each subject.

| SPR plus physiotherapy group | | Physiotherapy group | |
|---|---|---|---|
| *Before* | *After* | *Before* | *After* |
| 81.7 | 89.7 | 70.3 | 74.0 |
| 48.1 | 58.2 | 39.9 | 52.9 |
| 69.2 | 87.0 | 82.0 | 89.7 |
| 87.7 | 92.4 | 65.3 | 62.8 |
| 43.1 | 66.6 | 62.4 | 69.6 |
| 67.8 | 75.0 | 82.2 | 85.7 |
| 59.9 | 63.6 | 52.5 | 61.6 |
| 42.2 | 53.3 | 62.5 | 65.6 |
| 72.4 | 86.5 | 65.0 | 69.2 |
| 43.9 | 59.5 | 70.4 | 75.2 |
| 48.8 | 52.5 | 58.3 | 63.5 |
| 81.7 | 90.6 | 48.5 | 55.6 |
| 44.9 | 67.8 | 33.0 | 35.7 |
| 58.7 | 65.2 | 86.0 | 89.1 |

**Table C.8**   Norwegian Multicentre Study data
In the Norwegian Multicentre Study survivors of acute myocardial infarction were randomly allocated to either Blocadren or placebo (Hwang and Rodda, 1992). The table below shows the number at risk at the start of each month and the number of deaths within that month, over 34 months of study.

| Month | Blocadren At risk | Deaths | Placebo At risk | Deaths |
|---|---|---|---|---|
| 1 | 945 | 19 | 939 | 31 |
| 2 | 926 | 10 | 908 | 9 |
| 3 | 916 | 7 | 899 | 4 |
| 4 | 909 | 3 | 895 | 10 |
| 5 | 906 | 5 | 885 | 7 |
| 6 | 901 | 6 | 878 | 10 |
| 7 | 895 | 5 | 868 | 10 |
| 8 | 890 | 2 | 858 | 3 |
| 9 | 888 | 5 | 855 | 7 |
| 10 | 883 | 2 | 848 | 4 |
| 11 | 881 | 3 | 844 | 6 |
| 12 | 878 | 5 | 838 | 5 |
| 13 | 873 | 1 | 833 | 6 |
| 14 | 836 | 0 | 801 | 2 |
| 15 | 806 | 5 | 764 | 5 |
| 16 | 767 | 5 | 737 | 3 |
| 17 | 722 | 0 | 702 | 3 |
| 18 | 672 | 0 | 649 | 4 |
| 19 | 631 | 0 | 599 | 1 |
| 20 | 592 | 2 | 558 | 3 |
| 21 | 542 | 2 | 523 | 2 |
| 22 | 507 | 1 | 483 | 1 |
| 23 | 463 | 2 | 442 | 1 |
| 24 | 419 | 0 | 393 | 3 |
| 25 | 375 | 1 | 352 | 2 |
| 26 | 337 | 0 | 315 | 1 |
| 27 | 295 | 0 | 278 | 2 |
| 28 | 267 | 2 | 242 | 2 |
| 29 | 237 | 2 | 207 | 0 |
| 30 | 197 | 2 | 172 | 2 |
| 31 | 145 | 1 | 126 | 0 |
| 32 | 100 | 0 | 81 | 3 |
| 33 | 50 | 0 | 39 | 0 |
| 34 | 12 | 0 | 7 | 0 |

Reprinted from Peace (1992, p. 222), by courtesy of Marcel Dekker Inc.

**Table C.9**   Rheumatoid arthritis data
In the rheumatoid arthritis cross-over study of Hill *et al.* (1990) carried out at Leeds General Infirmary and described in Example 7.6, subjects were asked to record how many paracetamol tablets they took, to alleviate pain, over each of their 2-week treatment periods. The results appear below.

| *Ibuprofen–Aspergesic group* | | *Aspergesic–ibuprofen group* | |
|---|---|---|---|
| *Period 1* | *Period 2* | *Period 1* | *Period 2* |
| 2.400 | 2.133 | 2.462 | 0.857 |
| 2.667 | 0.400 | 1.429 | 5.846 |
| 1.571 | 1.571 | 0.000 | 3.429 |
| 4.142 | 4.571 | 0.286 | 0.400 |
| 0.733 | 1.429 | 0.143 | 0.286 |
| 3.000 | 1.142 | 7.571 | 6.714 |
| 2.667 | 3.067 | 0.000 | 0.000 |
| 0.000 | 0.000 | 0.000 | 0.000 |
| 1.571 | 0.000 | 1.538 | 0.615 |
| 1.857 | 2.857 | 6.143 | 7.143 |
| 0.000 | 0.000 | 2.933 | 3.143 |
| 5.385 | 5.571 | 0.000 | 0.000 |
| 0.000 | 6.923 | 0.857 | 0.923 |
| 3.000 | 2.000 | 1.140 | 1.710 |
| 0.000 | 2.267 | | |

**Table C.10**  Data from a sequential intervention study
For definitions of variables, see Exercise 7.8.

| Observation | m | n | S | T |
|---|---|---|---|---|
| 1 | 0 | 1 | 0 | 0 |
| 2 | 1 | 1 | 1 | 0 |
| 3 | 1 | 2 | 1 | 0 |
| 4 | 2 | 2 | 1 | 0 |
| 5 | 2 | 3 | 1 | 0 |
| 6 | 2 | 4 | 1 | 0 |
| 7 | 2 | 5 | 1 | 1 |
| 8 | 3 | 5 | 2 | 1 |
| 9 | 4 | 5 | 3 | 2 |
| 10 | 4 | 6 | 3 | 2 |
| 11 | 4 | 7 | 3 | 2 |
| 12 | 4 | 8 | 3 | 2 |
| 13 | 5 | 8 | 4 | 2 |
| 14 | 6 | 8 | 4 | 2 |
| 15 | 6 | 9 | 4 | 2 |
| 16 | 6 | 10 | 4 | 2 |
| 17 | 6 | 11 | 4 | 3 |
| 18 | 6 | 12 | 4 | 3 |
| 19 | 6 | 13 | 4 | 3 |
| 20 | 7 | 13 | 5 | 3 |
| 21 | 8 | 13 | 5 | 3 |
| 22 | 8 | 14 | 5 | 3 |
| 23 | 9 | 14 | 6 | 3 |
| 24 | 10 | 14 | 7 | 3 |
| 25 | 11 | 14 | 8 | 3 |
| 26 | 12 | 14 | 9 | 3 |
| 27 | 12 | 15 | 9 | 4 |
| 28 | 12 | 16 | 9 | 4 |
| 29 | 13 | 16 | 10 | 4 |
| 30 | 14 | 16 | 11 | 4 |

Reprinted from Peace (1992, p.195), by courtesy of Marcel Dekker Inc.

**Table C.11**   Epilepsy data
Braathan *et al.* (1997) give data for 19 children with epilepsy who participated in a prospective study concerning the duration of treatment with carbamazepine. These children were selected out for entry to a further study. Selected variables are given below: here the BO test is the Bruininks–Oseretsky test of motor proficiency.

| Child number | Diagnosis | Duration of treatment (years) | BO test (µmol/l) |
|---|---|---|---|
| 1 | PS | 1 | 22 |
| 2 | GTCS | 3 | 21 |
| 3 | GTCS | 3 | 32 |
| 4 | PS | 1 | 17 |
| 5 | BECT | 1 | 27 |
| 6 | GTCS | 1 | 30 |
| 7 | PS | 3 | 37 |
| 8 | GTCS | 1 | 19 |
| 9 | GTCS | 1 | 18 |
| 10 | GTCS | 3 | 21 |
| 11 | PS | 1 | 26 |
| 12 | BECT | 3 | 29 |
| 13 | GTCS | 1 | 23 |
| 14 | PS | 3 | 33 |
| 15 | PS | 3 | 10 |
| 16 | BECT | 3 | 27 |
| 17 | GTCS | 3 | 26 |
| 18 | GTCS | 3 | 27 |
| 19 | GTCS | 1 | 23 |

PS = partial seizures; GTCS = generalized tonic-clonic seizures;
BECT = benign partial epilepsy with centro-temporal spikes.

**Table C.12**  Ozone exposure data
When humans are exposed to high levels of ozone reversible changes in lung function occur. The data below show part of an investigation by Ying *et al.* (1990), who exposed 13  non-smoking men to 0.4 ppm ozone. This shows their lung function ($FEV_1$) before and after exposure, together with their age, height and weight.

| Subject number | Age (yr) | Height (cm) | Weight (kg) | $FEV_1$ Before | After |
|---|---|---|---|---|---|
| 1 | 22 | 170 | 68 | 4.52 | 3.92 |
| 2 | 22 | 178 | 73 | 5.21 | 4.14 |
| 3 | 26 | 163 | 61 | 3.10 | 2.27 |
| 4 | 31 | 188 | 89 | 4.25 | 3.16 |
| 5 | 27 | 170 | 72 | 3.19 | 2.81 |
| 6 | 30 | 173 | 66 | 4.24 | 2.23 |
| 7 | 28 | 185 | 73 | 4.41 | 4.29 |
| 8 | 27 | 185 | 76 | 4.30 | 4.20 |
| 9 | 22 | 188 | 75 | 4.76 | 3.50 |
| 10 | 24 | 190 | 91 | 4.38 | 2.71 |
| 11 | 23 | 178 | 57 | 4.49 | 3.19 |
| 12 | 18 | 180 | 66 | 4.66 | 4.17 |
| 13 | 26 | 185 | 68 | 5.08 | 5.13 |

**Table C.13**  Anorexia data

Ben-Tovim *et al.* (1979) report a case–control study to test the hypothesis that anorexic people tend to overestimate their true waist measurements. Eight anorexic women were identified from a hospital in-patient unit and compared with 11 non-anorexic adolescent schoolgirls. The outcome variable used to compare cases and controls was the body perception index,

$$\text{BPI} = 100 \times \frac{\text{perceived waist width}}{\text{true waist width}}$$

The data collected were as follows:

| Subject number | Waist width (cm) | | BPI |
|---|---|---|---|
| | True | Perceived | |
| Cases | | | |
| 1 | 22.6 | 29.5 | 130.5 |
| 2 | 19.2 | 30.6 | 159.6 |
| 3 | 21.9 | 31.1 | 142.0 |
| 4 | 23.4 | 28.1 | 119.9 |
| 5 | 22.9 | 32.7 | 143.0 |
| 6 | 19.1 | 37.1 | 194.0 |
| 7 | 21.4 | 32.9 | 153.7 |
| 8 | 28.3 | 33.5 | 118.2 |
| Controls | | | |
| 9 | 24.9 | 32.9 | 132.3 |
| 10 | 16.6 | 27.9 | 168.1 |
| 11 | 22.0 | 28.7 | 130.5 |
| 12 | 22.2 | 34.1 | 153.6 |
| 13 | 21.4 | 33.9 | 158.4 |
| 14 | 19.1 | 39.3 | 206.0 |
| 15 | 18.2 | 36.9 | 202.7 |
| 16 | 21.4 | 31.4 | 146.5 |
| 17 | 17.6 | 40.4 | 229.5 |
| 18 | 20.0 | 34.6 | 172.8 |
| 19 | 24.3 | 31.8 | 130.9 |

**Table C.14**  UK population data
The following table shows the size of the UK population at successive 10-year Population
Censuses:

| Census year | Population size (thousands) |
|---|---|
| 1801 | 11 944 |
| 1811 | 13 368 |
| 1821 | 15 472 |
| 1831 | 17 835 |
| 1841 | 20 183 |
| 1851 | 22 259 |
| 1861 | 24 525 |
| 1871 | 27 431 |
| 1881 | 31 015 |
| 1891 | 34 264 |
| 1901 | 38 237 |
| 1911 | 42 182 |
| 1921 | 44 227 |
| 1931 | 46 338 |
| 1951 | 50 525 |
| 1961 | 52 609 |
| 1971 | 55 515 |
| 1981 | 55 776 |
| 1991 | 57 801 |

**Table C.15**   Nasal cancer data

Breslow and Day (1987) give data on nasal sinus cancer mortality amongst Welsh nickel refinery workers, as reproduced below. Column 1 has age when first employed (1 = $<20$, 2 = 20–27.4, 3 = 27.5–34.9, 4 = 35.0–54.4 years); column 2 has year of first employment (1 = 1902–09, 2 = 1910–14, 3 = 1915–19, 4 = 1920–24); column 3 has duration of exposure to nickel compounds (1 = 0.0, 2 = 0.5–4.0, 3 = 4.5–8.0, 4 = 8.5–12.0, 5 = 12.5 or more years); column 4 has the number of deaths; and column 5 has the number of person-years. The five columns of data have been further split into three segments below.

| | | | | | | | | | | | | | | |
|---|---|---|---|---|---|---|---|---|---|---|---|---|---|---|
| 1 | 1 | 2 | 0 | 19406   | 2 | 2 | 2 | 1 | 528066  | 3 | 3 | 2 | 2 | 169654 |
| 1 | 1 | 3 | 0 | 70000   | 2 | 2 | 3 | 4 | 497481  | 3 | 3 | 3 | 1 | 111962 |
| 1 | 1 | 4 | 0 | 52836   | 2 | 2 | 4 | 2 | 279542  | 3 | 3 | 4 | 0 | 55060  |
| 1 | 1 | 5 | 0 | 33209   | 2 | 2 | 5 | 2 | 97982   | 3 | 3 | 5 | 1 | 840    |
| 1 | 2 | 1 | 0 | 2166    | 2 | 3 | 1 | 0 | 82886   | 3 | 4 | 1 | 0 | 679445 |
| 1 | 2 | 2 | 1 | 175294  | 2 | 3 | 2 | 0 | 253653  | 3 | 4 | 2 | 0 | 686531 |
| 1 | 2 | 3 | 0 | 179501  | 2 | 3 | 3 | 0 | 206343  | 3 | 4 | 3 | 1 | 458838 |
| 1 | 2 | 4 | 1 | 121217  | 2 | 3 | 4 | 2 | 111541  | 3 | 4 | 4 | 1 | 183701 |
| 1 | 2 | 5 | 0 | 77877   | 2 | 3 | 5 | 0 | 45434   | 3 | 4 | 5 | 0 | 42665  |
| 1 | 3 | 1 | 0 | 71400   | 2 | 4 | 1 | 0 | 1021139 | 4 | 1 | 2 | 0 | 14773  |
| 1 | 3 | 2 | 0 | 267774  | 2 | 4 | 2 | 1 | 1088072 | 4 | 1 | 3 | 0 | 36570  |
| 1 | 3 | 3 | 0 | 267714  | 2 | 4 | 3 | 0 | 869314  | 4 | 1 | 4 | 0 | 17290  |
| 1 | 3 | 4 | 0 | 210773  | 2 | 4 | 4 | 3 | 585779  | 4 | 2 | 1 | 0 | 3176   |
| 1 | 3 | 5 | 0 | 157445  | 2 | 4 | 5 | 0 | 250398  | 4 | 2 | 2 | 2 | 164801 |
| 1 | 4 | 1 | 0 | 279472  | 3 | 1 | 2 | 3 | 116939  | 4 | 2 | 3 | 5 | 56130  |
| 1 | 4 | 2 | 0 | 344109  | 3 | 1 | 3 | 1 | 262567  | 4 | 2 | 4 | 0 | 7258   |
| 1 | 4 | 3 | 0 | 315170  | 3 | 1 | 4 | 1 | 151760  | 4 | 3 | 1 | 0 | 34540  |
| 1 | 4 | 4 | 0 | 267320  | 3 | 1 | 5 | 1 | 32238   | 4 | 3 | 2 | 2 | 124253 |
| 1 | 4 | 5 | 0 | 176503  | 3 | 2 | 1 | 0 | 3824    | 4 | 3 | 3 | 1 | 68881  |
| 2 | 1 | 2 | 1 | 174418  | 3 | 2 | 2 | 3 | 330710  | 4 | 3 | 4 | 0 | 4382   |
| 2 | 1 | 3 | 2 | 521768  | 3 | 2 | 3 | 2 | 265273  | 4 | 4 | 1 | 1 | 354720 |
| 2 | 1 | 4 | 0 | 304922  | 3 | 2 | 4 | 3 | 90851   | 4 | 4 | 2 | 3 | 319077 |
| 2 | 1 | 5 | 2 | 142282  | 3 | 2 | 5 | 0 | 19540   | 4 | 4 | 3 | 0 | 141845 |
| 2 | 2 | 1 | 0 | 3831    | 3 | 3 | 1 | 0 | 49453   | 4 | 4 | 4 | 0 | 17203  |

**Table C.16**   Data sets from the text

In certain places in the text, data sets have been used which are too big to be written out in full. These, and the larger of the data sets which do already appear, are available electronically at http://www.reading.ac.uk/AcaDepts/sn/wsn1/publications99.html. The following is a list of the available data, showing a point of origin in the text and the order in which variables appear in electronic form. All data sets have been constructed in free format (that is, with spaces between the variables).

| Point of origin | Variables |
|---|---|
| Table 2.10 | As in the table. |
| Example 5.9 | Tenure (1 = owner/occupier, 2 = renter), CHD outcome (0 = no, 1 = yes), survival time (days). |
| Table 7.1 | As in the table. |
| Table 9.15 | As in the table. |
| Table 9.8/9.18 | Type of country (1 = industrialized, 2 = developing), sugar (kg/head/year), DMFT score. |
| Example 9.12 | HDL (mmol/l), age (years), alcohol (units/week), cholesterol (mg/day), fibre (g/day). |
| Example 9.14 | Fibrinogen (g/l), age (years), *H. pylori* status (0 = no, 1 = yes). |
| Example 10.10 | Age (years), death (0 = no, 1 = yes). |
| Example 10.11/11.8 | Cholesterol fifth, SBP fifth, CHD event (0 = no, 1 = yes), survival time (days). |
| Example 10.12/11.10 | Age (years), total cholesterol (mmol/l), BMI (kg/m$^2$), systolic blood pressure (mmHg), smoking (1 = never, 2 = ex, 3 = current), activity (1 = active, 2 = average, 3 = inactive), CHD (0 = no, 1 = yes), survival time (days). |
| Example 10.22/11.11/11.12 | Sex (1 = male, 2 = female), Bortner score, Bortner quarter, CHD (0 = no, 1 = yes), survival time (days). |
| Table 10.38 | As in the table. |

# Solutions to Exercises

1.1   (i) Prevalence.
      (ii) Possible reasons could include the following:
        • those with angina subsequently quit smoking;
        • deception amongst smokers;
        • many smoke cigars and/or pipes;
        • confounding with other factors (e.g. alcohol, obesity).
      (iii) Cohort study amongst those without coronary heart disease with questions to include amount of all tobacco sources (perhaps biochemically determined) and former smoking.

1.2   A control group is required. The disease is so rare that a case–control study is the best option. Also it would be better to question new patients as they are identified: there could be a bias due to survival.

1.3   A cross-sectional study is the only feasible design (although this is not ideal due to the possibility of the disease leading to altered drinking habits). Collect information on past and present drinking, possible confounding variables (e.g. smoking, age) and episodes of the relevant diseases. Might sample randomly from general practitioners' lists, which might provide information on disease.

1.4   An intervention study with each subject exposed to both settings. Ideally, the order of settings to be varied between subjects, and the measurements to be taken, for a particular subject, a good time apart.

1.5   (i) Shortcomings include the following:
        • no linkage of individuals;
        • no allowance for confounding variables (e.g. fluoride exposure);
        • different age ranges in the two variables;
        • no common control over survey administration;
        • small range of sugar consumption (since means are used).
      The data are analysed, and discussed further, in Chapter 9.
      (ii) A case–control study would be possible; a cross-sectional study might also be an option. Either way, it should record data from individual children on sugar consumption (possibly by source), oral hygiene and the condition of teeth. The case–control study might select cases as children with DMFT scores that exceed a certain level and controls as children with zero DMFT scores. Samples should be drawn from the general population. Although it would be easier and cheaper to select children from dental practices, results are then likely to be biased since only those children who seek dental help would be included.

2.1   (i) Bar chart. Median = 1.
      (ii) 0.569 (0.528, 0.611).

2.2    (i)

| | Marital status | | | |
|---|---|---|---|---|
| Education | Single | Separated | Married | Total |
| Males | | | | |
|    Illiterate | 9 | 4 | 122 | 135 |
|    Literate | 57 | 14 | 357 | 428 |
|    Total | 66 | 18 | 479 | 563 |
| Females | | | | |
|    Illiterate | 1 | 4 | 13 | 18 |
|    Literate | 13 | 18 | 70 | 101 |
|    Total | 14 | 22 | 83 | 119 |
| Total | | | | |
|    Illiterate | 10 | 8 | 135 | 153 |
|    Literate | 70 | 32 | 427 | 529 |
|    Total | 80 | 40 | 562 | 682 |

(ii) Test statistic $= 0.86$ ($p = 0.65$).
39.9 (36.2, 43.6).

2.3    All show positive skewness.

2.4    (ii)

| Variable | Minimum | Q1 | Q2 | Q3 | Maximum |
|---|---|---|---|---|---|
| Protein C | 80 | 92.5 | 109 | 143.5 | 188 |
| Protein S | 63.91 | 93.375 | 103.75 | 117.86 | 142.76 |

(iii), (iv)

| Variable | Mean | Standard deviation | Skewness |
|---|---|---|---|
| Protein C | 119.1 | 31.89 | 0.78 |
| Protein S | 104.912 | 19.2240 | −0.17 |

(v) Protein S is not highly skewed. Protein C is, but the negative reciprocal transformation removes most of this skewness (and will be used subsequently).
(vii) Protein C (after using the transformation): (103.8, 121.2).
Protein S: (98.76, 111.06).
(viii) (0.502, 0.798).
(x) Preliminary $F$ test statistic $= 1.62$ ($p = 0.29$).
Pooled $t$ test statistic $= 0.62$ ($p = 0.54$).
(xi) Wilcoxon test $p = 0.68$.

(xii) Preliminary $F$ test statistic (after transformation) = 1.21 ($p$ = 0.66).
Pooled $t$ test statistic (after transformation) = 2.41 ($p$ = 0.02).
Wilcoxon test $p$ = 0.03.

(xiii) Protein C, but not Protein S, varies with drinking status. Non-drinkers have higher Protein C.

(xiv) (−9.0, 17.0). Yes, since it includes zero.

(xv) $t$ test statistic = −1.31 ($p$ = 0.2). No evidence of a real difference.

2.5    (i) Test statistic = 0.04 ($p$ = 0.97).

     (ii) 0.06 (−2.40, 2.52).

     (iii) No effect.

2.6    The major features are as follows:
- The bulk of sugar intake is extrinsic.
- Extrinsic (and thus total) intake decreases with obesity.
- Intrinsic intake increases with obesity.
- Lactose intake is largely unrelated to obesity.
- Sugar intake patterns are very similar for men and women.
- Women derive slightly more energy from non-extrinsic sugar, and less from extrinsic sugar, than do men.

2.7    0.644 (0.532, 0.757).

2.8    (i) 0.196 (0.147, 0.245): many users are missed.

     (ii) 0.952 (0.914, 0.989): non-users are usually identified.

     (iii) 0.891 (0.809, 0.973): positive test is fairly reliable.

     (iv) 0.370 (0.317, 0.423): negative test is unreliable.

2.9    (i) 100 (ii) 80 (iii) 120.

2.10   For consistency, both the cigarette smoking groups and the orientation of smoking habit could be standardized. The best orientation would have smoking groups labelling the rows, since the major comparisons will be made between these groups and because the order of magnitude of the numbers differs (e.g. in Table 1.2).

3.1    (i) 0.100 (0.030, 0.170) and 0.033 (0.024, 0.042).

     (ii) 3.02 (1.42, 6.41).

     (iii) 0.111 and 0.034.

     (iv) 3.25 (1.42, 7.43).

     (v) Continuity-corrected test statistic = 6.83 ($p$ = 0.009).

     (vi) 0.079 (0.027, 0.214).

3.2    $p$ = 0.018 (one-sided). The more severe the asthma, the more willing are parents to provide adequate treatment.

3.3    (i) 2.40 (1.11, 5.15).

     (ii) 3.16 (1.04, 9.56).

     (iii) Continuity-corrected test statistic = 3.14 ($p$ = 0.08). Fisher's exact test is better (an expected value is below 5). The two-sided test (found from doubling the one-sided $p$ value) has $p$ = 0.09.

     (iv) 0.140 (0.039, 0.395).

3.4    (i) 0.343 (high) and 0.314 (low) for men; 0.386 and 0.275 for women.

     (ii) 1.09 (0.89, 1.35) for men; 1.40 (1.14, 1.72) for women.

     (iii) 0.521 and 0.457 for men; 0.629 and 0.380 for women.

     (iv) 1.14 (0.83, 1.56) for men; 1.65 (1.22, 2.24) for women.

(v) Continuity-corrected test statistics are 0.56 ($p = 0.46$) for men, 10.33 ($p = 0.001$) for women.

(vi) Factor IX seems to have an effect on CVD only amongst women.

3.5 (i) 21.25 ($p = 0.002$).

(ii) 16.04 ($p < 0.0001$).

(iii) 5.21 ($p = 0.39$).

Although some of the numbers here are small, there is evidence of an effect of gestational age on the chance of survival. Furthermore, there is a dose-response effect.

3.6 (i) 0.00194 (0.00165, 0.00223).

(ii) 0.869 (0.732, 1.031).

(iii) Test statistic $= 4.37$ ($p = 0.04$).

3.7 (i) 0.88, 2.64, 3.27, 1.85, 0.95, 0.16.

(ii) (2.65, 4.00).

(iii) 1.00, 3.00, 3.72, 2.11, 1.08, 0.18.

(iv) (2.61, 5.70).

4.1 Male doctors are slightly more likely to drink heavily and much more likely to commit suicide, but much less likely to die from lung cancer, than are other people. Causes may include stress, ready availability of lethal doses of drugs and desire to promote non-smoking. The age structure of the profession may differ from the general population; cause-specific death rates are very likely to vary with age.

4.2 (i) and (iii). Ideally we would want evidence relating $F$ to $C$ and $D$ to $C$, provided neither was a causal link. We might decide to play safe if only one relation had been established, particularly if it were $D$ to $C$. Database searches revealed two examples: (i) Winn *et al.* (1991); and (ii) Johansson *et al.* (1994).

4.3 There is no evidence of confounding or interaction.

4.4 (i) 8.67 and 15.06.

(ii) 11.24 and 11.99.

(iii) 96.4 and 102.7, 11.15 and 11.88.

(iv) The huge difference in crude rates is reduced to a small rural excess after allowing for age (rural areas have an older age structure).

4.5 (i) 1.95.

(ii) Continuity-corrected test statistic $= 16.53$ ($p < 0.0001$).

(iii) 1.88

(iv) Continuity-corrected test statistic $= 14.70$ ($p = 0.0001$).

(v) Whether or not smoking is accounted for, those occupations specifically selected really do constitute a high risk. There is little evidence of confounding by smoking.

4.6 (i) 0.444, 0.511 and 0.544 for deprivation groups I and II. 0.480, 0.453 and 0.572 for deprivation groups III and IV. There appears to be an effect of age, little effect of deprivation and a possible interaction (inverted patterns).

(ii) 1.01 (0.85, 1.21).

(iii) 1.01 (0.85, 1.21).

(iv) Test statistic $= 0.63$ ($p = 0.73$).

(v) 1.03 (0.71, 1.50).

(vi) 1.03 (0.70, 1.50).

(vii) Test statistic $= 0.64$ ($p = 0.73$).

(viii) Continuity-corrected test statistic $= 0.003$.

(ix)  Continuity-corrected test statistic = 0.001.

(x)  No effect of deprivation group; absolutely no evidence of confounding by age; no evidence of interaction.

4.7  (i)  1.24. (ii) 1.24. (iii) 1.05. (iv) 1.04.

(v)  Test statistic = 2.78 ($p$ = 0.10).

(vi)  Test statistic = 5.59 ($p$ = 0.23).

(vii)  Test statistic = 9.37 ($p$ = 0.40).

(viii)  1.39. (ix) 1.39. (x) 1.08. (xi) 1.07.

(xii)  Test statistic = 2.80 ($p$ = 0.09).

(xiii)  Test statistic = 5.15 ($p$ = 0.27).

(xiv)  Test statistic = 8.92 ($p$ = 0.44).

(xv)  Weak evidence of interaction with sex; no further interactions; age appears to be a confounding variable in the relationship between factor IX and CVD; the effect on CVD of factor IX (if the sex interaction is considered insubstantial) may be summarized by age-adjusted $\lambda_{MH}$ or $\Psi_{MH}$ (with 95% confidence intervals): 1.05 (0.91, 1.21) or 1.08 (0.86, 1.36), with the effect non-significant at the 5% level.

5.1  (i)

|  | None | Occasional | Light | Moderate | Heavy |
|---|---|---|---|---|---|
| Risk | 0.088 | 0.077 | 0.056 | 0.057 | 0.075 |
|  | (0.062, 0.114) | (0.065, 0.089) | (0.047, 0.065) | (0.047, 0.067) | (0.057, 0.092) |
| Relative risk | 1 | 0.88 | 0.64 | 0.65 | 0.85 |
|  |  | (0.63, 1.22) | (0.46, 0.89) | (0.46, 0.91) | (0.58, 1.24) |

Alcohol seems to confer some protection against death, particularly in the lower consumption groups.

(ii) Problems include:

• no measurement of prior consumption – the sick may reduce their consumption;

• no consideration of confounding variables – abstainers may be a special group (for example, because of religious beliefs) with dietary and other lifestyle consequences.

Alternative design:

• keep cohort design (experiments unethical) unless cost considerations imply a case–control approach;

• attempt to measure 'lifetime consumption'; certainly isolate the never-drinkers;

• measure potential confounders such as smoking, other aspects of diet, exercise, pre-existing medical problems, age, etc.;

• include women;

• depending upon study design and cost, possibly measure morbidity as well as mortality – could also split by cause.

5.2    (i)

| Time | $n$ | $e$ | $c$ | $q$ | $p$ | $s$ (95% CI) |
|---|---|---|---|---|---|---|
| 0 | 17 | 4 | 0 | 0.24 | 0.76 | 0.7647 (0.5631, 0.9663) |
| 6 | 13 | 1 | 2 | 0.08 | 0.92 | 0.7010 (0.4808, 0.9211) |
| 12 | 10 | 4 | 2 | 0.44 | 0.56 | 0.3894 (0.1311, 0.6478) |
| 18 | 4 | 2 | 1 | 0.57 | 0.43 | 0.1669 (0,[a] 0.3972) |
| 24 | 1 | 1 | 0 | 1 | 0 | 0 |
| 30 | 0 | | | | | |

[a] Rounded up.

(ii)

| Time | $s$ (95% CI) |
|---|---|
| 0 | 1 |
| 2 | 0.9412 (0.8293, 1[a]) |
| 5 | 0.7647 (0.5631, 0.9664) |
| 7 | 0.7059 (0.4893, 0.9225) |
| 12 | 0.4941 (0.2428, 0.7454) |
| 16 | 0.3953 (0.1299, 0.6607) |
| 20 | 0.2635 (0,[a] 0.5388) |
| 23 | 0.1318 (0,[a] 0.3604) |
| 28 | 0 |

[a] Rounded up/down.

(iv) (−0.548, 0.570): no evidence of a difference ($p = 0.97$).
(v) Continuity-corrected test statistic $= 0.004$ ($p = 0.95$).
(vi) Continuity-corrected test statistic $= 0.02$ ($p = 0.88$).
(vii) Test statistic $= 0.05$ ($p = 0.82$).

5.3    (iii) Literate, 0.4154 (0.2812, 0.5496); illiterate 0.2291 (0.1763, 0.2819); difference 0.1863 (0.0421, 0.3305). Literate people have a higher 12-month survival probability ($p = 0.0009$).
(iv) Continuity-corrected test statistic $= 24.01$ ($p < 0.0001$).

5.4    (i) 1.03: the effect seems to be small.
(ii) Problems could include:
   • 'healthy worker effect' (only relatively healthy men are employed);
   • use of deaths only;
   • confounding factors (such as age, smoking);
   • no account of dose;
   • 'base' population is not observed (for example, problems with withdrawals in the study population).

5.5

| Exposure | Rate (95% CI) |
|----------|---------------|
| < 3 | 0.877 (0.582, 1.232) |
| 3–10 | 0.576 (0.286, 0.967) |
| 10–30 | 0.906 (0.527, 1.388) |
| 30–100 | 0.923 (0.650, 1.245) |
| 100–300 | 0.755 (0.523, 1.030) |
| 300–600 | 1.385 (1.002, 1.830) |
| 600 + | 2.308 (1.532, 3.243) |

There is a large effect at very high exposures.

5.6   (i) 8.862 (8.175, 9.576); 4.529 (4.198, 4.873); 9.640 (9.071, 10.226).

(ii) 0.511 (0.458, 0.571); 1.088 (0.984, 1.203).

(iii) For women, Hai has about half the mortality rate, and Morogoro about the same rate, as Dar, after accounting for age differences.

5.7

| Category | Vitamin C | Vitamin E |
|----------|-----------|-----------|
| 1 | 1 | 1 |
| 2 | 0.93 (0.79, 1.08) | 0.95 (0.78, 1.14) |
| 3 | 0.96 (0.74, 1.20) | 0.91 (0.69, 1.14) |
| 4 | 0.79 (0.58, 1.02) | 1.01 (0.64, 1.40) |
| 5 | 0.76 (0.46, 1.08) | 0.92 (0.71, 1.14) |

There is a benefit of vitamin C, no effect of vitamin E.

5.8   (i) 3.28 (2.06, 4.99).

(ii) 3.14 (2.02, 4.87).

(iii) Continuity-corrected test statistic $= 26.50$ ($p < 0.0001$).

(iv) Test statistic $= 12.87$ ($p = 0.38$).

6.1   (i) 0.67 (0.52, 0.88).

(ii) Continuity-corrected test statistic $= 8.35$ ($p = 0.004$).

6.2   (i) 1.70 (1.16, 2.49).

(ii) Continuity-corrected test statistic $= 6.96$ ($p = 0.008$).

6.3

| Food item | Odds ratio (95% CI) | Test[a] | p value |
|-----------|---------------------|---------|---------|
| Breaded chicken | 1.53 (0.37, 6.35) | 0.05 | 0.82 |
| Any chicken | 0.33 (0.03, 3.55) | 0.17 | 0.68 |
| Egg rolls | 13.07 (2.61, 65.48) | 9.17 | 0.003 |
| Fried rice | 2.49 (0.62, 10.06) | 0.90 | 0.34 |

[a] Continuity-corrected.

Although the small numbers make precise inferences based on the above unreliable, egg rolls are clearly the most likely source of SE.

6.4    0.335 (0.088, 0.724).

6.5    Post-menopausal women who bleed are more likely to be thoroughly checked for the cancer. Hence post-menopausal oestrogen users are more likely to become cases. Possibly the evidence of bleeding may influence the diagnosis (false positive rate increased). Either way there could be bias against oestrogen.

6.6    (i)    2.43 (0.90, 6.57) and 1.26 (0.66, 2.43).

(ii)    2.40 (0.88, 6.55) and 1.31 (0.68, 2.51).

(iii) Risk appears to decrease with increasing age of mother; no evidence of confounding.

6.7    2.01, 0.69, 8.57: all closer to unity.

6.8    (i)    5.50 (1.20, 51.1).

(ii)    Continuity-corrected test statistic $= 4.92$ ($p = 0.03$).

6.9    (i)    2.06 (1.10, 1.13).

(ii)    Continuity-corrected test statistic $= 5.22$ ($p = 0.02$).

(iii) Issues to be addressed include:

  • confounding factors (e.g. alcohol, occupation);

  • coverage (e.g. not everyone holds a driver's licence or has a telephone);

  • association of driving with crime (e.g. are past criminals less likely to hold a licence?);

  • effect of death due to spinal injury;

  • fear of disclosure of information.

6.10    (i)    1.69 (1.08, 2.64).

(ii)    Continuity-corrected test statistic $= 4.68$ ($p = 0.03$).

6.11    (i)    2.00 (0.66, 6.02).

(ii)    Continuity-corrected test statistic $= 0.95$ ($p = 0.16$).

6.12    (i)    3.00 (1.61, 5.59).

(ii)    Continuity-corrected test statistic $= 11.89$ ($p = 0.0006$).

6.13    There is overmatching: loss of efficiency since cases and controls are likely to be similar in terms of potential risk factors. Alternatives might include age, sex and parents' smoking habits.

7.1    (i)    Continuity-corrected test statistic $= 2.78$ ($p = 0.10$). Use either relative risk or odds ratio (with 95% confidence limits): 1.55 (0.97, 2.49) or 4.05 (0.99, 16.57).

(ii)    Potential problem is change in lifestyle by non-experimental group. Some monitoring of their lifestyle before and after recruitment might be considered, with subsequent adjusted comparisons.

7.2    (i)    Continuity-corrected test statistic $= 0.11$ ($p = 0.74$).

(ii)    Fisher's exact test $p = 0.003$ (one-sided).

7.3    (i)    Test statistic $= 3.04$ ($p = 0.006$).

(ii)    6.13 (1.90, 10.34): difference increases.

7.4    (i)    Continuity-corrected test statistic $= 8.46$ ($p = 0.004$).

(ii)    (0.0176, 0.0860).

(iii)    1295 (439, 2150).

7.5    (i) Selected results:

| Time | Blocadren | | Placebo | |
|---|---|---|---|---|
| (months) [a] | s | se | s | se |
| 1 | 0.980 | 0.0046 | 0.967 | 0.0058 |
| 11 | 0.929 | 0.0083 | 0.892 | 0.0101 |
| 21 | 0.904 | 0.0099 | 0.850 | 0.0120 |
| 31 | 0.863 | 0.0162 | 0.807 | 0.0166 |

[a] End of month.

  (ii)  Blocadren always does better; 'curves' diverge over time.

  (iii) Continuity-corrected test statistic $= 13.30$ ($p = 0.003$).

7.6 (i) Cross-over.

  (ii) Parallel group (possibly sequential).

  (iii) Cross-over.

  (iv) Sequential (or a parallel group).

  (v) Cross-over.

7.7 (i) Wilcoxon test $p = 0.45$.

  (ii) Wilcoxon test $p = 0.71$.

  (iii) Wilcoxon test $p = 0.37$.

7.8 (i) Ganciclovir is effective (reject $H_0$).

  (ii) 'Open' boundaries: study *may* go on for a very long time.

7.9 Stratified randomization: possible prognostic factors are hospital, age, sex, surgical procedure and severity of illness.

8.1 (i) 198. (ii) 86.4% (iii) 11.5%.

8.2 (i) 694. (ii) 92.2%. (iii) 89.3%.

  (iv) Standard deviation of before–after difference must be less than 6.365 kg/m$^2$

8.3 14 884 (increase of 2752) and 16 542 (increase of 2998).

8.4 (i) Possible inclusion criteria are:

   &bull; women aged 18–40,

   &bull; sexually active,

   &bull; physically healthy.

 Possible exclusion criteria are:

   &bull; therapeutic use of OCs,

   &bull; medical conditions that may be worsened by OC use,

   &bull; recent pregnancy.

  (ii) 1006 and 1060.

  (iii) Twelve-month continuation percentage reflects lack of pregnancy and acceptability of OCs jointly. These effects might be separated. Adverse events could be monitored. Survival methods might be used to compare short-term differences and allow use of information from the withdrawals.

8.5 (i) 87.2%.

  (ii) Problems could include:

   &bull; memory errors,

   &bull; do not know the true value of $r$,

- definitions of 'serious' and 'old',
- ability to go out of the house may induce bias,
- cause and effect may be reversed,
- there may be effects of other prescribed drugs.

8.6   (i)   3268. (ii) 436.

(iii) Increases by 6356 when a cohort study is used; stays the same when a case–control study is used.

8.7   (i)   22.0%. (ii) 47.9%. (iii) 81.6%.

(iv) 28.2%. (v) 67.4%. (vi) 96.3%.

(vii) Given that diversity of employment is likely, so that several employment groups may be defined, it seems worth using all the potential controls. Even then, only large odds ratios are likely to be detected for very 'small' employment groups (although this fact certainly does not rule out considering them).

8.8   (i)   1.42

(ii)   Power increases, but with diminishing returns. For the lowest odds ratios in the range considered, the power is unacceptably low. Selected results:

| $\Psi \simeq \lambda$ | Power (%) |
|---|---|
| 1.30 | 66.5 |
| 1.35 | 78.2 |
| 1.40 | 86.8 |
| 1.45 | 92.6 |
| 1.50 | 96.2 |

9.1   $F$ test statistic $= 4.71$ ($p = 0.035$). This is the square of the $t$ statistic in Example 2.10, with the $p$ value unchanged.

9.2

| Source | SS | df | MS | F | p |
|---|---|---|---|---|---|
| Alcohol | 1130.31 | 4 | 282.58 | 0.74 | 0.57 |
| Error | 13282.58 | 35 | 379.50 | | |
| Total | 14412.89 | 39 | | | |

(i)   $F$ test statistic $= 0.74$ ($p = 0.57$).
(ii)   Using error MS: (77.20, 124.66).
(iii)   Using error MS: (−20.45, 46.67).
(iv)   Kruskal–Wallis test $p = 0.49$.

9.3   (i)

| Source | SS | df | MS | F | p |
|---|---|---|---|---|---|
| Areas | 2.3203 | 8 | 0.2900 | 8.33 | <0.0001 |
| Case–control\|areas | 0.4089 | 1 | 0.4089 | 11.75 | 0.0007 |
| Interaction\|main | 0.1675 | 8 | 0.02094 | 0.60 | 0.78 |
| Error | 7.4150 | 213 | 0.03481 | | |
| Total | 10.3117 | 230 | | | |

(ii) The percentage figures differ by area and by case–control (CHD) status (after allowing for area differences); there is no evidence of a differential effect of CHD status between areas.

(iii) Test for normality of the percentages.

9.4 (i) 1.8, 1.5, 0.5, 0.3.

(ii) Same as (i).

(iii) Should give a mean of 1 (the parameter $a$).

(iv) 0.3, 1.5, $-1.0$, $-1.2$

9.5 (i)

| Source | SS | df | MS | F | p |
|---|---|---|---|---|---|
| Diagnosis | 32.92 | 2 | 16.46 | 0.38 | 0.69 |
| Year\|diagnosis | 49.29 | 1 | 49.29 | 1.14 | 0.30 |
| Error | 650.21 | 15 | 43.35 | | |
| Total | 732.42 | 18 | | | |

(ii) The 15th child has an unusually low test result.

(iii)

| Year | Diagnosis | | | Adjusted Mean |
|---|---|---|---|---|
| | PC | GTCS | BECT | |
| 1 | 22.542 | 22.375 | 25.50 | 23.47 |
| 3 | 25.792 | 25.625 | 28.75 | 26.72 |

(iv) $F$ test (for interaction) statistic $-$ 0.09 ($p = 0.92$): no evidence.

(v) Combination SS $= 90.69$.

9.6 $\gamma$-glutamyltransferase is a good marker (especially for moderate to high alcohol consumption) which is affected relatively little by the other six variables.

9.7 (ii) 0.334.

(iii) 0.329: hardly any different. $p = 0.04$: more likely to be valid because of a better approximation to normality.

(iv) 0.381: would stay exactly the same.

(v) $y = 81.0 + 0.201x$.

$F$ test statistic $= 4.76$ ($p = 0.04$).

$r^2 = 11.1\%$.

(vi) No systematic pattern although three standardized residuals are noticeably lower than the rest (two are below $-1.96$; one other standardized residual is just above 1.96).

(vii) The line is reasonably straight, although the 'problem' standardized residuals noted in (vi) clearly fall off the line. This establishes approximate normality of the residuals, and justifies use of standard inferential procedures.

(viii) $t$ test statistic $= 7.13$ ($p < 0.0001$).

(ix) (58.0, 103.9).

(x) $t$ test statistic $= 2.18$ ($p = 0.04$). $2.18^2 = 4.76$ ($p$ value the same).

(xi) (0.015, 0.388).

(xii) (63.3, 138.9).

(xiii) (94.2, 107.9).

9.8    With outlier: $y = 49.55 + 0.966x$.

Outlier is ($x = 100$, $y = 183$).

Without outlier: $y = 61.06 + 0.818x$.

9.9    Problems include:

- small $n$,
- non-linear relationship,
- residuals are non-normal,
- some smokers may have smoked pipes and/or cigars, contributing to their cotinine.

9.10   No effect of age ($p = 0.87$), height ($p = 0.98$) or weight ($p = 0.64$). On this evidence we can ignore these variables in future studies, but to be sure we should look at joint effects (interactions).

9.11   (i) Cases, 145.1; controls, 166.5.

(iii) No. A one-sided test would miss the difference in the unexpected direction. Test statistic (with pooled s.d.) $= -1.52$ ($p = 0.15$).

(iv) BPI goes down as true width goes up. A common regression line looks likely.

(v) $F$ test statistic $= 0.59$ ($p = 0.45$).

(vi) $y = 338.1608 - 8.6375$ (true) $+ 7.1174$ (cc), where cc $= 1$ for cases and 0 for controls (other parametrizations will give different equations). Mean true width $= 21.3947$. Adjusted means are 153.4 (cases) and 160.5 (controls).

(vii) The exact answers depend upon the parametrizations used; with the same parametrization throughout the two slopes should be the same (in absolute value).

(viii) Adjustment has reduced the difference in means from 21.4 to 7.1, although the control mean is still higher. Age might be another possible confounder, especially as the controls are schoolgirls, whereas cases are (presumably) unrestricted in age (Ben-Tovim et al. (1979) show that the cases are 4.5 years older, on average).

9.13   Best model is *either* (with 12.2% explained)

(i) $y = 6.16 + 0.0271$(carbon monoxide) $- 0.00158$(cotinine),

*or* (with 6.5% explained)

(ii) $y = 6.12 + 0.0129$(carbon monoxide).

In (i) cotinine is only marginally non-significant at the usual 5% level ($p = 0.09$). The final choice depends upon the requirements of, and future use for, the model.

9.14   $r^2 = 99.1\%$, but residuals have a clear pattern (down-up-down): the linear model is inappropriate.

10.1   Estimates and confidence limits should be the same (apart from a minor degree of rounding error). $\Delta D = 6.038$ ($p = 0.01$), which is very similar to the test in Exercise 3.1.

10.2   (i) Age group 35–39 and never-smokers.

(ii) 2.66.

(iii) 0.11.

10.3   (i) 3.56 (2.06, 6.14).

(ii) $\Delta D = 2.4036$, $\Delta$d.f. $= 3$ ($p = 0.49$).

(iii) 3.78 (2.12, 6.72). Virtually no confounding.

(iv)

|  | Odds ratio (95% CI) |
|---|---|
| <0.8 | 1 |
| 0.8–0.89 | 0.17 (0.07, 0.41) |
| 0.9–0.99 | 0.12 (0.06, 0.24) |
| ≥1.0 | 0.07 (0.04, 0.16) |

(v) $\Delta D = 36.86$, $\Delta\text{d.f.} = 1$ ($p < 0.0001$).
0.47 (0.37, 0.60).
The chance of wheeze decreases as the liability index increases: the odds decrease by a factor of about a half for each step up the tabulated scale, after allowing for the effects of mould.

10.4  (i) All estimates should be the same (apart from a minor degree of rounding error). $p = 0.41$ (men), $p = 0.001$ (women).
(ii) Sex: 1.39, age: 1.08, age/sex: 1.07 (the same as in Exercise 4.7).
(iii) Sex: $\Delta D = 2.81$, $\Delta\text{d.f.} = 1$ ($p = 0.09$),
Age: $\Delta D = 5.09$, $\Delta\text{d.f.} = 4$ ($p = 0.28$).
(iv) $\Delta D = 2.45$, $\Delta\text{d.f.} = 4$ ($p = 0.61$).

10.5  (i) There is an effect of feeding ($p < 0.0001$ unadjusted and adjusted for sex) and sex ($p = 0.02$ unadjusted and $p = 0.03$ adjusted for feeding). The differences are constant across the sex groups ($p = 0.72$).

| Comparison | Odds ratio (95% CI) |
|---|---|
| Boys : girls | 1.37 (1.04, 1.80) |
| Bottle : breast | 1.95 (1.45, 2.64) |
| Mixed : breast | 1.64 (1.08, 2.51) |

(ii)

| Sex | Feed | Resid | Dev Resid | St Dev Resid |
|---|---|---|---|---|
| Boy | Bottle | 0.8742 | 0.1096 | 0.2462 |
| Boy | Mixed | −2.1175 | −0.5052 | −0.8579 |
| Boy | Breast | 1.2433 | 0.1922 | 0.3670 |
| Girl | Bottle | −0.8742 | −0.1342 | −0.2473 |
| Girl | Mixed | 2.1175 | 0.5896 | 0.8279 |
| Girl | Breast | −1.2433 | −0.2284 | −0.3707 |

No indication of a problem.

10.6  (i) $\Delta D = 2.76$, $\Delta\text{d.f.} = 1$ ($p = 0.1$).
(ii) $\Delta D = 3.37$, $\Delta\text{d.f.} = 1$ ($p = 0.07$).

10.7  (i) Report should conclude that AOX, SMO and ALC all have an effect when considered alone, but ALC is 'removed' by AOX + SMO. There is evidence of an interaction between AOX and SMO. Extra models would be those with the remaining interaction terms (to check for remaining interactions) and SMO + ALC (to check whether SMO alone 'removes' ALC and to see whether AOX is still significant after allowing for SMO + ALC).

| Effect | $\Delta D$ | $\Delta d.f.$ | p value |
|---|---|---|---|
| AOX | 98.24 | 2 | <0.0001 |
| SMO | 82.19 | 1 | <0.0001 |
| ALC | 39.61 | 3 | <0.0001 |
| AOX\|SMO | 54.15 | 2 | <0.0001 |
| SMO\|AOX | 38.10 | 1 | <0.0001 |
| AOX\|ALC | 74.48 | 2 | <0.0001 |
| ALC\|AOX | 15.85 | 3 | 0.001 |
| SMO\|AOX, ALC | 23.69 | 1 | <0.0001 |
| ALC\|AOX, SMO | 1.44 | 3 | 0.70 |
| AOX*SMO\|main effects | 29.19 | 2 | <0.0001 |

(ii)

| Antioxidants | Non-smokers | Smokers |
|---|---|---|
| Low | 1 | 1 |
| Medium | 0.69 (0.45, 1.06) | 0.51 (0.17, 1.48) |
| High | 0.40 (0.21, 0.78) | 0.16 (0.045, 0.54) |

10.8  (i) Answer should include
   • unsuitability of relative risk for case–control studies;
   • problems of confounding not addressed by chi-square;
   • loss of information when grouping continuous variables.
   (ii) Answer could include:
   • details of fitted model;
   • interpretation of $\beta$ coefficients;
   • significance testing by analysis of deviance;
   • SAS parametrization;
   • need for exponentiation of an estimate to obtain $\psi$.
10.9  Report should include results of significance tests and parameter estimates for fibrinogen (the variable of study). Fibrinogen is highly significant when considered alone ($p = 0.01$), of marginal significance ($p = 0.06$) when adjusted for LDL cholesterol and does not interact with LDL ($p = 0.76$). LDL-adjusted odds ratios (with 95% confidence intervals) are 1, 1.41 (0.75, 2.65) and 2.00 (1.11, 3.61). Answer could also discuss the linear effect of the log odds ratio over the three ordinal fibrinogen groups: odds ratio (95% CI) = 1.41 (1.06, 1.88) and $p = 0.02$.
10.10  Estimate (95% CI) is the same (to 2 d.p.), $\Delta D = 4.53$ ($p = 0.03$).
10.11  Estimates (95% CIs) are the same (to 2 d.p.), $\Delta D = 11.32$ ($p = 0.02$).
10.12  Odds ratio (95% CI) = 0.52 (0.30, 0.90), $\Delta D = 5.56$ ($p = 0.02$).
10.13  (i) Odds ratio (95% CI) = 2.99 (1.61, 5.57), $\Delta D = 13.14$ ($p = 0.0003$).

(ii) $\Delta D = 13.15$, $\Delta$d.f. $= 1$ ($p = 0.0003$). Odds ratio (95% CI) $= 3.09$ (1.63, 5.87). Virtually no confounding.

10.14 (i) Yes, because the disease is rare; any other type of study would require a huge sample.

(ii) No, relative risks cannot be calculated from case–control data because the denominator for each risk assessment is unknown. Instead odds ratios should be given, as approximate relative risks.

(iii) Modelling avoids the problem of small numbers after stratification. Separate analyses by age are not necessary; simply adjust for age in the analysis.

(iv) Neither suggestion is acceptable. There is an interaction, which means that the sexes are best looked at separately.

(v) Results of tests in an analysis of deviance table ($\Delta D$ with $\Delta$d.f. for raw and adjusted effects). Estimates (unadjusted and adjusted) with 95% confidence limits in a separate table or diagram.

11.1 Selected results:

| Time interval | Blocadren | Placebo |
|---|---|---|
| 0–1 | 0.0203 | 0.0336 |
| 10–11 | 0.0034 | 0.0071 |
| 20–21 | 0.0038 | 0.0040 |
| 30–31 | 0.0082 | 0 |

The hazard with placebo is generally higher.

11.2 (i)

| Interval | Person-time | Actuarial |
|---|---|---|
| 0–6 | 0.0421 | 0.0444 |
| 6–12 | 0.0147 | 0.0145 |
| 12–18 | 0.1379 | 0.0952 |
| 18–24 | 0.1429 | 0.1333 |
| 24–30 | 0.2500 | 0.3333 |

(ii)

| Interval | KM |
|---|---|
| 0–2 | 0 |
| 2–5 | 0.0196 |
| 5–7 | 0.0938 |
| 7–12 | 0.0154 |
| 12–16 | 0.0750 |
| 16–20 | 0.0500 |
| 20–23 | 0.1111 |
| 23–28 | 0.1000 |

The estimates are very different for this small data set.

(iii) $h(t) = 0.0571$.

(iv) $h(t) = 0.0126t^{0.7519}$

(v) LCH plot shows approximately a straight line with 45° slope. Hence, both assumptions are reasonable: an exponential will suffice.

(vi)

|  | $\Delta$ | p value | Hazard ratio |
|---|---|---|---|
| Weibull |  |  |  |
| unadjusted | 0.113 | 0.74 | 1.23 |
| adjusted | 0.015 | 0.90 | 1.08 |
| Cox |  |  |  |
| unadjusted | 0.032 | 0.86 | 1.12 |
| adjusted | 0.008 | 0.93 | 1.06 |

(vii) LCH plot shows approximately parallel straight lines. Hence both assumptions are reasonable.

11.3 (i) 0.49 (0.29, 0.81): abnormal significantly worse ($p < 0.05$). Hazard ratios would be the same.

(ii) Controlling for age, the sex interaction has $\Delta = 1.394$ ($p = 0.24$). Controlling for sex, the age interaction has $\Delta = 0.005$ ($p = 0.94$). Hence there are no interactions (so far as can be determined). The effect of platelets can be found uncontrolled, $\Delta = 37.79$ ($p < 0.0001$); controlling for sex, $\Delta = 3.922$ ($p = 0.05$); and for age, $\Delta = 6.277$ ($p = 0.01$). The model in (i) is not the best since age could be dropped: $\Delta = 1.82$ ($p = 0.18$).

11.4 (i) For education, $\Delta = 10.97$ ($p = 0.0009$). For the time-dependent covariate, $\Delta = 2.95$ ($p = 0.09$): no evidence of non-proportional hazards.

(ii)

| Comparison | Hazard ratio (95% CI) |
|---|---|
| Illiterate : literate | 1.50 (1.17, 1.93) |
| Female : male | 0.98 (0.77, 1.25) |
| Christian : Hindu | 0.98 (0.68, 1.42) |
| Muslim : Hindu | 0.97 (0.76, 1.23) |
| Sep/divorced : single | 0.80 (0.50, 1.29) |
| Married : single | 0.88 (0.66, 1.18) |
| Regional : local | 2.04 (1.56, 2.68) |
| Advanced : local | 1.77 (1.37, 2.29) |
| Age : one year less | 1.004 (0.996, 1.012) |

(iii) Best model is

$$\log_e \phi = \beta_1 x_1 + \beta_2^{(1)} x_2^{(1)} + \beta_2^{(2)} x_2^{(2)},$$

where $x_1$ and $\{x_2^{(i)}\}$ are dummy variables for education and tumour type, respectively. This is so because both education and type are highly significant ($p < 0.001$) in the presence of the other and no other variable is significant ($p > 0.1$) in the presence of these two.

11.5

| Exposure group | Relative rate (95% CI) |
|---|---|
| < 3 | 1 |
| 3–10 | 0.66 (0.33, 1.32) |
| 10–30 | 1.03 (0.57, 1.89) |
| 30–100 | 1.05 (0.64, 1.72) |
| 100–300 | 0.86 (0.52, 1.42) |
| 300–600 | 1.58 (0.98, 2.54) |
| 600 + | 2.63 (1.56, 4.44) |

| Effect | $\Delta D$ | $\Delta d.f.$ | p value |
|---|---|---|---|
| Categorical | 6 | 27.13 | 0.0001 |
| Linear | 1 | 22.34 | < 0.0001 |
| Quadratic[a] | 1 | 0.30 | 0.72 |
| Cubic[a] | 1 | 1.37 | 0.24 |
| Higher-order[a] | 3 | 3.12 | 0.37 |

[a] Compared to previous model in the list.

11.6  $\Delta D = 22.24$, $\Delta d.f. = 1$ ($p < 0.0001$).
3.04 (1.97, 4.71).

11.7

| Category | Vitamin C | Vitamin E |
|---|---|---|
| 1 | 1 | 1 |
| 2 | 0.93 (0.79, 1.09) | 0.95 (0.79, 1.15) |
| 3 | 0.96 (0.76, 1.23) | 0.91 (0.71, 1.17) |
| 4 | 0.79 (0.60, 1.05) | 1.01 (0.69, 1.48) |
| 5 | 0.76 (0.51, 1.15) | 0.92 (0.73, 1.16) |
| Trend : p value | 0.05 | 0.40 |

11.8

| Effect | $\Delta D$ | $\Delta d.f.$ | p value |
|---|---|---|---|
| Compensation | 18.77 | 2 | 0.0001 |
| Panel | 11.55 | 1 | 0.0007 |
| Panel\|compensation | 11.21 | 1 | 0.0008 |
| Compensation\|panel | 18.43 | 2 | 0.0001 |
| Interaction\|main effects | 7.73 | 2 | 0.02 |

All terms are required.

|          | Low                  | Medium               | High                   |
|----------|----------------------|----------------------|------------------------|
| London   | 10.14 (7.71, 13.34)  | 13.18 (8.19, 21.20)  | 26.32 (14.16, 48.91)   |
| Cardiff  | 2.96 (1.68, 5.22)    | 14.28 (8.46, 24.12)  | 17.24 (7.18, 41.42)    |

11.9   (i) Age: $\Delta D = 26.61$, $\Delta$d.f. $= 3$ ($p < 0.0001$).
       Year: $\Delta D = 35.06$, $\Delta$d.f. $= 3$ ($p < 0.0001$).
       Duration: $\Delta D = 15.12$, $\Delta$d.f. $= 4$ ($p = 0.006$).
   (ii) Age: $\Delta D = 37.38$, $\Delta$d.f. $= 3$ ($p < 0.0001$).
       Year: $\Delta D = 25.33$, $\Delta$d.f. $= 3$ ($p < 0.0001$).
       Duration: $\Delta D = 12.61$, $\Delta$d.f. $= 4$ ($p = 0.01$).
  (iii) Taking the first group as base and expressing the rest in rank order:

| Age                   | Year                | Duration              |
|-----------------------|---------------------|-----------------------|
| 1                     | 1                   | 1                     |
| 5.33 (1.22, 23.27)    | 1.86 (0.90, 3.84)   | 4.94 (0.63, 38.52)    |
| 11.96 (2.70, 52.96)   | 1.06 (0.42, 2.64)   | 5.76 (0.73, 45.58)    |
| 30.82 (6.66, 142.61)  | 0.32 (0.13, 0.79)   | 10.54 (1.29, 85.82)   |
|                       |                     | 16.74 (1.87, 149.82)  |

# References

Agresti, A. (1996) *Introduction to Categorical Data Analysis*. John Wiley, New York.

ALSPAC (1995) *A Guide to the Avon Longitudinal Study of Pregnancy and Childhood*, 3rd edn. Royal Hospital for Sick Children, Bristol.

Altman, D.G. (1991) *Practical Statistics for Medical Research*. Chapman & Hall, London.

Altman, D.G. and De Stavola, B.L. (1994) Practical problems in fitting a proportional hazards model to data with updated measurements of the covariates. *Statist. Med.*, **13**, 301–341.

Anderson, P., Bartlett, C., Cook, G. and Woodward, M. (1985) Legionnaires disease in Reading – possible association with a cooling tower. *Comm. Med.*, **7**, 202–207.

Armitage, P. (1955) Tests for linear trends in proportions and frequencies. *Biometrics*, **11**, 375–386.

Armitage, P. and Berry, G. (1994) *Statistical Methods in Medical Research*, 3rd edn. Blackwell, Oxford.

Armstrong, B.G. and Sloan, M. (1989) Ordinal regression models for epidemiologic data. *Am. J. Epidemiol.*, **129**, 191–204.

Ashton, J. (ed.) (1994) *The Epidemiological Imagination*. Open University Press, Buckingham.

Autier, P., Dore, J.-F., Lejeune, F.J. *et al.* (1996) Sun protection in childhood or early adolescence and reduction of melanoma risk in adults: an EORTC case-control study in Germany, Belgium and France. *J. Epidemiol, Biostatist*, **1**, 51–57.

Barbash, G.I., White, H.D., Modam, M. *et al.* (1993) Significance of smoking in patients receiving thrombolytic therapy for acute myocardial infarction. *Circulation*, **87**, 53–58.

Barker, N., Hews, R.J., Huitson, A. and Poloniecki, J. (1982) The two period cross over trial. *BIAS*, **9**, 67–116.

Basnayake, S., De Silva, S.V., Miller, P.C. and Rogers, S. (1983) A comparison of Norinyl and Brevicon in 3 sites in Sri Lanka. *Contraception*, **27**, 453–464.

Bates, D.M. and Watts, D.G. (1988) *Non-linear Regression Analysis and its Applications*. John Wiley, New York.

Belsley, D.A., Ku, H.E. and Welsch, R.E. (1980) *Regression Diagnostics: Identifying Influential Data and Sources of Collinearity*. John Wiley, New York.

Benichou, J. (1991) Methods of adjustment for estimating the attributable risk in case-control studies: a review. *Statist. Med.*, **10**, 1753–1773.

Benichou, J. and Gail, M.H. (1990) Variance calculations and confidence intervals for estimates of the attributable risk based on logistic models. *Biometrics*, **46**, 991–1003.

Ben-Tovim, D., Whitehead, J. and Crisp, A.H. (1979) A controlled study of the perception of body width in anorexia nervosa. *J. Psychosomatic Res.*, **23**, 267–272.

Berry, G. (1983) The analysis of mortality by the subject-years method. *Biometrics*, **39**, 173–184.

Birkes, D. and Dodge, Y. (1993) *Alternative Methods of Regression*. John Wiley, New York.

Bland, J.M. and Altman, D.G. (1986) Statistical methods for assessing agreement between two methods of clinical measurement. *Lancet*, **i**, 307–310.

Bland, M. (1995) *An Introduction to Medical Statistics*, 2nd edn. Oxford University Press, Oxford.

Bolton-Smith, C. and Woodward, M. (1995) Intrinsic, non-milk extrinsic and milk sugar consumption by Scottish adults. *J. Human Nut. Dietetics*, **8**, 35–49.

Bolton-Smith, C. and Woodward, M. (1997) Trends in energy intake and body mass index across smoking habit groups for men. *Proc. Nut. Soc.*, **56**, 66A.

Bolton-Smith, C., Woodward, M, Smith, W.C.S. and Tunstall-Pedoe, H. (1991) Dietary and non-dietary predictors of serum total and HDL-cholesterol in men and women: results from the Scottish Heart Health Study. *Int. J. Epidemiol.*, **20**, 95–104.

Bortner, K.W. (1969) A short rating scale as a potential measure of pattern A behaviour. *J. Chronic Dis.*, **22**, 87–91.

Box, GEP. and Cox, D.R. (1964) An analysis of transformations. *J. R. Statist. Soc. B*, **26**, 211–252.

Boyce, T.G., Koo, D., Swerdlow, D.L. *et al* (1996) Recurrent outbreaks of *Salmonella enteritidis* infections in a Texas restaurant: phage type 4 arrives in the United States. *Epidemiol. Infect.*, **117**, 29–34.

Boyle, P., Maisonneuve, P. and Doré, J.F. (1995) Epidemiology of malignant melanoma. *Br. Med. Bull.*, **51**, 523–547.

Braathan, G., von Bahr, L. and Theorell, K. (1997) Motor impairments in children with epilepsy treated with carbamazepine. *Acta Paediatr.*, **86**, 372–376.

Breslow, N.E. (1984) Elementary methods of cohort analysis. *Int. J. Epidemiol.*, **13**, 112–115.

Breslow, N.E. and Day, N.E. (1980) *Statistical Methods in Cancer Research. Volume I – The Analysis of Case-Control Studies*. International Agency for Research on Cancer, Lyon.

Breslow, N.E. and Day, N.E. (1987) *Statistical Methods in Cancer Research. Volume II – The Design and Analysis of Cohort Studies*. International Agency for Research in Cancer, Lyon.

Breslow, N.E., Day, N.E., Halvorsen, K.T., Prentice, R.L. and Sabai, C. (1978) Estimation of multiple relative risk functions in matched case-control studies. *Am. J. Epidemiol.*, **108**, 299–307.

Bristol, D.R. (1989) Sample sizes for constructing confidence intervals and testing hypotheses. *Statist. Med.*, **8**, 803–811.

Buck, C., Llopis, A., Nájera, E. and Terris, M. (eds) (1988) *The Challenge of Epidemiology. Issues and Selected Readings*. World Health Organization, Washington, DC.

Calle, E.E., Mervis, C.A., Wingo, P.A., Thun, M.J., Rodriguez, C. and Heath, C.W. (1995) Spontaneous abortion and risk of fatal breast cancer in a prospective cohort of United States women. *Cancer Causes Control*, **6**, 460–468.

Campbell, M.J. and Machin, D. (1993) *Medical Statistics. A Commonsense Approach*, 2nd edn. John Wiley, Chichester.

Campbell, M.K., Feuer, E.J. and Wun, L.-M. (1994) Cohort-specific risks of developing breast cancer to age 85 in Connecticut. *Epidemiology*, **5**, 290–296.

Casagrande, J.T., Pike, M.C. and Smith, P.G. (1978) The power function of the exact test for comparing two binomial distributions. *Appl. Statist.*, **27**, 176–180.

Chatterjee, S. and Price, B. (1991) *Regression Analysis by Example*, 2nd edn. John Wiley, New York.

Clarke, G.M. and Cooke, D. (1992) *A Basic Course in Statistics*, 3rd edn. Arnold, London.

Clarke, G.M. and Kempson, R.E. (1997) *Introduction to the Design and Analysis of Experiments*. Arnold, London.

Clayton, D. and Cuzick, J. (1985) Multivariate generalizations of the proportional hazards model (with discussion). *J. R. Statist. Soc. A*, **148**, 82–117.

Clayton, D. and Hills, M. (1993) *Statistical Models in Epidemiology*. Oxford University Press, Oxford

Clayton, D. and Schifflers, E. (1987a) Models for temporal variation in cancer rates. I: Age-period and age-cohort models. *Statist. Med.*, **6**, 449–468.

Clayton, D. and Schifflers, E. (1987b) Models for temporal variation in cancer rates. II: Age-period-cohort models. *Statist. Med.*, **6**, 469–481.

Cochran, W.G. (1977) *Sampling Techniques*, 3rd edn. John Wiley, New York.

Cochrane, A.L., St Leger, A.S. and Moore, F. (1978) Health service 'input' and mortality 'output' in developed countries. *J. Epidemiol. Comm. Health*, **32**, 200–205.

Cohen, J. (1968) Weighted kappa: nomial scale agreement with provision for scaled disagreement or partial credit. *Psychol. Bull.*, **70**, 213–220.

Cole, P. and MacMahon, B. (1971) Attributable risk percent in case-control studies. *Br. J. Prev. Soc. Med.*, **25**, 242–244.

Collett, D. (1991) *Modelling Binary Data*. Chapman & Hall, London

Collett, D. (1994) *Modelling Survival Data in Medical Research*. Chapman & Hall, London.

Conover, W.J. (1980) *Practical Nonparametric Statistics*. 2nd edn. John Wiley, New York.

Cook, R.D. and Weisberg, S. (1982) *Residuals and Influence in Regression*. Chapman & Hall, London.

Cornfield, J. (1956) A statistical problem arising from retrospective studies, in *Proceedings of the Third Berkeley Symposium on Mathematical Statistics and Probability* (ed. J. Neyman). University of California Press, Berkeley.

Coughlin, S.S., Benichou, J. and Weed, D.L. (1994) Attributable risk estimation in case-control studies. *Epidemiol. Rev.*, **16**, 51–64.

Cox, D.R. (1958) Two further applications of a model for binary regression. *Biometrika*, **45**, 562–565.

Cox, D.R. (1972) Regression models and life tables (with discussion). *J. R. Statist. Soc. B*, **74**, 187–220.

Cox, D.R. and Oakes, D. (1984) *Analysis of Survival Data*. Chapman & Hall, London.

Crombie, I.K., Todman, J., McNeill, G., Florey, C. du V., Menzies, I. and Kennedy, R.A. (1990) Effect of vitamin and mineral supplementation on verbal and non-verbal reasoning of schoolchildren. *Lancet*, **335**, 744–747.

Crowther, C.A., Verkuyl, D.A.A., Neilson, J.P., Bannerman, C. and Ashurst, H.M. (1990) The effects of hospitalization for rest on fetal growth, neonatal morbidity and length of gestation in twin pregnancy. *Br. J. Obstet. Gynae.*, **97**, 872–877.

Daly, E., Vessey, M.P., Hawkins, M.M., Carson, J.L., Gough, P. and Marsh, S. (1996) Risk of venous thromboembolism in users of hormone replacement therapy. *Lancet*, **348**, 977–980.

Day, N.E., Byar, D.P. and Green, S.B. (1980) Overadjustment in case-control studies. *Am. J. Epidemiol.*, **112**, 696–706.

Dean, A.G., Dean, J.A., Coulombier, D. *et al.* (1996) *Epi Info Version 6.xx*. Brixton Books, Llanidloes, Powys.

Ditchburn, R.K. and Ditchburn, J.S. (1990) A study of microscopical and chemical tests for the rapid diagnosis of urinary tract infections in general practice. *Br. J. Gen. Practice.*, **40**, 406–408.

Dobson, A.J., Kuulasmaa, K. and Eberle, E. (1991) Confidence intervals for weighted sums of Poisson parameters. *Statist. Med.*, **10**, 457–462.

Doll, R. and Hill, A.B. (1950) Smoking and carcinoma of the lung. Preliminary report. *BMJ*, ii, 739–748.

Doll, R. and Hill, A.B. (1952) A study of the aetiology of carcinoma of the lung. *BMJ*, ii, 1271–1286.

Doll, R. and Hill, A.B. (1964) Mortality in relation to smoking: ten years' observations of British doctors. *BMJ*, i, 1399–1410, 1460–1467.

Doll, R. and Peto, R. (1976) Mortality in relation to smoking: 20 years' observations on male British doctors. *BMJ*, ii, 1525–1536

Doll, R., Peto, R., Wheatley, K., Gray, R. and Sutherland, I. (1994) Mortality in relation to smoking: 40 years' observations on male British doctors. *BMJ*, **309**, 901–911.

Donner, A. (1984) Approaches to sample size estimation in the design of clinical trials – a review. *Statist. Med.*, **3**, 199–214.

Donner, A. and Li, K.Y.R. (1990) The relationship between chi-square statistics from matched and unmatched analyses. *J. Clin. Epidemiol.*, **43**, 827–831.

Dorman, P. J., Slattery, J., Farrell, B. *et al.* (1997) A randomised comparison of the EuroQol and Short Form-36 after stroke. *BMJ*, **315**, 461.

Draper, N. R. and Smith, H. (1981) *Applied Regression Analysis*, 2nd edn. John Wiley, New York.

Drews, C.D., Kraus, J.F. and Greenland, S. (1990) Recall bias in a case-control study of sudden infant death syndrome. *Int. J. Epidemiol.*, **19**, 405–411.

Du Mond, C. (1992) An application of the sequential probability ratio test to an unblinded clinical trial of ganciclovir versus no treatment in the prevention of CMV pneumonia following bone marrow transplantation, in *Biopharmaceutical Sequential Statistical Applications* (ed. K.E. Peace), Statistics, Textbooks and Monographs vol. 128. Marcel Dekker Inc., New York.

Duffy, J.C. (1995) Alcohol consumption and all-causes mortality. *Int. J. Epidemiol.*, **24**, 100–105.

Durkheim, E. (1951) *Suicide: A Study in Sociology*. Free Press, New York.

Emerson, S.S. (1996) Statistical packages for group sequential methods. *Am. Statistician*, **50**, 183–192.

Feinstein, A.R., Walter, S.D. and Horwitz, R.I. (1986) An analysis of Berkson's bias in case-control studies. *J. Chronic Dis.*, **39**, 495–504.

Fihn, S.D., Boyko, E.J., Normand, E.H. *et al.* (1996) Association between use of spermicide-coated condoms and *Escherichia coli* urinary tract infection in young women. *Am. J. Epidemiol.*, **144**, 512–520.

Fisher, R.A. and Yates, F. (1957) *Statistical Tables for Biological, Agricultural and Medical Research,* 5th edn. Oliver and Boyd, Edinburgh.

Flanders, W.D., DeSimonian, R. and Freedman, D.S. (1992) Interpretation of linear regression models that include transformations or interaction terms. *Ann. Epidemiol.*, **2**, 735–744.

Fleiss, J.L. (1981) *Statistical Methods for Rates and Proportions*, 2nd edn. John Wiley, New York.

Fleiss, J.L. and Levin, B. (1988) Sample size determination in studies with matched pairs. *J. Clin. Epidemiol.*, **41**, 727–730.

Fleming, T.R. and Harrington, D.P. (1991) *Counting Processes and Survival Analysis*. John Wiley, New York.

Forster, D.P., Newens, A.J., Kay, D.W.K. and Edwardson, J.A. (1995) Risk factors in clinically diagnosed presenile dementia of the Alzheimer type: a case-control study in northern England. *J. Epidemiol. Comm. Health*, **49**, 253–258.

Freedman, D., Pisani, R. and Purves, R. (1978) *Statistics*. Norton, New York.

Freedman, L.S. (1982) Tables of the number of patients required in clinical trials using the logrank test. *Statist. Med.*, **1**, 121–130.

Freiman, J.A., Chalmer, T.C., Smith, H. and Kuebler, R.R. (1978) The importance of beta, the type II error and sample size in the design and interpretation of the randomized control trial. *N. Engl. J. Med.*, **299**, 690–694.

Gardner, M.J. and Altman, D.G. (eds) (1989) *Statistics with Confidence – Confidence Intervals and Statistical Guidelines*. British Medical Journal, London.

Garrow, J.S. (1981) *Treat Obesity Seriously. A Clinical Manual*. Churchill Livingstone, London.

Gart, J.J. (1969) An exact test for comparing matched proportions in crossover designs. *Biometrika*, **56**, 75–80.

Gefeller, O. (1992) Comparison of adjusted attributable risk estimators. *Statist. Med.*, **11**, 2083–2091.

Goldstein, H. (1995) *Multilevel Statistical Models*. 2nd edn. Arnold, London.

Gore, S.M. and Altman, D.G. (1982) *Statistics in Practice*. British Medical Association, London.

Greenland, S. (1989) Modeling and variable selection in epidemiologic analysis. *Am. J. Epidemiol.*, **79**, 340–349.

Greenland, S. and Robins, J.M. (1985) Estimation of a common effect parameter from sparse follow-up data. *Biometrics*, **41**, 55–68

Greenwood, M. (1926) *Reports on Public Health and Medical Subjects*. No. 33, Appendix 1. HMSO, London.

Hanley, J.A. and McNeil, B.J. (1982) The meaning and use of the area under a receiver operating characteristic (ROC) curve. *Radiology*, **143**, 29–36.

Härdle, W. (1990) *Applied Non-parametric Regression*. Cambridge University Press, Cambridge.

Hastie, T.J., Botha, J.L. and Schnitzler, C.M. (1989) Regression with an ordered categorical response. *Statist. Med.*, **8**, 785–794.

Heinrich, J., Balleisen, L., Schulte, H., Assmann, G. and van de Loo, J. (1994) Fibrinogen and factor VII in the prediction of coronary risk. Results from the PROCAM study in healthy men. *Arterioscler. Thromb.*, **14**, 54–59.

Hill, J., Bird, H.A., Fenn, G.C., Lee, C.E., Woodward, M. and Wright, V. (1990) A double-blind crossover study to compare lysine acetyl salicylate (Aspergesic) with ibuprofen in the treatment of rheumatoid arthritis. *J. Clin. Pharm. Therapeutics.*, **15**, 205–211.

Hills, M. and Armitage, P. (1979) The two-period cross-over clinical trial. *Br. J. Clin. Pharm.*, **8**, 7–20.

Horwitz, R.I. and Feinstein, A.R. (1978) Methodologic standards and contradictory results in case-control research. *Am. J. Med.*, **66**, 556–564.

Hsieh, F.Y. (1989) Sample size tables for logistic regression. *Statist. Med.*, **8**, 795–802.

Hwang, I.K. and Rodda, B.E. (1992) Interim analysis in the Norwegian Multicenter Study, in *Biopharmaceutical Sequential Statistical Applications* (ed. K.E. Peace), Statistics, Textbooks and Monographs vol. 128. Marcel Dekker Inc., New York.

Iman, R.L., Quade, D. and Alexander, D.A. (1975) Exact probability levels for the Kruskal–Wallis test. *Selected Tables in Math. Statist.*, **3**, 329–384.

Infante-Rivard, C., Mur, P., Armstrong, B., Alvarez-Dardet, C. and Bolumar, F. (1991) Acute lymphoblastic leukaemia among Spanish children and mothers' occupation: a case-control study. *J. Epidemiol. Comm. Health.* **45**, 11–15.

Jennison, C.J. and Turnbull, B.W. (1990) Statistical approaches to interim monitoring of medical trials: a review and commentary. *Statist. Sci.*, **5**, 299–317.

Johansson, I., Tidehag, P., Lundberg, V. and Hallmans, G. (1994) Dental status, diet and cardiovascular risk factors in middle-aged people in northern Sweden. *Comm. Dent. Oral Epidemiol.*, **22**, 431–436.

Jones, B. and Kenward, M.G. (1989) *Design and Analysis of Cross-over Trials*. Chapman & Hall, London.

Kahn, H.A. and Sempos, C.T. (1989) *Statistical Methods in Epidemiology*. Oxford University Press, New York.

Kalbfleisch, J.D. and Prentice, R.L. (1980) *The Statistical Analysis of Failure Time Data*. John Wiley, New York.

Kaplan, E.L. and Meier, P. (1958) Nonparametric estimation from incomplete observations. *J. Amer. Statist. Assoc.*, **53**, 457–481.

Karkavelas, G., Mavropoulou, S., Fountzilas, G. *et al.* (1995) Correlation of proliferating cell nuclear antigen assessment, histologic parameters and age with survival in patients with glioblastoma multiforme. *Anticancer Res.*, **15**, 531–536.

Katz, D., Baptista, J., Azen, S.P. and Pike, M.C. (1978) Obtaining confidence intervals for the risk ratio in cohort studies. *Biometrics*, **34**, 469–474.

Kaufman, D.W., Helmrich, S.P., Rosenberg, L., Miettinen, O.S. and Shapiro, S. (1983) Nicotine and carbon monoxide content of cigarette smoke and the risk of myocardial infarction in young men. *N. Engl. J. Med.*, **308**, 409–413.

Kauhanen, J., Kaplan, G.A., Goldberg, D.E. and Salonen, J.K. (1997) Beer binging and mortality: results from the Kuopio ischaemic heart disease risk factor study, a prospective population based study. *BMJ*, **315**, 846–851.

Kay, R. (1984) Goodness of fit methods for the proportional hazards regression model: a review. *Revue Épidémiologie Santé Publique*, **32**, 185–198.

Kiechl, S., Willeit, J., Poewe, W. *et al.* (1996) Insulin sensitivity and regular alcohol consumption: large, prospective, cross-sectional population study (Bruneck Study). *BMJ*, **313**, 1040–1044.

Kitange, H.M., Machibya, H., Black, J. *et al.* (1996) Outlook for survivors of childhood in sub-Saharan Africa – adult mortality in Tanzania. *BMJ*, **312**, 216–220.

Kleinbaum, D.G., Kupper, L.L. and Morgenstern, H. (1982) *Epidemiologic Research: Principles and Quantitative Methods*. Van Nostrand Reinhold, New York.

Kramer, O.S. and Shapiro, S. (1984) Scientific challenges in the application of randomized trials. *J. Am. Med. Assoc.*, **252**, 2739–2745.

Kupper, L.L., Karon, J.M., Kleinbaum, D.G., Morgenstern, H. and Lewis, D.K. (1981) Matching in epidemiologic studies: validity and efficiency considerations. *Biometrics*, **37**, 271–291.

Kupper, L.L., Janis, J.M., Karmous, A. and Greenberg, B.G. (1985) Statistical age-period-cohort analysis: a review and critique. *J. Chronic Dis.*, **38**, 811–830.

Kushi, L.H., Fee, R.M., Sellers, T.A., Zheng, W. and Folsom, A.R. (1996) Intake of vitamins A, C and E and postmenopausal breast cancer. The Iowa Women's Health Study. *Am. J. Epidemiol.*, **144**, 165–174.

Kvålseth, T.O. (1985) Cautionary note about $R^2$. *Am. Statistician*, **39**, 279–285.

Last, J.M. (1995) *A Dictionary of Epidemiology*, 3rd edn. Oxford University Press, New York.

Le, C.T. and Zelterman, D. (1992) Goodness of fit tests for proportional hazards regression models. *Biom J.*, **5**, 557–566.

Lemeshow, S., Hosmer, D.W., Klar, J. and Lwanga, S.K. (1990) *Adequacy of Sample Size in Health Studies*. John Wiley, Chichester.

Leung, H.M. and Kupper, L.L. (1981) Comparisons of confidence intervals for attributable risk. *Biometrics*, **37**, 293–302.

Liddell, F.D.K. (1980) Simplified exact analysis of case-referent studies: matched pairs; dichotomous exposure. *J. Epidemiol. Comm. Health*, **37**, 82–84.

Liddell, F.D.K., McDonald, J.C. and Thomas, D.C. (1977) Methods of cohort analysis: appraisal by application to asbestos mining. *J. R. Statist. Soc. A*, **140**, 469–491.

Lilienfield, D.E. and Stolley, P.D. (1994) *Foundations of Epidemiology*, 3rd edn. Oxford University Press, New York.

Lin, J.-T., Wang, L.-Y., Wang, J.-T., Wang, T.-H., Yang, C.-S. and Chen, C.-J. (1995) A nested case-control study on the association between *Helicobacter pylori* infection and gastric cancer risk in a cohort of 9775 men in Taiwan. *Anticancer Res.*, **15**, 603–606.

Little, R.J.A. and Rubin, D.B. (1987) *Statistical Analysis with Missing Data*. John Wiley, New York.

Lowe, G.D.O., Rumley, A., Woodward, M. *et al.* (1997) Epidemiology of coagulation factors, inhibitors and activation markers: The Third Glasgow MONICA Survey. I. Illustrative reference ranges by age, sex and hormone use. *Br. J. Haematology*, **97**, 775–784.

Lunn, M. and McNeil, D. (1995) Applying Cox regression to competing risks. *Biometrics*, **51**, 524–532.

Machin, D. and Campbell, M.J. (1997) *Statistical Tables for the Design of Clinical Studies*. 2nd edn. Blackwell, Oxford.

Maclure, M. and Greenland, S. (1992) Tests for trend and dose response: misinterpretations and alternatives. *Am. J. Epidemiol.*, **135**, 96–104.

MacMahon, B. and Trichopoulos, D. (1996) *Epidemiology. Principles and Methods*, 2nd edn. Lippincott-Raven, Hagerstown, MD.

McCullagh, P. (1980) Regression models for ordinal data (with discussion). *J. R. Statist. Soc. B*, **42**, 109–142.

McCullagh, P. and Nelder, J.A. (1989) *Generalized Linear Models*, 2nd edn. Chapman & Hall, London.

McDonagh, T.A., Woodward, M., Morrison, C.E. *et al.* (1997) *Helicobacter pylori* infection and coronary heart disease in the North Glasgow MONICA population. *Europ. Heart J.*, **18**, 1257–1260.

McKinlay, S.M. (1977) Pair matching – a reappraisal of a popular technique. *Biometrics*, **33**, 725–735.

McKinney, P.A., Alexander, F.E., Nicholson, C., Cartwright, R.A. and Carrette, J. (1991) Mothers' reports of childhood vaccinations and infections and their concordance with general practitioner records. *J. Public Health Med.*, **13**, 13–22.

McLoone, P. (1994) *Carstairs Scores for Scottish Postcode Sectors from the 1991 Census.* Public Health Research Unit, University of Glasgow, Glasgow.

McMahon, J., Parnell, W.R. and Spears, G.F.S. (1993) Diet and dental caries in preschool children. *Europ. J. Clin. Nutrit.*, **47**, 794–802.

McNeil, D. (1996) *Epidemiological Research Methods.* John Wiley, Chichester.

Mantel, N. (1973) Synthetic retrospective studies and related topics. *Biometrics*, **29**, 479–486.

Mantel, N. and Greenhouse, S.W. (1968) What is the continuity correction? *Am. Statistician*, **22**, 27–30.

Mantel, N. and Haenszel, W. (1959) Statistical aspects of the analysis of data from retrospective studies. *J. Natl. Cancer Inst.*, **22**, 719–748.

Mason, D., Birmingham, L. and Grubin, D. (1997) Substance use in remand prisoners: a consecutive case study. *BMJ*, **315**, 18–21.

Matthews, J.N.S. and Altman, D.G. (1996) Interaction 3: How to examine heterogeneity. *BMJ*, **313**, 862.

Mawson, A.R., Blundo, J.J., Clemmer, D.I., Jacobs, K.W., Ktsanes, V.K. and Rice, J.C. (1996) Sensation-seeking, criminality and spinal cord injury: a case-control study. *Am. J. Epidemiol.*, **144**, 463–472.

Mehta, C.R., Patel, N.R. and Gray, R. (1985) Computing an exact confidence interval for the common odds ratio in several 2 × 2 contingency tables. *J. Am. Statist. Assoc.*, **80**, 969–973.

Mezzetti, M., Ferraroni, M., Decarli, A., La Vecchia, C. and Benichou, J. (1996) Software for attributable risk and confidence interval estimation in case-control studies. *Computers Biomed Res.*, **29**, 63–75.

Miao, L.M. (1977) Gastric freezing: an example of the evaluation of a medical therapy by randomized clinical trials, in *Costs, Risks and Benefits of Surgery.* (eds J.P. Bunker, B.A. Barnes and F. Mosteller). Oxford University Press, New York.

Miettinen, O.S. (1970) Estimation of relative risk from individually matched series. *Biometrics*, **26**, 75–86.

Miettenen, O.S. and Cook, E.F. (1981) Confounding: essence and detection. *Am. J. Epidemiol.*, **114**, 593–603.

Miller, C.T., Neutel, C.I., Nair, R.C., Marrett, L.D., Last, J.M. and Collins, W.E. (1978) Relative importance of risk factors in bladder carcinogenesis. *J. Chronic Dis.*, **31**, 51–56.

Millns, H., Woodward, M. and Bolton-Smith, C. (1995) Is it necessary to transform nutrient variables prior to statistical analysis? *Am. J. Epidemiol.*, **141**, 251–262.

Montgomery, D.C. and Peck, E.A. (1992) *Introduction to Linear Regression Analysis,* 2nd edn. John Wiley, New York.

Mood, A.M., Graybill, F.A. and Boes, D.C. (1974) *Introduction to the Theory of Statistics,* 3rd edn. McGraw-Hill, Tokyo.

Morgenstern, H. (1982) Uses of ecologic analysis in epidemiologic research. *Am. J. Public Health*, **72**, 1336–1344.

Moritz, D.J., Kelsey, J.L. and Grisso, J.A. (1997) Hospital controls versus community controls: differences in influences regarding risk factors for hip fracture. *Am. J. Epidemiol.*, **145**, 653–660.

Morrison, A.S. (1992) Risk factors for surgery for prostatic hypertrophy. *Am. J. Epidemiol.*, **135**, 974–980.

Morrison, C., Woodward, M., Leslie, W. and Tunstall-Pedoe, H. (1997) Effect of socioeconomic group on incidence of, management of, and survival after myocardial infarction and coronary death: analysis of community coronary event register. *BMJ*, **314**, 541–546.

Moser, C.A. and Kalton, G. (1971) *Survey Methods in Social Investigation*. 2nd edn. Heinemann, London.

Moss, A.J., Jackson Hall, W., Cannon, D.S. *et al* (1996) Improved survival with an implanted defibrillator in patients with coronary disease at high risk for ventricular arrhythmia. *N. Engl. J. Med.*, **335**, 1933–1940.

Office of Population Censuses and Surveys (1980) *Classification of Occupations, 1980*. HMSO, London.

Ornish, D., Brown, S E., Scherwitz, L.W. *et al.* (1990) Can lifestyle changes reverse coronary heart disease? The Lifestyle Heart Trial. *Lancet*, **336**, 129–133.

Parmar, M.K.B. and Machin, D. (1995) *Survival Analysis. A Practical Approach*. John Wiley, Chichester.

Parsonnet, J. (1995) The incidence of *Helicobacter pylori* infection. *Aliment. Pharmacol. Ther.*, **9** (Suppl. 2), 45–51.

Passaro, K.T., Little, R.E., Savitz, D.A. and Noss J. (1996) The effect of maternal drinking before conception and in early pregnancy on infant birth-weight. *Epidemiology*, **7**, 377–383.

Patel, P., Mendall, M.A., Carrington, D. *et al.* (1995) Association of *Helicobacter pylori* and Chlamydia pneumoniae infections with coronary heart disease and cardiovascular risk factors. *BMJ*, **311**, 711–714.

Paul, C., Skegg, D.C.G., Spears, G.F.S. and Kaldor, J.M. (1986) Oral contraceptives and breast cancer: a national study. *BMJ*, **293**, 723–726.

Peace, K.E. (ed.) (1992) *Biopharmaceutical Sequential Statistical Applications*. Statistics, Textbooks and Monographs vol. 128. Marcel Dekker Inc., New York.

Peace, L.R. (1985) A time correlation between cigarette smoking and lung cancer. *The Statistician*, **34**, 371–381.

Pearl, R. (1929) Cancer and tuberculosis. *Am. J. Hyg.*, **9**, 97–159.

Pearson, M., Spencer, S. and McKenna, M. (1991) Patterns of uptake and problems presented at Well Women clinics in Liverpool. *J. Public Health Med.*, **13**, 42–47.

Peterson, B. (1990) Re: ordinal regression models for epidemiologic data. *Am. J. Epidemiol.*, **131**, 745–746.

Peto, R., Pike, M.C., Armitage, P. *et al.* (1977) Design and analysis of randomized clinical trials requiring prolonged observation of each patient. II. Analysis and examples. *Br. J. Cancer*, **35**, 1–39.

Pike, M.C. and Morrow, R.H. (1970) Statistical analysis of patient-control studies in epidemiology. Factor under investigation an all-or-none variable. *Br. J. Prev. Soc. Med.*, **24**, 42–44.

Pike, M.C., Morrow, R.H., Kisuule, A. and Mafigiri, J. (1970) Burkitt's lymphoma and sickle cell trait. *Br. J. Prev. Soc. Med.*, **24**, 39–41.

Pocock, S.J. (1979) Allocation of patients to treatment in clinical trials. *Biometrics*, **35**, 183–197.

Pocock, S.J. (1983) *Clinical Trials: A Practical Approach*. John Wiley, Chichester.

Pollard, A.H., Yusuf, F. and Pollard, G.N. (1990) *Demographic Techniques*, 3rd edn. Pergamon, Sydney.

Pontiggia, P., Curto, F., Rotella, G., Sabato, A., Rizzo, S. and Butti, G. (1995) Hyperthermia in the treatment of brain metastates from lung cancer. Experience in 17 cases. *Anticancer Res.*, **15**, 597–602.

Poole, C. (1986) Exposure opportunity in case-control studies. *Am. J. Epidemiol.*, **123**, 352–358.

Pooling Project Research Group (1978) Relationship of blood pressure, serum cholesterol, smoking habit, relative weight and ecg abnormalities to incidence of major coronary events: final report of the Pooling Project. *J. Chronic Dis.*, **31**, 201–306.

Pounder R.E. and Ng, D. (1995). The prevalence of *Helicobacter pylori* infection in different countries. *Aliment. Pharmacol. Ther.*, **9** (Suppl. 2), 33–39.

Prescott, R.J. (1981) The comparison of success rates in cross-over trials in the presence of an order effect. *J. R. Statist. Soc. C*, **30,** 9–15.

Raffn, E., Mikkelsen, S., Altman, D.G., Christensen, J.M. and Groth, S. (1988) Health effects due to occupational exposure to cobalt blue dye among plate painters in a porcelain factory in Denmark. *Scand. J. Environ. Health*, **14**, 378–384.

Rawnsley, K. (1991) The National Counselling Service for Sick Doctors. *Proc. R. Coll. Physicians Edinburgh*, **21**, 4–7.

Robins, J.M., Gail, M.H. and Lubin, J.H. (1986a) More on 'biased selection of controls for case-control analyses of cohort studies'. *Biometrics*, **42**, 293–299.

Robins, J., Greenland, S. and Breslow N.E. (1986b) A general estimator for the variance of the Mantel–Haenszel odds ratio. *Am. J. Epidemiol.*, **124**, 719–723.

Rodrigues, L.C., Gill, O.N. and Smith, P.G. (1991) BCG vaccination in the first year of life protects children of Indian subcontinent ethnic origin against tuberculosis in England. *J. Epidemiol. Comm. Health*, **45**, 78–80.

Rose, G.A., McCartney, P. and Reid, D.D. (1977) Self-administration of questionnaire on chest pain and intermittent claudication. *Br. J. Prev. Soc. Med.*, **31**, 42–48.

Rosner, B. (1994) *Fundamentals of Biostatistics*, 4th edn. Duxbury, Belmont, CA.

Rothman, K. and Boice, J.D. (1979) *Epidemiological Analysis with a Programmable Calculator*, NIH Publications 79-1649. US Government. Printing Office, Washington, DC.

Rothman, K.J. and Greenland, S. (1997) *Modern Epidemiology*, 2nd edn. Lippincott-Raven, Hagerstown, MD.

Ruth, K.J. and Neaton, J.D. (1991) Evaluation of two biochemical markers of tobacco exposure. *Prev. Med.*, **20**, 574–589.

Ryan, B.F. and Joiner, B.L. (1994) *Minitab Handbook*, 3rd edn. Duxbury, Belmont, CA.

Sackett, D.L. (1979) Bias in analytic research. *J. Chronic Dis.*, **32**, 51–63.

Saetta, J.P., March, S., Gaunt, M.E. and Quinton, D.N. (1991) Gastric emptying procedures in the self-poisoned patient: are we forcing gastric content beyond the pylorus? *J. R. Soc. Med.*, **84**, 274–276.

SAS Institute Inc. (1992) *Master Index to SAS® System Documentation, Version 6*, 4th edn. SAS Institute Inc., Cary, NC.

Schlesselman, J.J. (1974) Sample size requirements in cohort and case-control studies of disease. *Am. J. Epidemiol.*, **33**, 381–384.

Schlesselman, J.J. (1982) *Case-Control Studies: Design, Conduct and Analysis*. Oxford University Press, New York.

Schoenfeld, D.A. (1983) Sample size formula for the proportional-hazards regression model. *Biometrics*, **38**, 163–170.

Scott, A. and Wild, C. (1991) Transformations and $R^2$. *Am. Statistician*, **45**, 127–129.

Scragg, R., Mitchell, E.A., Taylor, B.J. *et al.* (1993) Bed sharing, smoking and alcohol in the sudden infant death syndrome. *BMJ*, **307**, 1312–1318.

Seber, G.A.F. and Wild, C.J. (1989) *Nonlinear Regression.* John Wiley, New York.

Senn, S. (1993) *Cross-over Trials in Clinical Research.* John Wiley, Chichester.

Shaper, A.G., Wannamethee, G. and Walker, M. (1988) Alcohol and mortality in British men: explaining the U-shaped curve. *Lancet*, **ii**, 1267–1273.

Shewry, M.C., Smith, W.C.S., Woodward, M. and Tunstall-Pedoe, H. (1992) Variation in coronary risk factors by social status: results from the Scottish Heart Health Study. *Br. J. Gen. Practice*, **42**, 406–410.

Shryock, H.S., Siegel, J.S. and Stockwell, E.G. (1976) *The Methods and Materials of Demography*, condensed edn. Academic Press, New York.

Siemiatycki, J. (1989) Friendly control bias. *J. Clin. Epidemiol.*, **42**, 687–688.

Smith, W.C.S., Crombie, I.K., Tavendale, R., Irving, I.M., Kenicer, M.B. and Tunstall-Pedoe, H. (1987) The Scottish Heart Health Study: objectives and development of methods. *Health Bull. (Edinburgh)*, **45**, 211–217.

Smith, W.C.S, Woodward, M. and Tunstall-Pedoe, H. (1991) Intermittent claudication in Scotland, in *Epidemiology of Peripheral Vascular Disease.* (ed. F.G.R. Fowkes). Springer-Verlag, Berlin.

Snedecor, G.W. and Cochran, W.G. (1980) *Statistical Methods*, 7th edn. Iowa State University Press, Ames, IA.

Srinivasan U., Leonard, N., Jones, E. *et al.* (1996) Absence of oats toxicity in adult coeliac disease. *BMJ*, **313**, 1300–1301.

STATACorp. (1997) *Stata Statistical Software: Release 5.0.* Stata Press, College Station, TX.

Steel, R.G.D. and Torrie, J.H. (1980) *Principles and Procedures of Statistics. A Biometrical Approach*, 2nd edn. McGraw-Hill, New York.

Steinbok, P., Reiner, A.M., Beauchamp, R., Armstrong, R.W. and Cochrane, D.D. (1997) A randomized controlled trial to compare selective posterior rhizotomy plus physiotherapy with physiotherapy alone in children with spastic diplegic cerebral palsy. *Develop. Med. Child. Neurology*, **39**, 178–184.

Stephens, M.A. (1974) EDF statistics for goodness of fit and some comparisons. *J. Am. Statist. Assoc.*, **69**, 730–737.

Stolley, P.D. and Lasky, T. (1995) *Investigating Disease Patterns. The Science of Epidemiology.* W.H. Freeman, New York.

Storr, J., Barrell, E. and Lenny, W. (1987) Asthma in primary schools. *BMJ*, **295**, 251–252.

Strachan, D.P. (1988) Damp housing and childhood asthma: validation of reporting of symptoms. *BMJ*, **297**, 1223–1226.

Swan, A.V. (1986) *GLIM 3.77 Introductory Guide.* Revision A. NAG, Oxford.

Sylvester, R.J., Machin, D. and Staquet, M.J. (1982) Cancer clinical trial protocols, in *Treatment of Cancer* (ed. K.E. Halnan) Chapman & Hall, London.

Tarone, R.E. (1981) On summary estimations of relative risk. *J. Chronic Dis.*, **34**, 463–468.

Tetzschner, T., Sørensen, M., Jønsson, L., Lase, G. and Christiansen, J. (1997) Delivery and pudendal nerve function. *Acta Obstet. Gynecol. Scand.*, **76**, 324–331.

Tham, T.C.K., Collins, J.S.A., Molloy, C., Sloan, J.M., Banford, K.B. and Watson, R.G.P. (1996) Randomised controlled trial of ranitidine versus omeprazole in combination with antibiotics for eradication of *Helicobacter pylori*. *Ulster Med. J*, **65**, 131–136.

Thomas, D.C. and Greenland, S. (1983) The relative efficiencies of matched and independent sample designs for case-control studies. *J. Chronic Dis.*, **36**, 685–697.

Thomas, D.C. and Greenland, S. (1985) The efficiency of matching in case-control studies of risk factor interactions. *J. Chronic Dis.*, **38**, 569–574.

Thomas, D.G. (1975) Exact and asymptotic methods for the combination of $2 \times 2$ tables. *Comput Biomed. Res.*, **8**, 423–426.

Thomas, L.H. (1992) Ischaemic heart disease and consumption of hydrogenated marine oils in England and Wales. *J. Epidemiol. Comm. Health*, **46**, 78–82.

Thompson, W.D., Kelsey, J.L. and Walter, S.D. (1982) Cost and efficiency in the choice of matched and unmatched case-control study designs. *Am. J. Epidemiol.*, **116**, 840–851.

Thorpe, K., Greenwood, R. and Goodenough, T. (1995) Does a twin pregnancy have a greater impact on physical and emotional well-being than a singleton pregnancy? *Birth Issues Perinatal Care*, **22**, 148–152.

Tiku, M.L., Tan, W.Y. and Balakrishnan, N. (1986) *Robust Inference*. Marcel Dekker, New York.

Tunstall-Pedoe, H., Smith, W.C.S., Crombie, I.K. and Tavendale, R. (1989) Coronary risk factor and lifestyle variation across Scotland: results from the Scottish Heart Health Study. *Scott. Med. J.*, **34**, 556–560.

Tunstall-Pedoe, H., Woodward, M., Tavendale, R., A'Brook R. and McCluskey, M.K. (1997) Comparison of the prediction by 27 different factors of coronary heart disease and death in men and women of the Scottish heart health study: cohort study:*BMJ*, **315**, 722–729.

United Nations (1996) *Demographic Yearbook 1994*. United Nations, New York.

Ury, H.K. (1975) Efficiency of case-control studies with multiple controls per case: continuous or dichotomous data. *Biometrics* **31**, 643–649.

Wacholder, S. (1991) Practical considerations in choosing between the case-cohort and nested case-control designs. *Epidemiology* **2**, 155–158.

Wacholder, S. and Silverman, D.T. (1990) Re: 'Case-control studies using other diseases as controls: problems of excluding exposure-related diseases' (Letter). *Am. J. Epidemiol.*, **132**, 1017–1018.

Wacholder, S., McLaughlin, J.K., Silverman, D.T. and Mandel, J.S. (1992) Selection of controls in case-control studies. *Am. J. Epidemiol.*, **136**, 1019–1050.

Walter, S.D. (1980a) Berkson's bias and its control in epidemiological studies. *J. Chronic Dis.*, **33**, 721–725.

Walter, S.D. (1980b) Matched case-control studies with a variable number of controls per case. *Appl. Statist.*, **29**, 172–179.

Wangensteen, O.H., Peter, E.T., Nicoloff, D.M., Walder, A.I., Sosin, H. and Bernstein, E.F. (1962) Achieving 'physiological gastrectomy' by gastric freezing. *J. Am. Med. Assoc.*, **180**, 439–444.

Weiss, N. (1995) *Introductory Statistics*. Addison-Wesley, Reading, MA.

Whitehead, J. (1997) *The Design and Analysis of Sequential Clinical Trials*, 2nd edn (rev). John Wiley, Chichester.

Whittemore, A.S. (1983) Estimating attributable risk from case-control studies. *Am. J. Epidemiol.*, **117**, 76–85.

WHO MONICA Project (1994) Myocardial infarction and coronary deaths in the World Health Organization MONICA Project: registration procedures, event rates and case-fatality rates in 38 populations from 21 countries in four continents. *Circulation*, **90**, 583–612.

Williams, D.A. (1982) Extra-binomial variation in logistic linear models. *Appl. Statist.*, **31**, 144–148.

Wilson, D.C. and McClure, G. (1996) Babies born under 1000 g – perinatal outcome. *Ulster Med. J.*, **65**, 118–122.

Winn, D.M., Blot, W.J., McLaughlin, J.K. *et al.* (1991) Mouthwash use and oral conditions in the risk of oral and pharyngeal cancer. *Cancer Res.*, **51**, 3044–3047.

Wong, O. (1990) A cohort mortality study and a case-control study of workers potentially exposed to styrene in the reinforced-plastics and composites industry. *Br. J. Ind. Med.*, **47**, 753–762.

Woodward, M. (1989) A computer-based method for determining optimal sample size with medical applications. *The Statistician*, **38**, 313–318.

Woodward, M. (1992) Formulae for the calculation of sample size, power and minimum detectable relative risk in medical studies. *The Statistician*, **41**, 185–196.

Woodward, M. and Tunstall-Pedoe, H. (1992a) Biochemical evidence of persistent heavy smoking after a coronary diagnosis despite self-reported reduction. Analysis from the Scottish Heart Health Study. *Europ. Heart. J.*, **13**, 160–165.

Woodward, M. and Tunstall-Pedoe, H. (1992b) An iterative technique for identifying smoking deceivers with application to the Scottish Heart Health Study. *Prev. Med.*, **21**, 88–97.

Woodward, M. and Walker. A.R.P. (1994) Sugar consumption and dental caries: evidence from 90 countries. *Br. Dent. J.*, **176**, 297–302.

Woodward, M., Shewry, M.C., Smith, W.C.S. and Tunstall-Pedoe, H. (1992) Social status and coronary heart disease: results from the Scottish Heart Health Study. *Prev. Med.*, **21**, 136–148.

Woodward, M., Bolton-Smith, C. and Tunstall-Pedoe, H. (1994) Deficient health knowledge, diet and other lifestyles in smokers: is a multifactorial approach required? *Prev. Med.*, **23**, 354–361.

Woodward, M., Laurent, K. and Tunstall-Pedoe, H. (1995) An analysis of risk factors for prevalent coronary heart disease using the proportional odds model. *The Statistician*, **44**, 69–80.

Woodward, M., Lowe, G.D.O., Rumley, A. *et al.* (1997) Epidemiology of coagulation factors, inhibitors and activation markers: The Third Glasgow MONICA Survey II. Relationships to cardiovascular risk factors and prevalent cardiovascular disease. *Br. J. Haematology*, **97**, 785–797.

Woolf, B. (1955) On estimating the relationship between blood group and disease. *Ann. Human Genet.*, **19**, 251–253.

World Health Organization (1992) *International Classification of Diseases: 10th revision.* WHO, Geneva.

Yanagawa, T., Fujii, Y. and Mastuoka, H. (1994) Generalised Mantel–Haenszel procedures for $2 \times J$ tables. *Environ. Health Perspect.*, **102** (Suppl. 8), 57–60.

Ying, R.L., Gross, K.B., Terzo, T.S. and Eschenbacher, W.L. (1990) Indomethacin does not inhibit the ozone-induced increase in bronchial responsiveness in human subjects. *Am. Rev. Respiratory Dis.*, **142**, 817–821.

Youden, W.J. (1950) Index for rating diagnostic tests. *Cancer*, **3**, 32–35.

Zhang, J., Savitz, D.A., Schwingl, P.J. and Cai, W.-W. (1992) A case-control study of paternal smoking and birth defects. *Int. J. Epidemiol.*, **21**, 273–278.

# Index